ADVANCED NURSING AND HEALTH CARE RESEARCH

Quantification Approaches

Frank E. McLaughlin, RN., PhD, FAAN

Professor, Department of Nursing
School of Education
San Francisco State University
San Francisco, California

Leonard A. Marascuilo, MA, PhD

Professor, School of Education
University of California, Berkeley
Berkeley, California

1990

W.B. SAUNDERS COMPANY

Harcourt Brace Jovanovich, Inc.

Philadelphia / London / Toronto / Montreal / Sydney / Tokyo

W. B. SAUNDERS COMPANY
Harcourt Brace Jovanovich, Inc.

The Curtis Center
Independence Square West
Philadelphia, PA 19106

Library of Congress Cataloging-in-Publication Data

McLaughlin, Frank E.
  Advanced nursing and health care research : quantification
approaches / Frank E. McLaughlin, Leonard A. Marascuilo.
    p. cm.
  ISBN 0-7216-3098-7
  1. Nursing—Research. 2. Nursing—Research—Statistical methods.
I. Marascuilo, Leonard A. II. Title.
  [DNLM: 1. Nursing Research—methods. 2. Statistics—methods. WY
20.5 M478a]
RT81.5.M38 1990
610.73′072—dc20
DNLM/DLC
for Library of Congress
                                    89-70285
                                     CIP

Sponsoring Editor: Thomas Eoyang

ADVANCED NURSING AND HEALTH CARE RESEARCH:
Quantification Approaches ....ISBN 0-7216-3098-7

Printed in the United States of America

Last digit is the print number: 9   8   7   6   5   4   3   2   1

DEDICATION

The death of Dr. Leonard A. Marascuilo, while we were completing page proofs of this text, was an especially sorrowful occasion. He so wanted to see the text published and gain first-hand feedback from the consumers of our joint efforts. Dr. Marascuilo was a former teacher of mine, a dear friend, and a stimulating and challenging colleague over the twenty-five years of our relationship. Leonard was a marvelous teacher of statistics and research, and he produced many outstanding graduates of the Ph.D. program in the School of Education of the University of California at Berkeley. His contributions to the field of education in particular and to the social, behavioral, and health sciences in general will be long remembered, through the publication of five textbooks and over seventy theoretical and data-based articles as well as through inspiration provided hundreds of students over his twenty-eight years of teaching at the University of California.

PREFACE

In the past two decades, there has been a dramatic change in the role of the registered nurse. In addition to the functions of a nurse as a health care provider, a new role has emerged that has become the dominant focus of a number of nurses. Research on the delivery of health care has become an important part of the profession's social mission. In the United States alone, there are more than forty-five doctoral programs and more than 150 master degree programs in nursing. We decided to write this book to help prepare nurses to participate in the vital development of sound and defensible research. In particular our goals were:

(1) To describe and illustrate beginning and advanced research techniques and statistical procedures, with emphasis on the performance of research;

(2) To develop one extensive research example and use it throughout the text to illustrate quantitative methods;

(3) To provide less extensive examples that illustrate special issues in nursing research;

(4) To present new techniques and approaches not generally available to nursing researchers;

(5) To provide an understanding of selected research techniques used in other disciplines that have particular application to nursing and health care research issues; and

(6) To demonstrate the range and variety of quantification techniques useful for hypothesis testing.

The research texts presently available for classroom use are, for the most part, introductory. In addition, a number of these beginner texts emphasize the role of the nurse as an intelligent consumer of research done by others and do not offer sufficient depth in the techniques of research to enable individual nurses to conduct research on their own. One of the major reasons we took on the challenge of writing this book on instrumentation, measurement, and advanced statistical methodologies was to illustrate, provide, and introduce to nurses alternative strategies for conducting quantitative studies in nursing and health care settings.

Our experiences in teaching and consulting with graduate and experienced researchers led us to prepare an advanced text for masters and doctoral programs in nursing, one that explains in sufficient detail a wide range of quantification methods relevant for investigating nursing problems and health care issues.

Chapter 1 describes the role of the nurse in research and highlights the importance of the research enterprise in nursing. Also introduced in Chapter 1 is a major hypothetical research study concerned with preoperative preparation. Use of this hypothetical example is made throughout a number of later chapters in the text to illustrate the great array of quantitative models useful to address important nursing questions.

In Chapter 2, the relationship between hypothesis testing, propositions, and measurement is depicted. Instrument development is illustrated in Chapter 3. In addition, a number of measurement issues including reliability, validity, instrument construction, testing, and refinement are elucidated. In Chapter 4, the strengths and weaknesses of both experimental and quasi-experimental nursing research designs are depicted using various components of the preoperative teaching study.

Mailed questionnaires, personal interviews, and phone surveys are illustrated in Chapter 5. The advantages and limitations of these methods are examined. Probability and nonprobability sampling schemes are discussed in Chapter 6. Qualitative research assets and drawbacks are presented in Chapter 7. Content analysis leading to the quantification of qualitative data are also to be found in this chapter.

Moving from instrumentation and measurement issues, in Chapter 8 we begin a presentation of quantitative statistical methods with an introduction to graphing techniques and tabular procedures. Missing data and the treatment of outliers are discussed. Chapter 9 provides a review of elementary statistics, a topic which is assumed to have been covered in depth in previous courses taken by the student. The latter half of the chapter introduces planned and post hoc comparisons, the meaning and interpretation of statistical interactions, the analysis of variance, and an extensive exposition of the role of confidence intervals in nursing studies. Power is illustrated and guidelines are presented for determining sample sizes.

Chapter 10 provides a review of simple regression and correlation. From that introduction, advanced topics on part, partial, and multiple correlation and regression are illustrated. Stepwise regression is introduced, and dummy coding is employed for analysis of variance studies with unequal sample sizes. Dummy coding is also used to explicate analysis of covariance and a discussion of treatment variable interactions is presented.

The discussion begun in Chapter 10 is extended to Chapter 11, where multivariate methods are discussed with an emphasis placed on multivariate analysis of variance, linear discriminant analysis, canonical correlation, and factor analysis. In Chapter 12, the four nonstatistical multivariate models—path analysis, linear structural equations, multidimensional scaling, and cluster analysis—are examined as specialized topics. Chapter 13 provides an in-depth discussion of contingency tables for two or more dimensions and the use of the loglinear model is illustrated. Chapter 14 covers single subject methodology, a topic rarely covered in nursing research.

Finally, Chapter 15 provides directions for combining information across studies using meta-analysis techniques that can be used for secondary analysis of data. An array of procedures that can be employed on data reported in scientific reports, doctoral and master's theses, and internal agency or governmental studies is illustrated.

In writing a text of this magnitude we assumed that students have already completed an introductory course in inferential statistics and measurement and a course in nursing research methodology. As will be seen, knowledge of Chi-square, regression, and the analysis of variance are assumed as early as Chapter 3.

In addition, we decided that the emphasis of the pedagogical exposition should be primarily conceptual and not computational in illustrating the variety of quantification techniques depicted throughout the text. As will be seen, text formulas are definitional in form rather than computational. Instead, it is expected that consumers of the book will use existing personal computer and mainframe computer statistical programs or packages for data reduction and data analysis.

As might be expected, a book of this scope has required the work and efforts of many individuals besides our own. In particular, we want to thank the Department of Nursing, School of Education, at San Francisco State University and the Graduate School of Education at the University of California at Berkeley for making it possible for us to complete the writing of this manuscript. Special thanks go to Ms. Cheri Araki, Ms. Deborah Curtis, Ms. Barbara Nakakihara, and Mr. Thomas Little for running computer programs, duplication services, and typing. Further, gratitude is offered to Dr. Robert Slaughter and Dr. Donald Chambers, School of Nursing, University of California at San Francisco for consultation and assistance with use of the Crunch Statistical Software Package. A critique of a preliminary version of the text was offered by Dr. Betty Mitsunaga and doctoral students at the School of Nursing, University of Wisconsin at Milwaukee and their helpful efforts are recognized. Special mention is made of the outstanding efforts and constructive suggestions made by Dr. Patricia Busk, School of Education, University of San Francisco. The suggestions and revisions offered by Dr. Mark Wilson, School of Education, University of California at Berkeley were noteworthy. A very particular appreciation is also extended to our large panel of anonymous reviewers.

Finally, we wish to thank the Institut fur Psychologie and Padagogik at the Ludwig-Maximilans Universitat, Munich, Federal Republic of Germany for providing excellent office space, computer facilities, and secretarial assistance during our sabbatical leave in 1988. Our special thanks go to Dr. Kurt Mueller, Dr. Klaus Schneewind, Dr. Weiner Schobo, and to Frau Ursula Siebert. In conjunction with our sabbatical leave, Herr Dieter Riemerschmid greatly facilitated our introduction into Bavarian social and cultural life and offered every assistance in the completion of this text.

San Francisco and Berkeley, 1989
Frank E. McLaughlin
Leonard A. Marascuilo

CONTENTS

Chapter 1

DEVELOPMENT AND GENERATION OF NURSING RESEARCH

1—1 NURSE RESEARCHER: A NEW ROLE FOR THE CONTEMPORARY NURSE

Research in nursing has not had a long history. In recent times research has taken on an important role for the nursing profession. Most observers of the contemporary nursing scene would place the beginning of modern nursing research in the early 1950s. The initiation of the journal *Nursing Research* as the first research publication for the international disciple of nursing in 1952 was an important milestone in promoting research in nursing (Gortner and Nahm, 1977). The preeminent goal of the journal was to encourage original investigations about nursing practice through the publication of scientifically sound studies by nurses and others. The first research grant given by the Division of Nursing, originally housed in the National Institute of General Medicine Science, was awarded in 1955 (Stevenson, 1987).

Much of the research reported in the 1960s did not directly describe or explain nursing processes and interventions in immediate patient care encounters. University faculties, for the most part, were preoccupied with studies describing and evaluating different curricula patterns in undergraduate and graduate education. Furthermore, a number of studies appearing in the professional literature examined the personal and professional characteristics of nurses and their demographic and occupational employment and distribution patterns in the United States. The profession's preoccupation with educating nurses and with their employment and occupational characteristics precluded significant research into the nurse's functions in modifying, changing, or improving the health status of individuals and groups (Hardy, 1987).

In the 1970s, a shift in the focus of research became apparent to members of the profession. Increasing stress on developing health concepts and models in which to describe, explain, predict, and prescribe nursing theory and practice became apparent in the studies reported in *Nursing Research*, as well as in two new research journals, *The Western Journal of Nursing Research* and *Research in Nursing and Health*. Over time these three nursing research publications have grown in scope in terms of the type and sophistication of articles accepted for publication.

Found in the shifting priorities of nursing

research was the mandate, in response to national and private commissioned studies, for increased emphasis on the preparation of clinical specialists and nurse practitioners on the graduate level. Some believed that expert clinicians would provide the spark for identifying the salient, pressing, nursing research problems and issues of major professional concern and that this cadre of university-prepared clinicians would stimulate critical inquiry in many health care settings (Roy and Obby, 1978).

Furthermore, the demand for expert practitioners of nursing to provide leadership in the provision of quality nursing care in the nation's health care facilities became a dominant theme. Research training that included the development and execution of individual and group research studies became incorporated into the advanced clinical training of nurses at the graduate university level. The increasing focus found in the nursing research literature, including thesis and dissertation investigations, contained studies that examined the clinical processes through which nurses modify, change, or improve the health status or nursing care of discrete subsets of individuals, client aggregates, groups, and communities (Adams, 1983).

The establishment of the publication *Annual Review of Nursing Research* demonstrated that substantive domains of knowledge were emerging through the conduct of nursing inquiries, which required systematic analysis, synthesis, and critical appraisal. The *Annual Review of Nursing Research*, initiated in 1983, provided critical, integrative reviews of research in the various content areas of nursing (Werley and Fitzpatrick, 1984). For instance, in volume 2 of the *Annual Review of Nursing Research*, research was examined in the nursing practice area that pertained mainly to the family. Topics were pregnancy, anxiety, and maternal health; experiences of parenthood; health promotion and illness prevention; and coping with elective surgery among others. This attention to nursing research represented a step forward in which research became an integrated component of nursing practice.

The 1986 opening of the National Institutes of Health National Center for Nursing Research marked a new phase in the history of nursing research (Merritt, 1986). As a consequence, an important role is played through the federal government's centralization of research funding and training in the National Institutes of Health. In addition, it will continue to establish and organize the future direction for and funding of nursing research vital to the improvement of health care into the twenty-first century.

In the 1980s the value and importance of nursing research were recognized by the nursing profession and by society as a whole. The more than 45 existing doctoral degree and the 150 master's degree programs in nursing incorporated research training into courses as a core content area. This development was characterized by the acceptance and use of research as an adjunct to health practice and by the acceptance that research investigations must emanate from significant nursing practice problems. One challenge of nursing research in the 1990s will be to test and verify the competing theoretical descriptions, explanations, predictions, and prescriptions about nursing roles that modify, change, or improve the health status of people at home, at work, in clinics, and in hospitals throughout the nation and the world.

1-2 GETTING STARTED: PRELIMINARY CONSIDERATIONS IN INITIATING A RESEARCH STUDY IN NURSING

In the following section some of the means and processes by which a nursing problem is selected for investigation are illustrated. The number, scope, and complexity of such problems may well be as large as the number of nurses available to execute them; therefore it is impossible to examine all of them. Instead a very small set of nursing research problems are examined to illustrate particular theoretical, methodological, and statistical issues that arise in carrying out research in nursing. For continuity and for pedagogical purposes, we examine in some detail research that is well known in nursing. The preoperative preparation research cuts across a wide spectrum of individual nursing specialty interests, theoretical perspectives, and methodological preferences. With careful examination of this specific research area, guidelines emerge or are provided, which can be useful to others in pursuing their own research interests in nursing. In this chapter the focus is on one substantive research domain; however, in the chapters that follow, a selected number of other topics and studies are examined for generalization and expansion of underlying principles.

No exposition on nursing research or any research-based discipline can be complete; all presentations must be brief. Our presentation is no exception. Nursing research, like all research in the health sciences, can call on a multitude of research methodologies and design principles to achieve its goal. The focus of health care is directly concerned with human beings. Therefore, an extremely heterogeneous set of research models and techniques demands that the presentation merely scratch the surface of numerous available methods. In this text a limited number of the basic models are examined in detail. With a firm understanding of the main framework of research methods, the nurse interested in research studies should be able to consult other resources with understanding and go beyond the methods described in the pages of this book.

Research questions can be generated from many sources. In clinical nursing, many specific health care events and interpersonal experiences may generate questions for study for nurses working with patients, families, and medical and ancillary personnel. Problems with other professional working units within agencies and institutions and among diverse community health programs and institutions also can serve as sources of subjects for a nursing investigation. For instance, the adequacy of various instructional approaches used by nurses to educate adolescents about safe sex practices may be at issue. The perceived lack of an effective program may be so severe that a nurse facing the experience may decide to do something about it and thereby may produce an innovative teaching protocol that needs to be studied to determine whether it provides benefits to clients and to the nursing field in general.

In another setting, certain activity of a repetitive nature may be so ingrained into the profession that it is applied routinely and without justification. The repetitiveness or lack of logic of the activity may be an irritant or a source of discomfort or uncertainty regarding the effectiveness of the activity to the practicing nurse. A decision might be made to examine the existing practices or procedures for positive outcomes. The evaluation may lead to speculations about doing something differently from that which is being provided by current, accepted practice to improve the situation. Often, previous experiences with similar procedures may suggest an alternative solution to the problem at hand, which needs to be tested for possible application in the future in the original setting or other similar settings. In other cases, coworkers or other colleagues may suggest procedures that might be of assistance in studying and evaluating a specific question. These interactions may lead to the development of ways to research the problem and thereby may provide a method of resolution. Nurses who have been trained to critically read research reports and journal articles are likely to recognize similar problems identified in the literature. This literature may offer clues on how to treat the question of interest. Frequently, solutions and research findings offered in reference sources may or may not be of actual value in resolving a faced problem. As a consequence, a research study may well be in order to find a workable solution.

In some instances, discussions with colleagues, reliance on past experiences, and knowledge of recent research can help resolve a problem. In other instances, fostering a major effort to provide the solution to a problem may be impractical, economically unwise, or logistically unworkable. As a consequence, many problems identified by nurses remain at the identified but unresolved stage. Uncontrollable crucial factors and other countervailing forces may not support the initiation of a research study. Possible factors are an unsympathetic or non-supportive managerial structure, indifferent or antagonistic professional staff attitudes, financial constraints, and conflict between health care agency leadership and the board of trustees or community oversight constituencies, including elected officials and citizen representatives.

Some professionals prefer to limit the extent or the kinds of questions that can be researched. They argue that not all nursing questions can be investigated. We do not agree with this position. By definition, nursing is *the diagnosis and treatment of human responses to actual or potential health problems* (American Nurses' Association Social Policy Statement, 1980). This definition takes into consideration the broad variety of human responses to health and illness. We contend that the ANA definition encourages a broad spectrum of nursing research questions, theoretical perspectives, and methodological approaches. Many areas not thought to be traditionally within the purview of nursing research can be investigated using this recently promulgated national definition of nursing.

For example, the October 1987 United States stock market crash affected the health status of many persons. Depression and suicidal tendencies were seen in many as a consequence of losing their money or their jobs. Nurse practitioners caring for these persons could describe and classify the variety of behaviors presented by depressed suicidal clients and later depict treatment protocols based on a category system evolved from their clinical practice. A published descriptive typology of behaviors and symptoms demonstrated by stock market crash victims would assist other investigators interested in the same or similar behavioral manifestations and resultant health problems in other contexts.

Other catastrophic events such as the nuclear accidents at Three Mile Island, USA (1979) and Chernobyl, Russia (1986) also could be sources of a nursing research project on the immediate and prolonged nursing problems experienced by employees and citizens living near these plants. A cross-cultural investigation of how people treated health problems as a result of these events could be of interest and value to nurses and other health professionals. As another example, the health problems suddenly cast upon people living on the slopes of Mount Saint Helens, Washington, following the volcanic eruptions could be of importance to many. In fact, this event was investigated and reported by a nurse concerned with the bereavement process undergone by persons living in the area of the volcanic eruption (Kiger, 1984).

New, less dramatic areas for nursing research can be derived from cases of children involved in serious automobile accidents. Some parents have health insurance coverage for the victims, which pays for a major portion of health care, and others must rely on public tax-supported institutions for assistance. With the two groups, the following research question could be investigated: Do children receive the same type of health and nursing care, and is their recovery process the same, regardless of their parents' ability to pay? Another nursing research topic might be the health status and the quality of health care provided to undocumented nonwhite aliens and their dependents in contrast to the health and quality of health care of whites living in the southwest. The range of research questions that can be asked and studied by nurses is wide, and the ANA definition of nursing strongly supports a diverse set of ways in which nurses may choose to investigate important problems concerning the health of society.

1–3 PROBLEM IDENTIFICATION AND CRITICAL REVIEW OF A CLINICAL NURSING STUDY

In planning research it is necessary to identify the problem area. For example, Brooten, Brown, Hollingsworth, Donlen, and Tanis (1983) were interested in studying the efficacy of different nursing procedures that relieved postpartum breast engorgement experienced by multiparous and primiparous women. Breast engorgement occurred in many different manifestations in the nurse's everyday practice on hospital labor and delivery units. In a literature review, the investigators identified a few relevant nursing research reports that related directly to their interest in finding the best way to relieve the pain and discomfort felt by newly delivered mothers. However, a number of clinical reports were located which promoted, for one reason or another, a diversity of techniques including avoidance of breast stimulation, application of ice, use of various analgesics, use of compression binders, application of breast pumps, use of tight-fitting bras, and administration of a prolactin inhibitor such as bromocriptine mesylate to prevent, reduce, or control breast engorgement and to decrease pain and leakage. At this stage, the investigators had a variety of options to use in investigating their research question. A comparative study using a variety of treatment techniques would help to establish which, if any, of the identified nursing and pharmacological protocols, were superior in arresting or preventing breast engorgement following the delivery of a baby.

For a successful inquiry, it is imperative that the investigators establish and refine the actual research problem in clear, unambiguous, and specific terms. To achieve this goal, any research question must be formulated so that it identified two or more variables which can be related to each other. The variables must be identified and defined in such a way that leads to sound measurement of the variables with high levels of reliability and validity; these topics are described in Chapter 3. The variables must satisfy data properties that permit a quantification or statistical treatment of the data. The specification of the target population and study site(s) to be studied should be precise and delimited. Finally the time framework in which the investigation is to be carried out must be clearly described.

The research question for the study of Brooten and colleagues could be phrased in the following form: What is the best procedure to employ to prevent, reduce, and control postpartum breast engorgement and to decrease pain and leaking of colostrum and milk within the first 28 days following delivery of a live infant at a university hospital in the eastern United States? With a clear research question such as the latter, researchers should be able to formulate testable hypotheses of the possible effects of implementing different protocols to reduce, prevent, or control the increased breast swelling and resulting pressure and pain experienced by newly delivered lactating mothers.

In the Brooten study, the investigators would have liked to specify the direction in which they expected one or more of the treatment procedures to take when used on a group of newly lactating mothers. Often prior research can be used to assist and predict the direction in which treatment effects are to be expected. In the research study of Brooten and coworkers, prior research was inconclusive, contradictory, and lacking in number and quality. A basis for prediction of treatment effects was not there. Because of this poor state of knowledge development, the investigators chose not to establish predictions in advance. They specified a series of null hypotheses which stated that no difference was to be found with use of any of the previously mentioned pharmacological and nonpharmacological techniques. They hoped to reject these series of nondirectional or "straw-men" hypotheses.

To maximize the amount of information about the treatment with a fixed budget, the Brooten investigators were faced with the decisions of selecting the best possible research design that would rigorously test the efficacy of different breast disengorgement protocols. Methodologies using exploratory, descriptive, correlational, experimental, or field work designs could have been used. The investigators selected a four-group comparison, correlational, quasi-experimental design. (This design is discussed in Chapter 4.) The compromise made by the investigators was based on the premise that physicians would not allow patients to be randomly selected for administration of the prolactin inhibitor, bromocriptine mesylate. Consequently patients who received the medication for newly lactating mothers (first group) were established as an intact study unit to be compared with three other nonpharmacologically treated groups. Women selected for the three other comparison groups were randomly assigned to one of three treatment conditions: the second group received compression binders only, the third group received standardized tight-fitting support bras, and the fourth group was restricted to limited intake of fluids.

The researchers had to identify and select relevant variables that measured the outcomes for the four-group comparison study subjects. Data selected were daily determined chest circumference, breast tension, severity of breast pain, number and amount of pain medications administered, and amount and leakage of colostrum and milk. Each variable was tied to the treatment conditions either on a priori or theoretical reasons. After discharge from the hospital each of the 68 study subjects was contacted by phone to report on the same data collected by the nurse researchers in the hospital. This was continued for a time period up to 28 days.

The collected data were easily scaled. Using a standard rating category for each variable, these scales produced consistent assignment of numerical values, enabling a statistical model called the *analysis of variance* to establish whether the four groups were comparable prior to entering one of the four treatment conditions. This was done using classification variables such as age and number of births. (The analysis of variance is described in Chapter 9.) No statistically significant differences were found on these variables. In examination of the dependent measures of the study, it was found that the pharmacologically treated group was most effective in preventing, reducing, or controlling breast engorgement and diminishing pain compared with that of the three nursing procedures conditions. In the three non-pharmacologically treated groups, the group given compression binders appeared to yield superior results for decreasing breast swelling, leakage, and pain.

At the conclusion of the study, the investigators offered suggestions for nursing interventions based on the study results. On the basis of the study, a combination of bromocriptine mesylate in conjunction with a compression binder appears to be the preferred method of minimizing breast swelling, leakage, and pain following delivery of a live infant in a low risk labor and delivery population. This recommendation for treatment, however, would need to be tested on another study sample because the investigators did not specifically test the combination of medication, the prolactin inhibitor, and compression binder treatment together. Because each method was highly effective in symptom management or in reduction of engorgement, it could be inferred that if the drug and binder were used together, this combination approach would be superior to all other conventional treatment approaches.

In briefly examining the study of Brooten and associates (1983), several considerations must be highlighted in getting a research project successfully underway. The impetus for this study came from the clinical arena of obstetrical nursing. The research literature base for choosing one treatment method over another was inconclusive or contradictory. Given the relative lack of firm objective knowledge about the degree of effectiveness of each treatment, singly or in combination, it is surprising that the investigators chose a design testing cause and effect relationships, when other research designs such as exploratory-descriptive approaches presumably would have provided a more thorough description and analysis of the important factors affecting pregnancy, delivery, and the postpartum period (Lederman, 1986). Some investigators might view the preliminary state of knowledge as too tentative in this particular research area to launch as methodologically rigorous an investigation as embarked on by Brooten and associates (1983).

The criteria for research problem formulation are designed to assist researchers to clarify the precise nature of the variables to be studied and the conditions and limitations under which these variables are examined and tested. The imprecision and lack of clarity of research problem formulations are areas in which many investigations are found lacking. Exactitude and operational specificity must be established at the study's onset in order to answer the research questions successfully. The research principles discussed in the Brooten research example are reviewed more fully in the next section in the examination of preoperative teaching and preparation of patients undergoing surgical intervention.

The view that is expanded in this book is that a researcher should always seek to find a parsimonious explanation of any phenomenon of interest to nurses. A theoretically elegant formulation is always preferred over inexact, ad hoc speculations. In many respects, the work of Johnson and colleagues (1978a; 1978b) holds the most promise of suggesting a sound and highly applicable set of formulations about why a planned preoperative teaching program works with specific types of persons undergoing major surgery.

For pedagogical reasons, several chapters in this book are built around a hypothetical study of cognitive priming and description of physical sensations in conjunction with precise instructions about exercises and ambulation in three different experimental conditions. Three experimental conditions are identified and serve as the focus for describing a research design and statistical models for data analysis. The conditions are as follows.

Treatment One: Patients placed in treatment one receive information prior to surgery only. Audiotaped information is played for each patient, supplemented by written descriptions of the surgical patient's career throughout the inpatient unit prior to discharge.

Treatment Two: Patients placed in treatment two receive the same audiotape and written information as those in treatment one and in addition are exposed to a detailed description of the typical physical impressions and sensations experienced preoperatively and postoperatively. Exercise instructions and sensation descriptions are given preoperatively only.

Treatment Three: Patients placed in treatment three receive the same audiotapes and written materials as in treatments one and two as well as descriptions of sensations and physical impressions of what to expect. They also are given explicit instructions in deep breathing, coughing, and ambulation exercises preoperatively. In addition, treatment three participants have the sensations and physical impressions instructions and exercise instructions repeated on days one and two postoperatively.

At this point, we begin a discussion which will appear repeatedly as we proceed to describe research methodology for nursing. This research, if it even were to be addressed, would have to be done in hospital settings. Ideally, a researcher chooses the hospitals at random to ensure *external validity* (discussed in Chapter 4). In practice, this can almost never be achieved. Instead, a researcher must use hospitals that are willing to volunteer their site for research purposes. Few hospitals will do this. Thus, the actual sites used serve as a delimiting factor in this research, and, for that matter, all research in nursing and health care.

No two hospitals are identical. Staffs vary and their positions on health care practices vary. Patients differ in attitude, ethnic makeup, financial security, age and gender, and a host of other characteristics. Hospitals vary in age, type of equipment, standard operating procedures, board of director policies, and many other salient characteristics. All these factors are thought to affect patient recovery. Furthermore, we must not fail to mention the important impact that physicians have on patient care and recovery. Research must include this important factor. As can be seen, the uncontrollable variables that enter into any nursing study are numerous. The goal for the nurse researcher is to perform each study in the best possible manner in a setting that is not the best of all possible worlds.

1–4 EXAMPLE OF COMPLEXITY IN THE RESEARCH OF PREOPERATIVE INFORMATION GIVEN TO PATIENTS

Many nurses have been traditionally concerned with what happens to patients prior to surgery and immediately after surgery. A number of anecdotal and impressionistic reports appeared in the nursing literature in the 1960s and 1970s detailing various attempts and approaches to assist patients in preparing for and successfully coping with the surgical experience. The literature suggests, at least from our experience and clinical insight, that fortuitous and productive outcomes occurred which have a beneficial effect on hospital patients. For instance, showing each patient who is about to undergo surgery a view of the operating room and recovery area, the equipment, tubes, gadgets, TV monitors, and related instruments provides an opportunity to reduce anxiety and to get a better grasp of the events that he or she is soon to encounter. In addition to inspection of the procedures to be performed and knowledge of prospective series of events and of care takers, an explanation of what nurses, physicians, and others will be doing to help the patient after surgery are positive forces in the prognosis of many operative patients. Also, evidence suggests that recovery is precipitated if expectations for the patient's performance after surgery are communicated, including getting the person to breathe deeply and to cough with periodic assistance.

Although cited reports are compelling, caution should be exercised in following procedures or methods in a successful case. In some instances it would be imprudent to change practice based upon subjective accounts by individual personal testimony. The approaches described in the literature make a certain amount of empirical sense, although no objective data exist with which a dispassionate observer would feel comfortable. Even so, some initial efforts at collecting a series of objective data on comparative groups of patients were described in the late 1960s and early 1970s (Dumas and Johnson, 1972; Dumas and Leonard, 1963; Egbert, Battit, Welch, and Bartlett, 1964; Healy, 1968; Johnson, 1965; Johnson, 1966; Lindeman and Van Aernam, 1971).

With the introduction of objective outcome measures such as reducing the incidence of postoperative vomiting, a more coherent picture of the results of different preparatory procedures for presurgical conditions begins to take shape. In particular, some nurses began to speculate about the relationship of particular nurse-initiated activities with persons prior to surgery and the effects upon the postsurgical careers of specific subsets of patients.

Johnson and associates were concerned about the effects of different preparatory procedures and strategies on patients and the apparent lack of an underlying theoretical explanation of why some nurse actions worked and others seemingly had little or no discernible effect. In an early set of studies, Johnson noted while working as a surgical nurse that a review with patients of the actual sequence of events, including the kinds of sensations likely to be experienced, seemed to be reassuring and helped to speed the recovery of some patients. It was also apparent from early encounters with presurgical candidates that some persons were non-accepting or resisted much description or review of what was going to occur following surgery. These observations were then followed by an attempt to explain why some patients responded positively or negatively to preoperative information. Over a course of many studies, Johnson and associates evolved a set of theoretical statements and propositions having to do with the cognitive structuring of anticipated unpleasant physical and psychological events (Johnson, Fuller, Endress, and Rice, 1978; Johnson, Rice, Fuller and Endress, 1978). In addition to prior surgical nursing experiences, some of the work of Janis (1958) about stress and Leventhal (1970) on coping influenced Johnson in the formulation of a theory on coping strategies of surgical patients.

In the approximately 20 years devoted to the topic, Johnson has refined a number of postulates regarding surgical preparation of patients. A set of interrelated propositions have developed concerned with the provision of information to patients. The propositions detail the postoperative outcomes demonstrated by patients who are given explicit descriptions of the physical sensations happening before and after surgery. Subsequent propositions have been formulated about the integration of procedural information and physical sensation descriptions with planned deep breathing, coughing and ambulation exercises, and postoperative outcomes. It appears that the cognitive structuring undergone by patients to successfully cope with the physical and psychological assault resulting from surgical intervention is a requisite component for patient recovery. It is assumed that nurse-inaugurated discussions, exercises, and descriptions of future recovery experiences augments or strengthens the person's psychological and physical resources and capabilities. In essence, a psychological and physical road map of what is going to happen to you and your body and the part that you and care providers will play

to get you through the hospital experience is vital to postoperative recovery (Johnson, 1984).

One major difficulty in the preparation of patients undergoing physical and psychological trauma is the specification of which actions of the nurse or other care provider may be of direct assistance in helping persons cope successfully. The major studies performed in the 1970s and early 1980s are comparisons of groups of persons experiencing different types of presurgery and postsurgery preparation protocols (King and Tarsitano, 1982; Hill, 1982; Wells, 1982). The variability of hospital site characteristics, differing nurse attributes and patient qualities, and the variety of surgical procedures performed are major factors influencing study outcomes. To date it is difficult to state whether every person benefits from a sustained rehearsal of events prior to and following surgical intervention (Wilson, 1981). There are competing hunches about the mediating variables that significantly influence the success of any particular anticipatory guidance or teaching program with surgical patients (Johnson, 1984).

Another nursing dimension requiring theoretical formulation is the specification of desired outcomes for any particular cognitive priming format. That is, what combination of procedural, sensory, or psychological information is most effective in preparing patients for the stress of surgery and its aftermath. Variables that have been examined to account for postoperative outcomes include the number of requests for postoperative pain medications, the number and kind of postoperative complications such as infections, pneumonia, ruptured sutures, and similar conditions that follow surgery. Psychological attributes such as anxiety and mood states, degree of confusion or disorientation, and feelings of helplessness or powerlessness have been examined and related to patient outcomes. Placed on a continuum, the possible outcomes range from death to recovery. Because most positive outcomes are expected to be found at the recovery end of the continuum, many approaches have been used to specify desirable outcome states for a specific preoperative teaching program (Devine and Cook, 1983; Devine and Cook, 1986; Hathaway, 1986).

Complicating the choice of particular measures of success in preparing persons for surgery is the inability to understand exactly which cognitive forces are at work in helping a person to cope with a physically and psychologically threatening event. Some investigators have taken an atheoretical and pragmatic approach to the issue of preparing persons for surgery. They claim that it is not important to speculate about why a preparation program works; simply acknowledge that the program does work and do it. A variety of different psycho-educative programs have been employed within a wide array of settings, with different client groups, under different site and surgical interventions, with variable standardized and nonstandardized preparation packaging formats, which have resulted in numerous positive outcomes with no theoretical explanation for their success (Devine and Cook, 1983; Devine and Cook, 1986; Hathaway, 1986). The pragmatist who looks at the range of studies and findings and who leans to the atheoretical argument would simply find a program that suits the setting and temperament of those using it and proceed accordingly. This is not considered research in its typical scientific sense. It is a model not to be recommended.

The perfect nursing study is not possible. The study we will describe is probably among the best that can be done and, for that reason, it must never be forgotten that it is a *hypothetical* one. Its value is that the example provided exemplifies how a clinical nursing investigation might be performed to achieve desired scientific standards. The proposed design provides guidelines as to how to proceed even though in the real world and under the best of all circumstances, the study is most likely flawed. In any case the researcher should design the perfect study to be performed in the best of all possible worlds and then begin convert-ing the ideal study into the real study, which circumstances and budget allow. Most likely, the final study will not provide a clear-cut answer to the original research question but it will provide an answer that, combined with the findings of other investigations, leads to a set of conclusions that serve to improve nursing practice.

1–5 THE HYPOTHETICAL STUDY

The hypothetical study will be conducted in three hospitals. Suppose that a survey was made of acceptable hospitals and that eventually a selection of three was made from among those who agreed to participate. The three hospitals were selected from a master list of volunteer institutions in which over 200 abdominal surgical procedures are performed each year. The three institutions represent a range of primary, secondary, and tertiary health care organizations currently found in the United States. They are as follows:

One: Hospital One is a hospital in a rural setting,
Two: Hospital Two is a community based hospital located in a suburban locale,
Three: Hospital Three is a large teaching and research health science center in an urban area.

We now assume that after the setting for the research has been decided on, the *hypotheses* to be tested are formulated based upon theoretical expectations and the stated goals and objectives of the research (Fig. 1–1). These topics will be discussed later.

Figure 1–1. Experimental design of the preoperative teaching study.

Covariates	Independent Variables			Dependent Variables
Gender	*Hospital One*	*Hospital Two*	*Hospital Three*	Length of Stay
Age	Treatment One	Treatment One	Treatment One	Number of pain medications
Severity	Treatment Two	Treatment Two	Treatment Two	in first 24 hours
Education	Treatment Three	Treatment Three	Treatment Three	Number of pain medications
Provider				in second 24 hours
Family income				Number of postoperative
Weight				complications
Smoking history				Number of days at home
Alcohol pattern				
Drug use				
Exercise				
Uncertainty				

After the hypotheses have been stated in clear testable forms, the *dependent* and *independent* variables of the study must be *operationally* defined. For our hypothetical study, the dependent variables were derived from a concept encompassing key attributes of postoperative recovery following surgery:

1. Length of inpatient unit stay (number of days until discharged from the hospital). This variable measures the amount of time that the patient stays within the hospital. Length of stay directly measures the postoperative recovery course experienced by the patient. Fewer days in the hospital decreases the financial cost of care and enables patients to return home and recouperate quickly.

2. Number of pain medications requested within the first forty-eight hours after surgery. This variable measures the number of times the patient is experiencing pain and discomfort postoperatively, thus requiring the administration of drugs to reduce or control pain and discomfort during the critical first two days after surgery.

3. Number of postoperative complications experienced by the patient after surgery. This variable measures the postsurgical aftermath in terms of number of undesirable occurrences such as prolonged bleeding, elevated body temperature, presence of wound infection, bladder distention, bowel impaction, and other adverse consequences.

4. Number of days spent at home before the person was able to leave his place of residence unassisted. This variable measures the ability of the person to recouperate and resume activities of daily living including the return to gainful employment and resumption of daily adult functions and responsibilities.

It is hypothesized that the four dependent variables provide a direct measurement of the efficacy of the three surgical preoperative preparation programs. The hypothetical construct of postoperative recovery can be viewed on a continuum ranging from negative to positive outcomes. The negative or undesirable end of the continuum can be reasoned to include such observable events as death, permanent disfigurement, long-term immobility, inability to return home and resume normal functions of daily life such as going to work, prolonged psychological trauma, life-threatening postoperative complications, inordinate degrees of pain,

and the necessity of having additional surgery performed. The positive or desirable end of the continuum can be argued to include survival, minimal or no change in body image, early ambulation and good mobility, early hospital discharge with rapid resumption of all normal responsibilities, minimal or transient psychological discomfort, temporary or no postoperative complications, transient pain, and no additional surgery required.

The construct of postoperative recovery and its logically derived operational measurement provide different measures of the outcome or effectiveness of the three preoperative preparation educational programs. Treatment three patients (sensation descriptions and exercises preoperatively and postoperatively) in contrast to treatment one (procedural information) and treatment two patients (sensations and exercises preoperatively) are expected or predicted to have a shorter postoperative hospital stay, require less pain medications, experience fewer postoperative complications, recuperate more quickly, and thus leave home or return to work earlier.

Variables other than the independent variable also can have an effect on the dependent variables. Those confounding or extraneous variables are usually uncontrolled and often are referred to as *covariates*. Covariates can be considered as confounding independent variables that can mask the effects of the independent variables of primary interest. The effects of covariate variables must be examined, accounted for, or removed in any study. The undesired effects of covariates are usually treated statistically. The statistical control of covariates is described in Chapters 9 and 10 in which the analysis of variance and the analysis of covariance are depicted. The confounding independent variables (covariates) for this hypothetical study are the following:

1. Gender. Females are expected to recover more slowly than males.

2. Age (at last birthday). Older persons are expected to recover more slowly than younger persons.

3. Severity (presurgical status classified as mild, moderate, or severe). Persons with more severe health problems prior to surgery are considered higher surgical risks and are expected to recover more slowly than those with few significant or no health problems.

4. Education (number of years of completed schooling ranging from elementary to postgraduate level). The higher the educational level of the person, the more likely that he or she will benefit from the planned instructional program and will recover postoperatively.

5. Provider (coverage by private, third party health insurance or public tax-supported facilities and programs such as Medicare). Patients who do have not third party health insurance may delay needed surgery and thus may be expected to be at greater risk when surgery is ultimately performed.

6. Family income level (0 to $50,000 and above). The higher the income level, the quicker the person's postoperative recovery will be. Educational level is expected to strongly correlate with income level.

7. Weight (to the nearest pound). A relationship exists between the weight of a person and the speed of postoperative recovery. Persons above normal body weight preoperatively are expected to recuperate more slowly than those at or below normal body weight.

8. Smoking history (ranging from never having smoked to smoking more than one pack per day). Heavy smokers are expected to recover from surgery less quickly than nonsmokers.

9. Alcohol pattern (ranging from never having consumed alcohol to consuming more than two drinks per day). Heavy drinkers are expected to recuperate from surgery more slowly than nondrinkers.

10. Drug use history (yes or no). Persons who report recreational drug use are expected to recover from surgery more slowly than those who do not report drug use.

11. Participation in an exercise regimen (yes or no). Those persons who exercise regularly are expected to recover more quickly than those who do not exercise.

12. Psychological uncertainty about illness scale (mean = 50, with a standard deviation of 10). Those persons who report higher levels of uncertainty about their illness and surgical outcome are expected to recuperate more slowly than those who are less psychologically uncertain.

The data for the 246 patients of this hypothetical study are reported in Table B-1 (see Appendix) along with the coded categories used to define each measure. The selection of both independent demographic and classification variables and dependent or outcome variables was based on prior research reported in a variety of surgical teaching programs as well as the current federal/state fiscal reimbursement schedule aimed at decreased length of stay.

The particular research design selected for our invented study is a comparative experiment occurring in a naturalistic field setting. After participating in an informed consent procedure, persons agreeing to serve as research subjects are systematically assigned to one of the three treatment conditions described earlier. The statistical properties of systematic sampling are described in Section 6–14. Each research subject is exposed to a treatment protocol the afternoon or evening prior to surgery. The audiotapes, description of sensations and deep breathing, coughing, and ambulation exercises last approximately one half hour. The same treatment nurse works with all patients in the three experimental conditions within each of the three study institutions. A random sample of sessions is audiotaped as a check on the consistency of the *manipulated independent* variable of the study: the different operative teaching and preparation programs. Furthermore, two trained nurses independently observe and systematically rate the treatment nurse's verbal and nonverbal interaction with a patient for consistency with the operation teaching protocol for that specific condition.

The demographic variables are ascertained by reviewing the patient's hospital record. Preoperative status, smoking history, alcohol and drug use, and exercise patterns are gathered from the initial history and physical examination performed on all surgical patients. The uncertainty scale is administered as part of the admission and intake interview conducted on all patients to the institution. The outcome variables of length of stay, number of pain medication requests and administrations for the first 48-hour period after surgery, and number of postoperative complications (hemorrhaging, ruptured sutures, pneumonia or atelectasis, infections, elevated temperature, and similar clinical problems) are gained from a review of the doctor's progress notes and the nursing care plans or nursing notes and intershift and/or 24-hour written report. Information concerning the number of days from discharge to the time that the patient was able to leave home unassisted is determined by means of a telephone call to a responsible adult living at the patient's residence. If the patient lives alone, the report can be obtained by a visit to the residence.

1–6 SUMMARY

This chapter briefly traced the development of nursing research in the United States. The role of curriculum development, theory construction and evolution, research training of nurses, national publications, federal government policies and funding priorities, and advanced clinical training of nurses among other factors were identified as contributing to the continuing progress of nursing research. Next, preliminary guidelines were offered about the initiation and development of a nursing research project. Suggestions for problem formulation and development were offered. An obstetrical nursing research project example was employed to discuss the clinical impetus for the conduct of a study. A discussion of the evolution of another clinical research investigation was presented. The project described was that of a hypothetical study concerning the preoperative education and preparation by nurses of surgical patients undergoing abdominal surgical interventions. The steps and processes through which nurse investigators evolved a theoretical rationale and testing protocol for a series of studies investigating different intervention strategies using sensory information and educational material were reviewed. The choice of methodology, the selection of samples and study sites, the explication and definition of operational measures of the degree of effectiveness of different interventions were described. The use of theory and empirical indicators to devise and implement the research protocol were discussed.

The next chapter describes the use of nursing theory upon which to base a nursing research investigation.

REFERENCES

Adams, E.: Frontiers of nursing in the 21st century: development of models and theories on the concept of nursing, J. Adv. Nurs., 8: 41–45, 1983.

American Nurses' Association: Nursing: a social policy statement, Kansas City, MO American Nurses' Association, 1980.

Brooten, D., Brown, L.P., Hollingsworth, A.O., Donlen, J., and Tanis, J.L.: Relieving postpartum breast engorgement, Nurs. Res., 32: 225–229, 1983.

Devine, E.C., and Cook, T.D.: A meta-analysis of effects of psychoeducational interventions on length of postsurgical hospital stay, Nurs. Res., 32: 267–274, 1983.

Devine, E.C., and Cook, T.D.: Clinical and cost-saving effects of psychoeducational interventions with surgical patients: a meta-analysis, Res. Nurs. Health, 9: 89–105, 1986.

Dumas, R.G., and Johnson, B.A.: Research in nursing practice: A review of five clinical experiments, Int. J. Nurs. Stud., 9: 137–149, 1972.

Dumas, R.G., and Leonard, R.C.: The effects of nursing on the incidence of postoperative vomiting, Nurs. Res., 12: 12–15, 1963.

Egbert, L.D., Battit, G.E., Welch, C.E., et al.: Reduction of postoperative pain by encouragement and instruction of patients, N. Engl. J. Med., 270: 825–827, 1964.

Gortner, S.R., and Nahm, H.: An overview of nursing research in the United States, Nurs. Res., 26 (1): 10–33, 1977.

Hardy, M.A.: The American Nurses' Association influence on federal funding for nursing education, 1941–1984, Nurs. Res., 36: 31–35, 1987.

Hathaway, D.: Effects of preoperative instruction on postoperative outcomes: a meta-analysis, Nurs. Res., 35: 269–275, 1986.

Healy, K.M.: Does preoperative instruction make a difference? Am. J. Nurs., 68: 62–67, 1968.

Hill, B.J.: Sensory information, behavioral instructions and coping with sensory alteration surgery, Nurs. Res., 31: 17–21, 1982.

Janis, I.J.: Psychological Stress. New York, John Wiley & Sons, 1958.

Johnson, J.E.: Effects of nurse patient interaction on the patient's postoperative discomforts. Unpublished master's thesis. New Haven, CT, Yale University, 1965.

Johnson, J.E.: The influence of purposeful nurse-patient interaction on the patient's postoperative course. In Exploring Progress in Medical-Surgical Nursing A.N.A. 1965 Regional Clinical Conferences, 16–22, New York, American Nurses' Association, 1966.

Johnson, J.E.: Coping with elective surgery. In Werley, H.H., and Fitzpatrick, J.J., eds., Annual Review of Nursing Research, vol. 2, New York, Springer, 1984.

Johnson, J.E., Fuller, S.S., Endress, M.P., et al.: Altering patients' responses to surgery: an extension and replication, Res. Nurs. Health, 1: 111–121, 1978b.

Johnson, J.E., Rice, V.H., Fuller, S.S., et al.: Sensory information, instruction in a coping strategy, and recovery from surgery, Res. Nurs. Health, 1: 4–17, 1978a.

Kiger, S.: A reliability assessment of the SCL-90-R using a longitudinal natural disaster bereaved sample. In Communicating Nursing Research, 17, Boulder, CO, Western Commission on Higher Education in Nursing, 1984.

King, I., and Tarsitano, B.: The effect of structured and unstructured preoperative teaching: a replication, Nurs. Res., 31: 324–329, 1982.

Lederman, R.P.: Anxiety and conflict in pregnancy: relationship to maternal health status. In Werley, H.H., and Fitzpatrick, J.J., eds., Annual Review of Nursing Research, vol. 2, New York, Springer, 1986.

Leventhal, H.: Findings and theory in the study of fear communication. In Berkowitz, L., ed., Advances in Experimental Social Psychology, vol. 5, New York, Academic Press, 1970.

Lindeman, C.A., and Van Aernam, B.: Nursing intervention with the presurgical patient: the effects of structured and unstructured preoperative teaching, Nurs. Res., *20*: 319–332, 1971.

Merritt, D.H.: The national center for nursing research, Image, *16*: 84–85, 1986.

Roy, C., and Obby, S.M.: The practitioner movement: toward a science of nursing, Am. J. Nurs., *78*: 1698–1702, 1978.

Stevenson, J.S.: Forging a research discipline, Nurs. Res., *36*: 60–64, 1987.

Wells, N.: The effects of relaxation on postoperative muscle tension and pain. Nurs. Res., *31*: 236–238, 1982.

Werley, H.H., and Fitzpatrick, J., eds.: Annual Review of Nursing Research, New York, Springer, 1984.

Wilson, J.F.: Behavioral preparation for surgery: benefit or harm? J. Behav. Med., *4*: 79–102, 1981.

Chapter 2

NURSING SCIENCE:
The Interrelationship of Nursing Constructs, Concepts, Hypothesis Formulation, and Measurement

2 – 1   RESEARCH BASED ON NURSING THEORIES

The relationship of nursing theory, constructs, and hypotheses derived from propositions linking nursing concepts is described in this chapter. The emphasis in the discussion of theory development focuses on the identification and formulation of hypotheses that can be tested through different research strategies. Next, the identification of approaches taken by nurse researchers to the development of propositions linking different aspects of a particular theory in a research design is illustrated in terms of research on preoperative teaching. The empirical connections between the measurement of operational health care variables are illustrated. Linkages between independent and dependent variables enabling the testing and verification of health constructs are developed. The different levels of measurement of health care variables are elucidated. Finally, the relationship and development of

nursing theories through testing under varying scientific perspectives about nursing phenomena are discussed.

A meta-paradigm about the domain of nursing has evolved through the work of a number of nurse theorists and has been used to build theories about four interacting components: the client, the nurse, the health of the client, and the environment in which the nurse and client interact and function. A number of schools of thought in nursing theories have emerged which addressed the interrelationship of these four interacting components. Three major theoretical perspectives have been subsumed under a number of nurse theorists. The needs theorists (Abdellah, Beland, Martin, and Matheney, 1973; Henderson, 1966; Orem, 1971) conceptualized nursing functions as meeting unmet needs expressed through a hierarchical level based on Maslow's (1954) hierarchy of needs and Erikson's (1963) stages of human development (Meleis, 1985). The interactionist theorists (King, 1971; Orlando, 1961; Pater son and Zderad, 1976; Peplau, 1952; Travelbee, 1969; and Wiedenbach, 1964) focused their attention on the processes of nursing care and the ongoing interaction between nurses and their clients. Nursing functions emphasize individual and environmental interactions in which the nurse regulates, modifies, or changes forces that influence the adaptation, self-care capabilities, and well being of the person (Meleis, 1985). The *outcome* theorists (Johnson, 1980; Levine, 1969; Rogers, 1970; and Roy, 1976) conceptualized the outcomes of nursing care and the nursing process as directly affecting the harmony or stability of the individual and environment (Meleis, 1985). These theorists view the goal of nursing as maintaining harmony and stability and preserving energy or equilibrium. For them, the consequences of nurse interactions can be determined by examining the outcomes achieved by the client. Research based on these diverse theoretical positions has developed slowly because of incomplete degrees of clarity among theoretical constructs, propositional linkages, and operational measures needed to test, verify, and expand theory.

The major issue to address in the development of an investigation concerned with nursing events, processes, procedures, problems, and issues is the theoretical underpinnings on which an inquiry is based. The development of nursing theory is a relatively recent mandate in the discipline. A considerable body of theoretical formulations about nursing has been published within the past 30 years. Prior to the 1960s, most writings about nursing practices and processes were based on philosophical and value-laden imperatives directed to the performance of nursing activities, actions, and interventions. The field of nursing has evolved and expanded rapidly because of the impetus of revolutionary developments in science and medicine and the significant attention brought to questions affecting health care by doctorally trained nurse investigators. In the contemporary literature a tremendous profusion of investigative reports can be found, often based on theoretical notions and predictions about events of importance and interest to the practicing nurse of today. To advance and integrate the findings of many studies that often appear to be disparate and unrelated inquiries, the nurse researcher needs to identify, understand, and synthesize the interrelationships among the studies.

Making the connections between different studies is not easy. The difficulty stems in part from the undefined domain of nursing as a field of professional practice. This lack of a uniform definition has lead to ambiguous or competing definitions of nursing, both within and outside of the discipline (Schlotfeldt, 1987). As a consequence, the identification of nursing research is problematic and confusing. The publication *Nursing: A Social Policy Statement*, by the American Nurses' Association (1980), provided a major effort by the profession to clearly articulate the domain of nursing as "the diagnosis and treatment of human responses to illness or potential disruptions in health status."

The diverse opinions of other professions and of the public regarding what constitutes legitimate societal interests to be served by the nursing community seriously influence the research and theory construction and testing tasks of the profession. In addition, a question remains as to whether professional nurses should be seen solely as adjuncts to the medical profession or whether their role should be shared with legitimate independent and interdependent disciplines. Under the federal governmental reimbursement rules of 1983, the professional practice of nurses has been sharply affected. Health institutions are placing a specific dollar value on nursing care based solely on the minutes and hours spent by nurses in direct patient care. This industrial model of task analysis and time and motion description of nurse functions does not adequately or accurately account for the very important health activities performed for clients, families, aggregates and groups directed to patient teaching, psychosocial counseling, coordination of inpatient and outpatient care, and other indirect care functions.

Health care facilities have drastically limited patient length of stay because of federal government payment retrenchment. Because of government policy, quality health care is no longer a right for many citizens but a privilege for those who can afford third party health care insurance coverage. The United States national health policy promulgated through the Department of Health and Human Service under the federal political administration of 1980–1988 effectively redirected health care into two distinct levels of quality. One level is found in private, community or research-teaching institutions where large numbers of patients or their families can pay for their care. The other level of health care is provided in municipal or county tax-supported health care facilities that care for indigent persons or those whose health care insurance is insufficient or exhausted.

Nurses have had to recognize this new reality and redesign roles and functions in different federal reimbursement settings that more efficiently intervene in human responses to illness or potential disruptions in health status. The impact of these political and societal changes means that theories of nursing must be rethought, approached, and formulated in ways that permit the incorporation of revolutionary changes in health care provision mandated by the national health policies created in the 1980s and 1990s. In addition, nursing theories must be prepared to assimilate other political and economic changes that make an impact on nursing practice and that are sure to arise in the near future.

The preceding discussion briefly highlights how political socioeconomic forces can have an influence on the nursing field. Knowledge of these political and economic factors should heighten perceptions of the effects that they must have on developing sound theoretical nursing models. That is, the construction and testing of theoretical propositions concerned with nurse-initiated actions must relate in part to the perceived societal mandate given or logically assumed by nurses to be within their purview. For instance, testing different neurosurgical techniques on humans or removing impacted teeth would not be seen as being within the scope of contemporary nursing practice. A major war or catastrophic occurrence, however, would compel many health professionals to play roles not traditionally or conventionally associated with societal expectations. Under warlike or cataclysmic conditions, for instance, some nurses might find themselves doing selected surgical procedures traditionally viewed within the scope of a surgeon's practice. Therefore, theories should be formulated to permit, when necessary, the inclusion of these hypothetical expectations.

A number of branches in nursing exist in which there are clear overlaps with other disciplines, including medicine. For example, consider the case in which a client is experiencing grief over a loved one's death. Depending upon the context of the nurse-client relationship and the contract, other professionals may feel obligated to offer assistance also or intervene to reduce the grief experience. The attending physician, the unit consulting psychologist, the social worker, and the religious counselor, among others, may also view themselves as possessing a mandated role to talk with or counsel the grieving client. Depending on state licensure laws, institutional policies, and normally sanctioned customs, all the involved professionals may intervene collectively, singly, or not at all, and with varying degrees of success or respite to helping meet the client's particular needs. To build a theoretical explanation about grief without defining the roles of the participants would be unrealistic. As suggested by this example, the theory must recognize the fluid boundaries of professional discretion, action, and evaluation in many health care situations to arrive at propositions that can be used for evaluation, testing, and research.

2–2 CONTEMPORARY FORCES INFLUENCING NURSING THEORY DEVELOPMENT

The definition and construction of any theory are vast and complex. The world of the scientist entails an ongoing search to find descriptions and explanations of events, observations, and occurrences. The scientist is continually trying to find order and predictability in what appears to be chaos. The normative structure of science is one in which events can be named, described, classified, and predicted. In applied fields like nursing, the nurse also is seeking predictability in terms of anticipating the outcomes of a particular set of actions in patient care. For example, the use of diaphragmatic breathing and leg exercises is predicted to reduce the incidence of particular postoperative complications such as elevated temperature and pneumonia. The nurse using these procedures wants to state with a great deal of certainty that patients who receive these interventions will benefit in concrete terms. Furthermore, there is a cost quotient associated with the time that each nurse spends using these procedures with preoperative and postoperative clients. If the preparatory procedures are ineffective or result in more complications, an increased cost to the patients and to the institution results. If this were the case, the professional nurse's time might be spent more equitably on other activities with or on behalf of the client. Underlying these and associated issues of effectiveness and outcomes is the concern of relating actions to an explanation of the reasons why some treatments are effective and some are ineffective. Here the role of explanation and prediction comes to the fore.

2–3 FIVE APPROACHES USED BY NURSE INVESTIGATORS TO DEVELOP, MODIFY, OR EXPAND NURSING THEORIES

Multiple strategies are used to develop, modify, or expand theory in nursing. The preeminent arena for theory development is to be found in situations in which nurses engage in assessments and actions concerned with health and illness. Theory development opportunities occur in nurse interactions and transactions with clients and interpersonal support systems. Furthermore, the environmental contexts involving nursing processes and therapeutics greatly affect the practice of nursing and must be accounted for in the construction and testing of nursing theories. Also, it should be noted that theory creation and refinement takes place in nurse administrative, teaching, and consultative roles in health care delivery systems. According to Meleis (1985), five major strategies can be used by a nurse investigator to develop, modify, or expand theory in nursing.

1. Theory-Practice-Theory

Under the theory-practice-theory strategy, it is assumed that an investigator constructs a world view or approach to theory according to personal educational and life experiences. In turn, the particular theoretical persuasions held by the investigator to examine nursing practice is called upon as an aid to develop theory. This means that nursing practice is examined through theories and concepts developed through prior knowledge. Verified concepts are put into practice and used to shape perceptions of encounters in the nurse-patient care situation. These encounters are then used to generate alterations in the initial concepts so that a new

or modified theory is generated and tested. In time a new cycle is begun.

2. Practice-Theory

Under the practice-theory strategy, it is assumed that nursing theory evolves directly from observation of nurse practices and encounters. Here the nurse researcher observes new phenomena in the work scene, develops new concepts, and isolates properties of the concepts in the practice area. Categories emerge and are identified as meaningful to nursing practice. Concepts are labeled, relationships are developed, and propositions for testing are stated. Studies are performed and, based on the findings, recommendations for practice follow. The process undergoes a new cycle, and improvements are made to the theory and practice.

3. Research-Theory

Under the research-theory model, theories evolve from confirmed or refuted research findings. In particular, this strategy is used in synthesizing systematic research in a delimited nursing area. In these instances, there is general agreement in the nursing profession about the major concepts in the field. A science and body of knowledge about the particular nursing field are recognized and accepted. A nurse-conducted project that focuses on a manageable number of variables with patterns that are easily detectable and that allow for hypothesis testing can be generated. Facts and data are collected and used to verify or challenge research hypotheses that connect knowledge to what is already known and accepted as true.

4. Theory-Research-Theory

Under the theory-research-theory strategy, nursing research is based on theories that are developed by other disciplines but are given unique nursing perspectives. The process of theory verification is guided by the nurse investigator's knowledge of theories and research from other disciplines, clinical experience and wisdom, and extensive knowledge of the nursing domain under examination. Theories, research findings, and methods from other fields are synthesized. The nursing perspective employs these models to test propositions concerning health/illness questions. Finally, the original theory is reexamined, based on new research findings and evaluated as to the theory's significance to nursing. Application of theories from other fields to the field of nursing is emphasized under this model.

5. Modified Practice-Theory

Under the modified practice-theory strategy, theory development starts in the practice situation. Here the inquiring nurse brings to the clinical situation an educational and experiential background plus a theoretical bent. This model assumes that nurses are well prepared to explain phenomena through health-illness perspectives. Within this approach, experience, sensory, and intuitive data are attached to cognitive, affective, and inferential interpretations so that concepts evolve from complex constellations of impressions, perceptions, and experiences. Using this strategy, theory testing is refined through the deliberate recorded experiences and systematic observations reported by the nurse investigator.

2–4 DEVELOPING THEORETICAL NURSING PROPOSITIONS FOR TESTING

In most research reports, the project can be categorized either as *theory generating* or as *theory testing* in emphasis. Theory generating studies reflect the lack of theory in a particular substantive area. They are often justified on the basis of their potential for new theoretical formulations and hypothesis development which have significance for the specific content area. Theory testing investigations contain the theoretical or conceptual background to justify their study. The reasons why the research was undertaken are presented. Also given are rationales for how the study addresses a phenomenon not previously described or reported and how it fills in gaps in present knowledge or theory; the potential significance of the theory for nursing is also articulated. Concepts are stated and defined. Propositions contained in the concepts are logically deduced through a set

of reasoned statements that relate propositions to hypothesized relationships or conjectural statements, and then are tested.

The first step in theory formulation is the identification and classification of the major concepts. This may well be the most difficult part of any research study using human subjects. A concept like health, illness, nurse, environment, well being, pain, and so on, is described by words or a collection of words with the purpose of conjuring up a mental image to the person. Concepts are, for the most part, abstract mental inventions or creations that can be used to characterize or depict real experiences, observations, or occurrences. Most often concepts evolve from the constellations of impressions, perceptions, and knowledge experienced over time. After they are defined they can be placed in cause and effect statements of how they are related to one another.

Concepts provide a description about the properties of a phenomenon and are not the phenomenon per se. We provide meaning to our sensory, intuitive, and experiential data by attaching verbal labels or written descriptors that help us understand what we see and observe. The theorist or researcher must, as a consequence, attach cognitive, intuitive, and inferential meaning to concepts through the use of words or terms. With careful development through the application of words or terms to define a concept, a definition should eventually emerge which most accurately reflects underlying meaning and the sense of a concept for research purposes that is understandable to others.

Concepts can be either one-dimensional or multidimensional. For Fawcett and Downs (1985), nursing care is a one-dimensional concept that they term as *invariable*. To them it is either present or absent. Technically this actually represents a one-dimensional concept that is *dichotomous*; it has only two states. A one-dimensional concept can often be transformed into a multidimensional concept by defining the various *facets* that the concept possesses. For example, two facets of nursing care are acceptability and adequacy. Acceptability can be characterized along a continuum from high to low acceptability. At the same time, the same nursing care can be characterized along a continuum from excellent adequacy to poor adequacy. With refinements, each facet can be further partitioned into categories or discrete nonoverlapping states that might represent high, moderate, or low degree qualitative facets. Some facets can be scaled and some can only be described. Formal procedures have been developed to identify the facets of a concept. Some of the methods, namely, factor analysis and multidimensional scaling, are described in Chapters 11 and 12. Their importance to growth in nursing research is well established and is of interest and value to the investigator in nursing science.

Concepts can be classified on the basis of the extent of their observable or measurement characteristics. Concepts are either directly observable with empirical referents or highly abstract and referable to a complex, global property of some unobservable thought, feeling, or process that individuals experience (Kaplan, 1964). Height and weight are examples of directly observable concepts, and fear and anxiety are examples of highly abstract concepts. Willer and Webster (1970) classify concepts as either *observables* or *constructs*. Observables, on one hand, are immediately accessible to or very close to being immediately accessible to direct observation, measurement, and counting. Surgical nurse and postoperative abdominal surgical patients are examples of descriptive terms easily accessible to direct inspection and enumeration. Constructs, on the other hand, contain remote or highly abstract properties and therefore are not directly accessible to sense observation or impression such as sight, hearing, smell, taste, or touch. Pain and stress are examples of constructs. Constructs are thought to have greater usefulness because they can be applied to a wide spectrum of events, experiences, impressions, and intuitive insights. Finally, constructs can be logically connected in the formulation of research hypotheses and findings.

The second phase in theory formulation is the identification of the concepts to be connected or related to one another in a theory. Concepts are the basic building blocks of theories and for that reason must be precisely defined. Usually concepts are mutually exclusive with little or no overlap, so that the meaning of one concept may be distinguished clearly from the meaning of another concept. A well-defined concept is one which provides an unambiguous expression of the way that the concept will be used in a particular context. At any stage of theory development, some definitions of concepts are taken as understood and others are newly introduced to explain some aspects of proposed theory treated unsuccessfully or poorly explained by other theories.

Two types of definitions are needed to make a concept derived from a theory empirically testable. They are termed *constitutive* and *operational*. The constitutive or theoretical definition explains a concept with other descriptions that are intuitively meaningful. The concept of pain could be constitutively defined in terms of feelings of intense bodily discomfort, mental distress, apprehension, and unpleasant physical sensations. In this particular illustration, the concepts of bodily discomfort, mental distress, apprehension, and unpleasant physical sensations are used in place of the concept of pain. An operational definition of a concept provides an abstraction with observable meaning and measurement. It can include the activities needed to measure the concept or provide direction on how to manipulate it in a study. An example of an operational definition of pain could be the number of analgesic medications administered and recorded for a patient following or during the first 24 hours after surgery. Operational definitions link constitutively defined concepts to the real world by indicating how the concepts are measured.

Figure 2–1, taken from Fawcett and Downs (1985), depicts in schematic form the relationship between concepts such as preparatory information and its effects on a postoperative recovery study, operational definitions, and measurements or indicators of the concept(s). For example, the concept of preoperative information contains three operational definitions and indicators: audiotape of procedural information given each patient, audiotape and book of exercises and activities to be done by each patient before and after surgery, and audiotape of sensory information describing bodily sensations and experiences throughout the patient's surgical and postsurgical career. Figure 2–1 reveals that some concepts, such as preoperative information, possess more than one operational definition and measurement.

Upon completion of concept identification and operational definition specification, the opportunity is created for the formulation of a set of propositions that connect the concepts together in a theory. Propositions are declarative statements about one or more

General Model for Proposition in Nursing Research

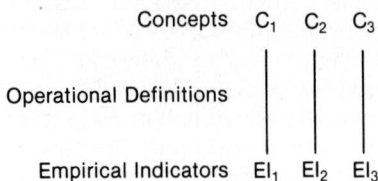

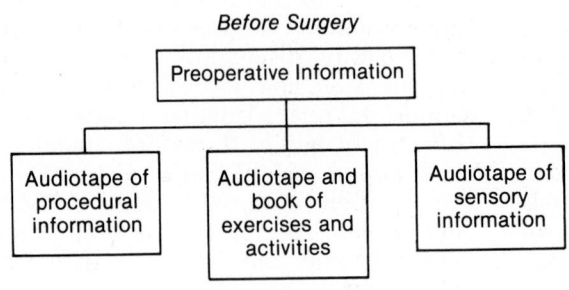

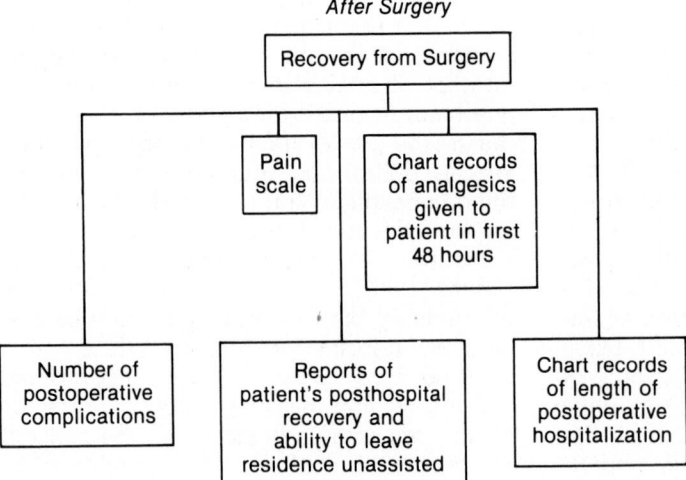

Figure 2–1. Linkage of concepts to operational definitions in a preoperative teaching study.

Adapted from Fawcett, J., and Downs, F.S.: The Relationship of Theory and Research, East Norwalk, CT, Appleton-Century-Crofts, 1985.

concepts and their interrelationship to one another. They can be described as indicating relational or nonrelational patterns. A nonrelational proposition is one that simply asserts the existence of a concept. "Human beings experience in the course of their life severe pain," is an illustration of a nonrelational concept. An example of a proposition that asserts the level of a concept is "Mr. Smith has severe pain in his left shoulder." This demonstrates a formulation of a relational concept depicting pain.

Relational propositions connect or tie together two or more concepts and are phrased in a declarative sentence that expresses an association between the concepts. Relational propositions specify patterns or degrees of covariation among concepts that are variables. Relational propositions can specify the recurrent existence of a phenomenon, the direction of a relationship between concepts, the shape or underlying probability distribution of a relationship between concepts, the strength or magnitude of the relationship between concepts, the symmetrical or nonsymmetrical nature of the relationship between two concepts, the concurrent and sequential relationship between concepts, the deterministic and probabilistic degree of certainty of occurrence relationship between concepts, the necessary and substitutable relationship between concepts, and, the sufficient and contingent nature of a relationship between concepts (Fawcett and Downs, 1985).

As examples of relational propositions consider the meta-analysis (discussed in Chapter 15) of 68 preoperative teaching studies performed by Hathaway (1986) involving the relationship of fear/anxiety, postoperative recovery, and preoperative procedural and sensory information and psychological coping strategies concepts. At the same time let us select propositions from the Devine and Cook (1983), Johnson et al (1978a, 1978b), Johnson (1984), and Ziemer (1983) reports which we also use to illustrate different types of relationship assertions.

Type 1. Simple Existence of a Relationship

It is reported by Hathaway (1986) that a relationship exists between preoperative instruction and fear and anxiety experienced by patients about to undergo surgery. Patients with preoperative instruction show less fear and anxiety than patients given no instruction. This proposition simply states that a relationship exists between the two concepts of preoperative instruction given and not given, and fear and anxiety.

Sometimes a proposition can indicate the level of the existence of a phenomenon. For example, patients demonstrate different levels of fear and anxiety before surgery. Here we see that some patients are more fearful and anxious than other patients about to experience the same surgical intervention.

Type 2. Direction of a Relationship

A proposition that shows the direction of the relationship is as follows. Persons given sufficient information about what may happen to them recover faster than those given inadequate or no information about the preoperative phase and postoperative recovery process. This proposition asserts that a positive relationship exists between the concepts of preoperative information and postoperative recovery.

Type 3. Shape of a Relationship

It is also reported by Hathaway (1986) that a relationship exists between preoperative information (procedural, sensory, and psychological) and postoperative outcomes, so that the average patient who receives preoperative instruction is at the 66th percentile of a similar group who does not receive preoperative instruction. This is a statement about group differences resulting from two different treatments given to patients about to undergo surgery.

Type 4. Strength of a Relationship

The following is a propositional statement that provides a statistical expectation about the strength of the relationship between preoperative and postoperative concepts and their operational measurements as reported by Hathaway (1986). A moderate (effect size of $\delta = .44$) positive relationship exists between preoperative instruction and postoperative outcomes. (See Chapter 15 for a discussion of effect size.)

Type 5. Symmetry of a Relationship

If the following propositions were true, they would represent symmetrical relationships. There is a positive relationship between preoperative information and postoperative recovery and vice versa. This is an example of a symmetrical relationship. If A, then B; and if B, then A. Unfortunately, this is not true. The following nonsymmetrical relationship has been established by Johnson and associates (1978a; 1978b). The positive relationship between preoperative information and postoperative recovery is nonsymmetrical. The proposition of Johnson and associates (1978a; 1978b) indicates that information given preoperatively hastens postoperative recovery; no claim is made about the effects of postoperative recovery on the provision of preoperative information. In this example, *time* precludes the reverse propositional statement as being true. Preoperative education must precede postoperative recovery. The following proposition, which is not from the preoperative preparation literature, may represent an example of a symmetrical relationship between concepts. Overweight men over the age of 50 have more health problems than underweight men over the age of 50. The reverse of the propositional assertion is underweight men over the age of 50 have fewer health problems than overweight men over the age of 50.

Type 6. Concurrent Relationships

If both concepts appear at the same time, the relationship is said to be *concurrent* or *coextensive*. An example of a concurrent relationship between propositions takes the following form. The presence of both procedural and psychological information in preoperative instructions is positively related to postoperative outcomes (Hathaway, 1986). It can be asserted that the relationship between types of preoperative instruction and postoperative outcomes exists and is concurrent.

Type 7. Sequential Relationships

If one concept appears prior to the other concept, the relationship between concepts is stated to be sequential. An example of a sequential relationship is the association between information given preoperatively and the length of postoperative hospital stay (Devine and Cook, 1983). Patients given preoperative training have shorter lengths of postoperative hospital stay than those given no preoperative training.

Type 8. Deterministic Relationships

Deterministic relationships state what always happens in a given situation. Such propositions assert the degree of certainty of its occurrence. These assertions are most often found in the physical and biological sciences and seldom in behavioral and health science fields, including nursing. An example of a deterministic relationship is that all patients exposed to preoperative teaching have no postoperative complications. To date the research literature does not support this deterministic relationship.

Type 9. Probabilistic Relationships

Probabilistic relationships are concerned with the chances or probabilities of some-

thing happening in a given circumstance. An illustration is provided in the following statement. Preoperative instruction accounts for 20% improvement in postoperative outcomes (Hathaway, 1986). A future study might predict that 25% to 35% of patients would show improvement.

Type 10. Necessary Relationships

In some theories, propositional relationships are labeled as being *necessary* relationships provided that the appearance of one concept A is required before a second concept B is observed. Concept B occurs, only if concept A occurs. An example of a necessary relationship is as follows. Information about sensations associated with surgery given preoperatively reduces postoperative distress (Johnson and coworkers, 1978a; 1978b). Necessary relationships cannot be modified. Concept A and only concept A must appear before concept B can happen.

Type 11. Substitutable Relationships

In some cases, concept C may serve as a substitute for concept A in bringing about the appearance of concept B. An example of a substitutable relationship between propositions is the following. Preparation in procedural information and psychological information or sensory information is related to postoperative outcomes. In a substitutive relationship propositional statement, some other similar concept such as sensory information replaces psychological information combined with procedural instruction to elicit the second concept of postoperative outcomes (Johnson, 1984).

Type 12. Sufficient Relationships

Relationships that are termed *sufficient* state that when concept A occurs, a certain other concept B will occur, regardless of any other circumstance. An example is as follows. Procedural, sensory, and psychological behavior information given preoperatively will reduce postoperative distress. The need for sensory information was offered as an example of a necessary relationship earlier in this discussion. Sensory information, however, is necessary for reduction of postoperative distress, but is not sufficient. Rather, three types of information (procedural, sensory, and psychological) are required to reduce stress (Johnson, 1984).

Type 13. Contingent Relationships

Relationships that are *contingent* state that when a given concept A occurs, a certain other concept B will occur, but only if a third concept C is present. An illustration is provided in the following. Provision of preoperative information leads to use of coping behaviors postoperatively, which in turn leads to a reduction of postoperative symptoms (Ziemer, 1983). Thus two concepts form a chain, and a third must be present for the expression of the second. Concepts A and B form a chain, but B will occur only when C is present.

Type 14. Complex Relationships

Devine and Cook (1983) suggest that a relationship exists between information given preoperatively and length of postoperative stay and also that it is negative, asymmetrical, and sequential and moderate in strength (average effect size, $\delta = .39$). Here several propositional assertions are made in one statement. First, the relationship is negative: Length of stay is short for preoperative preparation and long for no preoperative training. Second, it is asymmetrical because time does not permit or allow for training after the operation. Third, it is sequential, because of the time limitations. Fourth and last, the effect size is moderate.

2-5 RELATIONSHIP OF THEORETICAL PROPOSITIONS TO MEASUREMENT

Theories exist to provide explanations and connections between concepts. They can be used to guide research and, in turn, may be guided or reformulated because of research. The variety of strategies used by nurses to generate, develop, and extend theory suggests that a multidimensional approach is the most realistic tactic to be used in most nursing studies (Meleis, 1985). The five major theory development strategies (theory-practice-theory, practice-theory, research-theory, theory-research-theory, and modified practice-theory) described in Section 2-3 suggests that each strategy generates hypotheses to be tested. Hypothesis formulation entails a series of educated guesses or speculative statements about relationships among concepts and their operational measures. Meleis depicts the different ways in which theory can evolve. The five types of strategies also show that hypotheses to be tested in the nursing setting either can be deduced directly from prior research and theoretical expectations or can be inductively arrived at from intensive comparisons and contrasts of specific nursing interactions. All five approaches ultimately culminate in a set of research hypotheses that can be tested and verified or refuted with real data.

A nurse is constantly faced with the relationship that exists between practice and outcomes. For example, if a patient is given a postoperative pain medication, what objective and subjective events are expected as a consequence of the administration of an analgesic medication? Will the patient's blood pressure and other vital signs change in any predictable pattern? What will the patient verbally report to the nurse, two hours after the pain medication, that indicates that the medication is having a desired or undesired effect?

The nurse who administers many pain medications to many patients undergoing various types of surgical procedures observes a variety of responses to the administration of an identical dose of an analgesic. Some patients report mild cessation of pain; others report moderate cessation of postoperative pain; yet others report great relief. Still other patients may report no relief in the amount and type of pain experienced after pain medication administration. If a nurse begins to sort out the different characteristics of patients and types of surgical procedures that may account for the differential responses to similar pain medications, the first steps toward a research study are begun.

In some cases, a nurse may observe a pattern that explains some patients' response patterns. For example, patients who experienced orthopedic surgical procedures generally may be seen to have lesser cessations in pain occurrences than patients who have had general abdominal surgical procedures. Later, it may be further observed that in a specific surgeon's pyloric valvotomy procedure, postoperative patients experience less pain than patients of another surgeon. Again, an observant nurse could speculate on which factors may account for the differences. Could the differences result from some variation in surgical competency between the two surgeons? Or, could the difference be explained in part by the higher number of elderly Asian men in the first surgeon's case load as opposed to the few elderly Asian men in the second surgeon's case load? Or, could the noted differences be due to the fact that the same nurse performing the evaluation is also Asian and uses, in conjunction with the first surgeon's patients, a meditation technique that the elderly male patients view as appropriate to their cultural background? Obviously there are numerous competing hunches or hypotheses that can be generated from these nurse-patient encounters. The promising ones are worthy of empirical testing.

Examining the relationships between the different variables associated with pain medication effectiveness entails a speculation about the relationship of how one variable or group of variables may affect another variable or group of variables. The speculation often involves a cause and effect relationship between the variables. The causative variable is usually referred to as the *independent* variable, whereas the outcome is usually called the *dependent* variable. In the previous example, patient response to pain medication is the dependent variable. Possible independent variables that may explain patient responses to pain medications are surgeon competency, ethnicity, gender, and meditation. These four independent variables can be hypothesized to have an effect on the dependent variable, patient response to pain medication. This model is pursued in the following section. Readers who are already knowledgeable about independent and dependent variables and levels of measurement can pass over the remaining topics in this chapter or may read them in the context of a review.

2–6 INDEPENDENT AND DEPENDENT VARIABLES

All speculations between a variable or set of variables and some observable or set of actions that are put to the test in a research study involve a *seemingly* cause and effect relationship between two sets of characteristics. The presumed causative variables are referred to as the *independent* variables, and the outcome variables are referred to as the *dependent* variables. In some cases, the statement "A causes B," is a valid scientific statement. More often it is not. Consider the two statements:

1. The drug Lasix (furosemide) is a diuretic that causes the kidneys to remove excess water from the body.
2. Smoking causes lung cancer.

The first statement is a scientific fact. A patient retaining water in body cells will start urinating within 10 minutes following an injection of 40 mg Lasix (furosemide). The second statement is not a scientific fact even though the Surgeon General has decided that smoking is harmful to one's health. This latter statement is actually a correlational statement expressing an association between two variables. In essence, it says, "the risk of poor health is higher for people who smoke than it is for people who do not smoke." We know that it is not a cause and effect statement because not all smokers develop lung cancer or experience poor health and because many nonsmokers also develop poor health conditions and some even develop lung cancer.

For the first statement, the independent variable is the presence or absence of the drug. The dependent variable is the amount of fluid eliminated following the injection of the drug or a placebo. For the second statement, the independent variable is the act of smoking or not smoking. The dependent variable is the state of having poor or good health. Both statements appear to say that the presence or absence of the independent variable is associated with the presence or absence of the dependent variable. In the first case, the statement represents a cause and effect relationship. In the second case, the statement represents a correlational relationship.

This ambiguity exists in all statements between an independent and dependent variable that are put to empirical testing. Can the ambiguity be eliminated? Probably not. Cause and effect relationships are established on theoretical and not on empirical grounds. With a good theory, cause and effect relationships can be described and defended. Statistical methods applied to research data can be used to *support* or *challenge* the truth of a cause and effect relationship, but they cannot be used to prove the truth of a cause and effect relationship. Instead, statistical methods can be used to show *associations* between independent and dependent variables. This use of statistics is demonstrated repeatedly throughout the pages that follow.

The classic view of an independent variable is that the variable is manipulated by the investigator. An example of an independent variable from the hypothetical study discussed in Chapter 1 consists of the three different preoperative patient instructional preparatory programs assigned at random to the patients about to undergo surgery. The manipulation involves a protocol and a set of three different procedures applied to the patients. These procedures are predicted to have an effect on the four dependent variables: length of stay, number of pain medications, number of postoperative complications, and time spent at home before leaving residence on own. In this case, the treatment intervention is clearly manipulated.

In the complex health settings in which nurses work, many independent variables are not manipulated: that is, the variables cannot be controlled by nurses or other professionals. Patient gender and ethnicity and surgeon competency are characteristics that can have an effect on the number of pain medication requests. Under certain conditions they can be treated as independent variables and their hypothesized relationship to pain medication usage could be tested empirically. For example, a study could be set up to test the hypothesis that females recover from surgery faster than males. Here gender is not manipulated. It is determined at conception by chance factors.

Other examples of nonmanipulated independent variables abound in the research literature. Here are two examples in which a relationship of a nonmanipulated independent variable to an outcome variable is described.

1. Single men have more health problems than married men.
2. Surgical incisions heal faster on young people than on older people.

The first example illustrates a hypothesis of group differences. If $\overline{Y}_S$ is the mean number of health problems had by a group of single men over a given year and $\overline{Y}_M$ is the corresponding mean for married men, the statement implies that:

$$\hat{\psi} = \overline{Y}_S - \overline{Y}_M$$

is a number greater than zero. Such a hypothesis is tested by the Student t test which is reviewed in Section 9–6. The second example describes a correlational hypothesis. If X is used to represent the age at which a person receives a surgical incision and Y represents the number of days for the wound to heal completely, and if r_{XY} is used to represent the correlation between X and Y, the second statement implies that:

$$\hat{\psi} = r_{XY}$$

is a number greater than zero. This hypothesis also is tested by a t test reviewed in Section 9–6.

These two examples exhaust the kinds of hypotheses that relate an independent variable to a dependent variable. The first example provides a test of group differences and the second example provides a test of variable association. All empirical hypotheses can be stated either as a test of group differences or as a test of association. There are no exceptions, as will be seen when research methodology is presented in later chapters.

2–7 OPERATIONALIZING ABSTRACT HEALTH VARIABLES

After dependent and independent variables have been selected for study, methods must be generated for measuring them. In deciding how to test hypotheses, a measurement theory must be established. Measurement theory consists of a set of assumptions, methods, procedures, propositions, and practices that can be used to study the way that the world of theory is related to the world of observations. Measurement theory is always presumed to be operative whenever scientific concepts, hypotheses, and theories are used to frame a nursing research question or objective (Selltiz, Wrightsman, and Cook, 1976). The concept of pain requires operational indicators to determine whether it exists and in what amounts and its frequency and intensity. Behavioral indicators of pain are required to assess the absence or presence of the concept of pain. The concept of pain is an abstraction. Even though pain is given the following second definition in *Webster's New World Dictionary* (2nd edition, 1980), "a sensation of hurting, or strong discomfort, in some part of the body, caused by an injury, disease, or functional disorder, and transmitted through the nervous system," there is no clue as to how to measure its strength and depth.

For all of us, pain denotes an idea formed from personal observation and sensory experiences resulting from illness, accidents, and general stress. A concept like pain, is called a *hypothetical construct*. Everyone knows what constitutes pain, but no one is able to decide which of two patients experiences the greater amount of this hypothetical variable and universal human experience. The concept is labeled pain because pain shares a combination of essential properties or events that sets it apart from other occurrences in some qualitative or quantitative manner (Waltz, Strickland, and Lenz, 1984). Webster's definition does this but does not go far enough in providing a nurse with a means for its assessment.

Operationalization is the process of defining how a hypothetical concept such as pain is measured. In operationalization, the concept is redefined in explicit, unambiguous, observable terms and by specific operations that must be completed in order to measure pain. Operationalization is a part of practically every component of nursing activities and functions. The process of operationalization of a concept makes explicit the linkage of thought, sensation, and experience, for instance, by identifying how pain can be described and measured in concrete terms (Waltz et al, 1984). An example of operationalizing pain in the hypothetical preoperative instruction study is the definition of postoperative pain as the number of times that pain medication is administered for the first 48-hour period after surgery, as measured through the number of documented entries in the patient record. It can be inferred that the individual patient with no documented entries for pain medication experienced little or no postoperative pain in contrast to the person who had 12 documented entries for the first 48-hour period.

As might be expected, the concept of pain can be defined and measured in a variety of ways. We could simply question each patient every 4-hour period about whether or not pain is being experienced. Alternately, we could give the patient a mood checklist

and infer from his responses the degree of pain experienced. Perhaps a color chart could be used by asking a patient to describe preoperatively which color describes a typical or normal state as a baseline, and then ask the patient to identify which color describes the postoperative status. Or, we could ask family members or primary support system members to estimate the degree of pain experienced by a patient. Finally, all the above measurement approaches could be used to effect a multidimensional measure of the concept, pain.

A number of assumptions are involved in the preceding examples of measuring pain. First, it is assumed that all patients react equally to a given pain stimulus. This is false. Two persons experiencing the same pain respond in different ways (Geach, 1987). The assessment of pain is further complicated by the confounding of extraneous variables like age, cultural background, and gender, which prevent all patients from asking for pain medication postoperatively, even if their pain is severe and of equal intensity. For instance, young Hispanic men may view a request for pain analgesics as being in conflict with certain cultural values about masculinity and strength and, as a consequence, Hispanic patients may adopt a stoic stance and suffer in silence.

In measuring pain, assume that all patients are willing to tell the truth and are able to assess accurately their own pain experiences (Whipple, 1987). Furthermore assume that when a patient is asked about pain, the nurse, the patient, and the patient's significant other(s) will not behave in a manner that could produce a distortion or bias in the patient's response to questions about pain. Additionally, assume that for any of the above measures, questions asked or the measurement instruments employed are related to what the inquiring nurse had conceptualized or theorized as to what "pain" is about. In other words, the measurement of pain must be valid.

2–8 LEVELS OF MEASUREMENTS

In examining variables for the presence or absence of certain attributes of interest or in determining how much of an attribute such as pain is present, it is necessary to establish some *quantitative index* that is correlated with the underlying attribute. Where variables are defined in terms of quantitative estimations expressed as numerical values, the level of exactness must be decided on to be used to assess the variable in question. This leads to a discussion of *measurement* and *scaling* principles. But first it should be noted that a number of variables of interest to nurses do not lend themselves to measurement in terms of quantitative scales. Frequently qualitative measurement is all that can be achieved. Suffice it to say that many of the profound experiences that people face when ill are not amenable to easy measurement, examination, or analysis. The emotions of hope, fear, anger, abandonment, impending death, bodily and psychological threat and injury, and similar emotional states are difficult and in many ways impossible to measure quantitatively in any meaningful way.

Measurement can proceed on many levels. For example, it can be said that John is tall, taller than his father, in the 4th quartile of the distribution of adult male heights, or 6 feet 3 inches tall. Except for the first assessment, each assessment is a refinement of the one before. This hierarchy of refinement is a key point in measurement.

The point in considering levels of measurement is that when a researcher has to make decisions on measuring some psychological or physiological characteristic such as degree of pain following surgery, the objective is to obtain a measurement as high on the measurement classification scale as possible to obtain satisfactory indications of pain. This implies a hierarchy of scales. For measurement theorists the lowest level of measurement is simple naming and classification, with the highest level producing meaningful differences and ratios among observations. In simple terms, the hierarchy involves nominal, ordinal, interval, and ratio measurements.

A *nominal* scaled variable is one whose levels are described in verbal terms by indicating class exclusion or inclusion. Adults about to undergo surgery can be classified according to:

1. Gender:
   a. male
   b. female
2. Race:
   a. Asian
   b. black
   c. white
   d. other

3. Season of birth:
   a. winter
   b. spring
   c. summer
   d. fall

The states or categories of a nominal variable have no ordered or quantitative bearing on one another. For example, the classes of gender can be reordered as

4. Gender:
   a. female
   b. male

and the classes of race can be reordered as

5. Race:
   a. black
   b. white
   c. Asian
   d. other

There is no correct order, and so the classification is strictly nominal. Nominal variables are sometimes called *categorical* or *attribute* variables.

A parenthetical comment is made here about the nominal category of season of birth. The seasons of the year can be scrambled when speaking of health variables such as severity of heart attack, onset of gallbladder symptoms, and degree of pain experienced by patients following surgery. In some situations, however, the seasons of the year can be used to represent an ordered relationship. Measles, for instance, is seasonal in onset. If one were studying the prevalence and incidence of measles, the order of the seasons could not be ignored. Birth rates and death rates also reflect seasonal differences. A variable that is strictly nominal in one setting can be ordinal in another setting.

In the preoperative teaching study, there are a number of nominal classifications: men and women, exercisers and nonexercisers, drug users and nondrug users, levels of severity, and years of education, among others. The last two variables are examples of ordinal variables. For example, the classes of severity can be ordered as

6. Severity:
   a. mild
   b. moderate
   c. severe

Degree of education can be represented by the ordered classes as follows:

7. Years of education:
   a. less than 8th grade education
   b. 8th to 12th grade education
   c. more than a 12th grade education

Ordinal variables have an underlying nature of less to more. Here the goal is to set up a monotonic relationship between the characteristic and its measurement. A relationship between true pain and measured pain is monotonic if low levels of true pain correspond to low levels of measured pain and if high levels of true pain correspond to high levels of measured pain. Clearly, the goal of measurement is to maximize the correlation between true pain and measured pain. With ordinal variables, measurement theory does not seek to determine the pain distance between any two adjacent categories, nor can categories be defined that suggest that the pain differences among categories are equal. In trying to locate patients on a pain index from no pain to a little pain to much pain to a great deal of pain, it is possible only to locate a patient according to the four ordered categories and not according to precise quantitative units. If five patients were asked about their own amount of postoperative pain using the preceding four ranges of choices: no pain, a little pain, much pain, and a great deal of pain, it is possible only to locate each patient according to greater or less pain compared with locating the other four patients. The monotonicity of the scale holds, but its quantitative properties are unknown.

An interval variable is measured on a quantitative scale that can be discrete or continuous. Quantitative variables are those in which measurement is possible in both whole and decimal units. The number of pain medications that a patient receives is measured on a discrete scale with the classification or measurement possible in whole units (i.e., 0, 1, 2, 3 . . .). A patient receives either three or four pain injections in a 24-hour period. The patient does not receive 3.20 medications. Continuous variables can be conceptualized as representing a continuous progression from the smallest amount of the variable to the largest possible amount, with all decimals being a possible value for the variable.

To say that a variable has interval properties implies that equality of differences between paired observations on different parts of the scale represent equal differences in terms of the underlying hypothetical construct. Thus, if $d_{12} = X_2 - X_1$ is equal to $d_{34} = X_4 - X_3$, and if d_{12} and d_{34} represent equal changes between (X_2 and X_1) and (X_4 and X_3) on the underlying variable, the scale is said to have equal interval properties.

There is a misconception about what constitutes an interval scale. For example, consider four presurgery adult patients given the Stanford-Binet IQ test, and suppose that their tested scores are given by $X_1 = 95$, $X_2 = 105$, $X_3 = 125$, and $X_4 = 135$. For these data, $d_{12} = 105 - 95 = 10$, and $d_{34} = 135 - 125 = 10$, so that $d_{12} = d_{34}$. Does this mean that IQ is measured on an interval scale? It does if the difference in *cognitive ability* for subjects 1 and 2 is equal to the difference in cognitive ability for subjects 3 and 4. As we know, this is not true. The subject with an IQ of 135 is better able to solve cognitive problems at a higher level of performance than the subject whose IQ is 125, and the difference in behavior for these two superior persons is much greater than it is for the two subjects who are five points above and below the mean IQ of 100. The cognitive skills of subjects 1 and 2 are very similar, even though the patient whose IQ is 105 is slightly superior to the patient whose IQ is 95. The difference in performance for subjects 1 and 2 is considerably less than that for subjects 3 and 4. Although the numerical differences are equal on the measurement scale, the IQ scale does not possess interval properties for assessing cognitive ability on its *true* scale.

Human heights and weights are measured on an interval scale. The difference in height between two subjects whose heights are 65 and 69 inches, respectively, is identical with the difference in height of two other persons whose heights are 72 and 76 inches. In like manner, the difference in weight of two persons whose weights are 140 and 152 is identical to the difference in weights of two different persons whose weights are 190 and 202 pounds respectively. In both cases, the difference in weight is 12 pounds. Many physical measurements have interval scale properties, but most psychological variables do not.

We would like to present an example of a ratio scale but find that it is difficult because ratio scales are even rarer then interval scales. A ratio scale is one in which ratios have equal meaning. For example, the Stanford-Binet test lacks ratio properties because even for $r_{12} = 105/95 = 1.1053$, it cannot be concluded that subject 2 has 10.53 percent more cognitive ability than subject 1. Now consider, $r_{34} = 135/125 = 1.08$. We know that subject 4 is considerably brighter than subject 3, but the ratio suggests that subject 4 is brighter by only 8 percent; the ratio should be higher than that reported for subjects 1 and 2, who are very similar in cognitive ability.

Consider the variable Y—number of pain relievers administered over a fixed period of time. Possible values are (0, 1, 2, 3, 4, 5 . . .). This variable has both interval and ratio scale properties. For example, $d_{35} = 5 - 3 = 2$ and $d_{24} = 4 - 2 = 2$ represent 2 more administrations for relief. Also, $r_{12} = 2/1 = 2$ and $r_{24} = 4/2 = 2$ represent equal ratios. Relative to one administration, two represents twice as many, and relative to two administrations, four represents twice as many. Even so, as an index of pain this variable (y) may not represent a ratio nor an interval scale. In practice, we can never know for sure.

Ratio scales provide all the information that interval measures do. They possess one additional property: They begin from a true or absolute zero point. That is, obtaining zero on our hypothetical pain scale would have to indicate the total absence of pain. Classically, volume, length, and weight are defined as examples of ratio scales. For instance, in our preoperative study if one of our subjects weighs 100 pounds and another weighs 200 pounds, we can say that, based on the ratio scale characteristics, subject A weighs twice as much or is two times as heavy as subject B.

After this introduction, our discussion of selecting a scale for research purposes continues. As an example of the kind of reasoning that a researcher would follow in trying to set up the measurement of pain following an operation, the weakest type of measurement would be simply to ask the patient "Are you in pain?" The only acceptable answers are *yes* and *no*. Very few researchers would be satisfied with such a simplistic, dichotomous measurement of pain. The next step up the measurement scale is to try to measure pain with a set of ordered classes. Here, there are an unlimited number of nominal sets that can be used. We suggest some classes although we are sure that the experienced nurse can suggest even more appropriate or insightful ones.

Beginning with a simple set of classes, a patient might be asked, "How much does it hurt?" The patient may say, "It doesn't hurt at all," "It hurts a little," "It hurts a lot," or "I can't stand it." There are obvious weaknesses in that kind of question. One patient's response, "It hurts a little." may equal another patient's response, "It hurts a lot." It is not clear what is actually being measured each time a patient is quizzed. Another problem is that it may be impossible to establish measurement reliability (a psychometric property discussed in Chapter 3) for such an item. Although this item lacks acceptable measurement properties, it has face validity (a property discussed in Chapter 3), and it is amenable to higher level statistical analyses than the simple question, "Are you in pain?" The ordering of the classes places the measurement on a scale from low to high.

The next step up the measurement hierarchy would be to see whether a more reliable and valid set of classifications could be defined to measure pain, a set that provides a reference point for patients to compare with their present state of pain. Ideally one would like to have an absolute reference point. But such a model is probably not obtainable in a clinical situation of this kind. As a compromise, a relative reference point can be obtained for each postoperative patient. The patient could be asked, "Compared with your pain four hours ago describe whether the pain now is much worse, worse, the same, better, much better, or gone?" Measurement problems still exist with this question, but reliability checks are possible and more powerful statistical models are available for treating these kinds of ordered qualitative information.

Going another step up the measurement scale, the subject may be asked: "Think of the worst pain you have ever had and suppose, on a scale from one to ten, you give the worst pain experience a ten. How would you rank the pain you are having now?" Here the subject has to provide a number from one to ten. A great variety of statistical methods can be applied, provided that the responses satisfy the statistical assumptions of normality, equality of variance, linear relationships, and so on (discussed in Chapters 9 and 10).

In theory, one should be able to go even higher on a measurement scale. The measurement of the previous variable is most likely discrete. Most patients would respond with an integer such as two or seven; none would say 3.2579. The scale lacks continuity. About the only way to obtain a sophisticated measure of pain would be to use a physical measure of pain.

Suppose that a tuning fork measurement procedure were used to get a more precise indication from patients concerning the exact degree of pain. Further suppose that patients establish as a baseline the most comfortable and the most uncomfortable sound heard. For measurement purposes these two reference points could be located on a decibel scale that has the properties of continuous measurement. Then each patient could be asked to indicate at what sound level their pain could be located. The pain indicator could be located at an exact point between the two poles identified by the patient at the initial tuning fork exercise. Therefore, if a patient identified the most comfortable sound at 20 decibels and the most uncomfortable sound at 76 decibels, there is a continuous scale ranging between these two values. Even though the scale is continuous, a patient must identify the pain he associates with a particular sound level, of 61, for example, which is a discrete scale. This is an increasingly more precise measurement of pain reported by that patient. Even so there is no way to know whether or not this scale has interval or ratio properties.

The highest level of measurement is a ratio scale. In addition to being able to speak of equality of ratios, this type of scale has a meaningful absolute zero point. The ideal measurement of pain is probably a physiological measure that serves as an absolute index of pain. A chemical laboratory analysis of particular chemical properties associated with pain would be the ideal measurement. Such a chemical index would have an absolute reference point and patients could be placed on that scale for exact locations of pain. Patients tested who had a zero reference point would be stated to have absolutely no pain if such a test existed. The important characteristic is that statements like, "Mr. Jones is experiencing twice as much pain as Mr. Smith," or "The pain felt by Ms. Adams is one fifth the pain felt by Ms. Black," are possible. On a ratio scale, comparisons shown as fractions are interpretable.

Practice should suggest that interval and ratio scales are almost always unattainable. Consider some common scales and their properties. Body temperature as a measurement of health is not on an interval scale,

and because it does not have interval properties, it cannot have ratio properties. Arterial blood pressure diastolic readings used as measurements of clinical change are not made on an interval scale. Number of days in hospital after surgery has interval and ratio properties when treated as *days*, but may not have these properties when used to measure severity. Number of pain relievers treated simply as a *number*, has interval and ratio properties, but as a measurement of severity or level of pain, it probably does not.

Is there a summary for this discussion on nominal, ordinal, interval, and ratio scales? The answer is a resounding "yes." Most measurement can satisfy the property of *ordinality*; rarely can it achieve interval, and almost never achieve ratio properties. Many misconceptions about the need for scales exist. It is frequently said that *nonparametric* statistics are valid for nominal and ordinal scales and that *normal curve* statistics are valid for interval and ratio scales. This misconception should be corrected early. Statistical methods are not based on scale properties. Statistical methods are based on the nature of the probability distribution possessed by variables, whether on a nominal, ordinal, interval, or ratio scale. The next section shows how statisticians classify variables. The statistician's classification scheme is important when selecting statistical models for data analysis, hypotheses testing, and estimation of treatment effects.

2-9 STATISTICAL VARIABLES

Statisticians define variables as being either *qualitative* or *quantitative* in nature. The statistician's qualitative variable is equivalent to the psychometrician's nominal variable. Ordinal variables can also be qualitative and are referred to as ordered qualitative variables.

Quantitative variables are variables whose states are numbers. If the numbers consist of a countable set like {0, 1, 2, 3, . . .}, {36.2° C (97.2° F), 36.3° C (97.3° F), 36.4° C (97.4° F), . . .}, or {100 mg, 110 mg, 120 mg, . . .} they are said to be *discrete*. But if the numbers include the set of decimals, it is said to be *continuous*. For example, body temperature, in theory, is measured on a continuous scale extending from a dangerously low of 90° F to a life threatening high of 105° F. All decimals in this range are a possible body temperature. In the end, the statistical variables that a practicing nurse is most likely to encounter are unordered and ordered qualitative variables and discrete quantitative variables.

2−10 THE ROLE OF THEORY IN NURSING RESEARCH

During the past two decades, those who are in academic nursing or at the forefront of nursing research have concentrated their efforts on generating theories for nursing research. It cannot be said that all efforts have been fruitful or that the generated theories have provided acceptable levels of prediction and explanation for untested or new hypotheses. In fact, if these theories are scrutinized by scholars of the philosophy of science, probably only some could pass unscathed through the numerous canons of scientific rigor. To nurse researchers, this state of affairs comes as no surprise. Careful reading of the literature shows that nursing research has many discerning critics.

In the past, classical physics was often offered as an example of a discipline with an advanced set of theories that produced the best predictions and explanations for the variables and events included in its domain of study. Because of the high status given to physics in the hierarchy of science disciplines, the new emerging field of nursing theory has, in some instances, been held to the models used by physics and the natural and biological sciences. Use of these models to depict nursing theory development has met with little success. To use physics as a model or any of the natural sciences is to us undesirable and unproductive to the future of nursing research.

In examining classical physics, we note that it has had an extremely long history. Ancient Egyptians and Greeks had excellent working models of many physical principles and laws. Certainly, others before them also knew about the principles and laws of physics and the way discrete masses were effected by outside forces. Many physical laws were known and understood before Newton studied them and summarized the results on paper for others to read, understand, and use. Aristotle, Galileo, Copernicus, Kepler, and lesser known or remembered scholars

and investigators contributed to an understanding and knowledge of physical laws long before Newton. Even the drawings of Leonardo da Vinci preceded the writings of Newton; in his drawings and writings can be seen much of what we associate with Newtonian physics today. Although Newton may be considered an important figure in the development of mechanics, gravitational theory, and related components of modern physics, it must be remembered that he did not invent physics single-handedly. Much of physics was already known before he wrote the *Principia* (1687). Like Rome, modern physics, was not built in a day. It took centuries.

It is probably a true statement that all sciences have their beginnings in the observations of naturalistic events and processes. Most likely some specific type of event is seen by someone who recognizes that when event A appears, event B soon follows. If the observer possesses a high degree of intellectual and observational abilities together with critical insight and, if the sequence of events is seen over and over again, the observer may generalize from a series of discrete objective observations to a theoretical statement that seeks to connect event A to event B. If the theory adequately describes and explains some phenomena repeatedly, practice may lead to verifiable predictions and reasonable explanations of other events not originally included to join event A to event B. For a discipline like physics, many centuries of observations of events and processes preceded the effort of Newton and his followers to quantify the observed events through the postulation of mathematical relationships that showed how event A and event B related to one another.

Nursing is in the observational stage of development as a science. That it does not have sufficient observations reported in the literature on which to generate a theory like Newtonian physics is obvious. That nursing theories will never reduce to mathematical formulae is without question. Although there may be an immediate desire for strong nursing theories that explain and predict nursing processes and outcomes right now, delayed gratification has its advantages and often is its own reward.

Physics and the other natural and biological sciences are poor models for nursing to emulate. Newtonian physics represents a *grand* theory of physics. It is not the only grand theory in physics. Other grand theories are the quantum mechanics theory, relativity theory, weak gravitational theory, strong gravitation theory, the big bang theory, and many other specialized theories in use today to explain specific events and relationships that the physicist cannot presently explain under a single theory of physics. Thus, not even the "queen of sciences," functions within only one theory. If physics can abide and grow with multiple theories, so also can nursing.

Merton (1968) differentiates grand theories from middle range theories. To Merton, grand theories are the core theories of a science and are not testable because they represent conceptual frameworks. They are important because they are used to spawn middle range theories which in nursing research are practice-oriented. Suppe and Jacox (1985) suggest that most nursing theories are middle range theories.

In essence, our position is that some nurse theorists are prematurely concerned with identifying the grand theory or theories of nursing. We are convinced that no grand theory adequately represents the domain of nursing today. Our main reason for this belief is that the subject matter of nursing research is *people*. Each man and each woman is a unique person. The psychological make-up of each person is idiosyncratic to that person. The genetic background of each person is unique to that person. The physiological and biochemical processes associated with each person are specific to that person. Not even identical twins are truly identical. Building a body of knowledge that is sound across such a heterogeneous lot is like building a gigantic bridge across the Pacific Ocean from San Francisco to Hong Kong on piles driven into heterogenous mud.

Not even the theories of the most advanced behavioral science, psychology, comes close to imitating the theories of physics. Physicists can describe almost without error the exact path that a rocket shot into space will take if certain forces are known to be in operation during the time of the flight. Psychologists cannot predict with a high degree of accuracy what an adult male would do if suddenly attacked in a dark alley by a menacing robber aiming a gun at his chest and demanding that he give up his money or be killed.

For humans, exact predictions are unattainable. The extreme variability and unpredictability of human behavior guarantee that a single person theory about health and illness cannot be generated. Even the best theories of psychology are only statements about *mean* or *average* tendencies and not statements of expectations for individual behaviors. The theories of psychology are used to state expectations and predictions about average or group behavior only and are not theoretical propositions specific to one person's anticipated behavior. Individual differences across people cannot be eliminated.

As an example of a middle range theory, examine Johnson and associates' research on preoperative preparation of persons undergoing stressful events such as surgery (1978a; 1978b). The propositions developed from Johnson's research are general expectations about the response of *groups* or *aggregates* of patients who undergo a particular sensory, psychological, or procedural preparation program prior to surgery. The propositions do not predict or state the expectations for the performance or outcomes based on participation in a particular preoperative instructional program for a specific patient. The outcomes or consequences of participation in a particular preoperative teaching format are statements of expectations for the performance of a group or aggregate of patients. The research of Johnson and associates is not an imitation of the type of research encountered in physics. The theory is not for a specific person but for a *typical* person. The findings of Johnson and associates cannot be applied to all patients with equal success. Applications of the findings may work well in many cases and not so well in others. The theoretical propositions upon which the study is based cannot be construed to represent a grand theory. It represents a *middle range* theory.

Nursing must develop middle range theories and test propositions derived from these kinds of theories. These delimited theories, if sound, lead to findings in a contained and constrained sphere of professional interest. Findings based on theoretical expectations derived from middle range theories can be evaluated and selectively used in practice in a number of health settings. Research in nursing requires elementary theories to enable subsequent growth, development, and refinement of theoretical formulations for research, practice, and education. If grand theories are the preeminent goal sought by nurse theorists, nursing research will be significantly slowed because testable propositions are slow to emerge. This book describes research design procedures that can help the nurse investigator to develop, test, and reformulate theoretical expectations and propositions deduced from middle range nursing theories. Findings from markedly defined and prescribed domains of nursing concern and interest can lead to success in selective predictions and limited explanations of nursing findings in a delimited sphere of science. An illustration of this initial success is found in the preoperative preparation research domain.

It should not be concluded that the search for grand theories should be abandoned altogether. Wherever a sufficient body of research exists, attempts to generate grand theories should be pursued with vigor. At this time, not many avenues seem to be open for this development. In the limited research-based domains of nursing, the theoretical construction of grand theories should await the development of substantive middle range theories that have been tested and supported. As smaller, less comprehensive theories increase in number, dominant concepts and outcomes will resurface repeatedly and the common characteristic will be seen and recognized as being important. From the identification of these dominant concepts, the grand theories of nursing are eventually generated. For the most part, the time for the development of grand theories in nursing has not arrived. It is a project for the next generation of nursing researchers.

Meehl (1978) lamented the lack of evidence of cumulative science in the behavioral sciences, pointing out that psychology was the worst offender. According to Meehl, the history of psychology is overloaded with fads, fashions, and folderol. As an example, the whole sensitivity-encounter group movement in the 1960s promoted instant behavioral change as a consequence of participating in short one- to two-week workshops. Many businesses, governmental organizations, educational institutions, and community groups were intrigued by claims that interpersonal and organizational difficulties in their respective institutions could be solved through the intensive sensitivity-encounter small group methodology. Numerous organizations strongly encouraged employee participation in such programs. The programs offered to institutions and organizations were expensive and involved contractual arrangements enabling sensitivity group leaders to serve as consultants in a follow-up capacity with employees and their managers. Much was written in the professional behavioral science literature extolling the virtues of this planned change organizational and personal growth methodology. Substantive personality, small group, or planned change theory, theoretical propositions, or outcome research did not accompany this charismatic promotional venture.

Today, the sensitivity-encounter group bandwagon is a thing of the recently forgotten past. The research that was reported has not been continued and what was learned has not developed further significant research or more definitive knowledge about personal growth and organizational change. A science must have growth. If it cannot grow and be used to explain more and more phenomena, it is not a science. Knowledge in science must be cumulative and complementary. Nursing research should not fall into the pattern of fads, fashions, and folderols. The opportunities for research must be identified and pursued.

Suppe and Jacox (1985) provide six guidelines for the direction of research in nursing. They are summarized here.

1. Nurses interested in developing theories for nursing should become acquainted with the philosophy of science literature. In particular, doctoral students in nursing should be encouraged to take courses in the philosophy of science curriculum.

2. The development of middle range theories facilitates the formulation and testing of theories with a more limited focus and capability of being tested.

3. Taxonomies of nursing diagnosis should be viewed as a form of a grand theory. They should be used to generate middle range theories.

4. Multiple approaches to theory development and testing should be encouraged. Both qualitative and quantitative methods should be called on in achieving this goal of nursing research.

5. Theory development should include attention to methodology. Each theory must be tested either through qualitative or quantitative methods.

6. Careful attention should be given to recent developments in the evaluation of theory. As theories develop and are tested, they

should be evaluated and assessed to determine how well they provide means for growth and addition for new and novel nursing experiences.

We support these propositions and provide methods in the following chapters that should facilitate nursing research development and theory testing and reformulation.

2–11 SUMMARY

The interrelationships of nursing constructs, concepts, theoretical propositions, and hypotheses have been illustrated. The five different strategies identified in the work of Meleis, which a researcher can use in the development, evaluation, reformulation, and expansion of nursing theory, have been presented. The need to develop testable hypotheses based on operational measurements of concepts and constructs has been discussed. Examples of 14 types of research propositions were presented based on the preoperative teaching research literature. Approaches to the measurement of quantitative health care variables have been identified. The state of theory development and its expansion as a direct result of nursing research are areas in need of systematic and creative refinement and synthesis.

REFERENCES

Abdellah, F.G., Beland, I.L., Martin, A., et al.: New Directions in Patient-Centered Nursing: Guidelines for Systems of Service, Education and Research, New York, Macmillan & Co., 1973.

American Nurses' Association: Nursing: A Social Policy Statement, Kansas City, MO, American Nurses' Association, 1980.

Devine, E.C., and Cook, T.D.: A meta-analysis of effects of psychoeducational interventions on length of postsurgical hospital stay, Nurs. Res., 32: 267–274, 1983.

Devine, E.C., and Cook, T.D.: Clinical and cost-savings effects of psychoeducational interventions with surgical patients: a meta-analysis, Res. Nurs. Health, 9: 89–105, 1986.

Erikson, E.H.: Childhood and Society, New York, Norton, 1963.

Fawcett, J., and Downs, F.S.: The Relationship of Theory and Research, East Norwalk, CT, Appleton-Century-Crofts, 1985.

Geach, B.: Pain and coping, Image, 19: 12–15, 1987.

Hathaway, D.: Effects of preoperative instruction on postoperative outcomes: a meta-analysis, Nurs. Res., 35: 269–275, 1986.

Henderson, V.: The Nature of Nursing, New York, Macmillan & Co., 1966.

Johnson, D.E.: The behavioral system model for nursing, In Riehl, J.P., and Roy, C., eds., Conceptual Models for Nursing Practice, New York, Appleton-Century-Crofts, 1980.

Johnson, J.E.: Coping with elective surgery, In Werley, H.H., and Fitzpatrick, J.J., eds.: Annual Review of Nursing Research, vol. 3, New York, Springer, 1984.

Johnson, J.E., Rice, V.H., Fuller, S.S., et al.: Sensory information, instruction in a coping strategy, and recovery from surgery, Res. Nurs. Health, 1: 4–17, 1978a.

Johnson, J.E., Fuller, S.S., Endress, M.P., et al.: Altering patient's responses to surgery: an extension and replication, Res. Nurs. Health, 1: 111–121, 1978b.

Kaplan, A.: The Conduct of Inquiry, San Francisco, Chandler, 1964.

King, I.M.: Toward a Theory of Nursing: General Concepts of Human Behavior, New York, John Wiley & Sons, 1971.

Levine, M.: Introduction to Clinical Nursing, Philadelphia, F.A. Davis Co., 1969.

Maslow, A.H.: Motivation and Human Personality, New York, Harper & Row, 1954.

Meehl, P.: Theoretical risks and tabular asterisks: Sir Karl, Sir Ronald, and the slow progress of soft psychology, J. Consult. Clin. Psych., 46: 806–834, 1978.

Meleis, A.I.: Theoretical Nursing: Development and Progress, Philadelphia, J.B. Lippincott Co., 1985.

Merton, R.: Social Theory and Social Structure, New York, Free Press, 1968.

Newton, I.: Principia, London, English Royal Society, 1687.

Orem, D.E.: Nursing: Concepts of Practice, New York, McGraw-Hill, 1971.

Orlando, I.J.: The Dynamic Nurse-Patient Relationship, New York, G.P. Putnam's Sons, 1961.

Paterson, J.G., and Zderad, L.T.: Humanistic Nursing, New York, John Wiley & Sons, 1976.

Peplau, H.: Interpersonal Relations in Nursing, New York, G.P. Putnam's Sons, 1952.

Rogers, M.E.: An Introduction to the Theoretical Basis of Nursing, Philadelphia, F.A. Davis Co., 1970.

Roy, C.: Introduction to Nursing: An Adaptational Model, Englewood Cliffs, NJ, Prentice-Hall, 1976.

Schlotfeldt, R.M.: Defining nursing: a historic controversy, Nurs. Res., 36: 64–68, 1987.

Selltiz, C., Wrightsman, L.S., and Cook, S.W.: Research Methods in Social Relations, New York, Holt, Rinehart & Winston, 1976.

Suppe, F., and Jacox, A.K.: Philosophy of science and the development of nursing theory, In Werley, H.H., and Fitzpatrick, J. J., eds.: Annual Review of Nursing Research, vol.3, New York, Springer, 1985.

Travelbee, J.: Interventions in Psychiatric Nursing, New York, Springer-Verlag, 1969.

Waltz, C.F., Strickland, O.L., and Lenz, E.R.: Measurement in Nursing Research, Philadelphia, F.A. Davis Co., 1984.

Webster's New World Dictionary, ed. 2, Springfield, MA, G. & C. Merriam Co., 1980.

Whipple, B.: Methods of pain control: review of research and literature, Image 19: 142–145, 1987.

Wiedenbach, E.: Clinical Nursing: A Helping Art, New York, Springer-Verlag, 1964.

Willer, D., and Webster, M., Jr.: Theoretical concepts and observables, Am. Soc. Rev., 35: 748–757, 1970.

Ziemer, M.M.: Effects of information on postsurgical coping, Nurs. Res., 32: 282–287, 1983.

Chapter 3

INSTRUMENTATION, RELIABILITY, AND VALIDITY:
Selection, Design, and Evaluation of Nursing Measurement Instruments

3–1 GENERAL CONSIDERATIONS IN SCALE SELECTION

For any research study or evaluation project, it is recommended that instruments that have been developed to measure the interrelating concepts possess strong psychometric properties such as reliability and validity. The measurements generated by the instrument must clearly relate human behavior to the hypotheses of interest. If this cannot be done, the creation of a new measurement device becomes a necessity. The construction of a new research tool to measure a domain of interest is one of the most complex sets of activities an investigator can undertake. Therefore, if the research is not adequately funded and staffed by research methodologists and content specialists, it would be difficult and unrealistic to construct and validate research tools in a preliminary study or a final study. The instrument must be ready before the study is begun. Many investigators underestimate the time and effort required to develop a worthwhile and psychometrically sound instrument.

If the development of a measurement instrument must be undertaken, a reasonable first step in the selection of appropriate instruments is to consult general directories that list instruments specifically developed to measure a phenomenon pertinent to the scientific base of nursing. From this review, appropriate measurement instruments can often be selected that are directly related to the hypotheses of the study. Six excellent compendiums of educational and clinical nursing instruments are:

Annual Reviews of Nursing Research, vols. 1–6, New York, Springer, 1983–1988.
Frank-Stromberg, M., ed.: Instruments for Clinical Nursing Research, East Norwalk, CT, Appleton-Lange, 1988.
Reeder, L.G., Ramacher, L.G., and Gorelnik, S.: Handbook of Scales and Indices of Health Behavior, Pacific Palisades, CA, Goodyear Publishing Co., 1976.
Robinson, J.P., and Shaver, P.R.: Measures of Social Psychological Attitudes, Ann Arbor, University of Michigan Press, 1973.
Ward, M.J., and Lindeman, C.A.: Instruments for Measuring Nursing Practice and Health Care Variables, vols. 1 and 2, Washington, DC, DHEW (HRA-78-53 and 54), 1978.
Ward, M.J., and Fetler, M.E.: Instruments for Use in Nursing Education, Boulder, CO, WICHE, 1979.

Two extensive encyclopedias of general educational and psychological tests are:

Mitchell, M. J., Jr., ed.: Tests in Print 3, Lincoln, University of Nebraska Press, 1983.
Mitchell, M.J., Jr., ed.: The 9th Mental Measurement Yearbook, Lincoln, University of Nebraska Press, 1985.

Many psychosocial and physiological measurement instruments are in use today. Information about these instruments can be had from:

1. the research office of a school of nursing or nursing service staff development/program evaluation office,
2. the test librarian in the departments of psychology, sociology, and education,
3. other educational authorities in a local college or university, who may provide assistance in instrument identification or selection.

Standard test resources contain extensive information about tests, scales, and instruments used over different samples and in different settings. To assist the selection process of choosing the right instrument, test manuals often can be of help. Described in most manuals are the aims and purposes of each instrument, methods used to develop and refine scales and subscales, reliability and validity determinations, age and population groups, and other salient demographic and psychometric data. A number of instrument reference sources contain detailed critiques of many instruments and citations listing published reports using a particular test. Manuals for published tests describe explicit procedures for test administration. Often the wording of the items, the rules for scoring, the instructions given the person tested, the time limits, the amount of coaching, the encouragement allowed, and like considerations are specified in the manual for published tests, Standards for Educational and Psychological Testing (1985) by the American Psychological Association.

When a researcher has decided to use an existing research instrument, it is necessary to systematically evaluate the tool prior to data collection. Waltz and Bausell (1981) recommended the following major considerations in selecting an instrument:

1. What is the cost in dollars and energy of using the instrument?
2. What are the qualifications of the test developers in the area covered by the instrument?
3. Is the instrument development based on contemporary accepted measurement theory and concepts?
4. Is the purpose of the instrument clearly defined by the test developers?
5. Does the stated purpose of the instrument differ from the intended purpose(s) of the researcher?
6. If modifications are needed by the researcher, are they extensive and feasible?
7. Are the types of participants for which the instrument was developed clearly described?
8. Are the participants in the researcher's planned study different or similar to those for which the instrument was originally designed?
9. Are the objectives or rationale for each test item described in the instrument manual?
10. What is the nature or type of measurement scale used in the tool, and is it appropriately employed?
11. Are the scoring procedures clearly described so that the researcher can follow the identical rules established for the tool?
12. Are the test administration procedures

detailed explicitly enough that the researcher can follow the accepted procedure for administration?

13. Does the scale have nominal, ordinal, interval, or ratio properties, and what evidence is offered to support such scale properties?

14. What special training is required of the researcher in order to use the instrument properly?

15. What are the various steps and rationale described by the test developers in pretesting and modifying the instrument?

16. What reliability and validity procedures were employed to assess the psychometric properties of the instrument?

17. What are the necessary reliability and validity procedures required of the present investigator in order to strengthen the psychometric value of the research tool?

18. What critical independent evaluations of the instrument have been reported in the research literature?

19. What are the major strengths and limitations of the research instrument?

20. Does the instrument lend itself to meaningful statistical procedures for analysis?

When making a search through standard references for existing measurement tools, it may be found that no satisfactory instrument exists to test particular concepts about health or illness. To learn that an appropriate or theoretically precise instrument for a specific research question does not exist is an all too common experience of researchers in the health and behavioral sciences. Many paper and pencil instruments found in standard educational, psychological, and nursing reference sources were developed in the 1930s, 1940s, and 1950s. Frequently the concepts are time-bound and rooted in discarded notions about intelligence, sex roles, personality development, cultural influences, health and wellness, and similar considerations.

Exacting scholarly work is often required before embarking on the arduous task of instrument development. Being a productive researcher is much like being a successful detective. In reviewing the research literature, paying attention to the key names of investigators in like or parallel areas of concern can be greatly valuable and useful. The researchers who are studying events, proc-

esses, and clinical phenomena compatible or similar to that of a proposed nursing investigation may prove to be of value, especially if they have developed research tools that address the special requirements of the research question to be studied. Additionally, researchers with similar concerns may have come across an instrument that details their requirements and concomitantly may help in the study to be conducted. Often, this information can be ascertained through a telephone call, a letter, or a personal visit to the researchers who have studied similar questions.

Because researchers want to make their findings known to others, nurse investigators attend regional, national, and international conferences. Attendance at these conferences can be profitable because personal contact and direct discussion can be obtained on questions of mutual interest. If travel to a conference is not feasible, colleagues in attendance can obtain information by collecting abstracts and conference handouts. Sometimes audiotapes can be made with advanced planning by the speaker. This type of information gathering can be of great help in study planning and development.

3–2 MEASUREMENT OF A CONCEPT: PAIN AS AN EXAMPLE

Much of what nurses do centers on actions to assess and reduce patients' pain. But what is pain? A simple question but a hard one to answer. Over time, the measurement of pain has been attempted through the following four principle modalities (Jacox, 1977):

1. Self-reports of persons to predefined rating categories

2. Observations by trained observers using operationally defined behaviors from which the presence, absence, and relative intensity and duration of pain can be inferred

3. Physiological monitoring of body responses deemed to have correlates with pain experiences such as muscle reflex, nerve conduction, and evoked brain potential

4. Photogrammetry featuring film or videotape recordings that record and allow quantification of behavior reflecting pain experiences in children and adults.

None of these modalities has produced the perfect measurement of the concept of pain, probably because no total encompassing measurement exists (Franck, 1986).

Reports of the location, intensity, quality, onset, duration, coping responses, pain relief effects, and other like assessment indices are not, unfortunately, free from error. Random and systematic bias on the part of the respondent and the observer in the clinical situation can occur when pain is measured or recorded. For example, nurses often reflect a bias when making inferences about the amount of pain experienced by different types of patients.

Even when trained observers are used, bias in the measurement and evaluation of pain can occur. For example, the particular cultural background of the raters or observers can have important consequences as to whether pain is thought to be related to specific stereotypes such as old women who are widowed. As another example, nurses with northern European ethnic backgrounds as a group systematically underestimate pain occurrences with hospitalized persons more often than do nurses with southern European ancestry (Davitz and Davitz, 1981). In terms of empathetic responses to pain, Korean and Japanese nurses consistently infer the greatest patient suffering—both physical and psychological (Davitz and Davitz, 1981). Other biasing effects are certain to exist in other situations.

Neurophysiological measurement approaches have been used to provide apparent clearly interpretable measurements of pain. Blood pressure determinations, pulse monitoring, breathing respirations, and palpation to determine muscle tension have been the principal means to infer particular pain events with hospitalized persons. Although these procedures provide excellent noninvasive measurements, physiological estimation devices do not necessarily generate clearly interpretable measurements because many neurophysiological variables or factors can and do affect the measurements. Respiration may rise or fall, depending on specific insults to some body system such as a myocardial infarct. Other factors, however, such as elevated body temperature, medications administered, cultural background of the patient, and psychological makeup of the patient experiencing the pain attack may simultaneously affect respiration.

Plethysomographic recordings using very sophisticated measurements of abdominal tension are also fraught with confounding factors as measurements of postoperative pain. Placing sensors on particular muscle groups and eliciting continuous objective recordings on postoperative patients represents a highly advanced procedure for measuring physiological processes. Whether such a device provides a clear operational measurement of the concept of pain or whether it is measuring something else is still a dilemma. Baseline abdominal wall tension rates exist for all persons. Depending on a person's preoperative status, large differences in measurement can occur in short periods of time because of other factors. Thus, in addition to the variation between persons, measurement is confounded by variations within persons. Furthermore, many concurrent physiological events such as paralytic ileus, peritoneal inflammation, urinary retention, gas distention, responses to anaesthetic agents and medications, and other similar occurrences may be going on with postoperative patients. As a consequence, such measurements should be used with care.

The question may be raised whether it is irrelevant to be concerned with the cause of pain when a direct physiological recording demonstrating muscle tension in the abdominal wall can be derived and hence it can be inferred that such tension is the cause of a patient's pain. First, one patient's perceived discomfort level of abdominal tension may be another patient's tolerance or comfort level (Meinhart and McCaffery, 1983). Second, possible causes of tension in the abdominal wall are short-term ones. For instance, tension due to urinary retention is relieved easily when a patient urinates, and tension due to gas evaporates when a patient has a first bowel movement. Often changes in body position affect abdominal tension levels without any specific intervention (Menzel and Martinson, 1977). The crucial point to keep in mind regarding the preceding discussion is that no particular measurement approach is inherently superior to any other procedure, despite the high technology equipment available. In the end, it must be admitted that if the measurement cannot be related clearly to the concept or construct being evaluated or tested, it has no utilitarian or scientific value.

3-3 MULTIDIMENSIONAL APPROACHES FOR MEASURING PAIN

In developing a new instrument, begin with a definition of the construct or concept in question. Then every attempt is made to match the instrument's characteristic with the original definition. Because of the complexity and diversity of human hehavior in health and illness, impreciseness and ambiguity exist in the definition and specification of major health constructs and concepts. Thus, it has become necessary to take a multidimensional approach to the establishment of tests, scales, and instruments which identify, define, and describe the domain of human behavior represented in a particular construct encompassing health or disease states and responses. No single scale, instrument, or test can comprehensively capture or truly represent all key facets of a particular health construct; therefore, it is important for a nurse investigator to use a number of different measurement approaches to establish or test theoretical expectations or predictions of major research interest. The following discussion of research about the construct of pain exemplifies a varied approach to its measurement.

Johnson and associates (1978a; 1978b) used a multidimensional approach to estimate pain. Early reports describe work in a laboratory setting with healthy college age students. Students had blood pressure cuffs inflated on their arms to the pain threshold. Experimental groups were given distracting mathematics exercises to help cope with the pain induced by the cuff. The control group simply used whatever mental exercises they usually employed when coping with pain.

Likert scales (1932) were developed to ascertain the students' subjective reports of pain. A Likert scale is formed by adding a set of scores, usually integers, which are assigned to the ordered categories of a set of items. To obtain item scores, persons are asked to indicate agreement or disagreement to a range of ordered options for every scale item. Each ordered option is given a numerical score often ranging from 1 to 5. The sum of the scores of a person's responses to all separate items gives the total score, which is interpreted as reflecting an estimate of the dimension being measured. For more information on Likert scales, see Section 5-12.

In the study of Johnson and associates, two scales were developed to measure the relationship between physical intensity and distress. After a blood pressure cuff had been inflated to pain threshold, college students were instructed to think first about the intensity of the sensations or the physical feeling of the pain and to mark the sensation scale, with a number 0 to 10, with 0 labeled "no sensation," 5 labeled "medium sensations," and 10 labeled "maximum sensations." Subjects were then asked to think about how much the sensations distressed or bothered them. They were given the ordered options of no distress, slightly distressing, moderately distressing, very distressing, and extremely distressing. The findings revealed that both experimental and control groups reported high pain sensation; however, experimental subjects were less distressed than control subjects (Johnson and Rice, 1974). In this study with healthy young college students, it was demonstrated that an experimental intervention—distracting mathematical exercises—could help persons cope with pain, and that persons have equally painful experiences and yet report different responses to the same pain level. From these studies, Johnson and colleagues were stimulated to move their research into hospitals with patients experiencing pain.

The Johnson approach to the measurement of sensation and distress is based on the theoretical expectations or propositions about pain. Discrepancy about sensations to be experienced after surgery leads to increased distress among specific groups of patients. Increased distress in turn leads to increased use of postoperative analgesic medications to help patients cope with pain. In general, Johnson (1984) and Johnson, Christman, and Stitt (1985) have found that provision of concrete sensory information preoperatively enhances the patient's ability to cope postoperatively. Repeated research has shown that pretreatment exposure to painful stimuli or descriptions of the sensory experience of the painful stimulus produces a substantial reduction in pain perception (Geden, Beck, Hauge, and Pohlman, 1984).

Other investigators have approached the measurement of pain in different ways. Using an a posteriori approach, Melzack and Torgerson (1971) speculated that patients experience painful events differently in terms of both quality and intensity of the specific noxious stimuli. These medical researchers demonstrated that patients with different clinical pain describe their experience with reference to different adjectives. Hospitalized patients with different illnesses selected from extensive lists of adjectives those adjectives that particularly depicted the type and quality of pain experienced. Later, a series of psychometric evaluations of clinical pain yielded the McGill Pain Questionnaire (Melzack, 1975). This instrument allows persons to rate pain by way of a series of both qualitative and quantitative or intensity dimensions.

Stewart (1977) took another approach to pain assessment and developed a Stewart Pain-Color Scale. This assessment instrument presents a chromatic array of yellow-orange, red-black colors. A sliding pointer is set by the person being assessed to indicate the degree of redness that best represents that person's pain. Persons in high pain generally place the pointer in the red-black spectrum of the scale; those in low pain tend to place the pointer in the yellow-orange spectrum of the scale. It is noteworthy that the scale was used in a cross-cultural study with young children, for whom the color red was most associated with pain (Savedra, Tesler, and Ward, et al 1981).

3–4 DEVELOPING A PAIN SCALE: HYPOTHETICAL EXAMPLE

The preceding section is a background to the diverse ways in which investigators have conceptualized as well as attempted to measure a single construct, pain. For example, suppose that none of the available instruments are of value for a specific study. Generating a new scale might proceed as follows:

The scale constructor may generate a data base by recording discussions with patients, other care providers, and family members and persons significant to the patient. The different ways in which patients describe their pain could be recorded in an information file, preferably a computer file of a personal computer. A good data base can provide a wealth of information. For example, it could provide the primary adjectives used for specific types of surgery by patients and others. These adjectives could be used to help generate a pain scale. Also a good data base can provide other valuable information

that can at a later time help in the evaluation of the effectiveness of the resulting pain scale designed to provide valid measurements of pain. Thus, a well-documented data base can serve two major purposes in scale construction: the raw material to use in the scale and information to use in the evaluation of the scale.

Additional sources of information can be valuable in scale construction. Descriptions by nurses, physicians, and care providers of statements by patients of pain can be added to the data base to help interpret the meaning of a scale. Patient records can be examined and abstracted. These data can be used to provide a typology of pain descriptors made by patients over each 24-hour time period. Careful reading of patients' exact words and written comments can provide interpretations of what patients mean to convey when speaking about or describing their own pain. Logs of postsurgical patient care and systematic record keeping are also very useful in developing possible items to place on a proposed pain scale.

In examining comments about incisional pain, a wide array of descriptions are certain to be identified. These descriptions can serve as a basis of a new scale. For example, incisional pain can be described as follows: aches, twitches, pinches, stabs, sharp, pierces, shooting, gnawing, grinding, cramps, stitches in the side, smarts, stings, tingles, burns, on fire, sore, throbbing, colic-like, tummy ache, agonizing, grating, wince, racked, biting, excruciating, hurting, acute, tortuous, consuming, sore, irritated, inflamed, angry, red, festering, galled, chafing, rasping, harsh, prickles, scraping, itches, nauseating, rank, tender, slow, fast, spasms, punishing, roaring, sudden, unexpected, screaming, constant, gasping, numbing, pulsating, intermittent, severe, dull, intense, squeezing, blinding, and so on.

One way to compress this extensive information to a workable set of pain items is to identify the 10 descriptions most frequently used with midline incisional pain and the 10 adjectives most frequently identified with transverse incisional pain. Here it can be seen that computer data storage and special software can be used to greatly facilitate the frequency counting process. Computer storage and retrieval lead to faster, efficient, and correct counts.

Suppose that as a result of a frequency count, descriptions such as sharp, excruciating, hurting, harsh, spasm, inflamed, pulsating, screaming, severe, and blinding are most often described for midline abdominal incisional pain. Furthermore, suppose that descriptors such as burning, aching, pricking, sore, tingling, dull, itching, slow, irritated, and tender are most often stated to represent transverse abdominal incisional pain. These descriptions can be used to create a scale to measure pain. The 10 descriptions identified with midline incisional pain can be given to $N = 25$ patients to assess and rate according to specified rules. The responses can be used to build a scale to be used on other patients. The same procedure can be used for the 10 descriptions associated with transverse incisional pain. We describe scale construction for the midline incisional pain.

3−5 RELIABILITY OF A SCALE

A major first problem that needs to be examined by a person constructing a measurement instrument is how well the proposed scale generates reproducible data. If it does so with a high degree of precision, the scale is said to be *reliable*. Reliability is a psychometric property that all measurement instruments must satisfy (Stanley, 1971). The measurement of reliability is based on the assumption that any observation is the sum of two independent components. They are termed *error* and *true value*. Symbolically, it is assumed that

Observation = error + true score

In theory, these components can be measured. In terms of these components, the reliability is defined as:

$$\rho_{XX'} = \frac{\text{variance of the true scores}}{\text{variance of the observations}}$$

If the error variance is zero, the reliability coefficient, $\rho_{XX'}$ is equal to 1. Because the error variance is never equal to zero, the reliability is a number less than 1 but greater than zero.

In practice, reliability can be assessed in many ways. One set of methods is based on obtaining paired pieces of information on each test subject. These methods have assorted problems because differences between scores from one form to another form of the same instrument or from one occasion to a second occasion with the identical instrument can often be attributable to errors of measurement. Other reliability methods use internal properties of sets of response focusing on consistency or lack of consistency in responses. Different reliability coefficients and estimates of components of measurement error are based on various types of evidence. Because methods used to estimate reliability take into account different sources of error, an investigator planning to use a particular instrument must weigh the type of reliability evidence and decide whether the preponderance of information about a scale supports its use in a specific study (Standards for Psychological and Educational Testing, 1985).

We begin our discussion of reliability by examining test-retest reliability. First, however, we must briefly digress with a review of correlation theory and the Pearson product moment correlation coefficient. Correlation coefficients range across a scale of -1 to $+1$. A correlation coefficient of -1 means that increases in one variable are perfectly related to decreases in another variable. A correlation coefficient of $+1$ means that increases in one variable are perfectly related to increases in another variable. For reliabilities assessed via correlation coefficients, the term *related* means that the relationship is *linear*. A discussion of this type of relationship is presented in Section 10−1. Finally, if two variables are completely unrelated to one another, the correlation coefficient approaches or is equal to zero.

3−6 TEST-RETEST RELIABILITY

Test-retest reliability refers to a theoretical way to measure the reproducibility of a scale. In the abstract it is performed as follows. A group of subjects is given the instruments to complete. A score is found for each subject. A second test identical to the first test is given to each subject, and a second score is obtained. The Pearson product moment correlation coefficient between the two sets of scores is determined. Note that in practice such a procedure can never be applied. Test items on the first test become teaching items so that when the second test is given, the subjects respond with extra or additional knowledge. Thus, test-retest is a

①
$$r_{XY} = \frac{N\left(\sum_{i=1}^{N} x_i y_i\right) - \left(\sum_{i=1}^{N} x_i\right)\left(\sum_{i=1}^{N} y_i\right)}{\sqrt{N\left(\sum_{i=1}^{N} x_i^2\right) - \left(\sum_{i=1}^{N} x_i\right)^2} \sqrt{N\left(\sum_{i=1}^{N} y_i^2\right) - \left(\sum_{i=1}^{N} y_i\right)^2}}$$

②
$$r_{XY} = \frac{25(1400) - (169)(171)}{\sqrt{25(1459) - (169)^2} \sqrt{25(1383) - (171)^2}} = 0.9390 = 0.94$$

theoretical model. In practice, test-retest correlations are determined as follows. A test is created that is assumed to measure the construct, and each subject takes the test twice. The resulting set of scores are correlated. In general, in scale and instrument development, test-retest reliability coefficient estimates of +0.70 and higher are desired.

Here as an example, we want to determine whether the 10 most frequently nominated descriptors by patients with midline incisional pain are selected by patients upon repeated testing. In essence, we must address the issue of test-retest reliability. To test this property of the scale, two sets of observations are made by administering the pain scale twice to each patient over a period of time in which the intensity of the pain is stabilized. Because pain is expected to subside over time, it may not be possible to obtain data for a test-retest model. In practice, a test-retest reliability measurement is not an appropriate statistic if the time period between administrations of the scale is too long. The basic consideration justifying the use of a test-retest coefficient of reliability (stability) is that the subjects do not change substantially over time. If patients are tested on the first postoperative day and retested on the second day, the coefficient becomes an invalid measurement of reliability because the time period between testings is too long. For a reliable measurement of pain, the time period between testings must be short because pain is unstable and changes quickly over time. For variables that are known to be stable over time, such as cognitive ability, longer time intervals may be perfectly fine.

A possible solution to the measurement of pain is to administer the pain scale immediately before satisfying the patient's first request for a pain relief drug. The second testing can be performed just before the second dose is given. For many patients, the nurse should anticipate a reduction of reported pain between the two requests. If the reduction in pain were minimal between the two evaluations, the resulting measurement of reliability could be defended. Because the last assumption is almost certain to be false, test-retest reliability may not be justified. Even if it were justified, the theoretical definition of reliability is not usable. In place of the theoretical definition, statistical procedures are used to estimate reliability. The most common method is to correlate the two sets of observations using the Pearson Product Moment Correlation Coefficient.

There are many ways to compute a correlation coefficient. A formula for hand calculation use is given by equation 1 at the top of this page.

As an example of the use of this formula, suppose that the 10 descriptors are given on two occasions to 25(N) patients and that the results are as shown in columns labeled Pretest and Posttest in Table 3−1. Let x refer to the pretest and y refer to the posttest. Then

$$\sum_{i=1}^{25} x_i = 8 + 9 + \ldots + 1 = 169$$

$$\sum_{i=1}^{25} x_i^2 = 8^2 + 9^2 + \ldots + 1^2 = 1459$$

$$\sum_{i=1}^{25} y_i = 7 + 7 + \ldots + 0 = 171$$

TABLE 3–1 DATA USED TO DEMONSTRATE THE MEASUREMENT OF RELIABILITY AND VALIDITY FOR A HYPOTHETICAL PAIN SCALE

Observation	Pretest	Posttest	Odd	Even	Nurse 1	Nurse 2	Rank 1	Rank 2	Total	Days	Uncertainty	Ego Strength
1	8	7	4	4	3.0	3	10.0	9.5	34	6	1	20
2	9	7	4	5	5.0	4	20.5	15.5	34	9	1	30
3	1	3	0	1	1.0	2	3.5	5.5	14	3	0	80
4	6	7	3	3	3.0	3	10.0	9.5	27	5	1	50
5	2	4	1	1	1.0	2	3.5	5.5	18	5	1	20
6	10	9	5	5	5.0	4	20.5	15.5	42	9	1	30
7	0	1	0	0	1.0	1	3.5	2.0	11	2	0	60
8	6	7	3	3	2.0	3	7.5	9.5	28	5	1	40
9	9	9	4	5	5.0	4	20.5	15.5	37	6	0	70
10	8	9	4	4	4.0	4	13.5	15.5	36	9	1	80
11	0	2	0	0	1.0	2	3.5	5.5	11	4	0	30
12	10	9	5	5	5.0	5	20.5	22.5	43	8	1	20
13	9	9	5	4	5.0	4	20.5	15.5	39	7	1	50
14	8	9	3	5	4.0	3	13.5	9.5	35	7	1	40
15	10	9	5	5	5.0	5	20.5	22.5	43	9	0	60
16	10	8	5	5	5.0	4	20.5	15.5	40	6	1	30
17	10	9	5	5	4.0	5	13.5	22.5	37	7	1	50
18	9	7	4	5	5.0	5	20.5	22.5	35	8	1	40
19	4	5	3	1	2.0	1	7.5	2.0	23	4	0	60
20	10	9	5	5	5.0	5	20.5	22.5	41	9	1	70
21	8	10	4	4	3.0	4	10.0	15.5	32	7	0	60
22	9	9	4	5	4.0	5	13.5	22.5	35	6	1	50
23	10	10	5	5	5.0	4	20.5	15.5	40	5	1	20
24	2	3	0	2	1.0	2	3.5	5.5	12	3	0	70
25	1	0	0	1	1.0	1	3.5	2.0	14	4	0	80

$$\sum_{i=1}^{25} y_i^2 = 7^2 + 7^2 + \ldots + 0^2 = 1383$$

and

$$\sum_{i=1}^{25} x_i y_i = 8(7) + 9(7) + \ldots + 1(0) = 1400$$

so that equation 2, at the top of page 42, applies.

The scale shows a high degree of reliability. It indicates that the two tests share 94% of their total variance. It is also said that one test explains 94% of the variance in the other test. This concept is developed more fully in Section 10–3.

Squaring a reliability coefficient to obtain a measurement of explained variance is incorrect. Examination of the definition provides the reason for not squaring $\rho_{XX'}$. Even though we have denoted the correlation coefficient as r_{XY}, it must be emphasized that Y is actually the same variable as X but measured at a second time (Guilford, 1965).

Three "quick and dirty" tests can be done to see whether the use of the correlation coefficient is justified as a measure of test-retest reliability. One test is to compare the two means. The means should be equal because the same variable is measured both times. In this case,

$$\overline{X} = \frac{1}{N} \sum_{i=1}^{N} x_i = \frac{1}{25}(169) = 6.76$$

and

$$\overline{Y} = \frac{1}{N} \sum_{i=1}^{N} y_i = \frac{1}{25}(171) = 6.84$$

At least with respect to mean values, the assumptions of equality of means seems acceptable. In addition to equal means, the scales should also have equal variances or standard deviations. In this case, equations 1 and 2 as shown at the top of page 44 apply.

Here the assumption of equal variance is in question. The subjects are less variable on the second testing and, as a consequence, the test-retest reliability measurement of association is suspect. A researcher must pay particular attention to sample statistics when fundamental assumptions about the

①

$$S_X^2 = \frac{1}{N-1} \sum_{i=1}^{N} (x_i - \overline{X})^2 = \frac{N\left(\sum_{i=1}^{N} x_i^2\right) - \left(\sum_{i=1}^{N} x_i\right)^2}{N(N-1)}$$

$$= \frac{25(1459) - (169)^2}{25(24)} = 13.19$$

②

$$S_Y^2 = \frac{1}{N-1} \sum_{i=1}^{N} (y_i - \overline{Y})^2 = \frac{N\left(\sum_{i=1}^{N} y_i^2\right) - \left(\sum_{i=1}^{N} y_i\right)^2}{N(N-1)}$$

$$= \frac{25(1383) - (171)^2}{25(24)} = 8.89$$

nature of a measurement characteristic are suspect or violated. The most likely explanation for the violation of equal variance in this example is that subjects became sensitive at the first testing to the adjectives contained within the pain instrument, and consequently their performances on the second testing became more alike and less heterogeneous. The increased homogeneity of subject responses on the second test should caution the investigator that the instrument may be unreliable in the sense that the two forms are measuring different constructs and therefore needs to be reworked or discarded.

Finally a visual evaluation test is available by examining the scatter diagram shown in Figure 3–1. If the data seem to trace a straight line at a 45-degree angle, the correlation coefficient is a valid measurement of reliability. That is, the bulk of scores should rest on or be very close to the fit of the 45-degree line. In the case of the pain scale test-retest scatter diagram of pain score distribution of 25 patients, visual inspection reveals a clustering of scores on the upper right-hand and lower left-hand quadrants. Subjects at the upper end of the scale could only come down on retesting and subjects at the lower end of the scale could only go up on retesting because of the phenomenon of regression to the mean. (Regression to the mean is described in Section 4–6.) One of the major problems associated with this example is that the number of descriptors contained in the scale is 10. With such a small

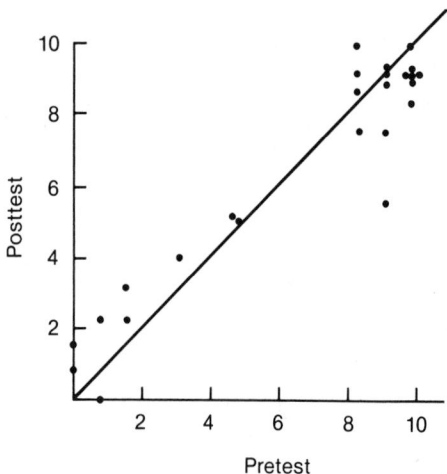

Figure 3–1. Scatter diagram of pretest and posttest score for 25 patients.

number of descriptors, subjects with scores close to zero or 10 had little room for change except to go up (low scoring subjects) and to go down (high scoring subjects). Again, the reliability of the pain instrument using a test-retest reliability model is in question. A different model of reliability should be used for these kinds of data.

3–7 PARALLEL FORM RELIABILITY

The test-retest reliability model can have a serious measurement problem. Patients may be sensitized or tuned in to the purposes of the investigation. Some may remember items from the first administration of the pain scale and provide the same responses regardless of intervention effectiveness, even though the second responses may not be what they actually feel or experience. The shorter the time interval between first and second administration of the same instrument, the greater the probability that patients will recall their initial responses and give it again.

The use of parallel forms of the pain scale may help to correct this problem. A major issue in the use of parallel forms is whether the two forms of the pain scale produce substantial agreement or consistency in the classification of patients. For example, one may wonder whether patients in great pain are differentiated on both forms from those who are not in pain. The typical method used to construct parallel forms of a measurement instrument is to create twice as many items as needed. Half of the items are placed on one form and half on the other.

Items can be assigned to the two forms in many ways. One procedure is to use a table of random numbers to create the two forms. The main disadvantage of this commonly used procedure is that by chance alone the two resulting scales may differ on a number of characteristics. For example, most of the negative descriptors may appear on one form. One way to prevent this problem is to pair the items on the basis of similarity and then use a random assignment procedure to place one member of each pair into one of the two parallel forms.

To be acceptable as a pain scale, a satisfactory coefficient of reliability or equivalence between both forms of the pain scale must be established. This is done by computing a correlation coefficient similar to that of a test-retest model. The only difference is that the pretest scores are replaced by the scores on one form of the test and that the posttest scores are replaced by the scores on the second form. The three tests recommended for testing the assumption of equality of means, equality of standard deviations, and the relationship between variables, which must approximate a 45-degree angle straight line, should be used in this situation as well (see Section 3–6).

As indicated, one way to generate two parallel forms of the pain scale is to use two sets of the original 67 descriptors. Recall that the 10 descriptors used were generated from the

same content domain and are thought to be relatively alike or homogeneous. One way to generate parallel forms is to randomly select two sets of items from the original list of 67 descriptors. To estimate the reliability coefficient of parallel forms of the pain scale, the two alternate forms are administered to the same patients on the same occasion or to the same patients on two separate occasions, provided the time difference is brief. If the two forms of the pain scale have high parallel form reliability, the Pearson Product Moment Correlation Coefficient will be close to +1.00 in numerical value, and the instrument will be said to have high parallel form equivalence.

3–8 SPLIT-HALF AND ODD-EVEN RELIABILITY

One of the major problems with the two previously described measures of reliability is that the order of presentation of the adjectives on the pain scale to the patients could have an effect on how they respond to the individual items contained in the scale. Presented in a different order, the responses might differ, and the total scores for any one patient could fluctuate, producing an unreliable measurement. One way to handle the problem is to generate two scores on each subject. An easy way to do this is to produce a test of the odd-numbered adjectives and a second test from the even-numbered adjectives. The resulting measurement of association is called an *odd-even reliability coefficient*. This can be done in a multitude of ways. The resulting correlation coefficient is often referred to as a split-half reliability coefficient. When we say split-half, we are not referring to the approach in which the first half of an instrument's items are compared with the second half of the items contained in the same scale. This procedure is not recommended because the latter half of the scale can be biased because of fatigue or boredom.

An example of an odd-even reliability coefficient is provided with the data of Table 3–1 with the columns of data headed Odd and Even. The odd score consists of the sum of the positive responses to the odd numbered descriptors (sharp, hurt, spasm, pulsate, and severe), whereas the positive responses to the even-numbered items are used to define the second score (excruciating, harsh, inflamed, scream, and blinding). In this case, $r_{odd, even} = 0.90$. This does not, however, measure the reliability of the test. It measures the reliability of half of the test. To obtain the reliability, it is necessary to use the Spearman-Brown Prophesy formula (Guilford, 1965):

$$r_{XX'} = \frac{2r_{odd, even}}{1 + r_{odd, even}}$$

For our example,

$$r_{XX'} = \frac{2(0.90)}{1 + 0.90} = 0.95$$

This indicates that 95% of the variance in each test is shared by the other test. As before, the three quick and dirty statistical tests described earlier can be used to test for stability (see Section 3–6).

One possible problem with this reliability model is that if an unfortunate choice of order is made, the measure will be biased. To avoid this complication it is suggested that random assignment of adjectives to the list be done before administration.

3–9 INTERNAL CONSISTENCY RELIABILITY FOR QUANTITATIVE MEASURES

The previously discussed methods suffer from a common weakness in that any coefficient may be confounded with order of presentation of items. One way to handle this problem is to determine all possible split-half correlations and use their average value as the reliability coefficient. Although such a suggestion makes sense, very few researchers would want to compute all the correlations just to determine a simple average. Even so, not all is lost for computing formulas exist that can be used with ease to obtain such an average correlation coefficient.

This measurement of association can be approached from many different angles. One way is to define association in terms of mean squares defined from a two-factor analysis of variance in which the factors are *items* and *subjects*. The analysis of variance is discussed in Chapter 9. In particular, the reliability coefficient is defined as:

$$\alpha = 1 - \frac{MS_{I \times S}}{MS_S}$$

where $MS_{I \times S}$ is the mean square of the interaction of the items with the subjects and MS_S is the mean square between the subjects. This measurement is called Cronbach's alpha (α) (1951). A computing formula, called Hoyt's formula (1941) can also be represented as,

$$\alpha = \frac{N}{N - 1}\left(1 - \frac{1}{MS_S}\sum_{i=1}^{N} MS_i\right)$$

where MS_i is the mean square for the i-th item or, in terms of our example, adjective. In practice, it is rarely computed in this form because the simpler ANOVA form is easy to use.

As an example of its use, consider the data of Table 3–2. The numbers in this table were generated by asking each patient to rate the adjectives as

1. no pain
2. mild pain
3. discomforting pain
4. distressing pain
5. unbearable pain

The scores for the 10 items were then totaled and reported in Table 3–1 in the column headed Total. The basic statistics required to determine α are presented in Table 3–3. This table was produced by CRUNCH (Bostrom, 1986) in terms of a two-factor analysis of variance. In terms of the statistics of Table 3–3, the measurement of reliability is given by

$$\alpha = 1 - \frac{MS_{I \times S}}{MS_S} =$$
$$= 1 - \frac{0.681}{12.1467} = 0.9440 = 0.94$$

This large value for α indicates a high degree of consistency in responses to the items. The 10 adjectives define a reliable scale of pain.

In the present instance of calculating coefficient α (alpha) we have another way of interpreting reliability. With our 10-item pain index scale, we really have 10 one-item instruments and each of which should behave in the same way as the total instrument (Fox, 1982). Thus, if postoperative patients are in

TABLE 3–2 RESPONSES TO THE 10 DESCRIPTORS PRESENTED AS LIKERT SCALE ITEMS RANGING FROM 1 TO 5

Obser-vation	Sharp	Excru-ciating	Hurt	Harsh	Spasm	Inflamed	Pul-sating	Scream-ing	Severe	Blind-ing
1	4	4	4	2	2	4	3	3	4	4
2	4	4	4	3	1	2	4	4	4	4
3	1	1	1	2	1	4	1	1	1	1
4	4	1	2	2	1	3	3	3	4	4
5	1	1	1	1	1	4	1	2	4	1
6	4	5	4	4	3	4	4	5	4	5
7	1	1	2	1	1	1	1	1	1	1
8	4	2	1	1	1	3	4	4	4	4
9	1	4	4	4	4	4	4	4	4	4
10	4	3	4	4	4	4	4	3	3	3
11	1	1	1	1	1	2	1	1	1	1
12	4	5	4	4	4	4	4	5	4	5
13	5	5	4	4	3	3	4	3	4	4
14	2	4	4	4	3	4	1	4	4	5
15	4	5	4	4	4	4	4	5	4	5
16	4	5	4	4	3	3	3	5	4	5
17	4	5	3	3	3	3	3	4	4	5
18	2	4	3	3	3	4	4	4	4	4
19	4	2	1	1	1	3	3	3	3	2
20	4	5	4	4	4	4	3	5	4	4
21	3	4	2	1	4	2	4	4	4	4
22	1	4	3	3	4	4	4	4	4	4
23	4	5	3	4	3	3	4	5	4	5
24	1	3	1	1	1	1	1	1	1	1
25	1	1	1	2	1	4	1	1	1	1

pain, all or most of the adjectives would most likely be selected and rated as high, thereby representing the pain state of the patient. If the patient is not in pain, none of or few of the descriptors should be nominated or rated with high values. In the case of our pain index, α measures the extent to which performance on any one of the 10 descriptors is a good indicator of performance on any other descriptor in our same pain scale (Waltz, Strickland, and Lenz, 1984). In this sense, α measures *internal consistency*.

Examination of the two formulas presented for α show how to raise the level of reliability or internal consistency of any proposed scale. Because MS_S is in the denominator of both formulas, an attempt should be made to maximize its value. This can be done by testing patients who cover the full range of the characteristic being measured. In our example, we have done this successfully because some subjects scored very low and some scored very high on the pain scale. The total pain scores ranged from 1 to 43, with 0 and 50 being the possible extremes. In our example, we did not find anyone at the upper limits of the range. From an operational point of view, the goal is to include in the construction process subjects who cover the full range of the variable being measured.

A second way to increase α is to decrease the size of the numerator. As suggested by the Hoyt (1941) formula, the standard deviations of the scores can be minimized for each item. Thus, items should have the same level of attraction for each subject. For example, note that the descriptor *excruciating* is given many 4 and 5 values and very few 1, 2, and 3 values. *Spasms* is also a descriptor that receives homogeneous ratings of 3 and 4 by most of the patients. Other homoge-

TABLE 3–3 STATISTICS FOR CRONBACH'S ALPHA*

Source	d/f	S of S	MS
Between subjects	24	291.40	12.1467
Within subjects	225	174.20	
Between adjectives	9	27.28	
A × S	216	146.92	0.6802
Total	249	465.60	

*Based on the Likert Scores of Table 3–2.

neous items with small standard deviations are *hurt* and *severe*. These kinds of items are excellent candidates for a pain scale.

As indicated by the analysis of variance model, another way to increase the value of α is to choose items that do not interact with the subjects. In practice this is hard to achieve because it requires some advanced knowledge on how subjects will respond to certain items. For the most part this condition seems to be satisfied for all of the subjects of Table 3–2. For example, subject one tends to rate all descriptors as 2, 3, or 4. Apparently no one provided, for example, nine values of 1 and one value of 5. In other words, each patient tends to respond similarly to each item on the list of 10 descriptors.

3–10 INTERNAL CONSISTENCY FOR DICHOTOMOUS VARIABLES

Sometimes subjects are asked to respond positively or negatively to each item. For example, each patient could be asked, "Is the pain sharp? Answer *yes* or *no*." This format could then be repeated for the remaining

nine descriptors to provide for each patient a score that covers the range of zero to 10. An example of this model is provided in Table 3–4. The analysis of variance table for these data is provided in Table 3–5. Coefficient α for these data is given by

$$\alpha = 1 - \frac{MS_{I \times S}}{MS_S}$$
$$= 1 - \frac{0.0978}{1.3000} = 0.9248 = 0.92$$

In this form, α is called the Kuder-Richardson 20 Formula. It is just a special case of Cronbach's α where the dependent variables are dichotomous instead of quantitative. Sometimes it is written as

$$KR_{20} = \frac{I}{I-1}\left(1 - \frac{1}{MS_S}\sum_{i=1}^{I} p_i q_i\right)$$

where p_i is the proportion of *yes* responses to the item i and

$$q_i = 1 - p_i$$

TABLE 3–4 DISTRIBUTION OF YES AND NO RESPONSES TO THE 10 PAIN DESCRIPTORS

Observation	Sharp	Excruciating	Hurt	Harsh	Spasm	Inflamed	Pulsate	Scream	Severe	Blinding
1	1	1	1	0	0	1	1	1	1	1
2	1	1	1	1	0	1	1	1	1	1
3	0	0	0	0	0	1	0	0	0	0
4	1	0	0	0	0	1	1	1	1	1
5	0	0	0	0	0	1	0	0	1	0
6	1	1	1	1	1	1	1	1	1	1
7	0	0	0	0	0	0	0	0	0	0
8	1	0	0	0	0	1	1	1	1	1
9	0	1	1	1	1	1	1	1	1	1
10	1	1	1	1	1	1	1	1	0	0
11	0	0	0	0	0	0	0	0	0	0
12	1	1	1	1	1	1	1	1	1	1
13	1	1	1	1	1	1	1	0	1	1
14	0	1	1	1	1	1	0	1	1	1
15	1	1	1	1	1	1	1	1	1	1
16	1	1	1	1	1	1	1	1	1	1
17	1	1	1	1	1	1	1	1	1	1
18	0	1	1	1	1	1	1	1	1	1
19	1	0	0	0	0	1	1	1	1	0
20	1	1	1	1	1	1	1	1	1	1
21	1	1	0	0	1	1	1	1	1	1
22	0	1	1	1	1	1	1	1	1	1
23	1	1	1	1	1	1	1	1	1	1
24	0	1	0	1	0	0	0	0	0	0
25	0	0	0	0	0	1	0	0	0	0

TABLE 3-5 STATISTICS FOR THE KUDER-RICHARDSON 20 MEASURE OF RELIABILITY*

Source	d/f	S of S	MS
Between subjects	24	31.20	1.3000
Within subjects	225	23.20	
Between adjectives	9	2.08	
A × S	216	21.12	0.0978
Total	249	54.40	

*Based on the scores of Table 3-4.

Another form of the Kuder-Richardson formula is called KR_{21}. By definition, KR_{21} is

$$KR_{21} = \frac{N}{N-1}\left(1 - \frac{\overline{X}(N-\overline{X})}{N(S_X^2)}\right)$$

It differs from KR_{20} in that $\overline{X}/N$ is used as a common value for each of the p_i of KR_{20}. For this formulation $\overline{X}$ is the mean of the total test.

3-11 INTER-RATER RELIABILITY: SPEARMAN'S RANK MEASURE OF CORRELATION

Sometimes patients are not able to respond to a personal interview or to a paper and pencil test, and so information on pain must be obtained from some other source. The typical source is the nurse who normally cares for the patient. Thus, an instrument that produces reliable measurements across different observers is needed. In this case, a reliable instrument is one in which classification or rating of patients into pain categories is consistent across nurses. For example, if one nurse classified a patient as having *mild* pain, a researcher wants to know that a second nurse classifying the same patient also reports the patient as having *mild* pain and not something else.

Suppose two nurses rate the 25 patients as shown in columns headed Nurse 1 and Nurse 2 of Table 3-1. One way to measure the between rater or inter-rater reliability is to rank the scores breaking the ties using mean ranks. The ranks are reported in Table 3-1 under the headings Rank 1 and Rank 2. The resulting correlation coefficient is called Spearman's ρ (rho) and is denoted by $\hat{\rho}_S$. The value of ρ is given by $\hat{\rho}_S = 0.82$. This indi-

cates a high degree of inter-rater reliability, at least as determined from the two nurses who did the rating. It is worth noting that the correlation coefficient determined from the original classification is given by r = 0.87. One might wonder why ranks are used when the data are already quantitative. One of the reasons is that the scale 1, 2, 3, 4, and 5 is discrete and covers a small range of values. Correlation coefficients are best for variables that cover a large range and that approximate the distribution of a continuous variable. For small scales with a small number of response values, Spearman's ρ is recommended. Sometimes more than two nurses can perform the pain ratings. In that case, Kendall's Coefficient of Concordance is used to estimate the reliability. The procedure is described by Marascuilo and McSweeney (1977).

3-12 INTER-RATER RELIABILITY: CHI-SQUARE STATISTIC AND CRAMER'S V

Sometimes inter-rater reliabilities are determined using Chi-square statistics based on frequency counts. This approach is recommended whenever the classes cannot be ordered. It would not be recommended for the data of Table 3-1 because Chi-square completely ignores any ordered relationship that might exist between an independent and dependent variable or sets of categories. For illustration only we show how reliability would be measured for unordered categories. Remember Chi-square should never be used for ordered categories (see Section 13-9).

First a two-dimensional frequency table is established like that of Table 3-6. Next

TABLE 3-6 INTER-RATER RELIABILITY FOR TWO NURSE RATERS*

	Category	C_1	C_2	C_3	C_4	C_5	Total
				Nurse Two			
	C_1	2	4	0	0	0	6
	C_2	1	0	1	0	0	2
Nurse One	C_3	0	0	2	1	0	3
	C_4	0	0	1	1	2	4
	C_5	0	0	0	6	4	10
	Total	3	4	4	8	6	25

*Based on the nurses' ratings of Table 3-1.

Chi-square is computed and then related to Cramer's V (1951). By definition, Chi-square is defined as

$$X^2 = \sum_{j=1}^{J} \sum_{k=1}^{K} \left(\frac{f_{jk} - F_{jk}}{f_{jk}} \right)^2$$

and Cramer's V is defined as

$$V = \sqrt{\frac{X^2}{NM}}$$

where M is equal to the minimum of $(J - 1)$ or $(K - 1)$. It is rarely computed in this form. One of the easier ways to use computing formulas is given by

$$X^2 = N \left(\sum_{j=1}^{J} \sum_{k=1}^{K} \frac{f_{jk}^2}{f_{j.}f_{.k}} - 1 \right)$$

where

f_{jk} = observed frequency in the j-th row and k-th column

F_{jk} = expected frequency for the f_{jk}

$f_{j.}$ = observed frequency in the j-th row

and

$f_{.k}$ = observed frequency in the k-th column.

For the data of Table 3–6, the equation at the bottom of this page applies. From this measure, the reliability coefficient is computed as

$$V = \sqrt{\frac{38.32}{25(4)}} = \sqrt{0.3832} \equiv 0.62$$

As we see, V = 0.62 is considerably smaller than $\hat{\rho}_S = 0.82$. This reduction is expected because V ignores the order on the categories. It should not be used on the data of Table 3–6.

3–13 INTER-RATER RELIABILITY: PERCENT AGREEMENT

In addition to using frequency measures based upon the Chi-square statistic to measure inter-rater reliability, some researchers prefer to use a more primitive or intuitive measurement based on counting the number of times two independent raters agree in assigning subjects to a set of mutually exclusive and exhaustive categories. This measurement is called the *percent agreement* between the two raters. For the data of Table 3–6, two independent nurses assigned 25 subjects to five mutually exclusive and exhaustive categories. As indicated by the diagonal frequencies, they agreed a total of nine times. Both nurses assigned two subjects to category one, two subjects to category three, one subject to category four, and four subjects to category five. For these two independent raters the percent agreement is given by

$$P = 1/25(2 + 0 + 2 + 1 + 4)$$
$$= 0.36$$

This is a low level of agreement and is at variance with the inter-rater reliability measurement computed in terms of a correlation coefficient. As shown in the next section, this measurement should not be used to measure inter-rater reliability.

3–14 INTER-RATER RELIABILITY: COHEN'S KAPPA (K)

Another measurement of percent agreement has been proposed by Cohen (1961). It is a corrected version of P, the percent agreement. It is corrected to account for the fact that two raters acting independently can produce a frequency table with a Spearman correlation coefficient of zero or a Cramer's V of zero. As an example, consider the data of Table 3–7. For these data the number of agreements is given by 81 + 1 = 82, so that

$$X^2 = 25 \left(\frac{2^2}{6(3)} + \frac{4^2}{6(4)} + \frac{0^2}{6(4)} + \ldots + \frac{4^2}{10(6)} - 1 \right) = 38.32$$

TABLE 3–7 INTER-RATER RELIABILITY USING ONLY TWO CATEGORIES*

		Nurse Two		
	Category	C_1	C_2	Total
Nurse One	C_1	81	9	90
	C_2	9	1	10
	Total	90	10	100

*Where P = 0.82 and V = 0.

the percent agreement is given by P = 0.82. For these data both Spearman's correlation coefficient (Section 3–11) and Cramer's V (Section 3–12) are equal to zero. In terms of the percent agreement, it would be concluded that a high level of inter-rater reliability existed, but in terms of the correlation coefficient an opposite decision would be made. Clearly, there is a problem. The explanation is that the numbers of Table 3–7 are based on the fact that 90% of the subjects are members of category one, whereas only 10% are members of the remaining category. Because 90% of the subjects belong to category one, the two raters are certain to place most of the subjects in category one and thereby show a high level of apparent inter-rater reliability. This example shows why some researchers use this measurement in journal articles and reports. It is usually high and provides a superficial and erroneous impression of significance. In this example, P = 0.82, and yet no relationship exists between the two sets of ratings.

Cohen's solution for this dilemma is to define a corrected percent agreement as

$$K = \frac{P - P_0}{1 - P_0}$$

where

$$P_0 = \sum_{c=1}^{C} P_{c.}P_{.c}$$

In this equation, P_0 is the probability of agreement, assuming that the characteristics under question are independent when viewed or evaluated by the two raters. For the data of Table 3–6,

$$
\begin{aligned}
P_c &= (3/25)(6/25) + (4/25)(2/25) \\
&+ (4/25)(3/25) + (8/25)(4/25) \\
&+ (6/25)(10/25) \\
&= 0.208
\end{aligned}
$$

With this correction,

$$K = \frac{0.38 - 0.208}{1 - 0.208} = 0.2171 = 0.22$$

Again, this result does not agree with the decisions based on the use of a correlation coefficient to assess inter-rater reliability. We recommend that Cohen's K be used rarely.

3–15 APPROACHES TO DETERMINATION OF VALIDITY

The preceding section dealt primarily with various techniques employed to garner support for the reliability of a scale. The next vital phase of test construction focuses on the question: what extent do the numbers obtained from a scale reflect true differences among the subjects rather than constant or random error among the subjects? A scale is said to be *valid* if it measures the characteristic under investigation. For any single measurement, an investigator must try to increase the scale's validity by reducing as much as possible its susceptibility to influences other than the dimension it purports to measure. The validity of an instrument is judged by the extent to which the scale results are compatible with other relevant evidence that is known to be correlated with the scale. Although evidence may be gathered in different ways, validity always refers to the degree to which the evidence supports the inferences that are made from the numbers generated by an instrument (Cronbach, 1971).

There are many ways to measure validity. The different means of accumulating evidence of validity have been usually organized under three major categories: *content-related*, *criterion-related*, and *construct-related* evidence of validity. The "use of the category labels does not mean that there are distinct types of validity or that a specific validation strategy is best for each specific inference or instrument use" (*Standards for Educational and Psychological Testing*, 1985). Some of these approaches to determining validity are considered in the following sections.

3–16 CONTENT-RELATED VALIDITY DETERMINATIONS

A preeminent concern in the construction of a new test resulting in numeric scores is to assess whether the items contained in the instrument represent the domain under study. In achievement test construction, curriculum authorities and knowledgeable educators who are familiar with the subject matter of a test are asked to generate a pool of possible test questions according to test specification. For example, a nurse educator may want to create a scale that measures quantitative reasoning in the calculation and administration of medications. One way to identify the items for the scale is to describe quantitative reasoning to 10 experts or teachers in this area. After the construct is described precisely and the universe or domain of content specified, each of the 10 authorities would be asked to create 5 test items that measure quantitative reasoning in drug calculation and administration. The 50 test or scale items would serve as the basis of the final scale to be constructed. It is conceivable that a total of 20 of the original 50 generated items would be retained to measure the construct of interest. As a final step all items generated are evaluated against the purpose and intent of the scale or test and accepted or rejected based on a priori guidelines.

The investigator in our pain example could choose a different strategy for generating items. A log can be kept of all postoperative pain descriptors furnished by patients and care providers through both verbal and written reports. After the descriptors are selected, expert judges such as groups of nurses who currently care for preoperative and postoperative surgical patients can be asked to examine the items to see whether they actually measure the construct.

We provide no example on evaluating *content* or *domain* validity because no objective criteria are readily available that can be easily used in providing descriptions of many clinical events concerning nurses. In contrast, achievement test content domains can be established and subject experts can be requested to assign test items according to preestablished categories. Also, algorithms or rules can be constructed to assure representativeness of domain content based on the guidelines suggested in Standards for Educational and Psychological Testing (American Psychological Association, 1985).

Evaluating content validity in some respects can be viewed as an art form, drawing heavily on intuitive and inductive powers of the test constructor and the evaluation of the items. Content validity in other respects is based on theory considerations and on how well the scale relates to the constructs that tie theory and scale together. In our case, the 10 descriptors seem to reflect important aspects of pain experiences. Certainly, descriptors such as joyful, happy, pleased, gay, contented, smiling, and other terms of good feeling, would not be used to define pain. These descriptions may help define a scale of well-being, but they logically would not have any bearing on the construct of pain.

In summation, the test developer must present a reasoned argument using logical, rational, and statistical evidence to support the construct represented and offer ways that the scale or test should and should not be used. Others planning to use the instrument must make their own judgment about whether the instrument assists in describing or predicting vital human behavior.

3–17 CRITERION-RELATED VALIDITY DETERMINATIONS: CONCURRENT AND PREDICTIVE

Another approach to validation of a scale or a test is to determine how well it works. If a scale works well, a user can make more accurate decisions with the help of the instrument than can be made without the instrument. In our example, we want to know whether the pain scale helps to differentiate patients who are in great pain postoperatively from those who are not. If the scale is a valid measurement of pain, its use can help a nurse to assess patient performance on other clinically relevant characteristics. With a valid scale of pain, several propositions or theoretical expectations can be stated. Patients who score high on the pain scale should, for instance, request and receive more analgesic medications than patients who place low on the instrument. Patients who score low on the pain scale should require significantly less direct nursing time than those high on the pain scale. Patients who place high on the pain scale and receive timely analgesic medication administration should require progressively less postoperative medication administration than those patients at the opposite pole of the scale. An instrument that helps nurses to distinguish individual patients on their present status on the above dimensions is said to possess *concurrent validity*. Placement on the pain scale is said to concur with some other relevant criterion measurements. In concurrent validity studies, the measurements are taken concurrently or contiguously with one another.

Consider the correlations between the nurses' ratings of Table 3–1 and the patients' total scores as defined by totaling the Likert scores of Table 3–2. The total score is reported in Table 3–1 as Total. If there is concurrent validity in these measurements, the pain scale and the nurses' ratings can be considered to be measuring the same construct. In this illustration, the correlations for each nurse with the patients' scores are given by r = 0.95 and r = 0.88, respectively. For the nurses' ranked data, the correlations are r = 0.92 and r = 0.88, respectively. These figures offer remarkably strong support to the concurrent validity of the pain scale. In reality, most measurements of concurrent validity are much lower than the values presented in this hypothetical illustration.

In other instances, one might be interested in *predicting some future* behavior of postoperative patients based on their reported level of midline incisional pain within the first 48-hour period following surgery. For example, in the absence of important clinical symptoms (elevated temperature, bleeding, infection, and similar clinical signs), one might wonder whether the reported level of discomfort on the pain scale is a good predictor of postoperative complications and unstable condition of the patient such as placement on critical list, administration of last rites, notification of kin, and similar untoward events.

If the length of inpatient hospital stay can be predicted from the patient's pain scores within the first 48-hour postoperative period, evidence of validity is supported. Or, if the number of days that the patient spends at home before venturing outside can be predicted from the patient's pain scores prior to hospital discharge, further evidence of validity is indicated. If the pain scale can adequately predict the above events by pinpointing patients who will differ in the future, the scale is said to possess *predictive validity*. With predictive validity, knowledge of patients' pain scores enables a nurse to predict important patient behaviors in the future.

As an example of predictive validity, suppose the length of stay in hospital for the 25 patients was shown in Table 3–1 under the heading, Days. The correlation coefficient of this outcome variable as predicted from Total 1 is given by r = 0.84. This represents a high degree of prediction. This value is certainly large enough to conclude that the 10 adjectives possess predictive validity.

As shown in the two examples to establish the criterion validity of the pain scale, both concurrent and predictive validity are expressed in terms of a correlation coefficient. In any case, the validity coefficient cannot exceed the square root of the reliability coefficient (Cronbach, 1971). It is easy to see why a validity coefficient cannot exceed the square root of the reliability coefficient. On the one hand a reliability coefficient is a measurement of association between a variable and itself. In the best of all possible worlds, $\rho_{XX'}$ should equal 1. It usually differs from 1 because of sampling variation. On the other hand, a validity coefficient is a measurement of association of a variable with another variable which is not itself. All correlations of X with another variable Y must be less than 1. Thus, no validity coefficient can exceed a reliability coefficient.

In the world of human behavior and health care, we realistically look for validity coefficients expressed in values reaching +0.40 and higher. Note that a correlation coefficient of −0.50 or greater in *numeric* value is indicative of validity. That the sign of the correlation is negative is not important because multiplication of each sign by −1 converts the correlation to a positive value. Negative correlations frequently reflect an inversion between scale scores and an external behavioral criterion measurement. One way to convert the correlation coefficient to a positive value is simply to reverse the order on the scales. For example, a Likert scale scored as

1. strongly agree
2. agree
3. indifferent
4. disagree
5. strongly disagree

and negatively correlated with a dependent variable can have the scoring reversed to

1. strongly disagree
2. disagree
3. indifferent
4. agree
5. strongly agree

and have an accompanying reversion in algebraic sign.

In some cases, however, a prediction might be made to a criterion measure, which should not be related to the instrument being validated. In that situation, validity coefficients between a range of +0.30 and −0.30 would be desired. The latter situation is discussed under construct validity, which follows.

3–18 CONSTRUCT-RELATED VALIDITY DETERMINATIONS: KNOWN GROUP, CONVERGENT, DISCRIMINANT, AND FACTORIAL

The most challenging task in the evaluation of a new scale is the demonstration of the *construct validity* of the scale. The importance of construct validity is that it provides the necessary linkage of theory with theoretical conceptualization. In validating a measurement of postoperative pain, we would probably be less concerned with the adequate sampling of descriptors or with relating resultant scores to a criterion. In a nursing investigation we would, however, be more interested in the extent to which the pain scale corresponds to a theory of pain that is acceptable or defensible on either a priori or empirical grounds. Construct validity can be approached in a number of ways, but logical analysis and the testing of relationships predicted on the basis of theoretical considerations must always be emphasized. Constructs are almost always explicated in terms of other constructs. In our pain scale example, the investigator must be in a position to specify, before data collection, predictions or theoretical expectations about how the pain construct will function in relation to other constructs.

In Chapter 1, we described a hypothetical study for preoperative teaching and preparation of patients for surgery. In Chapter 1, a psychological construct described as uncertainty was introduced as 1 of the 10 covariate measures. Uncertainty measures were obtained on each patient prior to surgery. Uncertainty is a cognitive construct and occurs in situations in which the decision maker is unable to assign definite value to objects and events or is unable to accurately predict outcomes. Uncertainty in illness states is characterized by ambiguity, complexity, inadequate information, and unpredictability. Perception of uncertainty has been shown to influence the stress experienced by hospitalized patients (Mishel, 1983a). When uncertainty was present, compliance with a treatment regimen was low. Uncertainty is also associated with problems in psychosocial areas of adjustment and is a predictor of posthospital discharge recuperation and functioning of specific categories of patients such as open heart surgery patients, postmyocardial infarct patients, and cancer patients (Mishel, 1983b; Mishel, 1984; Mishel and Branden, 1988).

A common approach to test construct validation is the *known group* or *contrast group technique*. In using this procedure specific groups that differ on a known characteristic are studied because they are expected to differ on the critical attribute. In validating the pain scale, we expect patients who are experiencing great pain on the third postoperative day (as opposed to those who are not) to differ on the uncertainty index. Those in great pain are expected to have significantly higher pain and concomitantly higher uncertainty scores compared with those with low pain, who are expected to have lower uncertainty scores. If the group difference prediction holds, the instrument is said to have passed another crucial validity test.

The more typical approach used in the known group validity method is to identify or select two independent groups of patients. Those in one group would be expected to have little or no pain while in the hospital, and those in the second group would be expected to have higher levels of pain. The pain scale would be administered to members in both groups. Patients in group one should have lower pain scales and patients in group two should have higher pain scores. As another contrast group comparison, patients who are having diagnostic workups with primarily noninvasive procedures, in contrast to patients on first day postoperative total hip surgery, would reasonably be expected to differ on pain score scales.

An example of construct validity using the known group technique follows. Prior to surgery each patient was given the *uncertainty* scale described in Chapter 1. Patients with a score below 50 were classified as having low levels of uncertainty. Those with scores of 50 or higher were classified as having high levels of uncertainty. The results were dummy coded and reported in Table 3−1 under the column *Uncertainty*. The dummy code of 1 represents high uncertainty, and a code of 0 represents low uncertainty. The correlation coefficient between the dummy uncertainty code and the total score is given as r = 0.60. This correlation coefficient is large enough to conclude that the instrument also has a high level of construct validity. This difference is reflected in the mean score for the two groups. For the low uncertainty patients the mean is 21.9, and for the high uncertainty patients the mean is 35.2. Parenthetically, correlation coefficients between the two variables in which one has been dummy coded as 0 and another as 1 are called *point biserial correlation coefficients*. These coefficients are used to measure the association between a quantitative variable and a dichotomous variable.

Convergent validity refers to evidence that different methods of measuring a construct yield similar results. In Section 3−2 the different ways in which investigators have attempted to measure pain was discussed. Because of ethical considerations it would not be feasible to administer several instruments to the same patients within the period of the first two postoperative days. A compromise could be found using healthy college students as study subjects for this phase of test validation of the pain scale. For instance, as in the study of Johnson and Rice (1974), one could have students report their pain levels using an inflated blood pressure cuff. Using a random order of instrument administration, students would be requested to report their pain levels on the McGill Pain Questionnaire (Melzack, 1975), the Stewart Pain-Color Scale (Stewart, 1977), and the developed pain scale. If the correlation coefficients between two or more sets of scores are high, it can be stated that the pain scale has *convergent validity*. Different instruments measuring the same construct are said to converge.

One must be careful at this stage. If the pain scale correlated at +0.90 with the McGill Pain Questionnaire, one would have to ask why a new instrument had to be developed when a well-known and much used

instrument was at hand. The inquiring nurse facing that dilemma would have to offer sound rationale for using the newly developed pain scale. Arguments such as ease of administration, low costs, ease of score interpretation, and like supporting factors would have to be compelling. If such a high correlation coefficient was obtained on the Stewart Pain-Color Scale, the counterarguments could be made by Stewart proponents. It could be argued that the Stewart scale had the advantage over the pencil and paper pain scale in that young children as well as different cultures can be tested using colors to represent pain states.

Another approach to convergent validity can be done by correlating nurse inter-rater data and the patient's self-report data. The nurse inter-rater scores of perceived level of pain experienced by postoperative patients can serve as external criteria with which to compare the patients' reported pain levels found in Table 3−1 as Total. There is high agreement or convergence among these ratings of pain. The correlations of Total, Total for Nurse 1, and Total for Nurse 2 are given by r = 0.95 and r = 0.88, respectively.

Another form of validity is to ascertain whether the instruments have *discriminant validity*. Discriminability refers to the ability to differentiate the construct being measured from other constructs. In our example with other pain instruments, we would look at the correlations of the different pain instruments. If the correlations are low to moderate, there is support that they do measure different aspects of the construct pain.

As an example of discriminant validity, the pain scale would not be expected to be related to a construct such as *ego strength*. The correlation between the Total score and ego strength is given by r = 0.29. Obviously the pain scale cannot be used to measure nor to predict ego strength.

Campbell and Fiske (1959) proposed a construct validation procedure known as the *multitrait-multimethod matrix method* for testing the concepts of convergence and discriminant validity. Measurements of the same trait derived from dissimilar data ought to converge, and measurements of different traits ought to diverge. When different constructs are being measured, we would expect low positive or negative validity correlation coefficients. If this occurs, we can say that the pain scale diverges or discriminates from instruments measuring other constructs.

Two types of variance are considered in the Campbell and Fiske measurement approach. The first measurement involves variability in a set of values resulting from individual or subject differences in the trait being measured. It is called *trait variance*. The second measurement involves variability resulting from individual differences in the patient's or subject's ability to effectively participate or respond to the particular type of measurement procedure used. It is called *method variance*. An illustration of the method occurs when two or more different types of pain measurements are gathered on the same patient.

For example, suppose one measurement uses a brief videotape of the patient apparently in pain; the second measurement records the patient's abdominal muscle reflex states, and the third measurement represents a nurse observer's rating of the degree of pain experienced by the patient. When the correlation coefficients are high among the three different pain variables, the measurements are said to have low trait variance because it appears that the three instruments are measuring a single unitary construct. But if the correlation coefficients are low among the different measurement approaches because the three methods are measuring different constructs, the three different variables are said to have high method variance.

The isolation or identification of trait variance from method variance is reported to be a noted strength of the multitrait-multimethod approach to validity determination (Waltz et al, 1984). Because the Campbell and Fiske method does not possess an externally valid criterion measurement for evaluation purposes, we do not recommend its use. The Campbell and Fiske method predates the evolution of present day sophisticated computer and statistical technical developments for multivariate methods like factor analysis, canonical analysis, discriminant analysis (see Chapter 11), and multidimensional scaling (see Chapter 12). The multitrait-multimethod matrix method can be viewed retrospectively as the "poor man's factor analysis."

In another approach to construct validity, a *factorial validity technique* is used. Factor analysis constitutes another means of looking at the convergent and divergent validity of a large set of items. The use of factor analysis depends on mathematically complex techniques as well as the nurse's strong intuitive grasp of the meaning of the clusters and factors identified in the analysis. The model is described in Chapter 11.

Factor analysis is essentially a method for combining clusters of related variables. Each cluster, called a factor, represents in theory a unitary attribute. The procedure is used to identify related variables and group alike or closely similar items that reflect some underlying attribute. Factor analytic procedures seek to relate many variables by showing their basic structure, how they are similar, and how they are different. The factor analysts also seek to name the components of the structure or underlying unities of the factors. Thus an investigator can discover or create categories and variables that subsequently can be tested (Kerlinger and Pedhazur, 1973).

The data of Table 3–1 were submitted to a factor analysis. The results are presented in Table 3–8, and the numbers are correlation coefficients of each variable with the factor generated by the mathematical algorithm associated with factor analysis. As indicated, each of the variables except ego strength is strongly correlated with the factor of pain. The lowest correlation is with ego strength ($r = -0.32$). All the other correlations exceed $r = 0.64$ in value. Because all correlations are large and close to one another, except for uncertainty and ego strength, it is highly probable that the pain scale possesses acceptable psychometric properties.

TABLE 3–8 CORRELATION COEFFICIENT OF EACH VARIABLE OF TABLE 3–1

Variable	Correlation Coefficient
Pretest	.99
Posttest	.93
Odd	.96
Even	.96
Nurse 1	.96
Nurse 2	.94
Rank 1	.93
Rank 2	.91
Total	.98
Days	.87
Uncertainty	.64
Ego strength	−.32

*With the first principal component based on all 12 variables.

3–19 SUMMARY

In examining the various ways in which an investigator explores the reliability and validity of a research instrument, it is important to note that evidence is accumulated from a variety of measurement techniques. No single technique is superior to any other technique. The progressive accumulation of information and research findings by the investigator developing the research tool and other investigators using the instrument can be used to support the reliability and validity issues associated with a measurement instrument. Although statistical procedures greatly aid an investigator in answering the various concerns about the types of reliability and validity contained in any single instrument, careful, logical analysis of findings from these diverse approaches help the investigator and those using the instrument to determine whether the instrument contains the essential psychometric properties of reliability and validity.

REFERENCES

American Psychological Association: Standards for Educational and Psychological Testing. Washington, DC: American Psychological Association, 1985.

Bostrom, A.: CRUNCH software, Oakland, CA, 1986.

Campbell, D.T., and Fiske, D.W.: Convergent and divergent validation by the multitrait-multimethod matrix, Psych. Bull., 56: 81–105, 1959.

Cohen, J.: A coefficient of agreement for nominal scales, Ed. Psych. Measurement, 20: 37–46, 1961.

Cramer, H.: Mathematical Methods of Statistics. Princeton, Princeton University Press, 1951.

Cronbach, L.J.: Coefficient alpha and the internal structure of tests, Psychometrika, 16: 297–334, 1951.

Cronbach, L.J.: Test validation. In Thorndike, R.L., Ed., Educational Measurement. Washington, DC, American Council on Education, 1971.

Davitz, J.B., and Davitz, L.L.: Inferences of Patients' Pain and Psychological Distress: Studies of Nursing Behaviors. New York, Springer, 1981.

Fox, D.J.: Fundamentals of Research in Nursing. New York, Appleton-Century-Crofts, 1982.

Franck, L.S.: A new method to quantitatively describe pain behavior in infants, Nurs. Res., 35: 28–31, 1986.

Geden, E., Beck, N., Hauge, G., et al.: Self-reports and psychophysiological effects of five pain-coping strategies, Nurs. Res., 33: 260–265, 1984.

Guilford, J.P.: Psychometric Methods, ed. 4. New York, McGraw-Hill, 1965.

Hoyt, C.: Test reliability estimated by analysis of variance, Psychometrika, 6: 153–160, 1941.

Jacox, A.K., ed: Pain: A Source Book for Nurses and Other Allied Health Professionals. Boston, Little, Brown & Co., 1977.

Johnson, J.E.: Coping with surgery. In Werley, H.H., and Fitzpatrick, J.J., eds., Annual Review of Nursing Research, vol. 2. New York, Springer, 1984.

Johnson, J.E., Christman, N.J., and Stitt, C.: Personal control interventions: short- and long-term effects on surgical patients Res. Nurs. Health, 8: 131–145, 1985.

Johnson, J.E., Fuller, S.S., Endress, M.P., et al.: Altering patients' response to surgery: an extension and replication, Res. Nurs. Health, 1: 111–121, 1978a.

Johnson, J.E., and Rice, V.H.: Sensory and distress components of pain: implications for the study of clinical pain, Nurs. Res., 23: 203–209, 1974.

Johnson, J.E., Rice, V.H., Fuller, S.S., et al.: Sensory information, instruction in a coping strategy and recovery from surgery, Res. Nurs. Health, 1: 4–17, 1978b.

Kerlinger, F.N., and Pedhazur, E.J.: Multiple Regression in Behavioral Research. New York, Holt, Rinehart, & Winston, 1973.

Likert, R.: A technique for the measurement of attitudes, Arch. Psych. No. 140, 1932.

Marascuilo, L.A., and McSweeney, M.: Nonparametric and Distribution-free Methods for the Social Sciences. Monterey, CA, Brooks/Cole, 1977.

Meinhart, N.T., and McCaffery, M.: Pain: A Nursing Approach to Assessment and Analysis. New York, Appleton-Century-Crofts, 1983.

Melzack, R.: The McGill pain questionnaire: major properties and scoring methods, Pain, 1: 277–299, 1975.

Melzack, R., and Torgerson, W.S.: On the language of pain, Anesthesiology, 34: 50–59, 1971.

Menzel, N.J., and Martinson, I.M.: Effects of electrical surface stimulation on control of acute postoperative pain and prevention of atelectasis and ileus in patients having abdominal surgery. In Batey, M.E., ed., Communicating Nursing Research, vol. 8. Boulder, CO, 1977.

Mishel, M.H.: Adjusting the fit: development of uncertainty scales for specific clinical populations, West. J. Nurs. Res., 5: 355–370, 1983a.

Mishel, M.H.: Parents' perception of uncertainty of their hospitalized child, Nurs. Res., 32: 324–330, 1983b.

Mishel, M.H.: Perceived uncertainty and stress in illness, Res. Nurs. Health, 7: 163–171, 1984.

Mishel, M.H., and Braden, C.J.: Finding meaning: antecedents of uncertainty and illness, Nurs. Res., 37: 98–103, 1988.

Savedra, M., Tesler, M., Ward, J., et al.: Description of the pain experience: a study of school-age children, Iss. Compreh. Pediatr. Nurs., 5: 373–380, 1981.

Stanley, J.C.: Reliability. In Thorndike R.L., ed., Educational Measurement. Washington, DC: American Council on Education, 1971.

Stewart, M.L.: Measurement of clinical pain. In Jacox, A.K., ed., Pain: A Source Book for Nurses and Other Allied Health Professionals, 1977.

Waltz, C.F., and Bausell, R.B.: Nursing Research: Design Statistics, and Computer Analysis. Philadelphia, F.A. Davis Co., 1981.

Waltz, C.F., Strickland, O.L., and Lenz, E.R.: Measurement in Nursing Research. Philadelphia, F.A. Davis Co., 1984.

Chapter 4

EXPERIMENTAL AND QUASI-EXPERIMENTAL DESIGNS

4-1 EXPERIMENTAL AND QUASI-EXPERIMENTAL DESIGN

After an investigator has defined a research area for study, established the constructs of interest, specified the hypotheses to be tested, and selected the instruments to be used in the investigation, the next task is to design the study that best addresses the research questions within the limitations of finances. To many, the ideal design is the classic or *true experiment* of the natural sciences. With human subjects, the ideal or true experiment may not be attainable because of individual differences in response to a single stimulus. In many instances, a researcher must employ a *quasi-experiment* that approximates a true experiment as closely as possible, given the constraints of money, time, space, personnel, and other resources. In this chapter, the primary elements of true experiments and quasi-experiments in nursing research are described. Also considered are the concepts of explained and unexplained variations in ex-

periments. The principles of random sampling and randomization to achieve the strict standards of an experiment are presented. Finally, the assumptions, logic, concepts, and principles of *internal* and *external* validity, two characteristics used in the evaluation of all experimental and quasi-experimental studies, are depicted and applied to specific research designs.

4-2 THE ROLE OF THE EXPERIMENT IN NURSING RESEARCH

It is easy to assume that reports of research in the nursing professional literature have been performed under the same ideal conditions that are believed to pervade research conducted in other disciplines. This misconception must be challenged immediately. It is not true of other disciplines and is not true of research in the domain of nursing science. A factor that contributes to this misconception is the editorial policies of nursing research journals. According to research publications, completed research must be described according to a preestablished rigorous format. For example, a number of research journals require the author to follow the third edition of the *American Psychological Association (APA) Publication Manual* (1983) for describing the outcomes of original investigations. Some persons who read research based on this rigorous reporting style could easily form the impression that the precise steps described in the completed manuscript were really those actually followed by the author or authors.

An investigator is seldom able to follow the linear progression established in the original research plan. In most cases, multiple compromises are forced on the researcher before the study can be brought to a successful conclusion. The actual performance of a research study almost always involves a much more dynamic set of activities than that implied by the typical static report that finally is published. In this chapter, the principles of an ideal, experimental research design are depicted. Strategies are offered to approximate the theoretical characteristics of a sound research design, when the conditions for a true experiment cannot be attained.

In the natural and physical sciences, the *experiment* is the research model of preference. In these disciplines, a body of knowledge based on facts and theories is used to generate new theoretical propositions that connect independent and dependent variables in meaningful ways. Traditionally, the experiment has been the major research model used to test new propositions. In the natural and basic disciplines, experiments are conducted in controlled settings, free of the environmental and interpersonal forces thought to predominate in much of social and behavioral research. For example, in a laboratory study of pain, a researcher should control ambient conditions such as temperature, atmospheric pressure, humidity, light, noise, colors, furnishings, motion, and other factors that could have an impact on the collected data. In addition, interpersonal factors like the physical presence of another person in the environment of a test subject can be controlled by placing the subject in a closed booth, devoid of all interpersonal contact.

An independent variable such as *sound* can be manipulated from an electronic console, far removed from any personal contact with each subject being observed. In this manner, it is assumed that the effects of different levels of sound on pain can be assessed, free of the effects of instrumentation variables and the interpersonal bias produced by a human tester. Of course, this assumption has been challenged in both basic and behavioral sciences. In this case, a challenge can be advanced to the use of a sound-proof room as a place to perform such a study, because what is observed in the sound-proof room may have no bearing on environments other than that room. In all research, the site of a study can change the characteristics of the response variable so that the original hypothesis is not tested.

It can never be assumed that a completed or published study is free of all measurement and human error. The possible interference of confounding forces must be entertained and assessed to determine how they might have acted on each human or animal subject who had taken part in an experiment. No researcher has been able to perform the perfect experiment; perhaps no one ever will. The best that can be realistically expected is that an experiment must approach ideal or desired research design characteristics.

Outside the research laboratory environment, comprehensive control of confounding variables is almost never possible. Problems can occur to foil an otherwise perfect research plan, even in the laboratory setting. Experienced researchers know that uncontaminated environments rarely exist in most classic laboratory research. For instance, in the pain and sound study, instruments may fail, electrical power may be cut off, and the ambient temperature may suddenly rise or fall. At the same time, a research subject under observation may have an adverse reaction to the colors of the booth. Dust or pollen in the booth may induce an allergic reaction, or the subject may have a psychophysiological response to being locked in a closed booth for an extended period of time. Even in the best of all possible worlds, laboratory research can be compromised by factors not under the control of the researcher. Yet, the experiment is the preferred model for scientific investigations. The reasons for the elevated status of the experiment are considered here.

The main purposes of science are to describe, explain, and predict phenomena of interest, and the best model to address those canons of science is the experiment. The experiment provides the preferred avenue for description because independent researchers, using the same methods, can provide similar descriptions of what is observed. Experiments provide the opportunity to replicate research findings by the same or other investigators. Theories to explain relationships among variables are best tested in experiments to verify that the relationships exist and best explained in a clear, precise, and unambiguous manner. No other research model has been proposed that achieves these goals as efficiently and effectively as the experiment. In a carefully controlled experiment, data are collected that either support or refute the hypothesized relationship among the independent (predictor) variables and the dependent (outcome) variables. Thus, the experiment serves as a scientific model that is used to evaluate how well a theory predicts a specified outcome.

In essence, an experiment is designed to test propositions that connect variables in a cause and effect relationship. Ideally this test is performed through the control of all variables except those of theoretical interest. The classic experiment has been described by Campbell and Stanley (1963). According to their description, a classic experiment has three components:

1. The random assignment of subjects to experimental conditions
2. At least one control group established in the study
3. Clear and unambiguous specifications of the manipulation of an independent variable

When these three components are satisfied, the study is called an experiment.

4-3 EXPLAINED AND UNEXPLAINED SOURCES OF VARIANCE IN THE EXPERIMENTAL STUDY

A researcher learns from all studies—experimental or observational—that the resulting data always vary across subjects. Variation is part of our world and is the subject matter of science in general and nursing in particular. Two major sources of variation are present in all studies. These are traditionally referred to as *explained* variation and *unexplained* variation.

Variation is encountered in research stud-

ies under two different modes. In an observational study, correlation coefficients are used to assess the degree of variation in a dependent variable that can be attributed to its association with an independent variable. This form of explained variation is discussed in Chapters 9 and 10. The second form of explained variance is encountered in an experimental study with multiple groups in which the variation in a dependent variable is associated with group membership. In this case, an analysis of variance statistical model is used to assess the relationship between explained and unexplained variation. The experimental sources of variation are important for the topics discussed in this chapter. The points about explained and unexplained variation are illustrated in the following hypothetical experiment.

Consider a study in which two groups of newly diagnosed adolescent diabetic patients are taught how to self-administer insulin by means of two different instructional programs, Method A and Method B. Method A involves lectures, films, and audiotapes and is essentially didactic. Method B involves experiential learning in which experienced adolescent diabetics, with professional guidance and support, offer informal counseling, discussion, demonstrations, and assistance. To evaluate the effectiveness of either instructional method, each adolescent is followed up for a three-month period. During that period, the number of times an adolescent experiences adverse effects through underdosage or overdosage of insulin administration is recorded. The hypothesis of interest is to ascertain whether the mean number of adverse adolescent diabetic insulin experiences is a function of one or the other educational method.

In this study, two major sources of experimental variations exist. The first source is associated with the particular characteristics of the subjects. It is independent of the group to which research subjects are assigned for training. This source of variation is often referred to as *variation due to individual differences*. It is also called chance variation, within group variation, error variation, and residual variation. Not all adolescents experience the same reactions to over- or underdosages of insulin. Over a three-month period, most experience no adverse effects. Others may have one or more experiences.

The second source of variation results from the *differences between groups* or train-

① (Unexplained Variation) = (Age Variation) + (Interaction of Method and Age) + (Residual Unexplained Variation after Age is Removed)

---

② (Residual Unexplained Variation after Age is Removed) = (Intelligence Variation) + (Interaction of Method and Intelligence) + (Interaction of Age and Intelligence) + (Interaction of Method and Age and Intelligence) + (Residual Variation)

---

ing programs. If one program is more effective than the other, this would be expressed with more adverse reactions among the adolescents assigned to that program. This source of systematic variation is called the between group variation, treatment variation, or explained variation.

The purpose of an experiment is to determine the magnitude and direction of the sources of variation. Future studies would be planned to minimize the unexplained experimental variation and maximize the explained experimental variation. This research goal or objective had been called the *minimax principle*, and it has been well articulated by Kerlinger (1973).

Here we show how the minimax principle is used to design a study to test the null hypothesis of no difference in mean values for Method A and Method B. If no other variables are included in the study, it can be shown that as a first phase in the design of the study,

(Total Variation) =
> (Explained Variation)
> > + (Unexplained Variation)

In this case the (Explained Variation) is identical, with the variation associated with the difference between the two methods. Thus,

(Explained Variation) =
> (Method Variation)

As a second phase in the design of the study, let us now examine the (Unexplained Variation) and try to determine the sources of variance that tend to make it large. Perhaps the most salient variable that is correlated with the number of adverse reactions experienced over the three months of the study is age of onset of diabetes. Young persons tend to be more physiologically unstable as diabetics. One way to assess the effect of age is to define a set of three age groups

such as 10 to 12, 13 to 15, and 16 to 18. These three groups are used to determine the amount of variation explained by the categorization of adolescent age. The source of variation for this variable is contained in the (Unexplained Variation). This source of variation can be partitioned as shown in equation 1 at the top of this page.

In the third phase, this new measure of unexplained variation is examined and another variable that might be associated with the dependent variable is identified. In this study, a second confounding factor might be the level of intelligence of those in the study. Adolescents with less than average intelligence could be expected to have more problems in learning how to assess their need for insulin and then to learn and demonstrate how to inject the insulin properly. The adolescents at this phase in the design of the study could be categorized as below or above average intelligence. With the introduction of this additional confounding factor into the design, more explained variation can be extracted. In particular, the partitioning of the variation described in equation 2 at the top of this page is possible.

If other confounding factors could be identified, they would be added to the design. As illustrated, the effect of adding extra explanatory factors to the design is that the residual or unexplained variation becomes *minimized* and the explained variation becomes *maximized*. In this example, the explained variation associated with Method is given by the equation at the top of page 62.

Other sources of explained variation are (Age Variation), (Intelligence Variation), and (Interaction of Age and Intelligence). More on this important topic is presented in Chapter 9 in the presentation of the analysis of variance.

In addition to the true experiments and quasi-experimental designs described in this chapter, a vast array of other designs exist

(Method Variation) + (Interaction of Method and Age) + (Interaction of Method and Intelligence) + (Interaction of Method and Age and Intelligence)

---

that are used in nursing and health care research. Some include the many forms of factorial analysis of variance designs with interaction effects and nested factors, including incomplete designs like Latin squares, fully crossed repeated measures designs, designs with covariates like the analysis of covariance, and multivariate designs. (The analysis of variance is discussed in Chapter 9, the analysis of covariance is discussed in Chapter 10, and multivariate techniques are described in Chapter 11.) Other designs can be found in Winer (1971) and Keppel (1973).

In the following sections, for simplicity most of the designs are described as if they contain only one control group and one experimental group. This is not the case in most nursing investigations. Whatever is reported for the simple two-group or prototype design can be extended directly to the more complicated design with blocking variables and many treatments.

4–4 RANDOM SAMPLING AND RANDOMIZATION: CORNERSTONES OF THE TRUE EXPERIMENT

The true experiment is one in which all variables except the independent variable are under the strict control of a researcher. Unfortunately, a true experiment with human subjects is rarely possible because control of all confounding experimental variables is impossible. Theoretical statisticians, led by the example of Sir R.A. Fisher (1925), have developed models that allow statistical control of extraneous variables. The least complex of these statistical models recommends that *simple random samples* be selected from the population of interest. A sample is said to be a simple random sample when

1. every element of the population has an equal probability of being assigned to the various experimental conditions of a study, and
2. assignment of each subject to the various experimental conditions is independent

of the assignment of all other subjects in the population.

Other sampling schemes are often used in nursing studies in which probabilities of selection are unequal for various persons and groups. Some of these models are described in Chapter 6 in which survey sampling methods are illustrated.

With human populations, random samples are almost never attainable because precise definitions of research populations are hard to specify. Procedurally, the specification of a random sample requires a list or roster of all possible subjects constituting or representing the population of research interest. In practice, these lists often do not exist. If such a list did exist, it would be used in the following manner.

Subjects of research interest are listed and given an identification number. The identification number starts at zero and ends when the population size is exhausted. In making the research subject identification and selection list, it is absolutely imperative that the rank order of a person on the list has no relationship to the dependent variable to be measured on each subject in the study. The assumed lack of an ordered relationship with the dependent variable makes random sampling workable with human subjects.

After the list of research subjects has been established, a table of random numbers is used to obtain samples for each of the study's experimental conditions. Random number tables are used because they have been constructed to satisfy the conditions required for random sampling. A table of random numbers minimizes the effects of possible confounding variables that could affect the experimental subjects in a study.

Random assignment of each subject to any one treatment group represents an equally likely and independent event. This method of assignment guarantees that all confounding variables are uniformly and equally distributed across all the experimental groups. Therefore, the resulting experimental groups are assumed to be similar on all variables not controlled by a researcher. No other research design possesses this inherent strength.

In health care studies, random samples for study are rarely available because subjects are often preselected on the basis of health status. Therefore, these samples fail to represent the population of interest. Often such samples are called *chunks* or *convenience* samples. The world of health care research is based on such convenience samples. To use these samples for generalizations is frequently inappropriate. The part of the population, used in most health care research, is not representative of the population to which inferences are made.

When random sampling is not possible, a researcher may have to make some compromises. A less efficient scheme in the creation of study groups may have to be employed, and alternative selection procedures often constrain the generalization of study findings.

Randomization strategies may be used with convenience samples. The designation of subjects to either a control or a treatment group can be performed through the use of a table of random numbers. Furthermore, a random number table can be used to assign groups of subjects to the various treatments under study. According to Marascuilo and Serlin (1988), "Randomization is the application of the principles of random sampling to a chunk from a population in which a number of equivalent groups are to be established whose differences from one another can only be attributed to chance."

To illustrate how a table of random numbers is used to established randomization samples from a convenience sample or chunk of a population, consider the preoperative teaching program described in Chapter 1. Each patient entering the hospital is assigned to one of the three treatments. Randomization can be achieved by selecting from the random number table a number between 1 and 9. If the number selected is 1, 2, or 3, the subject is assigned to treatment one. If the number selected is 4, 5, or 6, assignment to treatment two is made. If 7, 8, or 9 is selected, assignment to treatment three is made. If 0 is selected, another number is chosen. This method of subject assignment assumes that each person has a 33⅓% probability of being assigned to any one group, and each assignment is independent of all other assignments. It is important to note that the established three groups are very similar to one another on all possible confounding variables. This method of as-

signment assures uniformity across the samples. Thus, an investigator can defend conclusions about the effects of the independent variable (preoperative teaching method) on the dependent variable (patient outcomes), provided that competing explanations for the obtained differences are systematically entertained and then ruled out.

4-5 THE EXTERNAL AND INTERNAL VALIDITY OF EXPERIMENTS

Random assignment of subjects to experimental conditions is often confused with random sampling. In a study that uses random sampling, each member of the population has an equal chance of being included in the sample and each member is selected independently of all other members. If this model had been applied to the three teaching conditions in the preoperative surgery education program described in Chapters 1 and 2, the study would have had the increased probability of possessing the property of *external validity*. In practice, a study is said to have external validity if the findings observed in the study can be generalized to the population from which the samples were randomly drawn. This type of sampling is rarely, if ever, conducted because of the great cost encountered in trying to select a random sample.

In a true experiment using random samples, questions of external validity are not a major issue provided that no changes or unusual events transpire during the course of the experiment. This statement unfortunately is not applicable to a true experiment based on the randomization model of assignment of subjects to experimental conditions. Because a chunk has served as the basis of the randomization, external validity can be defended only if the chunk reproduces the population in all details. In general, chunks do not do this.

In addition to randomly assigning subjects to treatment conditions, treatment conditions can also be randomly assigned to different sets of randomly selected subjects. Both random assignment procedures produce a study that may be weak in external validity but strong in *internal validity*. A study is said to have internal validity if the results can be attributed to the independent variables in the study and not to some other extraneous or confounding variables. This means that the treatment alone produced the observed differences and that the differences cannot be attributed to other confounding causes. In an experiment, the investigator must show that the changes in the dependent variable are caused by or associated with the changes in the independent variable and not to any other variable. In the true experiment, this is not an issue provided that the subjects are randomly selected from the population, but this may not be true for a study based on randomization of a chunk.

From this discussion, it can be concluded that without random sampling a study cannot possess the necessary foundation on which to build a case that external validity is a strong feature of the designed experiment. If the grounds for external validity cannot be established, at least the researcher can use a randomization assignment procedure to create the framework necessary to justify claims for internal validity.

Most experiments in nursing research use convenience samples and thus lack external validity. This is not necessarily the case for internal validity when randomization procedures are used. Internal validity can be achieved but frequently at great expense. It should be noted that neither random sampling nor randomization was used in the preoperative teaching study. Instead, a systematic sampling scheme was adopted. (For a discussion on systematic sampling see Section 6–14.) In most cases, systematic sampling is the most feasible procedure to use in a health care setting. The basic assumption in using this sampling model is that patients arrive over time at the hospital with conditions that are uncorrelated or independent of the treatment to which each is assigned. This assumption is justified because

1. there is no reason to believe that the health conditions of people arriving one after another have a systematic relationship to the three educational programs,
2. the type and severity of health care problems of patients are randomly distributed in the general population of those possessing abdominal problems necessitating surgery, and
3. the assignment of patients to each of the three treatments is independent of their health condition.

4–6 THREATS TO THE INTERNAL VALIDITY OF AN EXPERIMENT

Even in a well-designed study, events occurring before and during the course of an investigation may seriously threaten the internal validity of the study. In light of this possibility, we must be concerned about possible competing explanations and threats to internal validity for the preoperative teaching findings. Campbell and Stanley (1963) and Cook and Campbell (1979) list a number of conditions that must be satisfied before internal validity can be assumed. Some of these confounding conditions have been identified as history, attrition, selection, maturation, instrumentation, regression, testing, interaction with selection, diffusion or imitation of treatments, compensatory equalization of treatments, compensatory rivalry by respondents receiving less desirable treatments, and resentful demoralization of respondents receiving less desirable treatments. One way to reduce the effects of these confounding influences is to establish comparison or control groups for the group receiving the intervention. If no comparison or control group is established, these confounding variables can serve as competing explanatory causes for the obtained experimental findings.

Other threats to internal validity may be of importance in certain specialized situations. Let us examine these threats to internal validity in relationship to the preoperative surgery teaching study. Some of the threats and examples given may seem unlikely in a nursing research study but are presented here to illustrate the type of threats to internal validity that could be encountered.

Even when agreement has been reached with a health care agency about the conduct of a nursing study, events may transpire during the course of the investigation that are unknown to the researcher. Agreements reached at the onset of a long-term experiment tend to dissipate when there are changes in key agency administrative personnel. Furthermore, written agreements tend not to be disseminated to actual patient care units where studies are conducted. Therefore, researchers need to be constantly vigilant and to make frequent checks to ensure that a study is operating according to plan. Vigilance is also necessary to identify the many factors operating during a study that could seriously undermine the integrity of the research. We describe some of these here for the preoperative teaching study.

1. History

History effects refer to events occurring during the course of the study between and within the three experimental teaching methods that may have influenced the final outcome of the research. In an experiment it is presumed that the events occurring over the passage of time among the three conditions during the course of the investigation are identical. Such an assumption in a health care setting is frequently tenuous. For example, suppose that in one of the three hospitals used in the study, the surgical staff changed after one month and introduced a radical technique for gallbladder surgery. At first, it might be thought that this constitutes a threat to internal validity. This may or may not be the case. It would not be a threat if the effects of the change were the same across all three treatment conditions at that hospital. The introduction of a new surgical procedure at only one hospital would certainly bias the treatment comparisons across the hospitals. That is, the patients in the hospital experiencing the change in surgical technique may have different mean values on such dependent variables as length of stay, postoperative complications, number of pain medications, and number of days at home before leaving unassisted. However, it would not jeopardize the study within that one hospital with respect to the treatment comparisons, provided that the new surgical procedure did not favor any one of the three preoperative training conditions. If the new surgical procedure favored one training condition, then comparisons across hospitals are confounded. If an analysis of variance were performed on the independent variable, this threat to internal validity would be seen as a hospital by treatment interaction.

Another instance in which history can be a significant threat to internal validity across the treatments is encountered when a change occurs in the assignment of registered nursing personnel in one hospital to one of the three treatment groups. For example, suppose that a functional model of nursing care was changed to a primary model of nursing care for patients in treatment one. This historical event could be an important confounding factor in the study with respect to both the treatment comparisons and the hospital comparisons. Again, this would be identified by a hospital by treatment interaction.

2. Attrition

A differential loss of subjects is a serious threat to internal validity. It can confound the results and make the comparisons between groups less than meaningful. As a study progresses, the dropping out of subjects is a perennial problem for all research extending over time. It is a particularly serious problem when the subjects are systematically leaving one study condition in comparison with the other conditions. Random attrition, though not desirable, is a less serious threat to internal validity. In longitudinal studies, the problem is most acute. The longer the study lasts, the greater the probability of losing subjects before the final data are collected. Lost subjects are costly in time, money, and scientific rigor. Subjects can be lost because of death, accidents, change of address, reduced motivation to continue to participate, and changes in health status. Some factors lead to subject attrition. Factors within a study that can contribute to subject dropout are the amount of time required of the subject, the frequency of times required for data collection and follow-up, the personal threat and discomfort that a person may experience as the study progresses, and the complexity of the study. In health care research, side-effects of drugs and medical procedures can lead to dropping out. As indicated, the list of reasons for differential research subject dropout is large.

The effects of differential dropout can be assessed by performing a small study of those who drop out and why they drop out. This can be achieved by selecting a small random sample of the dropouts. The dropouts can be reached by means of a phone interview or a short mail questionnaire that inquires about the reasons for their leaving the study. For example, in the preoperative teaching study it might be learned that subjects dropped out of treatment one in one hospital because of information revealed to them. They discovered that two other educational programs were available and that they had been assigned to the least favorable one. Because of their resentment, they refused to cooperate and continue with the treatment. This information can be used to suggest possible explanations for the findings.

In the preoperative surgical teaching study, dropout of subjects is not a problem mainly because the dependent measures were unobtrusive and could be obtained directly from hospital and nursing records. One of the variables could have been a problem, that is, the number of days at home before leaving unassisted. In our hypothetical example, data were obtained on all 246 subjects. In most other similar studies, this information would not be so easily obtainable.

It is conceivable that in at least one of the three operative teaching programs, some patients may choose not to continue participating because of experiencing personal discomfort or threat as a consequence of the teaching program. Hence, differential subject loss in one of the treatment conditions could compromise the internal validity of the study. Consider also the threat to internal validity caused by the introduction of a new surgical procedure at one of the hospitals. This historical event could lead to attrition from the study. It could happen that the surgical procedure on gallbladder patients in one of the teaching conditions could lead to greater postoperative discomfort, thus inducing a lack of cooperation among those patients. Even though patients were available for data collection, it would have to be concluded that the treatment had not been applied because of their refusal to continue.

3. Selection

Selection bias occurs when certain types of persons are collectively assigned to one group in a study or when treatments are assigned to preexisting groups that may differ. The first type of bias can happen when a researcher selects the most severely ill patients, as they enter the hospital, and places them in the control condition. The less severely ill subjects are placed in the experimental treatment condition. It is clear that such an assignment creates a bias in the study in favor of the experimental treatment condition. In the second case, bias can be introduced when patients are physically grouped according to severity in a hospital unit. Consequently, if the treatments are assigned to the preestablished groups with the experimental treatment assigned to the patients with the less severe conditions, bias is introduced. In both cases, it is seen that selection bias favoring the experimental treatment condition can occur when random assignment is not applied.

In the preoperative surgical teaching study, selection bias is not an initial issue because of the way patients were assigned to the three treatment conditions. Selection bias, however, can be introduced into the study at a midway point. With three different treatments in operation at one hospital over a considerable period of time, the medical and nursing staff would most likely form opinions about which is the most effective treatment. On this basis, some physicians might request that particular patients be placed in the treatment group assessed as being most effective. A corollary set of events could occur. The professional nursing staff could recommend particular patients for the favored treatment group.

To maintain the integrity of the study, such requests must be denied. At the time of data analysis a post hoc stratification of patients on the basis of physician and nurse evaluation of patient-treatment fit could be made. Patients who are classified as being in a favorable or unfavorable fit for a particular teaching program could be examined. This post hoc stratification could provide information on why the various teaching programs were successful or unsuccessful with certain types of patients in each of the treatment groups.

Selection bias could have been a problem in the preoperative teaching study if in a given hospital the first third of the incoming patients had been assigned to treatment one, with the second third to treatment two, and the last third to treatment three. Selection bias would have occurred if the patients had come into the hospital on the basis of some factor that is related to the treatment. For example, incoming patients in treatment one could have had less severe conditions and less complicated surgical procedures; these factors would make their postoperative recovery smoother and less complicated than that of patients in the other two treatment conditions. If experimental treatment one were the least effective treatment, the selection bias would support the alternative proposition that the treatment is effective when in fact it was not an effective treatment.

4. Maturation

Maturation is a serious threat to internal validity if the effects of variables like mental age, height, weight, hunger, fatigue, and similar developmental and dispositional states are systematic and orderly over a period of time. It is conceivable that in some situations it is difficult to determine whether the improvement observed over a period of time can be attributed to the treatment or to maturational changes or to the interaction of both treatment and maturational influences. Maturation is a particular issue in all growth and development studies, especially when young children or aged persons are studied.

In health care research, maturational problems can arise in longitudinal studies on chronic diseases such as arthritis, diabetes, many forms of cancer, and arteriosclerotic cardiovascular diseases. Boredom, fatigue, and motivation appear to be particular issues encountered in longitudinal studies. In addition, many degenerative neurological diseases such as multiple sclerosis, myasthenia gravis, and other similar conditions possess considerable maturational influences. In these cases, control or comparison groups that are as similar to one another as possible must be established at the initial phases of the study. If a preponderance of patients with these chronic or degenerative diseases exists in one group, the progressive developmental disease changes over time may affect the outcome of the study in unexpected and detrimental ways. If this occurred, a post hoc stratification of patients according to type of illness could be carried out and the data analysis could incorporate this dimension of patient differences. The findings from this analysis could be used to assess the effectiveness of the three different training programs with respect to this disease stratification.

In the preoperative surgical teaching study, differential maturation should not be a problem because of the way subjects have been assigned to the three treatment conditions in each hospital. Length of treatment is so short that long-term maturation problems should not be encountered. The fatigue and stress experienced by patients postoperatively could be a factor in one of the three treatment conditions if the condition placed extreme demands on energy levels of patients or their coping capacities.

5. Instrumentation

In all studies the researcher must choose appropriate instruments to assess the impact of the dependent variables. Instrumentation problems are often encountered in the repeated measures pretest-posttest design when the measurement properties of the posttest differ from that of the pretest. This phenomenon is operative primarily when using such instruments as scales, balances, or weights that may wear out in the process of being used repeatedly. Instrumentation is also prevalent in studies using interviewers or observers when they become fatigued over the course of the study. Measurements late in the data collection phase may not provide either valid or reliable information. If the effects of instrumentation are constant for all groups, bias results, but such effects do not confound or threaten the internal validity of the study. However, differential instrumentation across groups does threaten the internal validity of the study.

For example, in a study designed to assess the effectiveness of a pain intervention program, instrumentation problems would arise if the pretest given to the subjects were a self-report inventory and the posttest were a galvanic skin response measure. The two tests are different and each measures what is unique to each instrument; the information may not necessarily overlap. Instruments used to measure dependent variables may change during the course of a study. For example, scales may become out of balance or galvanic skin response measurements may become less accurate because of frequent use; or, the reverse may occur so that the measurements over time become more accurate.

In the preoperative surgical teaching study, instrumentation is not a problem because no instrument was used more than once. Instrumentation errors can be introduced if the record keeping at the three hospitals varies in such a way as to favor one institutional setting over another. This could introduce bias in treatment comparisons across the three hospitals. Comparisons within a hospital would not be compromised.

6. Statistical Regression

It is well known that short fathers tend to have short sons and that tall fathers tend to have tall sons. It is not generally known, however, that short sons are generally taller than their fathers and that tall sons are typically shorter than their fathers. This tendency of sons' heights to be nearer to the center of the height distribution is called *regression to the mean*. This regression to the mean is an outcome of the correlation that exists between two variables. This property of correlated variables is easy to explain and is the model for linear regression theory, which derives its name from the tendency of variables to regress to the mean of a distribution.

To help understand this concept, consider the intelligence quotients between parents and their offspring. In particular, consider the relationship between mothers and daughters. It is generally believed that the correlation coefficient of the IQ between mothers and daughters is given by r = 0.50 and that the mean IQ is 100. Suppose that it is known that a mother has an IQ of 120. Because of the regression phenomena, it is known that the best guess of the daughter's IQ is given by

$$100 + 0.5(120 - 100) = 100 + 10 = 110.$$

The predicted IQ of the daughter is closer to the mean IQ of 100 because the correlation coefficient measures the amount of the regression. As another example, suppose a mother has an IQ of 90. The best estimate for the IQ of her daughter is

$$100 + 0.5(90 - 100) = 100 - 5 = 95.$$

Again the predicted IQ of the daughter is closer to the mean of 100 than is the IQ of the mother.

Regression provides one of the most serious threats to internal validity. Consider a baccalaureate program in nursing in which two groups of nurses are to be evaluated on their knowledge of pharmacology. Group one consists of students who have had prior work experiences in health care, whereas group two consists of students who entered a nursing program directly from high school. Suppose that both groups of students are given a pretest on knowledge of pharmacology. Because of previous work experience, the mean score for the group one students was greater than the mean score of the group two students. After the pretest, both groups of students were instructed in a common classroom with a single instructor. Upon completion of the course, a pharmacology posttest was administered to all students. Assuming that the treatment effect is the same for both groups, one can make a prediction about the relationship between the mean scores for each group on the posttest. Students with prior work experience are expected to regress downward to the mean score of the total group, whereas students directly admitted from high school are expected to regress upward to the mean of the total group. Thus, although the mean difference on the pretest may be large, favoring the nurses in group one, the mean difference on the posttest tends to be smaller, suggesting that students fresh out of high school gained more from the instruction than did the students with previous work experience. This simple explanation is in error because the reduction in the difference in the means can be attributed to the expected regression of scores toward the mean of the total group. As indicated by this example, regression to the mean appears whenever compared groups are different in mean values on a variable correlated with the criterion.

For this situation a possible solution exists. Both groups of students can be divided into two groups by using a table of random numbers. One half of the students from each group can receive the training in the fall semester. The two groups trained during the fall semester can serve as the experimental groups and the two remaining groups to be trained during the spring semester can serve as the corresponding control or comparison groups. For the evaluation, all four groups would have to be given the same criterion test used at the end of the fall semester. Students in the experimental group with previous work experience would be compared with their counterparts who receive training in the spring semester. The same type of comparison can be made for the students admitted directly from high school. Finally the differences of the means for the two types of students would be compared in what is referred to as a repeated measures or pretest-posttest design (Keppel, 1973).

As another example of regression effects being a threat to internal validity, consider the operation of a mental health clinic in which incoming patients are given a battery of tests such as the Minnesota Multiphasic Personality Inventory (MMPI) before being assigned to psychotherapy treatment. Following treatment, the MMPI is readministered and, as expected, the patients show improvement. It would be tempting to say that the treatment produced the improvement, but that may not be the case at all. Patients who enter a mental health clinic are under psychological stress. Their scores on the MMPI reflect this stress by being low and indicative of mental pain or discomfort. On the second testing, whether or not they receive treatment, regression theory predicts an improvement in test scores. This always happens and it cannot be concluded that the psychotherapy treatment produced the increases. Regression to the mean could be the only apparent factor required to explain the improved test scores. Regression manifests itself most when groups have been selected because of their extreme scores. Therefore, true change can be confused with observed change.

For this example, there exists a partial solution in use of the analysis of covariance discussed in Chapter 10. For the solution, a comparison group could be selected at a different site where clients are undergoing a different type of treatment. The other clinic may have a treatment program that uses psychotropic drugs. The analysis of covariance provides a statistical means to control for initial group differences on the pretest. The solution is not perfect but in some cases may generate results that have limited usefulness.

Consider designing a study to assess the effects of the three treatments in the preoperative surgery teaching program on pain following surgery. Suppose patients were assigned to the treatment based on their responses to the pain inventory developed in Chapter 3 by a nurse researcher. Patients with the highest pain scores are assigned to one treatment program, patients with the moderate pain scores are assigned to a second treatment program, and patients with the lowest pain scores are assigned to a third treatment program. On subsequent testing, it is found that scores of subjects in the high pain group show that pain has been reduced, scores of subjects in the moderate group remain about the same, and scores of subjects in the low pain group demonstrate higher levels of pain. On this basis, it could be concluded that the treatment assigned to the high pain patients was the most effective, whereas the treatment assigned to the low pain patients was the least effective. It could be argued that the treatment given to the high pain group actually lowered their levels of pain, whereas the treatment given to the low pain group actually increased their pain.

Of course, these decisions are in error because the entire set of findings can be explained in terms of the regression to the mean phenomena. Even if nothing is done to the high pain patients, regression theory predicts a reduction in their pain level for the second or postoperative test. At the same time, regression theory predicts an increase in pain scores for the low pain group even if nothing happens to them. In the postoperative surgery teaching program, regression is not a threat to internal validity. Subjects are not selected on the basis of high or low scores on a pretest concerning the treatment to which they are to be assigned.

On the basis of this discussion, one may form the impression that extreme groups should not be used in research. Such an impression is wrong. Most of the patients whom nurses see and work with are almost assuredly representatives of extreme groups. If that is the case, how is the problem of regression to the mean to be avoided? Another solution is to rank order the subjects on the basis of a pretest or some preestablished index, and then set up matched pairs or sets (three or more matched subjects) that are randomly assigned to two or more different treatment conditions. Under this type of assignment, which is called blocking on a variable that is correlated with the dependent variable, the effects of regression work uniformly across all the groups. If the subjects are taken from the top of a distribution, they all regress downward together, and if they are taken from the bottom of a distribution, they all regress upward.

For example, suppose the first 30 patients entering the hospital were assessed using the pain inventory of Chapter 3. They could be blocked in 10 groups of 3 and assigned at random within each block to one of the three pain reduction programs. This could be repeated with each subsequent group of 30 patients. Although this controls regression effects, it introduces data analysis issues that require further considerations. See Marascuilo and Serlin (1988) for a discussion on randomized block designs. Please note that this design makes use of the minimax principle described in Section 4–3.

7. Testing

Testing can be a threat to internal validity in that the process of measuring may sensitize some subjects to the hypotheses tested by a study and may heighten the possibility of responding negatively or favorably to treatment. Testing is a problem when a reactive measurement is used. A *reactive* measurement alters, modifies, or affects the variable under study. The MMPI is an example of a reactive measurement because a subject who completes the MMPI can be changed simply by answering the questions.

Testing is of special concern when the test situations are novel, dramatic, or particularly unique to the subject. For example, giving students an achievement test in a nursing curriculum is an accepted and normative activity. Placing a student on a stage in front of an audience and asking for a demonstration of some psychomotor skills would be considered a very novel set of circumstances for nursing student subjects. Students in the latter situation would be more likely to recall their performance and on posttesting may attempt to mimic or model their behavior or do the complete opposite based on their pretest performance. In addition, accuracy of self-reports may increase with familiarity with the instrument.

In the instances of patient research, giving a patient a self-report inventory upon admission to a hospital unit, in conjunction with all the other tests performed, would be considered a less novel circumstance than asking the patient to use a color chart to indicate pain tolerance levels. Again, in the latter circumstance, patients would be more likely to recall their responses to the color chart and attempt to recapture their pretest performance. Using color charts in a hospital setting would not be a traditional patient expectation and would most certainly sensitize the patient to a unique set of circumstances for repeated testing. In itself, sensitization to a pretest is not harmful to a study if the effects are uniform across all treatment or study groups. The danger or threat to internal validity occurs if the sensitization is different in different groups.

Some investigators have addressed the issue of test sensitization by using parallel forms of the same test for pretest and posttest observations. Parallel or alternate forms of the same instrument have been constructed which possess adequate psychometric properties like reliability and validity and measure the same construct using different sets of items for two or more versions of the same test. An example is Speilberger's State-Trait Anxiety Test. This instrument measures the typical characteristics a person possesses in terms of baseline anxiety in interpersonal situations and situational characteristics in transactions with other persons. Items that test either dimension (state or trait) have been identified through various psychometric procedures, and two forms have been constructed to measure the same construct. In order to handle the effects of test presentation, half of the subjects in the control and experimental groups on pretest would be selected randomly to receive form A and half the control and experimental subjects would receive form B. On posttest, the administration of forms would be reversed.

In the preoperative surgery teaching study, the effects of testing are not present. Only an uncertainty instrument is used, and it is used only once prior to surgery. It is administered in the routine admission procedure environment where other tests are conducted on each patient.

8. Interaction with Selection

Under this threat to internal validity a researcher must be concerned with selection factors interacting with history, maturation, and instrumentation. This is a serious problem if an historical event has impact on one or more groups but not on all of the study groups.

Selection-history interaction can be a problem in the preoperative surgery teaching study in that three different hospitals are being used. In this case, the investigators would need to be concerned about any unique history in one or more hospitals which might affect the outcome measurements. For example, if during the course of the study one of the hospitals was purchased by a national for profit health care corporation, the effects on the staff and patients could be significant. When a corporation takes over an existing enterprise, top administration generally is changed, and commensurate changes occur at each lower level of personnel. Furthermore, the health care corporation may decide to cut costs by instituting restrictions on certain categories of patients and curtail or eliminate less profitable surgical procedures. These staff changes and patient admission restrictions and curtailment of surgical procedures may be implemented at different points in the course of the study. These changes may have differential impact on one or more of the treatment groups and thus affect the outcome measurements for the affected group or groups.

Selection-maturation interaction occurs when different groups are maturing at different rates. This problem can occur in the preoperative surgery teaching study if, by some quirk of fate, one of the treatment groups were overrepresented with older, severely ill patients. Younger patients are expected to recover more rapidly than older patients. Thus, if one group had a large number of older patients, the study would be compromised because the length of time in hospital would be increased, the number of postoperative complications would be expected to increase, and the length of time at home before leaving unassisted would increase. If these untoward events did occur, it would not follow that the experimental treatment was necessarily ineffective. The obtained results may be solely a reflection of an overabundance of older, severely ill patients in one particular treatment group. A possible way to handle this problem is do a post hoc stratification or blocking of the patients according to age, using the minimax principle of Section 4–3. Comparisons can be made between the treatments controlling for age.

Selection-instrumentation interaction occurs when an instrument influences the performance of groups differentially. Suppose that a nursing instructor gave a pretest and posttest in a sophomore nursing course and noticed that students who obtained low scores showed dramatic increases on the posttest, whereas students with high scores on the pretest showed small gains on the posttest. One explanation for this finding is that the posttest possessed a *ceiling*. A test is said to have a ceiling if many students obtain scores near the maximum possible score so that the true ability of the top students is

not assessed. If the test had been longer or if the items tested more content areas, the top students identified by the pretest could have obtained higher scores. If one treatment group contained more high-scoring students and a second treatment group contained more low-scoring students, then a selection instrumentation interaction may occur. The same problem could be encountered in the reverse situation in which a test contains a *floor*.

9. Diffusion or Imitation of Treatments

Diffusion or imitation of treatments is a significant problem in health care research. It occurs when a treatment applied to one group becomes applied inadvertently to a different treatment group. For instance, in its most common form, diffusion is found when subjects in one group discuss their treatment with patients in a different treatment group and then adopt on their own the treatment of their informant. In the nursing setting, it can also occur when nurses observe what they perceive to be a successful or more effective treatment in one group and impart knowledge of the preferred treatment to a different treatment group with patients who then put it into practice.

Diffusion or imitation of treatments can be a problem in the preoperative surgery teaching study. Patients in treatment one, in which information alone is given to patients, could discuss their preoperative teaching with patients in treatment two, in which patients receive information and instructions in exercises and deep breathing. Patients in treatment one may on their own adopt exercise and deep breathing activities without informing the researchers. In contrast, nurses could observe patients in both treatments one and two and note that patients in treatment two are having greater success. Without the knowledge of the researchers, these nurses may advise the patients in treatment one to exercise and breathe deeply after surgery. In both situations, treatment one could appear to be a better treatment than it really is.

Researchers in health care settings have to be particularly aware of the issue of imitation and vigilant in monitoring both patients and nurses during the course of a study. Of course, in a study of this nature, the nursing staff on the surgical units would be informed about the study and the different treatment programs given to patients. It is assumed that the permanent nursing staff would not consciously interfere or subvert the intended outcomes of the study. In present day health care, however, large numbers of temporary nursing personnel are being employed. Difficulties in providing communication to temporary workers is a constant dilemma. It is conceivable such personnel might casually observe the different treatment programs and, on their own, adopt a preferred or seemingly more effective intervention program with patients undergoing surgery.

10. Compensatory Equalization of Treatments

Compensatory equalization of treatments is related to diffusion of treatment in that the adoption of another treatment upon an already existing one is deliberate and usually follows an administrative decision. Consider the preoperative surgery teaching study. The perception from hospital administration may be that one of the treatments is patently inferior to the other treatments. Key administrators, physicians, or nurses may make a conscious effort to compensate for the less desirable preoperative teaching program. For instance, physicians may decide to become involved more directly in preoperative teaching to compensate for the perceived inadequacies of one of the preoperative teaching programs. Or, the nursing service administration may decide to institute a new standardized teaching program through the allocation of additional nurses to participate in preoperative instructions.

The problem can occur in the testing of new drugs. For example, consider a *double-blind study* in which two different drugs are being tested on patients with pneumonia. In a double-blind study neither the patients nor the administrators of the drug know which drug each patient is receiving. If the effects of one of the drugs is dramatic, it is seen by patients, administrators of the drugs, and the research team engaged in the study. In such situations, it is not uncommon to find demands for the use of the apparently effective drug on all patients. When this happens, the entire study is aborted. Sometimes, the decision may have been a correct one.

11. Compensatory Rivalry by Respondents Receiving Less Desirable Treatments

When members of one treatment group realize that they represent the underdog and are not expected to be the most successful group, compensatory rivalry occurs. In this instance, the subjects decide to turn the tables on the researcher and work harder to be more successful. In some cases, their motivation to succeed can be of such magnitude that they actually outperform the major treatment groups under study. This effect is seen more often in curricular research in nursing education programs and less frequently in studies at health care centers. It is difficult to see how this threat to internal validity would work in the preoperative surgery teaching study.

12. Resentful Demoralization of Respondents Receiving Less Desirable Treatments

Resentful demoralization for the classic control-experimental group study occurs when the research subjects are not told that they will do poorly; however, they perceive their performance as less than satisfactory. Eventually they find out that they are in a control group, not a desired experimental group, and they become resentful. In this case, instead of being motivated to fight back and win, these subjects do not put out any effort to succeed or improve. They view their status in their treatment condition as a negative reality and therefore they live up to it. This explanation is based on Festinger's self-fulfilling prophecy (1964).

As an example, consider a study of overweight adult males who are randomly divided into two groups following a diagnosis of hypertension and are placed on two different weight reduction diets. During the course of the study, some of the subjects in the second group discover that subjects in the first group are losing weight, whereas subjects in the second group are not losing weight. As a consequence, the subjects in the second group become demoralized and give up dieting. It is not surprising to find that the behaviors conform to the self-fulfilling prophecy.

This threat to internal validity does not

seem to be an issue in the preoperative surgery teaching study. None of the patients was told that any one treatment would be more helpful than any other, so that the likelihood of the development of this threat to internal validity is low.

4–7 THREATS TO THE EXTERNAL VALIDITY OF AN EXPERIMENT

Even when a study passes the tests for internal validity, a researcher must still treat the problem of external validity, that is, whether the findings found in the sample can be extended to the population of interest. If random sampling has been employed in the selection of experimental subjects and if the study has internal validity, it has external validity as well. Random sampling with internal validity is one way to guarantee external validity. But is it the only way? The answer is "no," and here we illustrate cases in which external validity can be entertained in the absence of random sampling.

Four threats to external validity have been described by Campbell and Stanley (1963). Some threats are interaction effects of selection biases and treatment, reactive or interaction effects of pretesting, reactive effects of experimental procedures, and multiple treatment interference. These four threats to external validity are examined in light of the preoperative teaching study.

1. Interaction Effects of Selection Bias and Treatment

An interaction effect of selection bias and treatment is said to exist when the sample of subjects responds as a group more favorably or less favorably to a treatment. The uniform response may be a function of some particular characteristic(s) internal to each subject. A strong tendency exists for all to react in a single specific manner with the treatment.

For example, suppose that in the preoperative teaching study most patients in treatment three (sensory and procedural information given pre- and postoperatively) possessed strong tendencies to deny or repress their feelings about the impending surgery. These patients routinely cope with

stress, negative experiences, or perceived adverse outcomes by denial or repression (sensitizers versus repressors) psychological mechanisms. This type of person is not acceptable as a representative of the population to which an inference or generalization is to be made. If persons with this personality type are admitted to a teaching program, they can produce negative results because they are psychologically set not to benefit from the program. They actually tune out their internal psychological equilibrium toward threatening information, and they resist attempts to help them cope with the anticipated pain. As a consequence, these persons constitute a group that is predestined to produce unfavorable findings and most certainly to have a less favorable response to any preoperative training program, no matter how well conceived or taught. Fortunately, this situation could not happen in the study described in Chapter 1. Randomization procedures guarantee that these types of persons will be equally distributed among the three study conditions.

2. Reactive or Interaction Effect of Pretesting

Giving a pretest may limit the generalizability of the experimental findings. A pretest may increase or decrease the sensitivity of the experimental subjects to the treatment conditions so that they are no longer like the subjects to which a generalization is to be made. A potential pretest interaction in the preoperative teaching study exists because the uncertainty scale was administered to all research subjects. If one of the treatments interacted with the items on the uncertainty scale, external validity could be compromised.

3. Reactive Effects of Experimental Procedures

Reactive effects occur when some experimental procedure affects all subjects in such a way that they are no longer like the subjects in the population to which the generalization of study findings is to be made. For example, if, in the preoperative teaching study, it had been decided to use television camera and videotape feedback with all patients, it is possible that many patients across the three treatment conditions would be motivated to participate with extra vigor in the program. The increased attention paid to them during filming and showing of their own performances is enough to significantly alter their behavior and responses to the three treatments. As suggested by this example, the subjects in the sample have been changed so much that they are no longer like the subjects in the population which an investigator would like to generalize.

4. Multiple-Treatment Interference

Multiple-treatment interference occurs when the same subjects are used repeatedly for two or more treatments and when the effects of the previous treatments are not erasable. The findings may be generalized only to persons who experience the same sequence of treatments. The prime example of the potential for this problem is in drug studies in which multiple drugs are administered in sequence. After-effects may confound the findings with drugs administered late in the sequence. This problem does not exist in the preoperative teaching study because each patient was given only one treatment.

Before closing this discussion on external validity, our position is that a researcher can help to alleviate the problems associated with external validity by providing as near a comprehensive description of the sample as possible. By this is meant that a researcher should supply to the reader information on the distribution of gender, age, ethnicity, income, education, health status, social class indicators, occupational status, life-style practices, personality indicators, and any other salient characteristics that the researcher can obtain and synthesize. This information should not be reported just to increase the size of the report but to *define* the population to which inferences can be made. In almost all cases, it will not be the target population of interest but it is an abstract population that is identical to the sample itself. With a careful description of the sample any reader can draw his or her own inferences about the variables and treatments and how they make an impact on a universe of subjects exactly like the subjects used in the investigation.

In addition to a complete description of the sample the investigator should provide a clear and complete description of the sites in which the study was performed. Can a study on pain conducted in a undergraduate university nursing class produce results that would be obtained on patients in a university teaching hospital intensive care unit? Obviously the answer is "no." As indicated, there are particular settings and sites where nursing research studies are conducted and where a high probability exists that new findings may not be replicable elsewhere.

Unusual historical events that apply to all subjects should be described in as much detail as necessary so that the reader can evaluate their possible effect on the findings. Suppose that a nursing research project was conducted in the close environment of the Three Mile Island Atomic Plant incident. Here, generalizability is clearly compromised. Events of this nature should be mentioned in the report.

From our perspective, the request for a comprehensive (1) description of the research subjects, (2) portrayal of the setting in which the research was executed, and (3) depiction of the unique historical or atypical events occurring during the course of a study applies equally to both true experiments and quasi-experiments. It is perhaps even more incumbent on researchers who use quasi-experimental designs to marshal evidence that the study possesses external validity. Some quasi-experiments can be shown to have the potential capacity of demonstrating external validity.

In planning a true experiment, a researcher is advised to use the minimax principle, which produces a minimal amount of unexplained variation and a maximum amount of explained variation. Although this is an ideal theoretical goal of experimental design, it is very hard to put into practice.

Let us reexamine the adolescent diabetic teaching program. The minimax principle mandates that a researcher should identify variables expected to be correlated with the dependent measurement. In this study, some possible confounding variables are age of onset of diabetes, gender of the subjects, birth order, and history of diabetes in the family. For example, fewer adverse reactions might be expected among adolescents with diabetic family members. This knowledge could be built into the study by grouping the adolescents into a group with no history of diabetes and a group with a history of diabetes. This blocking could be done with the other variables thought to be related to the dependent variable. The purpose of the blocking or the stratification is to provide an avenue that removes the variance associated with these sources so that they become explained components of variation. This is often not done because it is very difficult to identify the most important variables in advance. When the variables can be identified, they should be used to plan and design the study.

4–8 TRUE EXPERIMENTAL DESIGNS FOR NURSING RESEARCH

Much of the original thinking about experimental design dates from the work of R. A. Fisher (1925; 1966) and was expanded on by Kempthorne (1951), Cochran and Cox (1957), and other statisticians. The issues associated with quasi-experimental designs go back to the seminal work of Campbell and Stanley (1963). In this publication, three prototypes of experimental designs are described.

1. The Pretest-Posttest Control Group Design

Schematic number 1, at the bottom of this page, is a representation of the pretest-posttest control group design with only two groups.

This design can be extended to cover more than two groups. In some cases treatment

two corresponds to *no* treatment. In this sense, no treatment is synonymous with *control* group.

The pretest-posttest control group design in its simplest form consists of two groups generated by random sampling or by randomization. One group receives an intervention and one group does not. In addition, both groups are given the same pretest and posttest. The prediction is that the intervention will affect the measurement on the posttest. History, attrition, testing, and interaction with history and maturation could be problems if they operate differently in the two groups. A careful researcher would take measures to see that they do not or, if the interaction is inferred to have occurred, the researcher would take corrective measures and the impact would be considered in a discussion of the study's findings.

Possible threats to external validity are interaction of pretesting and treatment conditions, interaction with historical events, and reactive effects of the experimental procedure. Again, if a researcher is prepared and always on guard for the possible introduction of these threats, measures can be taken to minimize their effect upon external validity.

2. The Posttest-Only Group Design

Schematic number 2, at the bottom of this page, is a representation of the posttest-only group design with two groups.

The posttest-only group design is similar to the pretest-posttest design except that no pretest is given. The threats to internal validity in this design are the same as those in

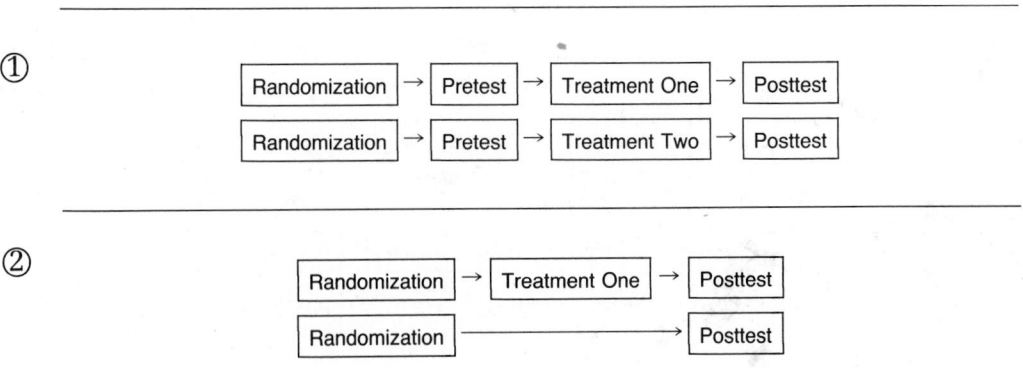

the pretest-posttest design except that testing is no longer an issue. Obviously, without a pretest, subjects cannot be sensitized by the pretest instrument affecting their posttest performance. Because there is no pretesting, this threat to external validity does not exist. The possibility of the three remaining threats to external validity should be recognized and evaluated.

3. The Solomon Four-Group Design

The schematic at the bottom of this page is a representation of the Solomon four-group design. This design can be extended to cover more than one treatment.

The Solomon four-group design is a combination of the *pretest-posttest control group design* and the *posttest-only group design*. If history, maturation, and attrition interact with any of the four groups, internal validity can be compromised. This design allows a researcher to assess the main effects of testing and the interaction of testing and treatment. It is particularly effective for assessing the interaction effect of pretesting and treatment. However, the three remaining threats to external validity could happen and could compromise the findings.

One of the main advantages in the use of a true experiment, in addition to its potential for high levels of internal and external validity, is that it provides a very sophisticated means of assessing the practical and theoretical findings of a study on the basis of explained and unexplained variation as described in Section 4–3. The standard statistical procedures used to evaluate true experiments are the analysis of variance and nonparametric analogs. (Some of these methods are illustrated in Chapters 9, 10, and 11.) A measurement of the amount of variation in a dependent variable that can be attributed to one or more independent variables and a measurement of the amount of variation that is unexplained are obtained in the analysis of variance. After these statistics are generated, the real world meaning of any statistically significant finding can be assessed. This property of true experiments is examined in Section 9–9.

4–9 QUASI-EXPERIMENTAL DESIGNS FOR NURSING RESEARCH

In this section is a description of how selected quasi-experimental designs can be evaluated and assessed on how well they achieve internal validity. A quasi-experiment is one that does not meet at least one of the three conditions required for a true experiment. We review these conditions here.

1. There is no randomization in the assignment of subjects to treatment groups.

2. There is no control or comparison group established in the study for assessing the effects of the treatments.

3. There is no manipulation of an independent variable by the experimenter.

Under condition one in a quasi-experimental design, naturally occurring *intact* groups, such as groups of patients or classes of students, are used as the subjects of a study. Under condition two, comparisons are made *within* each subject in a naturalistic setting and baseline or pretest data are used to assess the treatment in terms of the posttest data. In essence, each subject serves as his or her own control. Under condition three, a naturally occurring event in the world of the patient or personnel, such as type of nursing care assignment or the insti-

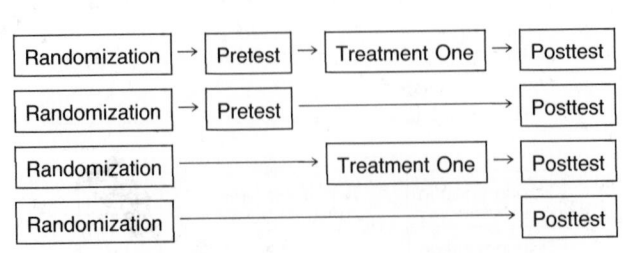

tution of an educational staff development program, serves as the *unmanipulated* independent variable of the study.

The presentation that follows is concise because every research study has its own problems related to site, staff, and resources. Our goal here is to suggest guidelines that can be used in the critical evaluation process which varies from study to study (Trochim, 1986).

Example 1. Use of Intact Groups Without Randomization

A schematic representation of intact groups without randomization design with only two groups is as follows:

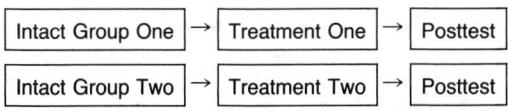

This design can be extended to cover more than two groups and can be modified by adding a *pretest*. This type of study occurs when two patient care units are set up in the same health care center or in different centers. One group is given the new treatment. The other group is given the old or standard treatment. Outcome measurements are taken and decisions are made about the effects of the treatment.

As an example, consider an alternative design to the preoperative surgery teaching study. Suppose that each treatment is used only on a given surgical floor, so that the study is carried out on three different floors in the same institution. This study is illustrated in Figure 4–1. Before this study is executed, the investigator must determine what threats to internal validity would occur if this design were to be employed. Some threats are as follows:

1. *History* could be a serious problem if the nursing staff during the course of the study implemented a different type of nursing care on one of the floors. If the nursing staff changed on one of the floors, internal validity would be compromised. It should be noted that this type of threat is not restricted to quasi-experimental studies. It is also a problem for the finest designed study based on random assignment of subjects to treatment. Any change in staff is harmful, whether the study is a true experiment or a quasi-experiment.

2. *Attrition* could be a serious problem if the more critical surgical cases were placed on a given floor with an increase in the number of complications and deaths on that particular surgical service. In this case, the issue of attrition can be addressed. With the adoption of random assignment of patients to the three surgical treatment floors, the effects of attrition based on severity would be equally distributed and hence would not pose a threat to internal validity.

An alternative to random sampling would be to group the patients according to levels of severity in blocks of three. The first patient entering the hospital with a given severity level could be assigned to floor one, the second entering patient to floor two, and

Independent Variable	Covariates		Dependent Variables
Surgical floor A; experimental preop teaching program #1	Gender Age Severity Education		Length of inpatient unit stay No. of pain medications within first 48 hours of surgery No. of postoperative complications No. of days spent at home before leaving unassisted
Surgical floor B; experimental preop teaching program #2	Provider Family income Weight Smoking history	SURGERY	
Surgical floor C; experimental preop teaching program #3	Alcohol usage Drug usage Exercise regimen Uncertainty		

*Nonrandom assignment of hospital patients to surgical floors.

Figure 4–1. Quasi-experimental design: intact groups without randomization*

the third entering patient to floor three. This process would be repeated for every block of three patients with similar severity status. The assignment makes use of the minimax principle.

3. *Selection* could be a factor because the manner in which patients are assigned to the three surgical services is not based on random assignment. The same procedures used to handle the bias from differential attrition can be used here to reduce the bias resulting from systematically placing certain categories of patients on one service as opposed to another.

4. *Maturation* could be a problem confounded by the selection process if older or younger patients are sent to different floors for preoperative preparation and postoperative recovery. This problem can be alleviated by random assignment.

5. *Instrumentation* could be a problem if the record-keeping behavior of medical and nursing staff were particularly deficient on one or more of the three surgical units. This threat could be a problem even in a carefully controlled true experiment. For both a true experiment and a quasi-experiment, this problem can be controlled by the constant vigilance of the researchers to ensure that good records are maintained. If this were not possible, an alternative would be to prepare forms on which physicians and nurses can record the appropriate information according to preestablished coding criteria and record-keeping rules and protocols. These forms, in addition to serving a research purpose, would also become part of the patients' permanent medical record.

6. *Regression* may be an issue if all the serious (major) cases went to one surgical floor and all of the mild (elective) cases went to another surgical service. This problem can be handled in exactly the same way as that suggested for selection and attrition.

7. The effects of *sensitization* of subjects to testing does not seem to be an issue in this specific hypothetical investigation.

8. *Selection interactions* have been discussed under maturation and regression.

9. *Diffusion of treatments* probably would not be a problem, provided that the patients on the various surgical floors had no opportunities to communicate with one another.

10. *Compensatory equalization* of treatments could be a problem if the nursing staff of the various floors exchange information about their various surgical teaching programs. If nurses, in one of the three teaching programs, perceived their program as less desirable, they might compensate by incorporating features of the more desirable programs that filter down to the patients. This is not an exclusive problem of quasi-experiments; it is also a problem for a study using a true experiment. Here a routine of spot checking of events and nurses' behavior is required if this problem is to be eliminated.

11. *Compensatory rivalry* does not seem to be an issue in this study.

12. *Compensatory demoralization* could be a problem if the nurses on one floor perceived their teaching method to be inferior to the other teaching methods and became discouraged about their instructional method's effectiveness. This slump in nursing morale also could be a problem in a controlled experimental study. The research team may be faced with nurse behaviors that suggest loss of faith in a particular teaching program. The researchers must strongly reemphasize that until the study is completed no one can objectively state which treatment is truly the more effective.

If a quasi-experimental study passes the tests of internal validity, a potential exists for an argument supporting its external validity. A delineation of the characteristics of the research subjects, a description of the setting where the study was conducted, and a clear narrative depicting the historical events transpiring during the course of the investigation greatly contribute to external validity assessment.

Example 2. Use of Intact Groups in Which the Treatments Are Defined in a Temporal Manner

The schematic at the top of page 79 is a representation of intact group design in which treatments are temporally defined with two groups. This design can be extended to cover more than two groups and can be modified by adding a *pretest*.

As an example, suppose that we study the effects of three different preoperative surgical teaching programs in one unit of one institution. This study is illustrated in Figure 4–2. Study groups are defined in terms of

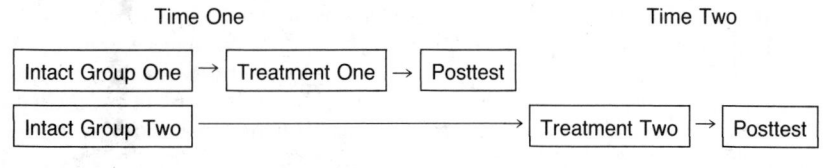

the week in which they enter the hospital. Some patients may stay less than one week and some may stay more than one week. Most are expected to stay less than one week. Study group one consists of all patients who enter the hospital during the first week of the study and who meet all criteria for being placed in one of the three teaching programs. Study group two is defined as patients entering during the second week. Study group

Covariates	Week	Teaching Program 1		Teaching Program 2		Teaching Program 3	
			Preoperative				
Gender	1	S_1	Dep. Var.†				
Age		.	1				
Severity		.	2				
Education		.	3				
Provider		S_{10}	4				
Family income							
Weight	2			S_{11}	Dep. Var.†		
Smoking history				.	1		
Alcohol usage				.	2		
Drug usage				.	3		
Exercise regimen				.	4		
Uncertainty				.			
	3			.		S_{21}	Dep. Var.†
				S_{20}		.	1
						.	2
						.	3
						.	4
						.	
	4	S_{31}	Dep. Var.†			.	
		.	1			S_{30}	
		.	2				
		.	3				
		.	4				
		.					
	5	S_{40}		S_{41}	Dep. Var.†		
				.	1		
				.	2		
				.	3		
				.	4		
				.			
	6			S_{50}		S_{51}	Dep. Var.†
						.	1
						.	2
						.	3
						.	4
						.	
						S_{60}	

*Nonrandom assignments of hospital patients to one surgical floor.
†Dependent Variables:
1, Length of stay
2, No. of pain medications in first 48 hours
3, No. of postoperative complications
4, No. of days at home

Figure 4–2. Quasi-experimental design intact groups defined according to week admitted to hospital.*

three uses patients entering during the third week. At week 4 the process enters another cycle. The cycles are repeated until 80 patients are observed under each of the three treatments. For the data analysis, patients of weeks 1, 4, 7, 10 . . . are grouped together, patients of weeks 2, 5, 8, 11 . . . are grouped together, and patients of weeks 3, 6, 9, 12 . . . are grouped together. In Figure 4–2, 10 subjects per week are represented. In practice, the numbers vary from week to week for most hospital settings.

In this study, some threats to internal validity are not important. These are maturation, instrumentation, regression, sensitization, interactions, compensatory rivalry, and resentful demoralization. For example, the time period encompassing the intervention is too short to see the effects of maturation in this design. Because no pretest is performed on study subjects, there are no opportunities for instrumentation, regression, sensitization, and interaction to occur. Compensatory rivalry and resentful demoralization cannot occur because different treatments occur on different weeks with different sets of study subjects.

1. *History* could be a problem because the three treatments are not in operation simultaneously. For example, if a major historical event occurred, the patients associated with that unusual event could be removed from the study. This would in effect reduce the sample size, provided that the investigator had not anticipated such an occurrence. One solution is to extend the time of the study by adding extra weeks to accumulate the necessary number of patients for each treatment to enable conclusive evaluations.

In any case it cannot be assumed that the effects of history will be comparable across the three conditions. If some unusual set of events occurs during one week of the study, its effect can be carried along across the three groups as the study continues. As an example, suppose that the nursing care is changed from a functional nursing model to a primary nursing model. After this model of nursing care is instituted, it continues throughout the course of the study and is experienced by patients in all three treatment groups. As another example, changing the surgical procedures midway through the study is not a serious threat to internal validity because its effects will be experienced by patients in each of the three treatment conditions.

Dangers always exist when the same treatment staff is engaged in the application of a series of different treatments over the course of the study period. The ability and capacity of the nursing staff to change preoperative teaching programs each week with different sets of patients are major limitations in this particular design. Even under the best of circumstances, the carry-over effects from one teaching program to another by the same set of nurses is an important methodological issue. Some nurses develop strong preferences for one or more of the different educational programs. Other nurses are severely challenged to change to another educational program as a consequence of the specific serial design of the study.

One component of this study that needs attention is the collapsing or pooling of information across the weeks of the study. Note that in Figure 4–2 treatment one is observed during weeks 1, 4, 7, 10 . . . . Data analysis requires that the information for these weeks be pooled. Before this is done, an analysis can be performed across the weeks to show whether the data are homogeneous. If they are homogeneous, the data can be pooled. If the data across weeks are heterogeneous, they can be discarded, provided that the researcher demonstrates that the unusual data are associated with some atypical historical event.

2. *Attrition* is less of a problem because each cycle involves only one week of time for each treatment. For example, a contaminated piece of equipment routinely used in surgery may lead to a higher incidence of postoperative infections over a very short period of time. This increased incidence of infections would probably be recognized quickly, and corrections would be implemented. The patients involved with this contamination could be removed from the study and the time period for the study extended. Thus, the effects of attrition on one treatment group might be noticeable for a short period of time. It is not a serious threat to internal validity because of its short duration and the removal of tainted subject data from the analysis.

3. *Selection* might be a particular problem when a surgical team schedules a large number of serious cases for a particular week or when their scheduling patterns of complex surgeries coincide with one particular preoperative teaching cycle. In most situations, selection is not a serious problem because

there is no reason to believe that particular types of patients would come to surgery in the same cycle as the rotation of the treatments.

4. *Diffusion* or *imitation of the treatments* could be a problem because nursing staff could change quickly. Recall as to which treatment was in operation for a particular week could be blurred. Also, there is the added problem of patients undergoing surgery during one week and then remaining in the hospital the following week when study treatments are changed. These changes could be problems for the nursing staff in trying to remember which treatment was given to particular assigned patients.

The color coding of patients' records might help to reduce the possible confusion over which treatment each patient was receiving. The color code for each patient in a particular preoperative teaching program could be indicated on the door of the room, and each patient's chart could also be color-coded according to research treatment. Another potential problem could exist in situations in which patients from different treatment groups are assigned to the same room. Patients would be able to see different teaching programs in operation, and they could discuss their own training with one another.

5. *Compensatory equalization* of treatments could occur if the administration decided that one treatment was less favorable than the others. To compensate for the inequalities, the nursing administration could provide more and better able nurses to coincide with the implementation of the perceived less effective treatment. Like example 1, it might be possible to present a case supporting external validity for a study like this.

Example 3. The Case in Which an Intact Group is Compared with an External or Standard Group

The schematic at the bottom of this page is a representation of an intact group compared with an external group. This design can be extended to cover more than two groups and can be modified by adding a *pretest*.

This design is useful for studies in which an outside standard is available and is used instead of a comparison group. It should not be confused with the *one-shot design without a control group*. The classic one-shot study design involves the specification of an independent variable that is applied to either an intact group or to one constructed on the basis of a randomization process. In such a study, there is complete absence of control and no internal validity. History, attrition, selection, maturation, instrumentation, statistical regression, and testing all are threats to internal validity for this study. For this reason, it cannot be recommended for nursing research. According to Issac and Michael (1985), no provisions for objective scientifically valid comparisons exist in this design. This is not true for the design we now describe.

Suppose that an inquiring nurse reads a research report detailing the effects of structured and unstructured preoperative teaching, for example, that of Lindeman and van Aernam (1971). In this report, extensive data are presented describing the positive effects of a structured preoperative teaching program in one midwestern hospital. Considerable information is available in the report on the preoperative teaching program and where it can be purchased. Furthermore, a good description is provided about the patient characteristics, types of surgeries performed, types of dependent measures taken, and procedures followed throughout the course of the study. With these types of information, it should be possible to replicate the study at another institution using the objective data of the original study as a *standard of comparison* for the new investigation.

The limitation of this particular approach is that most published research is too concise to be useful in generating the conditions and outcomes necessary for a standard. Some studies may not contain as much de-

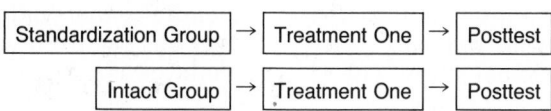

tailed information as needed to use as a standard. It may be necessary for the inquiring nurse to have considerable communication with the original researcher to attain precise enough information on which to base a new study. Other problems in using a standard external to the research subjects exist. There is never any guarantee that the outside standard is truly applicable to an innovative experimental program nor to the subjects participating in the study. If the outside standard is taken from a study conducted a number of years before the present study, the relevance and applicability of the variables, measurements, and corresponding statistics of the original research standard can be called into question. The passage of time and the acquisition of new knowledge and technical developments in nursing practices may suggest that the original study is not currently germane to the present historical health care scene.

Threats to internal validity that may cause problems are examined here.

1. *History* is a consideration in any study—a controlled experiment or a quasi-experiment. A prudent researcher will make sure that a running log is kept of events that happen during the course of an investigation. There is no way to tell what events are going to play an important role in the progress of a study and so keeping a log can be helpful in interpreting the results upon completion of the data analysis. In a longitudinal study, the research team can meet and summarize each week's happenings and place them in a permanent record that can be referred to at a later time.

2. *Attrition* could be a problem if some severely ill patients were not able to put the treatment program into practice and thereby dropped out of the study. Thus, attrition would compromise the findings so that comparisons with the original study would be biased, because the new study would not contain the proper proportions of severely ill patients as were contained in the original study. Another source of attrition could be encountered if patients refused to participate following surgery because they did not want to practice the preoperative training schedule.

3. *Selection* could be a problem if the patients in the new study were radically different from those in the original study. The researcher would be required to make a comparison of the types of patients and kinds of surgeries performed during the period of the original study and ensure that the new study group is similar to the group used as the standard. For example, it is imperative that distributions of gender, age, race, severity, types of surgery performed, and other pertinent independent variables are shown to be similar across the new study group and the original investigation.

4. *Maturation* should not be a serious threat to internal validity in this particular design if the groups are similar, as shown by all the pertinent classification variables. It would definitely be a problem if the groups differed, for example, in age or severity.

5. *Instrumentation* should not be a problem unless the measurements that were produced changed over time because of malfunctioning of the instrument or changes in calibration from baseline to maximum performance, assuming that the new research team is using the same procedures and instruments as those used by the original research team. Another possible instrumentation issue is that the new investigation may not scrupulously follow the record data extraction format used in the original investigation. This is of particular concern when medical records and nurses' notes are the basis of measurement for important dependent variables.

6. *Statistical regression* would be a problem if the new group represented an upper or lower group with respect to some variable that is correlated with the dependent measures. That is, regression would be a problem if the new study group differed from the one used in the original published research report. For example, if the new group has more severely ill patients than those in the original study, regression toward the mean would be certain to operate. Other extreme groups defined by differences in preoperative status such as health history, cardiac risk factors including smoking history, alcohol and drug usage, and other variables could produce regression effects that would compromise the findings.

With the use of an outside standard comparison group, one is in a better position to defend external validity provided that the study has been shown to possess an acceptable level of internal validity.

4–10 OTHER DESIGNS FOR NURSING RESEARCH

In the previous section, we scratched the surface in describing designs that are encountered in nursing research. These examples are only a few of the hundreds that can be found in the nursing and health care research literature. Each research question requires its own design. Although common elements may exist that pervade the designs usually encountered, each research question is unique and as such requires a particular methodological approach. In this section, we describe some of the common elements and designs that are incorporated into nursing and health care research. The description is selective but not exhaustive.

Other quasi-experimental designs described by Campbell and Stanley include the following:

1. Interrupted Time Series Designs

The schematic shown at the bottom of this page is a representation of an interrupted time series design. In this design observations are taken over time under treatment one. After a certain a priori selected point, treatment two is instituted and similar observations are taken. In some cases, treatment one is actually a control condition in which no treatment is applied. In single subject research the observations taken under treatment one are referred to as *baseline*, whereas the observations taken under treatment two are referred to as *intervention*. If the treatment has an effect, the mean for treatment two is expected to exceed the mean of treatment one. In single subject research, an often encountered expectation is that the mean of treatment one will be larger than the mean of treatment two. This type of expectation is desired when an undesirable mode of behavior is to be extinguished.

The prototype of an interrupted time series design consists of a longitudinal follow-up of one group of subjects over a long period of time. During the first part of the study subjects are observed repeatedly over baseline. An intervention is imposed and continued observations are made on the subjects. An example of such a study is one in which the length of the workday is changed from 8 hours to 12 hours. In such a study, a group of nurses would be scheduled to work an 8-hour day, and the amount of unscheduled hourly sick leave would be measured weekly for a period of 28 weeks. At the end of this baseline period, the work shift would be changed to 12 hours per day, and the same dependent variable, hours of unscheduled sick leave, would be measured. A test would then be made of the two sets of data to determine whether the change in hourly work schedule increased or decreased use of sick leave. Statistical procedures for analyzing these data are provided in Chapter 14 on interrupted time series (single subject designs).

There are situations in which interrupted time series models can be shown to have external validity, provided that the study can be shown to have internal validity. An intuitively appealing example in which external validity seems to be satisfied are the studies made of automobile accident deaths following the decision to reduce highway speed limits to 55 miles per hour. In these studies it was shown that traffic fatalities decreased. Recently, some states have removed this barrier to speeding and have experienced an increase in automobile accident fatality.

2. Counterbalanced designs

A counterbalanced design involves at least two independent variables, for example, three hospitals (H_1, H_2, and H_3) and three treatments (T_1, T_2, and T_3). If each treatment is measured within each hospital the study is said to be counterbalanced. This means that each classification of one of the variables is measured with each classification of

Treatment One	Treatment Two
Test 1 Test 2 Test 3 . . .	Test 1 Test 2 Test 3 . . .

the other variable. A schematic representation of this type of design is as follows:

Treatment One	Treatment Two	Treatment Three
Hospital 1	Hospital 1	Hospital 1
Hospital 2	Hospital 2	Hospital 2
Hospital 3	Hospital 3	Hospital 3

Another example of a counterbalanced design is one in which there are two groups of subjects usually assigned on the basis of a randomization process. Subjects in group one receive treatment A first and then are given treatment B. Subjects in group two receive treatment B first and then are given treatment A. In terms of the evaluation of the 8- or 12-hour workday, a researcher could perform a counterbalanced design study by establishing two groups of registered nurses, one group agreed to work an 8-hour work shift during the first 28 weeks. The second group of nurses would work 12 hours a day during the same period. At the end of the 28-week period, the work shifts would be reversed for the two groups. Usually these kinds of studies are analyzed using the analysis of variance (described in Chapter 9).

3. Different Sample Pretest-Posttest Design

The schematic shown at the bottom of this page is a representation of the different sample pretest-posttest design with only two groups.

The prototype of the different sample pretest-posttest design in its simplest form consists of two groups of subjects which are not randomly assigned to treatment but already exist in a group as a unit. Randomization is introduced through the random assignment of the independent variable to the two intact groups of subjects. With respect to the 8- or 12-hour workday study, it may be difficult to assign different nurses to different work shift

lengths at the same time. Instead, it may be administratively feasible to randomly select different units within a hospital and to assign each intact patient care unit to either an 8- or a 12-hour work shift schedule for a specified period of time. If the study can be replicated a number of times either in the same institution or over a number of different sites, the study findings have a better chance of being generalized (Trochim, 1986).

4. Regression Discontinuity Design

The prototype of the regression discontinuity design involves a single group of subjects who are measured on an independent variable and then partitioned according to some cutoff point. A post hoc investigation is then made of the two groups to determine whether the two groups differ markedly at the cutoff point. As an example, consider a study in which the independent variable is weight of adult males and the dependent variable is the weight of the same adults measured three months later. In this investigation, an experimental drug, which is a genetically derived enzyme that controls the storage of triglycerides in the fat cells of vessel walls, is to be used on adult males whose weight exceeds 200 pounds. For the study, 100 adult males are recruited and all those whose weights exceed 200 pounds are given the synthetically derived enzyme medication (lipoprotein lipase) to take over a three-month period.

According to the regression discontinuity theory, no treatment effect would be represented by the familiar scatter diagram of Figure 4–3 but if there were a treatment effect, the scatter diagram would look like Figure 4–4. With no treatment effect, one regression line would continue without break across the cutoff point of 200 pounds. With a treatment effect, there would be two regression lines, one for the males with weights be-

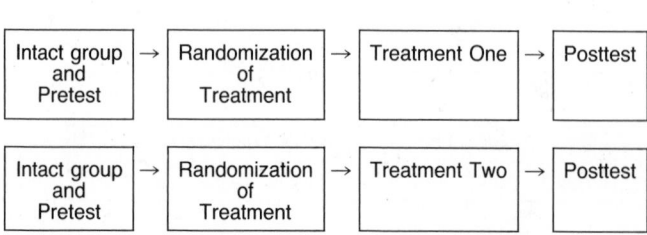

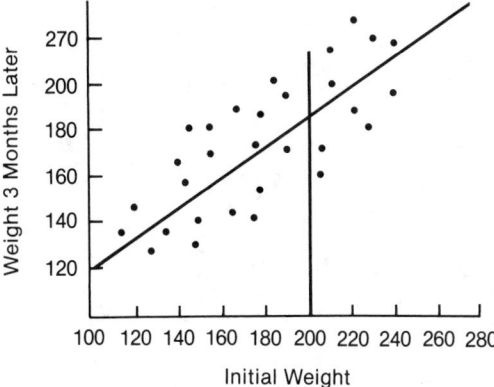

Figure 4–3. Regression discontinuity without treatment effect.

low 200 pounds and one for the males with weights above 200 pounds. The effects of the treatment would be measured by the difference in the two regression lines at the cutoff point of 200 pounds. The statistical procedures for evaluating the effects of the treatment are described by Marascuilo and Serlin (1988).

5. Retrospective Studies

Another set of procedures that should be known to the inquiring nurse are those used by epidemiologists. The epidemiology approach has some similarities to the detective tracking down a missing person. For example, the earlier studies on the association of smoking to lung cancer made use of a research scheme that was based on ruling

out explanatory causes. One model used is the *retrospective* study. In a retrospective study, people with a disability are interviewed after the fact. Two problems with retrospective studies are the accuracy of recall during the interview and a tendency to focus on answers that are supportive of the hypothesis under study.

For example, consider a retrospective study of a group of adult males with a known diagnosis of lung cancer. Members of the study were given an extensive questionnaire in which their past history on the use of cigarettes, cigars, and other tobacco products was obtained. In addition, a history was obtained on the use of coffee, tea, sugar, meat, fats, and other dietary products. Other questions dealt with possible pollutants in the environment, such as source of fuel to provide heat, location of the respondent's home, materials that the subjects used at work and at play, plus questions dealing with many other possible suspected causes and contributing factors to the incidence of lung cancer. The epidemiology approach is based on the systematic ruling out of the presumed causes one by one through demonstrating that each suspected factor has no association with the incidence of lung cancer. The factors that show an association are suspected of being the etiological factors. With this model, coffee, alcohol usage, burning of soft coal, and all the other factors investigated were ruled out. The one major exception was tobacco usage, with cigarette smoking presumed to be the most important causative agent for lung cancer.

6. Prospective Studies

Another model used by epidemiologists more frequently is the *prospective* study, in which a cohort of subjects are identified and then given an extensive questionnaire to complete about their health and living styles. Afterward they are followed up for a number of years to see how their health status progresses. An example of such a study is one in which the independent measurement is a life-style modification program with borderline hypertensive males. Instead of placing the subjects on antihypertensive drugs, subjects meet in groups monthly for one year to discuss changing their eating patterns, exercise regimens, smoking and drinking behavior, and stress management. At the

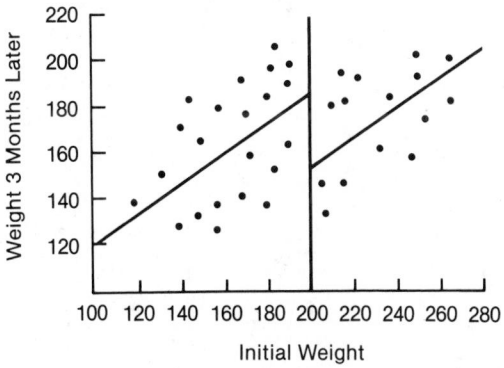

Figure 4–4. Regression discontinuity with treatment effect.

end of the year, the subject's blood pressure status is evaluated to see how effective the treatment has been. If the subjects have been able to modify their life-style patterns so that their diastolic blood pressures are below 90 mm of mg for the greater part of the year, the treatment is said to have been a success.

It should be noted that prospective studies can be modified by including more than one treatment group. For example, in the hypertension study half of the subjects could be given beta blockers and the other half could be given a placebo. Thus, the prospective study is turned into an experiment. For a critique of retrospective and prospective studies see Feinstein (1988).

4–11 SUMMARY

In this chapter the ideal research design has been described in terms of the classic or true experiment. The strengths of experimental research were identified. Also described are alternative research models called quasi-experiments. These are used to approximate an experiment when the constraints of money, time, space, personnel, and other resources preclude performing a true experiment. The concepts of explained and unexplained variation in relationship to true experiments are described and illustrated. Also shown was how these concepts are used to design an experiment. Furthermore, the roles of random sampling and randomization to achieve the standards of a true experiment were presented. The characteristics of internal and external validity were elucidated with specific examples to identify successful attributes of both true experiments and quasi-experiments which meet various validity criterion expectations.

REFERENCES

American Psychological Association: Publication Manual, ed. 3. Washington, DC, American Psychological Association, 1983.

Campbell, D.T., and Stanley, J.C.: Experimental and quasi-experimental designs for research and teaching. In Gage, N.L., ed. Handbook on Teaching. Chicago, Rand McNally, 1963.

Cochran, W.G., and Cox, G.M.: Experimental Designs. New York, John Wiley & Sons, 1957.

Cook, T.D., and Campbell, D.T.: Quasi-experimentation: Design and Analysis Issues for Field Settings. Boston, Houghton Mifflin, 1979.

Feinstein, A.R.: Scientific standards in epidemiologic studies of the menace of daily life, Science, 242: 1257–1263, 1988.

Festinger, L.: Conflict, Decision and Dissonance. Stanford, Stanford University Press, 1964.

Fisher, R.A.: Statistical Methods for Research Workers. Edinburgh, Oliver and Boyd, 1925.

Fisher, R.A.: The Design of Experiments, ed. 8. Edinburgh, Oliver and Boyd, 1966.

Issac, S., and Michael, W.B.: Handbook in Research and Evaluation: For Education and the Behavioral Sciences, ed. 3. San Diego, EDITS, 1985.

Kempthorne, O.: Design of Experiments. New York, John Wiley & Sons, 1951.

Keppel, G.: Design and Analysis: A Researcher's Handbook. Englewood Cliffs, NJ, Prentice Hall, 1973.

Kerlinger, F.N.: Foundation of Behavioral Research. New York, Holt, Rinehart, & Winston, 1973.

Lindeman, C.A., and Van Aernam, B.: Nursing intervention with the presurgical patient—the effects of structured and unstructured preoperative teaching, Nurs. Res., 20: 319–332, 1971.

Marascuilo, L., and Serlin, R.: Statistical Methods for the Behavioral Sciences. New York, Freeman, 1988.

Trochim, W.M.K.: Advances in Quasi-Experimental Design and Analysis. San Francisco, Jossey-Bass, 1986.

Winer, B.J.: Statistical Principles in Experimental Design. New York, McGraw-Hill, 1971.

Chapter 5

SURVEY RESEARCH METHODOLOGY AND QUESTIONNAIRE CONSTRUCTION FOR NURSING RESEARCH

5-1 HISTORY AND DEVELOPMENT OF SURVEYS: NURSING RESEARCH IMPLICATIONS

Sample surveys are currently among the more important basic research methods of the social, behavioral, and health science fields. They have applied utility for health care issues and concerns of professional nursing today. The sample survey is a relatively new research model that has come into prominence within the past 50 years for learning about social processes. Sample surveys consist of standardized approaches to the collection of information from individuals, households, and larger social entities such as schools, hospitals, and social and health care agencies by the questioning of systematically identified samples of individual subjects (Rossi, Wright, and Anderson, 1983, p. 1). The principal mode in which information is gathered is through questionnaires and/or interview schedules either in person, by mail, or by telephone.

Three basic technical developments come together to constitute the core of the sample survey method we know today. First, satisfactory and workable techniques have been developed which enable investigators to draw representative samples to produce unbiased estimates of important population parameters. Second, sufficient experience has been gained to make it possible to write questionnaires and interview schedules that ascertain valid and reliable answers to a variety of vital topics. Third, developments both in data processing and in inferential statistics now make it possible to calculate and evaluate with ease significant relationships among variables contained in complex phenomena.

Surveys have a long tradition in the United States. Starting in 1790, when Congress mandated a national census of all residents every 10 years, Americans have been accustomed to periodic surveys every decade that request such data as type of residence, number of persons living in the household, yearly income, educational level of household, and other information of importance in describing a national profile. Such a profile aids in planning social programs and allocation of national and regional resources. The United States census is one of the few surveys in which the universe is the sample. That is, every household is queried, not a sample of households representative of the universe.

The nursing profession has had long-term experience with surveys. The continuous need to document the state of nursing at different points in this history of the field have been greatly aided by survey data. Samples of nurses have been used for many questions concerned with education and labor force participation. For example, M. Adelaide Nutting reported in 1896 on the working hours of student nurses in training schools. Using information collected from a number of nursing schools, this courageous educator was able to document the long hours that student nurses were expected to work (56 to 60 hours in patient care, exclusive of any formal instruction in a one-week period). Undaunted by hospital administrators and phy-sicians, she tried to rally the Society of Training Schools to correct wide abuses in student "training" (Nutting, 1896, p. 39).

Numerous surveys have been conducted about the discipline of nursing, which were funded in the early and middle 20th century by private foundations and philanthropies. The Rockefeller, Carnegie, Kellogg, Russell Sage, and Johnson foundations among others all have funded major studies concerned with nursing using survey methods and sampling strategies. Later, the federal government, principally through the United States Public Health Service, The National Institute of Mental Health, the Bureau of Maternal Health, among many other federal agencies, has commissioned comprehensive studies dealing with the adequacy and number of nursing personnel in all types of health care roles and settings. Also funded by federal agencies were investigations detailing specific educational preparation needs and forecasting major trends in health care which were thought to have an impact on nurse performance. Major federal and state policies directly stem from survey data funded both by governmental and private sources. It should be apparent that crucial decisions that specifically affect nurses are made on the basis of information collected from surveys.

5–2 STRENGTHS AND LIMITATIONS OF SURVEYS: WHEN TO DO THEM AND WHEN NOT TO DO THEM

The ease with which important descriptive data are collected for all segments of a population is both the strength and the limitation of surveys. The ability to accurately portray salient characteristics of representative samples that relate to a larger population is an important advantage of surveys. The savings in time, money, and other material resources by using elements of a universe of persons or larger social aggregates from which to estimate important parameters of a populace behavior, attitudes, values, health beliefs, and health-illness attributes is the touchstone of this methodology.

The ease with which surveys can be launched by inexperienced persons also has contributed to the disrespect surveys have in the minds of many persons. It has been estimated that about 32 million households were contacted for survey data and that 100 million interviews were conducted in 1983 (National Research Council, 1983). Surveys are considered by the novice as rather easy to do. Asking questions is the most natural way to get information. It is an everyday part of life. We are constantly asking questions and in turn answering them. Because many adults have participated in a vast array of interviews or answered questionnaires, it seems all too facile to some to launch a survey whenever there appears to be a need for information.

A well-done survey is an extensive and potentially expensive undertaking. Too often, an investigator may find after completing a survey that it need not have been done at all; the information was already available from a source not investigated earlier. Unfortunately it follows that the investigator simply did not know how to get the appropriate information or to seek the appropriate resources for help. As an illustration of this calamity, a well-known nursing administrator prepared a grant application with a fixed deadline, which sought support to expand nursing services in a home health care program. Information about the particular community that the home care program was to service was to be obtained from a survey. Initially, the local public health department health care plan was examined for relevant information for a comprehensive community health profile. The data available were assessed as out of date. A survey of 25 representative health agencies and key personnel was commenced. About three months later, the desired information began to emerge. Meanwhile, vital time was lost and the grant deadline was missed. In this situation, the nurse administrator neglected to determine which federal and state agencies collect recent descriptive community data. Contrary to reports of dismantling, the regional Health Service Area was still in operation and had just completed an update on the comprehensive health care plan in which the home health nursing agency was to be inaugurated. The crucial data required for the administrator to fashion a realistic model for home health nursing were available. Much waste and duplication of activity happened. This occurs all too frequently. The inquiring nurse is advised to know about available resources and to find the people and facilities who know whether new information is

needed and can therefore be used appropriately.

In other situations, the selection of a survey design may not even be the best approach to solving a problem or answering a particular set of questions. For some studies, direct observation or measurement may be superior to retrospective questioning of individual respondents. If a nurse administrator is concerned about the quality of the staff development educational programs offered, direct observation of different educational programs may provide better information than sending out a 15-page questionnaire to all 500 nursing staff members. Field experiments in which the nurse administrator devises a scenario and then records staff members' responses to the contrived situation may be of great assistance in pinpointing problems. As an example, mock code blue cardiac resuscitation exercises with teams of nurses and physicians may identify difficulties in conducting the resuscitation procedure more clearly than sending out questionnaires to elicit staff responses to determine the issues.

Another helpful investigative procedure is content analysis of existing documents of an organization and the community served by its programs in contrast to asking people about their recollections of the past. Rather than conducting in-depth interviews, systematic perusal of organizational newsletters, committee minutes, newspaper articles, and other written records may be sufficient to develop an organizational profile and to show changes over time. All these methods have their drawbacks. The point is that it should not be automatically assumed that a brand new questionnaire is the only means of providing an answer to every immediate problem or long-term issues (Sheatsley, 1983, p. 195).

Even when a questionnaire or an interview schedule is the most feasible technique, one still must ask whether it can do the job. People simply may not have the information or cannot recall it. Frequently, patients are asked to evaluate technical components of their care. For instance, it would be foolish to ask a patient whether the sutures used to sew up a wound were the best under those circumstances. Information should be gathered from surgeons and operating room nurses, who would be more qualified to make this judgment. Additionally, asking people about events removed from present experience, such as childhood medical history, is subject to excessive recall error. Similarly, information obtained by asking someone to predict future behavior or courses of action such as asking a staff nurse his or her plans three to five years from now is likely to contain considerable margins of error.

Other considerations are the willingness of people to respond truthfully to the questions in the questionnaire or interview schedule. The social climate has changed considerably in the last 30 years regarding what constitutes acceptable social discourse. People are more open to discussing topics such as sexual behavior, political beliefs, religious views, and a host of topics that were not open to public discussion in the recent past. There are still areas in which it is questionable whether people will respond accurately. Topics such as alcohol and drug use, various sexual practices, alternate sexual preferences, cheating on income taxes, gambling, child payment support history, euthanasia, obesity, physical handicaps, child and spouse abuse, dreams, mental illness, mental retardation, incest, bestiality, terminal illness, undocumented legal alien status, criminal or arrest record, and disfiguring diseases, among other socially, legally, and ethically sensitive areas are at present survey topics that require special care and ingenuity to obtain satisfactory data. Sometimes a little thought can show that a questionnaire is simply not worth the available time and budget, because some persons either do not have or will not easily reveal the information that the inquiring nurse needs (Sheatsley, 1983, p. 196).

In the interview and questionnaire approach, heavy reliance is placed on the *verbal reports* from persons for information about their experiences and for knowledge of their own behavior. The person's report may or may not be taken at face value. This is the crux of the issue in questionnaires and interviews. Some persons may lie, distort, or unwittingly fail to provide factual relevant data when questioned. The surveyor is at the mercy of the respondent's willingness to accurately volunteer information that is relevant to the purpose of the inquiry. It is acknowledged that in everyday life we must, in order to function, accept at face value most of the information offered. We accept many verbal reports as valid in order to survive and operate in an efficient, orderly manner in our jobs, personal life, travel, and leisure activities. Through life experiences, however, we all learn to weigh and sift verbal statements when the person's motivation or the pressure to which the person is exposed prevents a candid report; in these circumstances we are not likely to give it much credence.

Nevertheless, every person has a unique opportunity to observe himself or herself. To the extent that a person can and will communicate knowledge about himself or herself, this provides the inquisitive nurse with information that could otherwise be obtained only by more time-consuming methods or not at all. Despite the inherent weaknesses of self-reports, it is frequently both possible and useful to get the person's own account of his or her feelings, perceptions, values, beliefs, opinions, and attitudes toward events and people in their environment (Selltiz, Wrightsman, and Cook, 1976, pp. 293–294).

In many instances a nurse administrator would not choose to launch a full-fledged sample survey. If the administrator is faced with limited resources and only two or three staff members who are able to assist, the best solution is to limit the questions to a few pertinent areas and not to depend on a formally constructed interview or questionnaire schedule, particularly when the resulting data will not be treated statistically. In interviewing key community leaders about a nursing care program, standardized questionnaires may inadvertently narrow the discussion and prevent full exploration of each community representative's views. Instead, the nurse administrator might advantageously prepare a brief interview guide and list perhaps a dozen crucial questions with appropriate probes listed under each. This ensures that all obvious areas are covered, but allows room for the nurse administrator to probe the unexpected response or to follow leads that could be easily over-looked with a formal interview schedule. Such interviews can be taped, classified generally into several categories, and analyzed qualitatively rather than statistically.

If the nurse investigator requires a large sample and needs the services of a number of interviewers and if the data are to be treated statistically, a standardized questionnaire or interview schedule must be developed. The choice of either approach has both advantages and disadvantages. In a questionnaire, the information obtained is limited to the written responses to prearranged questions. In an interview, the opportunity exists for greater care in communicating questions and in eliciting information. In addition, the interviewer has the opportunity to observe both the person being questioned and the total situation in which the interview is being conducted (Selltiz et al., 1976, p. 294).

5–3 ESTABLISHING THE GOALS AND HYPOTHESES TO BE TESTED USING SURVEY DATA

The primary consideration in the design of any survey, no matter how modest or extensive in scope, is the specification of the goals to be met by gathering and analyzing information. For in-house data gathering purposes, particularly for collecting information for administrative decision making, often some persons are tempted to bypass the necessary process of thinking through and writing explicit operational goals and survey objectives. Goals provide direction and guidelines on which to fashion the questions to be asked of respondents.

Seldom are investigators able to dash off acceptable operational objectives in one or two "think-tank" sessions. It is disturbing to see or experience the slap-dash questionnaires, telephone queries, and mailed instruments that are seen far too frequently. The most frustrating activity that an experienced survey researcher faces is the request to consult on a survey project when the data has already been collected and the survey goals are nonexistent. In many situations, the investigator or survey team is overwhelmed with a morass of facts, figures, graphs, verbatim transcripts of interviews, completed interviews, and questionnaire schedules. Often direction on how to study and report the data is lacking. At this point, the consultant is then asked to help the team make sense and derive meaning from these various data sources. This may prove to be an impossible task. The consultant must ask the person requesting assistance, "What were the goals and objectives to be served and how do the data collected address those goals?" Not infrequently, this is the moment of truth for all concerned. The pain and discomfort evident in the seekers of help when the consultant is extracting this crucial informational variable is something to behold. In the end, the

consultant is almost certain to wish that the investigator or survey team had asked for assistance prior to the initiation of the project. Much time, money, and intellectual despair could probably have been saved and a sound survey project could have been launched if the objectives had been stated before questionnaire construction and data collection.

In conjunction with establishing goals and objectives in a substantive survey design, it would be expected to see an analytical or conceptual framework shaping a study's design. Furthermore, the hypotheses or research questions would be expected to be clearly and operationally stated in ways that connect dependent and independent variables in a logical mode. The analytical framework directly influences the questions asked and the hypotheses to be tested.

In later sections of this chapter, various questioning strategies and scaling procedures are described. Many examples deal with eliciting nurses' attitudes, opinions, beliefs, and behaviors concerning strikes and other work stoppage actions. If a formal survey were to be started concerning, for example, nurses' attitudes toward strikes in San Francisco, California, one would have to specify in advance the goals to be met, the analytical/conceptual model to be adopted, and the hypotheses to be tested with the data collected from the survey instrument. Various goals could be offered, depending on the particular needs and requirements of the sponsoring organization or individuals. The associations of San Francisco hospitals might want to survey nurses' attitudes toward strikes as a basis for renegotiation of a new two-year union contract. Such information could provide the basis of being either generous or miserly in the rounds of union contract renegotiations. Likewise, the collective bargaining agents for nurses might commission a similar survey in order to determine how favorable a contract could be negotiated, if large numbers of their members would support a strike action. Previous research might suggest to the survey designers in the above instance that certain models of worker behavior, including satisfaction and dissatisfaction, are predictors of employee attitudes and behavior, particularly to collective actions such as strikes, worker pay levels, and grievance actions taken at the institutional level of the organization (Hetherington and Rundall, 1983, p. 192).

5–4 ILLUSTRATION OF THE USE OF A CONCEPTUAL FRAMEWORK IN A SURVEY

Concepts that could be useful in developing the theoretical framework in one particular survey of professional nurse satisfaction and health care organizational structure can be found in the work of Hage (1965). He defined four aspects of organizational structure as being critical to organizational functioning typically found in a bureaucracy such as hospitals. They are formalization, centralization, stratification, and complexity. Hage formulated an axiomatic theory of organizations in which seven propositions (dealing with formalization and productivity, formalization and efficiency, centralization and formalization, stratification and job satisfaction, stratification and productivity, stratification and adaptivity, and complexity and centralization) and 21 corollaries were specified in terms of measurable variables and testable relationships. These constructs were used to define testable hypotheses and to provide guides for questionnaire development.

For instance, consider the corollary that states that the higher the stratification in a hospital, the lower the sense of job satisfaction. Match this formulation with the following corollary. The higher the stratification, the higher the centralization and formalization to be found in a hospital, and the higher the formalization and centralization in a hospital, the lower the job satisfaction.

In order to construct a question that would measure worker perceptions of the aforementioned concepts, some definitions should be specified. *Formalization* refers to the degree to which the norms of a social system are explicit and enforced (Hetherington and Rundall, 1983, p. 185). Another way to look at formalization is the amount of discretionary behavior allowed an employee in a hospital. *Centralization* contains three components: the extent to which an employee defers to a supervisor's powers and control, who in the organization makes important decisions, and the relative amount of influence that the various status groups in the organization have at their disposal (Hetherington and Rundall, 1983, pp. 186–187). *Stratification* concerns the distribution of rewards within the organization and the chances for upward mobility. Communication patterns in highly stratified organizations are seen to be primarily top–down in the form of direc-

tives. From these definitions a survey investigator would have to develop operational measurements of each of the three concepts identified: formalization, centralization, and stratification.

In testing the relationship between formalization and job satisfaction, for instance, one question to ask is,

> How many times do you need to check out with your immediate supervisor, the progress of your work shift assignment?
> (a) Frequently
> (b) Often
> (c) Occasionally
> (d) Rarely
> (e) Never

The responses to this question could be used to test the hypothesis that the frequency with which the professional registered nurse must confer with an immediate supervisor lowers the nurse's job satisfaction with the position. As this example shows, each concept and the hypotheses derived from each concept would have to have particular survey questions identified and developed to test specific stated relationships.

5–5 SURVEY PROPOSAL GUIDELINES

The first and hardest task in any survey is to differentiate the irrelevant factors from the factors that are relevant to the problem that the survey is expected to address. This task is facilitated by providing a conceptual or analytical framework to guide the survey. Most surveys begin with a vague notion of the kinds of information required. The vague notions need to be developed before proposals can be submitted and funding obtained. It is expected that a systematic literature review has been conducted in conjunction with the writing of a survey proposal. The investigator should find out what work has been done on the same or similar problems in the past. The proposal also should identify in the literature review the factors that have not yet been studied by other investigators. In addition, the present survey proposal would be expected to describe how the survey can build on what has already been done in the problem area.

Further help with what should be included in the survey can be gained from conversations with colleagues and knowledgeable persons in the area. New ideas may be suggested, assumptions challenged or altered, and assistance garnered in clarifying doubtful points. Discussions with a variety of persons representative of different elements in the nursing community often present the investigator with a different reality and provide a sharp attack on preconceptions, biases, and blind spots. This exercise frequently is most humbling but is a necessary activity to obtain a realistic grasp of what the true focus of the survey and the questionnaire should be.

A questionnaire should provide the requisite data in a timely and cost-effective manner. Data provided too late to be of real use or an instrument that causes the researchers to run out of money before the analysis and final report are completed is a poor questionnaire, no matter how well it seemed to serve project objectives or test study hypotheses. Budgets have to be realistically developed to do justice to the survey and the adequacy of obtained results. Living within time and money constraints is a reality for everyone, including research staff and investigators. Timetables must be established and rigidly adhered to in order to accomplish the task at hand. Time and costs affect all aspects of surveys and impose a limit on the number of questions asked, the number of interviews to be conducted in person or by telephone, and the length of the interviews. Realistic anticipation of these and sundry expenses greatly enables the researcher to fashion the most useful instrument possible within these crucial constraints (Sheatsley, 1983, pp. 201–202).

5–6 QUESTIONNAIRE AND INTERVIEW METHODS: STRENGTHS AND LIMITATIONS

Of the two main methods to collect data, the questionnaire is generally less expensive than in-person or telephone interviews. The use of questionnaires requires less skill than personal interviews; questionnaires are frequently mailed or handed to respondents with a minimum of explanation. Questionnaires can be administered to large numbers of persons simultaneously. Interviews call for one to one questioning. In theory, more information can be gathered quickly by questionnaires than by face-to-face or telephone interviews. The questionnaire offers a standardized stimulus situation: standard instructions, standard wording, standard order

of questions and areas probed, and standard response categories. Thus uniformity of one measurement situation to another is ensured. Also the anonymity of questionnaires enables persons to respond more freely in areas in which they might feel threatened or open to public censure, ridicule, or disgrace. Furthermore, the mode of questionnaires places less pressure on persons, and they can respond at a pace that is comfortable for them. Interviews can place considerable pressure on a person to answer quickly concerning topics that are uncomfortable for the respondent; some distortion in answers may occur because the interviewee may not be able to handle silence or searching probes. For situations in which very sensitive questions are probed, the randomized response method can be employed to extract pertinent information (Warner, 1965). This model is described in Section 6–18.

Because it is structured, the questionnaire is useful in situations in which a high degree of consistency is required for descriptive or comparative purposes. The printed format of the questionnaire makes it ideal for the inclusion of scales involving ordering of responses that are more accurately portrayed by print or graphics and for questions that require the informant to rank or compare numerous items or to select responses from among a complex response set (Waltz, Strickland, and Lenz, 1984, p. 275).

It has been estimated that, for purposes of filling out a simple questionnaire, at least 10% of the adult American population is illiterate. For major American cities inhabited by significant numbers of persons for whom English is not the primary language, the illiteracy estimate is considerably higher. In some respects, the questionnaire is appropriate only for those who possess considerable formal education. Even many college graduates have little facility for writing and of those who do, few have the patience or motivation to write as fully as they might speak. The burden of writing or of maintaining interest is great enough to limit the number of questions that may be asked and constrain the fullness of the responses (Selltiz et al., 1976, p. 296). It should also be observed that the questionnaires are written mainly by educated persons who have a special interest and knowledge about the survey's topic. Surveyors usually consult with other educated and knowledgeable persons; therefore, it is much more common for questionnaires to be overwritten, overcomplicated, and too demanding of the respondent than to be over-simplified, superficial, and not demanding enough (Sheatsley, 1983, p. 200).

Interviews can be conducted with almost all segments of the population. They yield a better sample of a population because many persons are willing to talk and cooperate when all that is required is a conversation between two people. Many enjoy the attention and talking with others who are polite, attentive, and cordial and give the informant an hour or two of total undivided interest, respect, and regard. Interviews afford flexibility and provide immediate opportunity for clarification of meaning and identification of misunderstandings. Furthermore, interviews enable an investigator to pursue requests for intricate evaluation of events or persons and to explore particularly sensitive topics in depth. The interview also provides access to specific segments of society from whom written response cannot be gathered (Waltz et al., 1984, p. 274).

Unfortunately, the advantages accruing to the interview format make it a costly procedure in terms of personnel and material resources. It costs money to hire and train interviewers. The transcription of responses from audiotapes is also costly. An hour's tape recording of an interview with an articulate informant can take anywhere from three to six hours of a transcriber's time. The time commitment is considerable for both parties in the interview. Interviews frequently must be conducted at night or on weekends. Extensive logistical arrangements must be made to get informant and interviewer together. Often, the interviewer must travel considerable distances and into areas where personal safety is an issue. Other problems include the inability to provide anonymity, difficulty in achieving uniform administration across informants, and the potential for interviewer bias (Waltz et al., 1984, p. 274). Finally, interviews are inefficient and not recommended for use when intelligence about important events must be gathered from large samples of a particular universe of persons or social aggregates.

5−7 QUALITIES OF A GOOD QUESTIONNAIRE

The construction of a good questionnaire is an art. It is very hard to tell someone how to devise a sound interview or questionnaire schedule. We recognize an excellent protocol when we see it but it is often problematic to tell someone how to construct one. For example, if a team of persons were given the task of constructing a questionnaire with a particular research question and specific hypotheses, each questionnaire would contain different items and areas addressed, probes employed, use of open- and closed-ended questions, and lengths of time for instrument completion. Yet, it is possible that all completed instruments do justice to the inquiry and a good case could be made for the adoption of each.

A well-designed questionnaire should meet the objectives of the inquiry, obtain the most complete and accurate information possible, and do so within reasonable limits of time and resources. To mandate that the questionnaire meet the research objectives of the study seems patently gratuitous. Unfortunately, many instruments fail this preeminent criterion of a good questionnaire or interview schedule construction. It is not unusual to overlook key content areas because one is presumably studying an area in which much uncertainty exists and little objective data is readily at hand.

All researchers quickly learn that when data are being analyzed, gaps appear. Some questions thought to address key issues turn out to be useless, whereas other questions, which in retrospect most certainly should have been included, were not included. One way to forestall apparent gaps in content is to develop an outline of each question and to identify how that particular question addresses the research questions and hypotheses. In addition, specify how each question is to be qualitatively and quantitatively analyzed. Among other things, this laborious exercise quickly identifies project staff prejudices and pet interests. If honestly and carefully done at this preliminary stage, significant revisions in the instrument will most certainly occur. Constant revisions are required as consultant advice is sought. Further examination and reexamination of pertinent literature will most certainly identify areas that must be included. Finally, repeated pretesting of the instrument with target audiences will highlight additional areas that should be addressed. It is not unusual for a questionnaire or interview schedule to be revised 10 to 15 times before embarking on the parent study.

It is apparent that a good questionnaire provides the most complete and accurate information possible. Often, this may not happen because the respondents intervene in the process. They may misunderstand the question or reject the premise upon which the question is based. They may simply refuse to answer. They may lie or attempt to conceal their actual behavior or attitudes. The questions may be so far beyond their comprehension that they may answer randomly rather than confess their ignorance. When all these things occur, we have to judge the questionnaire as inadequate, no matter how well it met the surveys' objectives and purposes. A good instrument avoids the above pitfalls by encouraging truthful, frank and reliable information about the informant's attitudes and behaviors, no matter how sensitive the topic.

5-8 WHAT QUESTIONS TO ASK AND HOW TO ASK THEM

In deciding to ask questions, three dimensions should be considered:

1. the content of the question
2. the question, defined as the verbal stimulus to which the respondent is exposed
3. the provision for answering, which refers to the response that the respondent is expected (or, in some techniques, what the respondent is permitted) to produce (Fox, 1982, p. 216)

Questioning involves sampling. The investigator is not able to ask every possible question, assuming that all possible questions for any given area could be identified. One needs to decide the content of the questions. Content domains can be described as

1. content directed at establishing facts,
2. content directed at beliefs about what the facts are,
3. content directed at ascertaining feelings,
4. content directed at discovering standards of action,
5. content directed at present or past behavior,
6. content directed at conscious reasons for beliefs, feelings, policies, and behavior (Selltiz et al., 1976, pp. 299–307).

It is useful to develop a full blueprint of the various content areas in which questions covering specific situations are needed. With the areas identified, the researcher can turn to the sampling process, particularly to deciding what proportion of the questioning time will be allocated to each aspect of the content. The identification of all possible areas for questioning and the consideration of proportional allocation of time are often ignored. Yet they form the base from which the content or domain validity of the research tool can be identified.

The clear specification of goals and objectives and unambiguous hypotheses to be tested are the important precursors of asking the right questions in the survey. After the goals are specified, question writing can begin. The prime characteristic of a question is that it must be clear. The intent of the question and the type of information requested must be precise and obvious to the person being questioned. The question must be phrased in words and terms familiar to the respondent. The information being sought must be requested in nontechnical language and language free of the jargon used by health professionals. In the case of children, physical or emotionally handicapped persons, and those who do not speak or read English with facility, this requirement is foremost.

When educational and technical background differences between interviewer and informant are considerable, great pains should be taken to ensure that the language, vocabulary, and nuances of the questions can be understood and reasonably answered. Nurses and other health providers are particularly challenged to state questions in clear and unambiguous terms because of their extensive technical and professional expertise. Reviewing past observations of professional colleagues querying patients without gaining satisfactory data because of the differences in backgrounds of health providers and patients should underscore the importance of forming good questions. In phrasing questions the journalistic imperative should be followed: Keep it short and keep it simple!

A second characteristic of a good question is that it seeks only one piece or bit of information. A common pitfall in seeking information from respondents is to ask for several bits of information in the same question. This is confusing to many persons. These questions pose interminable problems for the investigators trying to make sense out of the response. Asking a client in the same question to describe a physical symptom, as well as whether he slept last night and what he wants for lunch is certain to confuse the informant. You may get a response to all three items, to two, or to one contained in the original question. When three different pieces of information are sought, three questions should be asked.

The third characteristic of a good question is that it does not lead or bias the respondent's response. It is an error to suggest to the informant that certain responses are more acceptable than others or that certain answers are more desirable. The differences in status, such as nurse versus patient, adult versus child, teacher versus student, may inadvertently shape the response unless the investigator is finely tuned to such social controlling processes. It is important to make the respondent aware that any position is acceptable and that the interviewer is not just seeking agreement to positions handed down by the investigator.

In the wording of questions it is always important to specify alternatives and not to load the alternatives responses. For example, if the introduction of the question starts with, "Don't you agree that . . . " or "Isn't it obvious that . . . ," it suggests that one response is more desirable than another. Instead, phrasing a question with this introduction does not lead the respondent: "Some people think that . . . others have the following view . . . what is your position?"

A fourth characteristic of a good question is linguistic completeness and grammatical consistency. Asking vague, ambiguous questions leads to all kinds of difficulty. If an item asks "What is your income?" answers will come in all sorts of terms. Income will be reported in hourly pay, weekly salary, monthly or annual earnings, and similar terms. If subjects are to be classified on income, it is necessary to specify what *income* means, for example, total family income, income before taxes, during the last calendar year, including income from all sources. The question "How long have you lived here?" elicits equal difficulties in interpretation. Does the investigator mean how long have you lived at this address, in this neighborhood, in this city, state, region?

Double-barreled questions such as "How satisfied are you with your salary and hours at the hospital where you work?" elicit confusion. If the nurse who is asked that question is satisfied with the salary but unsat-

isfied with the work shifts, how is that person going to answer? It would be difficult for the respondent to reply in terms of very satisfied, fairly satisfied, somewhat dissatisfied, or very dissatisfied. The survey should ask two questions, not one. Other areas of questions containing grammatical inconsistencies occur when the alternative responses overlap. "Are you generally satisfied with your job, or are there some things you don't like about it?" should not enable the nurse respondent to agree with more than one. The nurse should be able to respond truthfully "yes" or "no" to both alternatives.

5—9 OPEN-ENDED AND CLOSED-ENDED QUESTIONS

In considering the actual questions to be asked, the nurse investigator has to choose between *open-ended* or *closed-ended* questions or sets of questions. Open-ended questions ask for replies in the respondent's own words: "What do you like most about working at this hospital?" No answers are suggested. Closed-ended questions ask informants to choose from two or more categories. Following is an example.

> Which one of four statements comes closest to your opinion?
>
> (1) I mostly like working at this hospital.
> (2) I sometimes like working at this hospital.
> (3) I sometimes dislike working at this hospital.
> (4) I mostly dislike working at this hospital.

The advantage of open-ended questions is that they allow the informant to answer entirely unprejudiced by any alternatives suggested by the interviewer. They also reveal what is most important to respondents, what things are uppermost in their minds. For example, one could ask an open-ended question:

> What do you like least about working at this hospital?

Or, one could ask a closed-ended question:

> Here are five things nurses have told us they don't like about this hospital. Which one do you like least?

In response to the open-ended question, many informants may mention something not on the list of five choices. If the closed-ended question had been asked their actual opinions would not have been known. Another group of nurses might give one answer on the open-ended question and a different one on the closed-ended question, because the list reminded them of something they had not thought of when they answered the open-ended question.

Closed-ended questions suggest answers that respondents may not have thought of or they prompt responses that do not reflect the person's thinking about the factor being questioned. No matter how skillfully devised, closed-ended questions force respondents into response categories that are at times not truly reflective of their position. Nuances and shades of meaning are lost in closed-ended questions. In answering open-ended queries, a person can add qualifications, reshape particular meanings, and emphasize the forcefulness of his or her views. Specific disadvantages are, however, associated with open-ended questions. They elicit a great deal of irrelevant and repetitious responses. Highly verbal persons can be especially difficult to control and to keep to the point. Frequent awkward pauses occur as informants grope for thoughts and words. A skillful interviewer is challenged to keep respondents on track, to clarify their answers, to provide pertinent examples that illustrate their views, and to elaborate on sensitive or complex topics. Persons differ greatly in their ability to be verbally cogent and precise. Differences in response to open-ended queries may reflect differences in ability to articulate present viewpoints as well as real differences in shades and intensity of opinions.

Open-ended questions take more time for the respondent and cost more money to collect and analyze. Coding these responses on a questionnaire is an extensive process; issues of reliability and validity constantly come to the forefront in agreement about categories and classification schema. With open-ended questions, interviewers must be trained to know what constitutes an acceptable answer. They must spend more interviewing time probing and recording. Coders must be trained and supervised; constant rechecking is a must. Use of closed-ended questions avoids these problems. For a variety of sound reasons—time, money, interviewer variability, response variability, coding, and analytical problems—the nurse investigator using any large scale survey is advised to close up as many questions as possible. Open-ended questions are used only

1. when there are too many categories to be listed or foreseen,

2. when the respondent's spontaneous uninfluenced reply is desired,

3. to build rapport during interviews, following a long series of closed-ended questions, which may make informants feel that they have no chance to express themselves, and

4. in an exploratory interview and pretest, when the researcher wants to get some idea of the parameters of an issue with a view of closing up the questions later (Sheatsley, 1983, p. 208).

5–10 DEVELOPING RESPONSE CATEGORIES FOR QUESTIONNAIRES AND INTERVIEWS: SCALING CONSIDERATIONS

Open-ended questions permit respondents to frame their own responses. Closed-ended questions permit researchers to specify the answer categories most suitable to their purposes. Many questions form natural dichotomies.

Do you belong to the nurses' association?
(1) yes (2) no

Did you attend the strike vote meeting?
(1) yes (2) no

Often the nurse investigator sorts the sample into two groups, such as those who were active in the strike and those who were not, or those who approve of the issue and those who do not approve, or those who are particularly knowledgeable about an issue and those who are ignorant of it.

Often, the natural dichotomy provides a poor response distribution. If you ask patients, "Are you satisfied or dissatisfied with the nursing care you received in the hospital," only about 10% to 20% express dissatisfaction. Most indicate that they are satisfied. People are reluctant to criticize nurses, doctors, and other professional experts. They probably receive as good a care as they anticipated or know. Patients frequently have no point of comparison regarding what constitutes good nursing care. They possess no baseline or exacting standard of nursing care. If patients anticipate further hospitalizations, they may be extremely reluctant to be censorious of nursing actions. If they are really unhappy, they may switch hospitals if further assistance is needed in the future. But if one asked,

How satisfied were you with the nursing care you received in the hospital?
(1) very satisfied
(2) somewhat satisfied
(3) somewhat dissatisfied
(4) very dissatisfied

the marginal distribution will look like 50% very satisfied, 35% somewhat satisfied, 10% somewhat dissatisfied, and 5% very dissatisfied. The first two groups (1 and 2), which became combined in the dichotomous version may well turn out to be different (3 and 4) in terms of their characteristics, behavior, and other attitudes.

It is frequently useful to divide people into more than two categories; hence the popularity of five-point scales such as strongly agree, agree, undecided, disagree, and, strongly disagree. A five-point scale provides flexibility in that all five groups can be examined in terms of responses to other questions or other variables collected in the hospital from records or other sources. It is also easy to collapse such data when wanting to look at the two major groups: agree versus disagree. In general, scales with more than 5 or 6 discriminations are resented by informants who cannot make such fine determinations. Furthermore, with more categories the research investigator has problems associated with small sample size and analysis based on parametric models (Sheatsley, 1983, p. 209).

A large element of judgment is involved when the investigator places a respondent on a rating scale on the basis of the person's observed behavior, answers to open-ended and closed-ended questions, or other responses. In an effort to devise procedures that would make it possible to place informants on a scale with less likelihood of error, carefully standardized questions must be constructed. In this approach respondents do not directly describe themselves in terms of their positions on the issues in question. Rather, they express their agreement or disagreement with a number of statements directly related to the issue. On the basis of these responses they are assigned a score. In the process of standardizing the question-

naire, the investigator has established a rationale for interpreting scores as indicating varying degrees or levels in relation to the issue. The scale must differentiate people who are at different points along an issue. In other words, scale items must also allow shades of differentiation between both extremes or contrasting positions.

5–11 DIFFERENTIAL SCALES GENERATED FROM QUESTIONNAIRE ITEMS

The manner in which a scale differentiates respondents to questionnaires depends on the particular approach taken to scale construction and the method chosen to score each item on the scale. In some scales, the items can be chosen to form a gradation of such a nature that a person will probably agree with only one or two items. These items correspond to the informant's position on the issue, and are most likely in opposition to statements on either side of those selected. Such scales are called *differential scales*.

A differential scale consists of a number of items whose positions have been determined through ranking or rating procedures performed by independent expert judges. Judges are directed to react to the items independent of their own attitudes or views and to rate each statement according to the degree of favorability or unfavorability that they believed to be expressed by the items. The judges are instructed to place items reflecting extreme views on an issue at either end of a pole or in two distinct categories. All items reflecting intermediate views are to be assigned between the two extreme positions and scaled accordingly. Items for which no agreement or low agreement is reached are discarded. Later, numerical scale values are assigned the remaining items. The assigned numerical values are based on a dimension that might be favorable-unfavorable, and characterized as representing a continuum underlying a concept or construct.

For example, to develop a differential scale (known as a Thurston Scale) of nurses' opinions toward strikes as a collective-bargaining technique, a large set of items would have to be generated. Miller (1983) recommends 50 to 300 judges and several hundred items for rating. For example, one could have an item such as,

> Nurses' strikes are a threat to patient safety and welfare. Where would you place this item?

This item would be given to approximately 200 judges who would be asked to assign the item to the following scale:

Unfavorable 0 1 2 3 4 5 6 7 8 9 10 Favorable

The median score assigned by the 200 judges to this item is then treated as the *item score*. In this example, this item might be assigned a scale value of 1 or 2 in unfavorability toward a strike. Another item might be worded,

> Nurses strike to attain improvements in patient care. Where would you place this item?

Again the 200 judges would be asked to rate this item on the 11-point scale.

Unfavorable 0 1 2 3 4 5 6 7 8 9 10 Favorable

This statement probably would be assigned by most judges to category 9 or 10. In addition, in the determination of the median scale value assigned to an item by the judges, each item would be examined for variability in scale scores. If the semi-interquartile range were to be large, the item would not be included in the scale. The final set of items (usually between 20 and 30) would be distributed along a favorable to unfavorable continuum, using the judges' median values to determine final scale values for all items. An example of this type of scale and questionnaire is shown in Figure 5–1.

In this example, a 22-item scale has been produced from a larger pool of items. The items have been selected so that the median

values range from a value close to 10. Ideally one would chose items for which the distance between adjacent medians is equal to the range of the scale divided by the number of items in the scale. In this case, one would want the distance between contiguous items to be about 11/22 or .50. Thus, the scale values for the 22 items would be given by numbers very close to .50, 1.00, 1.50 . . . , 10. These numbers would be used to scale each nurse.

The scale values for the items selected by each nurse would be averaged and used as the nurses' scale values. For example, suppose that a specific nurse endorsed 5 of the 22 items. Suppose that the scale values of the 5 selected items are given by 4.5, 7.0, 8.5, 9.0, and 10. The mean value of these items is 7.90. This is treated as the nurse's scale score and it can be inferred to represent a favorable attitude toward the strike as a collective bargaining procedure.

The differential scaling technique is a very time-consuming and methodologically complex procedure. It requires large numbers of expert judges. Many have questioned whether the judges can be as dispassionate and as unbiased as proponents claim they are in scaling items. Many of the areas in which scales might be developed by nurses are emotionally charged and fraught with strong and conflicting views. For instance, euthanasia, no codes, and abortion, among many other such health care issues, can seriously jeopardize any person's objectivity. Furthermore, the measurement assumptions underlying this procedure are open to serious question. Claims are made that interval scale characteristics represented in the technique are not supportable (see Section 2–8

The following 22 statements are expressions of attitudes of using grievance procedures, work stoppages, or strikes to gain pay increases, improved working conditions, and better patient care. Please read each item and select the ones that best reflect your position on these issues. You may check as many items as you please.

(1) Formal in-house discussions with management to solve nurse grievances may lead to satisfactory resolution.

(2) There are justifiable reasons for professional nurses to engage in a strike.

(3) Because of uncompromising management positions, a decision to strike by professional nurses may be justified.

(4) There are occasions when a strike is the only option that professional nurses have to improve situations.

⋮

(21) Nurses' strikes are a threat to patients' safety and welfare.

(22) Nurses strike to attain improvements in patient care.

Figure 5–1. Example of a differential scale based on 22 items.

for the authors' position on scaling assumptions).

Also, if a person's responses scatter widely over noncontiguous items, the person's score is not likely to have the same meaning as a score with little scatter. The scattered responses may indicate that the informant has no attitude or that the attitude is not organized in the manner assumed by the scale. There is no a priori reason to expect that all persons have attitudes, beliefs, opinions, and similar dispositional states toward the same thing or that behavioral predispositions are the same for all (Selltiz et al., 1976, p. 415).

5–12 SUMMATED SCALES GENERATED FROM QUESTIONNAIRE ITEMS

Another major scaling approach to measuring attitudes, opinions, values, views, beliefs, and so on, are to be found in *summated scales*. The most widely used summated scale is the Likert scale (1932). Generally a Likert scale consists of a number of declarative statements or questions that require the informant to state a viewpoint on a topic. Informants are asked to indicate the degree of agreement or disagreement with the views contained in each statement or question. The most commonly encountered set of responses and scoring procedures used in a Likert scale item is

Response Category	Endorsement of the Item	
	Positive	Negative
(a) strongly disagree	1	5
(b) disagree	2	4
(c) undecided	3	3
(d) agree	4	2
(e) strongly agree	5	1

As an example, consider measuring attitudes toward nurses filing a formal grievance procedure against a health facility. If an item is written so that *strongly agree* represents a positive endorsement of using a grievance procedure, the item uses the positive endorsement numbers. If the item is worded so that *strongly disagree* represents a positive endorsement, then the item uses the negative endorsement numbers. For example consider the following two items.

1. Nurses who file a grievance should be promoted.
   (a) strongly disagree   1
   (b) disagree   2
   (c) undecided   3
   (d) agree   4
   (e) strongly agree   5

2. Nurses who file a grievance should be fired.
   (a) strongly disagree   5
   (b) disagree   4
   (c) undecided   3
   (d) agree   2
   (e) strongly agree   1

If a nurse responds (e) to question 1 and (a) to question 2, the total score for these two items is 5 + 5 or 10, the highest level of support for grievance procedures. But a nurse who responds (a) to question 1 and (e) to question 2, would be scored as 1 + 1 or 2, the lowest level of support for the grievance model.

In developing summated scales, the first step is to generate a large number of items or statements that clearly reflect favorable and unfavorable views toward the issue under consideration. Extreme views that all persons would endorse or not endorse should be avoided. Wide variability is desired in items, which spread individual responses over a continuum of favorability-unfavorability to the issue under review. Equal numbers of positively and negatively worded statements should be incorporated into the scale to prevent biasing responses or to avoid a response set.

Different opinions are held about the appropriate number of categories or alternative responses to be included in a Likert scale. Likert used five categories; others prefer a 7-point scale. There is also a difference of opinion about the use of a midpoint category called "uncertain," "undecided," "don't know," or "can't respond." Some argue that the inclusion of this response option makes the task less objectionable to people who cannot make up their own minds or who have no strong feelings or views about a specific item contained in the scale. Others feel that the use of this undecided category encourages fence-sitting, or the tendency not to take sides or to commit oneself to topics of a sensitive nature. Still others omit the undecided category and use either a 4- or 6-point category option to ensure that respondents take a position on each statement contained in the scale.

A number of standard response options have been developed by experienced survey specialists to summated scales. Again, depending on the number of response categories selected these options can fit many survey topics. Some examples are as follows:

1. Response categories useful in measuring peoples' satisfaction with amounts of a product, actions, positions, and other aspects. Examples are staffing levels, work productivity expectations, salary and fringe benefits, and similar indices. The response categories for this type of item are the following:
(a) too many
(b) more than average
(c) about right
(d) less than average
(e) too little

2. Response categories useful for comparisons of past events or with expectations for future events. Examples are comparisons of past work or school performance level with future levels, professional career options and like comparisons. The response categories for this type of item are the following:
(a) very much better
(b) slightly better
(c) about the same
(d) slightly worse
(e) very much worse

3. Response categories useful in determining frequency of many kinds of activities such as promotional opportunities for staff, amount of patient education conducted by nurses, number of physician-nurses joint conferences, and similar events. The response categories for this type of item are the following:
(a) always
(b) very often
(c) often
(d) not often
(e) never

4. Response categories useful for behavioral indicators of activities or frequency of activities such as voting in union elections, initiation of new patient care programs, participation in community education programs, and other similar events. The response categories for this type of item are the following:
(a) always
(b) most of the time
(c) about half of the time
(d) some of the time
(e) never

5. Response categories useful as a measure of the probability of the respondent's action such as going out on strike, joining a union, adopting a new nursing practice and similar courses of future action. The response categories for this type of item are the following:
(a) much more likely
(b) more likely

(c) no difference
(d) less likely
(e) much less likely

Depending on how many categories are used, scores are assigned to reflect degree of favorability toward the concept being measured. In general, the higher the score for all items relating to a concept, the more favorable the respondent's view or position regarding the concept. In Chapter 3, we provided an example of a summated pain scale possessing five response options with no midpoint (uncertain) response category. A disadvantage of a summated scale is that a person's total score may at times have little meaning, because many patterns of response to the various items may produce the same score. Because a summated scale often provides a wide range of response categories, the criticism has merit. It is reasonable to suppose that two similar total scores based on different combinations of item responses may reflect different views, attitudes, or other behavioral indicators toward the issue under consideration. This drawback can be addressed through careful item analysis to identify clusters of items that differentiate between subgroups of respondents and/or correlate with other relevant indicators in the total survey. Factor analytic procedures also can identify unidimensional scale items that represent an underlying attribute or concept (see Section 11–8). Summated scales such as Likert scales appear to involve considerable work but they are actually quite powerful because they provide an ordering of people on the characteristic being measured. An example of a Likert type scale is shown in Figure 5–2.

For example, a nurse who chose the following set of responses: (1) b, (2) d, (3) a, . . . (10) c, would be given the following Likert score

$$Y = 4 + 2 + 4 + \ldots + 3 = 30,$$

which is right on the midpoint of the scale that ranges from 10 to 50.

5–13 CUMULATIVE SCALES GENERATED FROM QUESTIONNAIRE ITEMS

Cumulative scales are another technique used in some surveys. Cumulative scales,

The following 10 questions seek your views regarding working conditions in this hospital following the initiation of the union contract. Please read each question and select the response that best reflects your position on these issues. Circle the letter that best corresponds or reflects your answer to each separate question.

(1) Since the nursing staff joined a union, how often do you vote in union elections?
    (a) always
    (b) most of the time
    (c) about half of the time
    (d) some of the time
    (e) never

(2) Since the nursing staff joined a union, how would you describe the working conditions in this hospital?
    (a) very much better
    (b) slightly better
    (c) about the same
    (d) slightly worse
    (e) very much worse

(3) Since the initiation of the union contract, how would you describe the amount of personnel available to provide patient care?
    (a) too many
    (b) better than average
    (c) about right
    (d) less than average
    (e) too little

⋮

(10) Since the new contract has been in operation, how often do notices for nursing promotions appear in the monthly hospital newsletter?
    (a) always
    (b) very often
    (c) often
    (d) not often
    (e) never

Figure 5–2. Example of a Likert scale used to measure views about working conditions in a union contract hospital.

like differential and summated scales, are made up of a series of items with which informants indicate agreement or disagreement. In a cumulative scale, the items are related to one another in such a way that ideally a person who replies favorably to item 2 also responds favorably to item 1; another investigative subject who replies favorably to item 3 also would be expected, under the scaling assumptions for the scale, to respond favorably to both items 1 and 2. Thus all respondents who answer a given item favorably should have higher scores on the total scale than those who answered that item unfavorably. The person's score is computed by counting the number of items answered favorably. This score places the person on the scale of favorable-unfavorable dimension provided by the a priori-derived relationship of the particular items to each other.

To evaluate unidimensionality, a technique based on Guttman (1944) provides a scalogram display of individual items arranged in a column and ordered from left to right according to subject selection from the most to the least selected or endorsed item. Individual research subjects are shown as rows and organized or ordered from top to bottom according to total score, from the highest to the lowest score. A perfect unidimensional scale would reveal on visual examination an orderly stepwise progression of selected scale items for individual test subjects and the scaled items. An example of a Guttman scalogram is provided in Figure 5–3. In this example, 25 subjects are listed according to their total score on the scale. In making the scalogram, the items are rank ordered on the basis of their item endorsement. In this example, item 1 received the most endorsement with 20 of the 25 subjects showing agreement, and item 10 received the least endorsement with only 3 subjects showing agreement. In ranking the subjects, a hierarchy of listing is made with subjects showing the strongest identification with the Guttman scale listed above subjects who deviate from the theoretical expectations predicted by a Guttman scale. In this example, subjects 1,

Item Number											
Subject	**1**	**2**	**3**	**4**	**5**	**6**	**7**	**8**	**9**	**10**	**Score**
1	1	1	1	1	1	1	1	1	1	1	10
2	1	1	1	1	1	1	1	1	1	0	9
3	1	1	1	1	1	1	1	0	1	1	9
4	1	1	1	1	1	1	1	1	0	0	8
5	1	1	1	1	1	1	1	0	0	0	7
6	1	1	1	1	1	1	1	0	0	0	7
7	1	1	1	1	1	0	1	1	0	0	7
8	1	1	1	1	1	1	0	0	0	0	6
9	1	1	1	1	0	1	0	0	0	1	6
10	1	1	1	1	0	0	0	0	0	0	4
⋮											
24	0	0	0	1	0	0	0	1	0	0	2
25	0	1	0	0	0	0	0	0	0	0	1
Total	20	17	15	13	10	9	8	5	4	3	

Figure 5–3. Example of a scalogram used to evaluate a Guttman scale.

2, 4, 5, 6, 8, and 10 meet the theoretical expectations associated with a Guttman scale. Subject 3 has a total score of 9 and did not endorse item 8, but did endorse items 9 and 10 that are higher up in the Guttman hierarchy of items. This subject is said to be nonscalable. These exceptions to theoretical expectation can be easily seen in the scalogram.

The deviation from theoretical expectations can be summarized in a statistic called the *coefficient of reproducibility*. The coefficient of reproducibility is defined as 1 minus the proportion of exceptions. In particular,

$$R = 1 - E/T$$

where E equals the number of errors in endorsement or the number of favorable responses that do not fit the expected pattern, and T is the total number of all possible endorsements. For S subjects and I items,

$$E = E_1 + E_2 + \ldots + E_I \text{ and } T = IS.$$

In our example,

$$T = 10(25) = 250$$

and

$$E = 0 + 0 + 2 + 0 + 0 + 0 + 2 + 0 + 2 + 0 + \ldots 8 = 30$$

so that the coefficient of reproducibility is given by

$$R = 1 - 30/250 = .88.$$

A coefficient of 1.00 means that the response pattern for any particular or specific scale score can be reproduced perfectly. When the reproducibility coefficient falls below a desired range of .9 to .8, the Guttman scalogram visual display can be used to help identify scale items that do not conform to theoretical expectations. When the questionable or outlier items are removed, the coefficient of reproducibility is reestimated until an acceptable coefficient is established (Dawis, 1987). Ideally the reestimation procedure should be based on a new sample of subjects. Using the same subjects to reevaluate the scale is suspect because such a model can capitalize on idiosyncrasies in the data. If statistical tests were available for the evaluation, the procedure based on using the same subjects in a post hoc manner is sure to maximize the errors generated by poor type I error control.

An illustration of a 10-item Guttman Scale is shown in Figure 5–4. The items of this scale are designed to reflect a fictitious cumulative scale detailing nurses' views about strikes. A nurse who disagreed or disapproved of strikes as a collective bargaining tool for professional nurses would probably disagree with all 10 statements and would most likely be assigned a score of zero. Nurses who viewed strikes as essential collective bargaining tools would probably agree with all 10 statements and would be assigned a score of 10.

There are rather complex theoretical assumptions underlying the use of a cumulative or *Guttman scale* (1944). First, the Gutt-

The following 10 statements are designed to seek your views regarding grievance procedures and strike actions in this hospital following the initiation of the union contract. Please read each statement carefully and select the response that best reflects your position on each issue. To each statement circle (a) *agree* or (d) *disagree* option. Do not leave any statement unanswered.

Option

a d   (1) Formal in-house discussions with management to solve nurse grievances may lead to unsatisfactory resolution.

a d   (2) There are justifiable reasons for professional nurses to engage in a strike.

a d   (3) Due to uncompromising management positions, a decision to strike by professional nurses may be justified.

         ⋮

a d   (10) There are circumstances for which a strike is the only option for a professional nurse to improve situations.

Figure 5–4 Example of a Guttman type scale designed to measure desire to participate in formal grievances and strikes against a health facility by nurses.

man scaling procedure offers no guidance for the selection or generation of items that are likely to form a cumulative scale. Second, response patterns are supposed to be reproducible. That is, if the above contrived scale is given to another set of subjects, the response pattern found in one sample needs to be the same or nearly the same as that found in the second sample. In many cases this does not happen. Some persons may pick item 2, skip item 3, and pick item 4 thus violating a central premise that the views held about an issue can be placed in a hierarchical relationship and that individual selection of items on a Guttman scale will reflect that ordered relationship. Third, Guttman or cumulative scales assume that the concept underlying the scale items are unidimensional. Much of what contemporary health care research is concerned with involves multidimensional phenomena. Also, any item scale may be unidimensional for one group of persons but not for another. The experience of different groups can lead to either multidimensional patterning or unidimensional patterning. In practice, the cumulative scale, though an interesting measurement approach, is a methodologically complex technique infrequently used in surveys of today, particularly when multidimensional scaling and multivariate procedures are required.

Until recently the Guttman scale approach was primarily of academic interest and could not be applied with ease. Today the use of a Guttman scale is facilitated by the number of computer programs available in commercial computer packages like SPSS (1986) and BIOMED (Dixon, 1983). It should be noted that disagreements exist among psychometricians concerning the correct procedure for determining the coefficient of reproducibility. For a discussion of this topic, see Mueller (1986).

5–14 SEMANTIC DIFFERENTIAL SCALES GENERATED BY QUESTIONNAIRE ITEMS

Another scaling technique of value in surveys is to be found in the *semantic differential technique.* Osgood, Succi, and Tannenbaum (1957) described the technique as useful for measuring the sociopsychological meaning of concepts or objects to a person. It may be thought of as a series of attitude scales. It is structurally very similar to a set of graphic rating scales. The subject is asked to rate a given concept like 12-hour work shifts, work stoppages, primary nursing, mandatory continuing education, clinical promotional ladder, and so on, on a series of 7-point bipolar scales (Mueller, 1986). The bipolar scales include adjective pairs such as: (1) fair–unfair, (2) clean–dirty, (3) good–bad, (4) important–unimportant, (5) strong–weak, (6) heavy–light, (7) large–small, (8) active–passive, (9) fast–slow, (10) hot–cold, and so on.

The subject's response can be used to determine whether for that particular person, two concepts are alike or different. For instance, what are the similarities or differences when a nurse is requested to rate "the nurse I am" versus "the nurse I would like to be." The investigator can draw a word profile of the meaning of these two concepts to the same nurse informant. Similarly, by comparing a group of nurses' responses to a given concept it can be determined where similarities or differences exist. The semantic differential technique is highly flexible and easy to use. Practically any concept can be rated. There is considerable flexibility in the development of bipolar scales.

The Osgood and colleagues (1957) book contains a large listing of bipolar adjectives developed in their original research. Later investigators have modified or added additional sets of adjective pairs (Snider and Osgood, 1969). When choosing items for a scale, be careful that the adjective pairs selected realistically relate to the concept being rated. For instance, the adjective pair red–green appears to be unrelated to the concept "strike." If respondents believe that the adjective pairs are frivolous, particularly regarding concepts that have great emotional or political significance to the person, an investigator may get resistant or hostile responses or the respondents may not complete the instrument.

It is also advisable to weigh whether the adjective pairs are measuring the same concept or an underlying dimension of the concept. Through extensive research, Osgood and colleagues (1957) identified three major clusters or dimensions of the adjective pairs, labeled *evaluation, potency,* and *activity.* The most important dimension is the evaluative cluster, which contains adjective pairs like valuable–worthless, good–bad, fair–unfair, clean–dirty, and similar evaluative pairs. Potency adjectives include such bipolar pairs as large–small, strong–weak, heavy–light. Examples of activity adjective sets are active–passive, fast–slow, hot–cold.

At times these three clusters must be considered separately because the informants' personal evaluative rating of a concept such as "strike" may be independent of the activity or potency rating. Two nurses who associate high levels of activity with the concept strike may have divergent views with regard to how valuable a strike may be. Some controversy exists as to whether three independent clusters are represented in the adjective sets used to date. Many investigators ignore the original descriptions and achieve a global estimate of the respondents' responses to a specific concept. For others, responses are analyzed through various factor analytical procedures, and the underlying dimensions are named according to the investigative

groups' particular view as to what is truly contained in the identified clusters. Some investigators advocate use of the evaluative dimension alone. Still others pay particular attention to the underlying dimensions said to be contained in a particular adjective set and carefully include adjectives representing all three dimensions and analyze the data accordingly. Finally, if a group of adjective opposite pairs are used with no particular theoretical construct in mind, it is a mistake to associate the construct with the semantic differential format. If the adjectives are not working together to measure a particular theoretical construct, they are not measuring anything of special conceptual or empirical importance (Mueller, 1986).

The scoring procedure for the semantic differential technique is similar to that used for Likert scales. Scores from 1 to 7 are assigned to each bipolar scale response. Typically, the positively worded adjectives are assigned higher scores (5,6,7) and negatively worded adjectives would be assigned lower scores (1,2,3). Adjective pairs are randomly reversed to prevent response bias. Subgroups of scale responses associated with the same dimension can be summed up to yield a total score. A note of caution is raised at this point. Osgood and colleagues (1957) suggested that the measuring instrument is not completely comparable across concepts. The meaning of the particular scales and their relation to other scales varies considerably with the concept being judged. "Strong" may be appropriate in judging a "strike" but not in assessing a new procedure for recording patient data labeled "Problem Record." It is sometimes difficult to develop rating scales that provide a consistent measurement of the underlying dimensions independent of the concepts being judged (Selltiz et al., 1976).

An illustration of a semantic differential scale used to assess nursing strikes is provided in Figure 5–5. If the positive end of each bipolar adjective pair is scored 7 and the negative end scored 1, then the score for a nurse who placed X's as shown in Figure 5–5 is given by

$$Y = 3 + 3 + 2 + 4 + 1 + 2 + 3 + 1 + 3 + 4 = 26$$

With a minimal scale value of 10, a maximal score of 70, and a middle score of 40, it can be concluded that this particular nurse re-

The following 10 bipolar adjectives are designed to seek your evaluation regarding strike actions in this hospital following the initiation of the union contract. Please examine each set of adjectives carefully and select the response that best reflects your view of a strike in terms of the scale represented by each set. For each adjective set, check 1 of the 7 *intervals* that best represents your evaluation. Do not leave any statement unanswered.

STRIKE

	1	2	3	4	5	6	7	
good					X			bad
kind					X			cruel
clean						X		dirty
beautiful				X				ugly
unsuccessful	X							successful
false		X						true
wise					X			foolish
negative	X							positive
important					X			unimportant
dark				X				light

Figure 5–5 Example of a semantic differential scale to assess the meaning of a strike to nurses.

spondent holds a negative or less favorable attitude toward the utilization of a strike.

The semantic differential technique is a versatile procedure. Many respondents, including older children, enjoy items using this approach. This technique also provides a good alternative to more traditional scales such as the dichotomous yes–no variety or the agree–disagree Likert technique. The important point to keep in mind when determining what and how to measure a set of concepts is the variety of techniques available. One can present a compelling survey using the preceding scales and examples of questions through creative synthesis of the diverse measuring approaches depicted.

5–15 MULTIDIMENSIONAL SCALES GENERATED FROM QUESTIONNAIRE ITEMS

Multidimensional scaling techniques are a set of procedures that can be used to represent spatially the interrelationship among a set of objects with reference to health and illness constructs and concepts. The data generally are a set of numbers that consists of a dimensional configuration or visual map of scale items representing empirical indicators of concepts and constructs. The principal use of these procedures is an effort to uncover, describe, and interpret the underlying structure connecting numerous scale items and thereby to create conceptual order and empirical meaning (Fitzgerald and Hubert, 1987). Because many nursing and health care concepts are multidimensional,

a discussion of the appropriate scaling procedures to be used is in order. However, a thorough discussion must wait until a basic understanding of multivariate data reduction and analytical procedures is established. The topic will be pursued in Chapter 12.

5–16 TELEPHONE SURVEYS IN NURSING RESEARCH

Researchers are increasingly making use of the telephone for social, behavioral, educational, and health care studies. The increasing difficulty that investigators have had in gaining access to large city populations, partly because of the concerns of many inhabitants about physical violence, personal safety, and crime, has forced many survey researchers to seek other avenues of entrée. Furthermore, federal and private funding agencies have become more reluctant to fund projects heavily based on personal interview methodology. Telephone surveys cost less than interviews performed in person. Finally, the advent of technical procedures for computer-assisted telephone interviewing (CATI) has provided an impetus to use telephone survey methodology.

Miller (1983) suggests that the major reservations and problems with telephone surveys are being resolved rapidly. For instance, the overall coverage of telephones in the United States is about 90%, and sample sizes reachable by phone begin to approximate levels characteristically reached in typical mail surveys. The bias in statistics begins to shrink because 9 of every 10 households can be reached by phone. Household occupants in the survey can be identified, demographic information elicited, and respondents selected at the time of the call. Important sample characteristics can be more accurately and easily gathered and classified during the phone interview than from outdated directories or lists. Refusals to participate are a little higher than found in personal interviews but are at an acceptable level today. Finally, rechecking of information elicited first by phone queries and later verified through personal interviews suggests acceptable consistency when the same information is compared (Miller, 1983).

Increasingly, selection of samples in phone surveys is done through random-digit dialing (RDD). Random dialing refers to the selection of telephone numbers listed in a telephone book, a professional directory, or a telephone listing of subjects by specific categories such as members of civic, fraternal, or political groups and similar special sample aggregates. In general, a set of randomly chosen digits corresponds to working telephone numbers. Random samples of survey subjects can be gathered quickly. To be highly effective and cost-effective, RDD must use an up-to-date roster of survey subjects with an accurate description of attributes required for survey selection and participation. In tandem with CATI, a rapid selection of subjects and questioning of respondents can take place. Prerecorded introduction of the survey, its purposes, and treatment of information is presented as a standard stimulus to all telephone respondents. Furthermore, the ability to use many different closed-ended questions allows the data to be easily coded with predefined response categories, often directly onto a computer program for data reduction and statistical analyses. A detailed description of stratified random design and cluster designs used in RDD is provided by Groves and Kahn (1979). (See also Sections 6-10 and 6-12 for surveys using stratified random and cluster sampling designs.)

5-17 MAILED QUESTIONNAIRES IN NURSING RESEARCH

Mail surveys as a data collection technique are coming into vogue after a period of high use and subsequent disuse due to low response rates and other methodological problems. Mail questionnaires have a desirable appeal. After providing the addresses of research participants, all the tedious work of locating respondents is assumed by the United States Postal Service. The cost of mailing first class materials is the same throughout the United States; therefore, it is not more expensive to perform a national mail survey than to do a local survey. This is not true when trained interviewers must be flown to and housed and fed in different parts of the country to do a national survey or when a regional survey is being used. To keep expenses down, most major survey organizations employ local field staff.

If mail surveys reached their potential in practice, it would be doubtful that either face-to-face or telephone interviews would be used today. Users of mail surveys, however, have been hampered by low response rates. Furthermore, current and complete listings of the general public do not exist. Samples drawn from telephone directories, utilities lists, professional directories, and similar listings are usually incomplete.

Hope is not abandoned for mail surveys. Dillman (1978) has developed the Total Design Method (TDM), which employs the application of a standard set of mail procedures that achieves good response rates. Twenty-eight studies have used the TDM in its entirety and have produced an average response rate of 77% (Dillman, 1983, p. 360). These studies have used questionnaires containing from 1 to 26 pages, with the average length being 10 pages (Dillman, 1978). The TDM consists of two parts:

1. identifying and designing each aspect of the survey process so that they may affect response in a way that maximizes response rates; and,
2. organizing the survey effort in a way that assures that the design intentions are carried out in complete detail.

Manipulation of all aspects of a survey requires consistency. A basic assumption underlying the TDM is that a person is most likely to respond to a questionnaire when the perceived costs to the respondents are minimized, the perceived rewards are maximized, and the respondent trusts that the expected rewards will be delivered (Dillman, 1983, p. 361). All efforts directed toward potential respondents are aimed at stimulating the timely return of accurately completed instruments. Whether the respondents return the questionnaires depends on the overall evaluation they make of the survey rather than an isolated reaction to specific aspects of the survey.

Dillman proposes seven components in mailed questionnaire design:

1. The questionnaire is designed as a booklet, usually 6½ by 8¼ inches reduced from the originally typed version.

2. Resemblance to advertising formats is studiously avoided. The booklets are printed on white paper which is slightly lighter (16 versus 20 lb.) than that used in advertisements to reduce mailing costs.

3. No questions are printed on the first page, which is used for an interest-provoking title, a neutral but eye-catching illustration, and necessary instructions to respondents.

4. No questions are allowed on the last page. It is used to invite additional comments and to express appreciation to participants.

5. Questions are ordered so that the most interesting and topic-related questions (as explained in the accompanying letter) come first; potentially objectionable or sensitive questions are placed later and those requesting demographic information are placed last.

6. Specific attention is given to the first question; it should apply to everyone, it should be interesting, and it should be easy to answer.

7. Each page is formatted with great care. Lower case letters are used for questions and upper case letters are used for answers. To prevent respondents from skipping items, each page is designed so that whenever possible respondents can answer in a straight vertical line instead of moving back and forth across the page. Overlap of each question is avoided from page to page, especially on back to back pages. Transitions are used to prevent disconcerting surprises in much the same way that a face-to-face interviewer would warn of changes in topic. Only one question is asked at a time. Visual cues—arrows, indentations, spacing—are used to provide direction.

The TDM implementation process is as specific as that for questionnaire construction and formatting:

1. A one-page letter (on 10⅜ by 7 in. stationery) is prepared. It explains

a that a socially useful study is being conducted,

b why each respondent is important,

c who could complete the instrument.

The cover letter also promises confidentiality in conjunction with an identification system used to facilitate follow-up mailings. The mail questionnaire has no interviewer to stimulate interest in it or to compensate for any of its inadequacies. Therefore, the cover letter must do a superb selling job. It makes or breaks the survey!

2. The exact mailing date is added to the letter, which is then printed on the sponsoring agency's letterhead. Using official stationery informs the respondent that the survey is associated with a legitimate enterprise. In many instances, the status and prestige of the sponsoring organization sells the social usefulness of the project.

3. Individual names and addresses are typed on the printed letters in matching type, and the researcher's name is individually signed with a blue ballpoint pen using sufficient pressure to produce a slight indentation. Every effort must be made to ensure that the respondent perceives the letter to be individually prepared and that it does not appear to be a form letter prepared for a mass audience.

4. Questionnaires are stamped with an identification number, the presence of which is explained in the cover letter.

5. The mailout packet, consisting of a cover letter, questionnaire, and business reply stamped envelope (6⅜ by 3½ in.) is placed into a monarch size envelope (7⅜ by 3¾ in.) on which the recipient's name and address have been individually typed (address labels are never used) and first class postage affixed.

6. Exactly one week after the first mailout, a postcard follow-up reminder is sent to all recipients of the questionnaire.

7. Three weeks after the first mailout, a second cover letter and questionnaire are sent to all nonrespondents.

8. Seven weeks after the first mailout, a second cover letter complete with the original cover letter and replacement questionnaire is sent by certified mail.

Dillman assures those who follow exactly the above questionnaire design and mailing and follow-up procedure that their return rates will be in the 70% to 80% range. The typical problems as well as shortcuts that survey researchers have taken in the past have been well identified and handled in the above outlined procedures. A nurse planning to use a mailed questionnaire would be well advised to heed Dillman's carefully planned and worked-out mail survey technique. In reviewing these steps it should be manifestly clear at this juncture that it is impossible to throw a questionnaire together in a day or a week. Whether the instrument is to be administered in person, by telephone query, or through the mails, great care must be exercised at all stages to ensure that the instrument asks the pertinent questions and provides a response format that participants find convenient, interesting, and engaging.

5–18 ADVANTAGES AND LIMITATIONS OF MAIL AND TELEPHONE SURVEYS

Despite the best efforts and most carefully implemented protocol, mail surveys have distinct limitations. One major issue is the difficulty of accessing a representative sample of a particular population. Traditionally, telephone directories, city directories, driver's license files, utilities lists, and subscription and periodical lists have been employed. The chief problem with telephone directories is that many persons do not have telephones and many of those who have telephones, particularly in urban areas, pay fees to have their telephone unlisted. It has been estimated that up to 30% to 40% of persons in large cities do not have listings in directories. Also those with listings may have telephone answering machines, which preclude telephone queries or follow-up.

Professional directories frequently contain up-to-date listings of specialized populations such as doctors, nurses, social workers, psychologists, clergy, and others. Many professionals, however, do not belong to national, regional, or local associations. Furthermore, depending on the purposes of the survey, professional associations are protective of members and the perceived turf of their respective constituencies. McLaughlin and colleagues (1978) found it difficult to get national and regional listings of physicians in the American Academy of Family Practice Directory. The study's purposes were to compare the performance of nurse practitioners with that of physicians in the assess-

ment and treatment of chronic illnesses. When listings were finally forthcoming, McLaughlin's investigative group found that about 20% of physicians listed had moved in the previous year. In many cases, mail soliciting participation was not forwarded because no other address was listed with postal authorities.

Another disadvantage of mailed surveys is that a larger proportion of those who refuse to be surveyed are probably persons with lower education and negative response sets. Another problem is the difficulty of handling certain kinds of questions such as open-ended items. Responses to open-ended questions in mail surveys are likely to be terse, difficult to interpret, and more likely than closed-ended questions to be omitted. Questionnaires that must rely principally on open-ended responses should be carried out by some method other than through the mails. Still another difficulty with mail questionnaires is the time it takes to set up and follow through (a minimum of two months), particularly along the explicit lines advocated by Dillman (1978).

5–19 SUMMARY

It should be clear that there are no simple, rigorous rules for questionnaire design, question writing, scaling of items, and the interpretative rules used to fashion meaning from diverse informant responses. Each survey presents new opportunities and different challenges. Each instrument is part of an overall research design, with its own particular goals and objectives and special sample characteristics. The mode of data collection and analysis is specific to the project's mission. Because of the instrument's being developed to meet overall survey objectives and not to control it, the wide variety of survey purposes dictates that the rules be flexible. In the end, a good survey instrument is the product of hard intellectual effort over a sustained period.

REFERENCES

Dawis, R.V.: Scale construction, J. Couns. Psych., *34*: 481–489, 1987.

Dillman, D.A.: Mail and Telephone Surveys. New York, Wiley-Interscience, 1978.

Dillman, D.A.: Mail and other self-administered questionnaires. In Rossi, P.H., Wright, J.D., and Anderson, A.B., eds., Handbook of Survey Research. New York, John Wiley & Sons, 1983.

Dixon, W.J., ed.: BMDP Statistical Software. Berkeley, CA, University of California Press, 1983.

Fitzgerald, L.F., and Hubert, L.J.: Multidimensional scaling: some possibilities for counseling psychology, J. Couns. Psych., 34: 469–480, 1987.

Fox, D.J.: Fundamentals of Research in Nursing. New York, Appleton-Century-Crofts, 1982.

Groves, R.M., and Kahn, R.I.: Surveys by Telephone. New York, Academic Press, 1979.

Guttman, L.A.: A basis for scaling quantitative data, Am. Sociol. Rev., 9: 139–150, 1944.

Hage, J.: An axiomatic theory of organizations, Administr. Sci. Q., 10: 289–320, 1965.

Hetherington, R.W., and Rundall, T.G.: The social structure of work groups. In Shortell, S.M., and Kalunzy, A.D., eds., Health Care Management. New York, John Wiley & Sons, 1983.

Likert, R.: A technique for the measurement of attitudes, Arch. Psychol., no. 140, 1932.

McLaughlin, F.E., et al.: Primary Care Judgments of Nurses and Physicians, vols. 1–4. Springfield, VA, National Technical Information Service, 1978–79.

Miller, D.C.: Handbook of Research Design and Social Measurement. New York, Longman, 1983.

Mueller, D.J.: Measuring Social Attitudes: Handbook for Researchers and Practitioners. New York, Teachers College Press, 1986.

National Research Council: Survey Measurement of Subjective Phenomenon, vols. 1 & 2. Washington, DC, National Academy Press, 1983.

Nutting, M.A.: A statistical report of working hours in training schools. New York, Proceedings of the American Society of Superintendents of Training Schools, 1896.

Osgood, C.E., Succi, C.J., and Tannenbaum, P.H.: The Measurement of Meaning. Urbana, University of Illinois Press, 1957.

Rossi, P.H., Wright, J.D., and Anderson, A.B.: Handbook of Survey Research. New York, John Wiley & Sons, 1983.

Selltiz, C., Wrightsman, L.S., and Cook, S.W.: Research Methods in Social Relations. New York, Holt, Rinehart & Winston, 1976.

Sheatsley, P.B.: Questionnaire construction and item writing. In Rossi, P.H., Wright, J.D., and Anderson, A.B., eds., Handbook of Survey Research. New York, Academic Press, 1983.

Snider, J.G., and Osgood, C.E., eds.: Semantic Differential Technique: A Sourcebook. Hawthorne, NY, Aldine, 1969.

SPSS Inc.: SPSS* User's Guide, ed. 2. New York, McGraw-Hill, 1986.

Waltz, C.F., Strickland, O.L., and Lenz, E.R.: Measurement in Nursing Research. Philadelphia, F.A. Davis, 1984.

Warner, S.L.: Randomized responses: a survey technique for eliminating evasive answer bias, Am. Statist. Assoc., 60: 63–69, 1965.

Chapter 6

SURVEY SAMPLING METHODS FOR NURSING RESEARCH

6–1 THE ROLE OF SAMPLING IN NURSING RESEARCH

After the primary problems encountered in defining constructs and designing methods for measuring the qualities and quantities of the concepts for nursing research, the next most difficult problem facing the nurse investigator is that of choosing a sample to observe, measure, and use for estimating and testing hypotheses about population characteristics. In this chapter, we examine sampling techniques associated with probability and nonprobability selection schemes for nursing studies using survey sampling methods. In addition, principles of ethics and informed consent are examined. The randomized response technique which has been developed for studying sensitive and embarrassing behaviors in human populations is illustrated. Finally, an example of a survey sample and procedure for estimating the costs of conducting a mail survey is provided.

6-2 ETHICAL CONSIDERATIONS AND INFORMED CONSENT PRACTICES

At the forefront of nursing research are the constant issues associated with confidentiality of subject response and informed consent. These topics have a significant history, which begins with the heinous medical experiments conducted on political prisoners in German concentration camps and prisoners in American prisons and also on patients in mental hospitals (Smith, 1977). Because of the inhumane treatment given to unwilling and unknowing subjects, a number of national and international organizations such as the United States Department of Health and Human Services (DHHS) and the United Nations World Health Organization (WHO) have formulated directives on the role which health personnel and health organizations *must* assume in the conduct of research on both humans and animals (Katz, 1972). Foremost in the United States are the guidelines developed by the National Institutes of Health, DHHS on the protection of the rights of humans in the conduct of biomedical research. These guidelines apply equally to the conduct of basic medical and behavioral science research in health care organizations and academic institutions.

Every health care organization that receives federal funds must file a statement with the DHHS as to the procedures and processes followed by that organization in both the review and conduct of all human and animal research performed by personnel representing the health organization. In addition, these guidelines apply to all facilities owned, operated, or leased by the organizations. As a basic minimum, each organization must establish an Institutional Review Board (IRB) composed of reputable health researchers and practitioners from diverse disciplines, a biomedical ethicist, a lawyer skilled in legal medical issues, clergy, and patients or patient representatives (Gortner, 1981).

The Institutional Review Board, which is most often called the Committee on Human Research in health facilities is charged with the formal review of all research applications and all research conducted under the auspices of the institution. All research applications must be accompanied by an informed consent protocol which details the following in laymen's terms:

1. the purposes of the project
2. the risks versus the benefits accruing to the patient or research participant
3. the freedom of the patient or participant to withdraw without adverse effects at any time during the history of the project
4. the name, address, and telephone numbers of the principle investigator and staff
5. provisions for the research investigator's signature and the patient's or legal guardian's signature
6. provision for the signature of a witness verifying that the signature was freely given.

Stringent guidelines for informed consent procedures are available from health agencies, research organizations, academic institutions, and funding agencies to be followed when human subjects are the source of experimental or research data. These guidelines are especially strict and carefully worded with respect to children and to persons who are mentally ill, incarcerated, or unconscious. No study using human subjects should be conducted that does not consider these ethical and legal issues, problems, and their contingencies. It should be noted that exemptions to the stringent requirements mandated by the Institutional Review Board exist. For example, administrative surveys or evaluation of educational programs which are normally part of the quality assurance process in health and educational institutions typically do not fall within the purview of the Institutional Review Board. It is a wise and prudent procedure, however, to submit all evaluative and administrative survey protocols for review and to have them officially acknowledged in writing as not needing IRB approval or surveillance.

Careful thought must be given to the wording of informed consent documents. In many nursing investigations, it is recommended that a research nurse seek the services of a biomedical ethics expert or of a professional lawyer who is knowledgeable in biomedical research issues. In all instances, before a research proposal is submitted for review, an Institutional Review Board should have the opportunity to check the proposal to see whether informed consent is adequately covered and whether the safeguards to confidentiality are sound, defensible, and possible so that the study can be undertaken and successfully completed. Protection must be guaranteed for all participants and all personnel involved in working on the study. Finally, the organization that is funding or sponsoring the study must be protected against future ethical and legal actions resulting from breach of confidentiality or resulting from bodily harm or psychological trauma to participants. Sources of information on informed consent procedures are:

1. American Nurses' Association: Human Rights Guidelines for Nurses in Clinical and Other Research, Kansas City, MO, American Nurses' Association, 1975.

2. Code of Federal Regulations: Title 45. Part 46, Washington, DC, January 26, 1981.

3. United States DHHS: The Institutional Guide to DHEW Policy on Protection of Human Subjects, Washington, DC, US Government Printing Office, 1971.

4. US National Commission for the Protection of Human Subjects of Biomedical and Behavioral Research: The Belmont Report: Ethical Principles and Guidelines for the Protection of Human Subjects of Research. DHEW Publication Number (05) 78-0012, Washington, DC, US Government Printing Office, 1978.

Each project extending over a period of one year must be reviewed annually to see that the informed consent procedures are followed. All significant problems identified by the research investigator must be addressed, and acceptable remedies must be offered by the investigator and concurred with by the committee in the annual review. The Institutional Review Board is charged with the responsibility of notifying the administration of the health care organization and the federal funding agency about violations compromising the bodily welfare or psychological integrity of research subjects. Projects are halted, funds withdrawn, and personnel disciplined when major infractions occur and are not remedied in good faith and in a timely, ethically sound manner.

To illustrate some of the principles identified in the preceding discussion, let us examine a hypothetical study of the sexual practices of bisexual men. The confidentiality protocols and informed consent procedures must be stringently developed without question in order to preclude the identification of sample members of the general society of family, work, church, police, law agencies, banks, military, government agencies,

and health and welfare agencies. Names and addresses of bisexual men on a roster provide a potentially dangerous document for blackmail and social censure. If placed in the wrong hands, a document of this sensitive nature could ruin the lives of many men by persons who have religious, social, or political opposition to bisexual behavior. Also at issue are the possible dangers of exposing respondents to high risks of psychological trauma or bodily harm.

6–3 NONPROBABILITY SAMPLING SCHEMES

An examination of the research literature in nursing science may lead one to believe that the greatest number of studies in nursing research makes use of nonprobability sampling schemes in *observational* settings. Observational studies include correlational studies, exploratory investigations, descriptive studies, hypothesis generating studies, and field research. Typically, these types of studies are performed on nonprobability samples, which are frequently referred to as *chunks* or *convenience samples*.

An example of an observational study using a chunk sampling scheme is described here. Consider a study in which the main interest centers on nurses' attitudes to caring for patients who are human immune virus-positive (HIV-positive). One way to obtain a sample for this type of study is to identify a hospital or nursing care center that is known to treat a large number of patients who are HIV-positive. After a health care site known to be experiencing a large number of cases has been selected, a sample of study subjects can be gathered from the patients.

Suppose that several units in a large tertiary hospital (research teaching hospital) are chosen to be the focus of the study. One problem with the study is that the selection factors that bring patients to the site are unknown and so there is no way to know whether the admitted patients represent a cross-section of all HIV-positive adults. As a consequence, the resulting patients to be observed represent a mixed group of HIV-positive persons for which generalization of chunk sample findings to a population is problematic.

For this hypothetical study, suppose that

the independent variables are knowledge of the HIV status of the patients and treating nurses. This type of study represents a *two-factor fully crossed design*, consisting of patients who are either aware or not aware of their HIV status and nurses who are either aware or not aware of the HIV status of the patients. This design is illustrated here.

Two by two factor design of HIV status awareness by nurses and patients.

| | | Awareness by Nurse | |
		Known	Unknown
Awareness by Patient	Known		
	Unknown		

Suppose that the dependent variables of the study consist of the number and types of nurse and patient verbal encounters. The observational protocol will note whether nurses are supportive, compassionate, sensitive, open, and helpful in assisting patients to cope with their presenting health problems.

In a study of this type, one could make full use of the patients that are admitted to the patient care unit over a specified time period. In theory a researcher could impose the four conditions of the design upon the patients by using a random process assignment scheme, but in practice such a study could not be performed today because of ethical considerations and informed consent procedures.

Data could be collected for this study by a participant observer who accompanies a nurse in the performance of typical nursing duties in the unit. For nurse-initiated encounters, records can be kept of the amount and type of interaction between the nurse and specific patients. In like manner, it can be noted when patients initiate interpersonal actions with specific nurses. Types of interpersonal transactions can be recorded. Verbatim conversations and comments between nurses and patients need to be transcribed. These data can be used to generate hypotheses about nurse behavior and knowledge of HIV health status by nurses and patients. On the basis of the collected data, the following research propositions can be tested and examined:

1. The communication styles of nurses who are aware of the HIV status of patients differ from the communication styles of nurses who are unaware of the HIV status of patients.

2. The communication styles of patients who are aware of their HIV status differ from the communication styles of patients who are unaware of their HIV status.

3. There is a statistical interaction between nurses' awareness of patients' HIV status and the patients' awareness of their own HIV status.

In this particular investigation, the study most likely possesses internal validity but not external validity. The study should be extended to other settings to learn whether the same findings can be reproduced with patients in other cities and with patients who represent different social and ethnic groups. In addition, the study should be reproduced in nonteaching and nonresearch health care settings to see whether the findings are applicable to other health care settings. With repeated investigation, nonprobability sampling schemes can be used to make inferences or draw conclusions about independent and dependent variables in nursing research.

Another example of a nonprobability approach is the use of a convenience sample such as that described in Chapter 1 for the preoperative teaching study. In this study, the convenience sample is transformed into a randomized sample by using probabilities to assign subjects to three different treatments. The advantage to this type of investigation is that a researcher has the opportunity to defend internal validity but not necessarily external validity (discussed in Chapter 4). In this case, a convenience sampling scheme is probably the only method of collecting data that can be used to test the hypotheses under investigation. In fact, it might be the best type of sample to use for this kind of investigation.

Another example of the use of a convenience sampling in nursing research is provided in the *snowballing technique*. With this type of sampling, an initial group of subjects is obtained for study. These subjects are then asked to nominate or identify similar subjects for inclusion in the study. An example of such a study is one in which:

1. the *sample frame* or list of subjects is nonexistent,

2. the members of the population are few in number, and

3. the subjects are not easily identified in the universe of interest.

An example of a study that satisfies all three conditions that support the decision to use a snowball sampling technique is one in which AIDS (acquired immunodeficiency syndrome) researchers want to sample bisexual men. Researchers ask the following two questions:

1. What are your sexual practices with both men and women?

2. Do you and your partners practice safe sex?

First, a list of bisexual men that can be sampled does not exist. Second, in a fixed local area, like a suburban bedroom community adjacent to a large city, the absolute number of population members is likely to be small. Third, because of contemporary social mores, bisexual behavior is generally perceived as a departure from acceptable community standards, making the identification of bisexual men difficult.

One way to obtain a snowball sample is to place ads in local newspapers announcing the purposes of the study and asking for bisexual men to volunteer information about their sex practices. Other subjects may be referred to the study through professional solicitations by mail or telephone contact with psychotherapists, sex counselors, and self-help groups in the community. The immediate respondents will be few in number. One way to snowball the sample is to ask the initial set of respondents to contact friends and acquaintances known to be bisexual and suggest that they join the study as informants on sexual practices. With the expanding network of contacts, a large enough sample can be generated.

The problem with this type of nonprobability sampling and with all nonprobability sampling is that bias is fairly certain to exist in the data. In this illustration, all the information is obtained from men who are willing to speak about very personal and intimate experiences, which are generally treated as private information by most persons. Checking the veracity of the statements may be difficult, expensive, or impossible. A researcher might develop a set of interrelated questions that can provide cross-checks to specific answers. Although biased estimates of sexual behavior may be generated, common and uncommon practices can be identified, described, classified, and correlated with other factors in the lives of the informants. Most likely internal validity is compromised in such a study; however, the information should be useful in opening other avenues for research and investigation which could eventually result in saving human lives.

Another nonprobability sampling scheme that is frequently encountered in nursing research is the *quota sampling method*. With this sampling procedure, a researcher specifies the number of subjects to be included in each category or class that defines the independent variable of the study. For example, a researcher may decide that a study involving single men, single women, married men, and married women should be made with 50 subjects in each group. To achieve this goal, subjects would be sampled until 50 are in each group. If no probability selection rules are used to define or identify the sample members, the problems of bias remain. There is no way to know whether the sample is *representative* of the groups to which inferences are to be drawn.

An important message is in these examples for the nurse researcher who uses nonprobability sampling or nonrandomization of subjects to experimental conditions. Statistical tests rarely can be applied to the data and used to generalize from the sample to the universe of interest. Immediately the question is raised: What can a researcher do to extract usable information from a nonprobability sample? From a statistical inferential point of view—very little. All statistical procedures that involve hypothesis testing are based on probability models. If the sampling does not involve probability models, formal statistical tests are not valid.

In the nonprobability sampling schemes, descriptive methods come to the forefront. With nonprobability sampling, a researcher is thoroughly justified in providing means, medians, standard deviations, ratios, correlation coefficients, percentages, and similar descriptive statistics to summarize the resulting data. Graphical methods like those seen in Chapter 8 can also be called on to provide visual displays of data and demonstrate relationships among variables in the sample. All verbal descriptions about the sample are valid, provided that (1) they describe the sample in unambiguous terms and

(2) another interpreter can arrive at the same conclusions when making an independent assessment of the specific sample data.

Using these descriptive measures to test inferential hypotheses about group differences or to assess the statistical significance of the correlations between variables is not justified. Description is the method of analysis for these kinds of studies, and the only method that can be done with justification.

Evaluation of nonprobability sampling models should not be viewed as opposition to their use. In much of nursing research only these kinds of studies can be done because sensitive issues are often involved in health studies or because small populations are difficult, if not impossible, to sample. Yet, these populations must be studied if nursing knowledge is to grow and advance.

Simple random sampling, a topic discussed in Section 6–5, is not always necessary for inference making if it can be shown that the sample is a good descriptor of the population from which it is said to be a member. This means that a researcher who uses a nonprobability sampling has the added responsibility of providing in a report or journal article a *detailed description* of the sample. This way each reader can assess the findings individually and can bring information to the analysis which the original researcher may not have had. (For more on this and related topics, see the articles by Serlin, 1987, Serlin and Lapsley, 1985, and by Kruskal and Mosteller, 1979.)

With nonprobability quota sampling schemes, a researcher can sometimes justify a statistical test of a hypothesis, provided that the inference is limited or constrained by the principle of internal consistency. That is, it is possible to make a statistical analysis of the sample, to test hypotheses about the sample, and to draw conclusions about the sample, but not about the population.

Such analyses are referred to as *conditional analyses*, and the statistical tests are referred to as *conditional tests*. Many nonparametric tests are conditional tests.

As an illustration in which a conditional test can be applied, consider a study on the use of contraceptives by single men and women and married men and women. In this study, suppose that each subgroup is sampled until 50 members are selected. After each of the four quotas are satisfied, each member is asked:

> Who assumes the responsibility in deciding whether or not to use contraceptives when having sex? I do ___ . My partner does ___ .

Results might be as shown in Table 6–1. The hypothesis to be tested on these data is

$$H_0: P_1 = P_2 = P_3 = P_4$$

where P_g = proportion of subjects who say "I do" in group g, where g = 1, 2, 3, and 4.

If this sample of 200 subjects were randomly selected from the separate four populations under the study, the Karl Pearson Test of Homogeneity (described in Section 13–2) would be performed and a direct inference to the four populations could be made on the basis of this test. Because we are not assured of population representation, that is not possible. The Karl Pearson test can be justified as a conditional test that applies directly to the specific 200 subjects sampled via the quota sampling scheme. If the Karl Pearson test leads to a rejection of the hypothesis, a researcher is justified in concluding that the proportions of respondents who say "I do" differ across the four groups of subjects in the study. In any case, however, the conclusion cannot be extended to the four populations. Any conclusion must be a conditional conclusion that is valid only for the members of the sample.

TABLE 6–1 RESPONSES OF SINGLE MEN AND WOMEN AND MARRIED MEN AND WOMEN*

Response	Single Men	Married Men	Single Women	Married Women
I do	30	10	40	5
My partner	10	40	10	45
Total	50	50	50	50

*Responses to the question, Who makes the decision to use contraceptives?
   I do ___ . My partner does ___ .

6–4 PROBABILITY SAMPLING SCHEMES

Besides survey sampling models, the use of probability sampling schemes for nursing research is difficult to attain. To use a probability model a researcher must have an up-to-date roster of the entire population from which to select the sample or samples. Such rosters are frequently nonexistent in the study of human populations. Thus, a number of alternatives have been proposed to overcome the problems encountered by not having a roster in advance of sample selection. In this section, we describe a few procedures that can be used to generate probability samples in very specific settings involving either experimental or observational research.

In the preoperative teaching study, probability samples can be assigned to one of three experimental treatments by using a randomization device such as the flipping of coins, the rolling of a die, or the use of a table of random numbers. Suppose that the decision to assign a patient to a particular treatment is to be based on the role of a die. After a subject is admitted to the study, a die is rolled and the number appearing on top is used to assign the subject to a specific treatment group. If a one or a two appears, the subject is assigned to treatment one. If a three or a four appears, the subject is assigned to treatment two. Finally, if a five or a six appears, the subject is assigned to treatment three. Thus, each subject has one chance in three of being assigned to any one of the three treatment groups. Because the tosses of the die are independent, the requirements of probability sampling are immediately satisfied. For a probability sampling, all assignments must be independent and the probabilities of assignment must be equal for all subjects.

In an observational study concerned with the changing roles of men's and women's responsibilities in child rearing activities, a nurse investigator chose to observe the naturally occurring behavior of two-parent families with one child when leaving or returning to a car at a shopping mall. The investigator picked one day per week at random and one hour between 9 AM and 9 PM for observation at random. Thus, each day had one chance in seven of serving as an observation period and each hour had one chance in twelve of serving as an observation period. One hundred two-parent, one-child families were observed during the course of the randomly selected day–hour periods. The researcher hypothesized that the division of responsibility for monitoring the child's leaving and returning to the car would be equally shared. Operationally this means that about 50% of the women were expected to hold the child's hand and 50% of the men would do likewise when leaving and returning to the car. In practice, it was observed that about 80% of the women held the child's hand when leaving and returning to the car, regardless of the sex of the child.

Here, probability sampling has been introduced by selecting days and hours at random using a table of random numbers. The independence of the observations might be an issue, but does not represent an important consideration in this instance. It is difficult to identify a systematic biasing mechanism that would produce a nonprobability sample in this type of study. The behavior of each family is presumably independent of all other families that enter the mall. It may be true that the observational units represent similar middle class families, but by cutting across all 12 hours of the day, 7 days of the week, a probability sampling of the users of the mall should be guaranteed.

As these examples illustrate, a researcher often must use ingenuity to produce a probability sample for nursing studies. In the following sections, we detail the classic probability schemes usable when a roster is available for selecting samples from a population of research interest. Many principles described in the subsequent sections can also be used by a nurse researcher in selecting samples to study using various research strategies and designs discussed in other chapters of the text.

6–5 SIMPLE PROBABILITY RANDOM SAMPLING FOR ESTIMATING A POPULATION MEAN

We begin the discussion on sampling procedures by first discussing *simple random sampling*. Simple random sampling serves as the common denominator of all probability sampling schemes. Other sampling procedures are based in one form or another on the principles of simple random sampling. Although simple random sampling is rarely used, understanding it aids in evaluating other sampling methods that are more commonly used in survey research. Much of what appears in the remainder of this chapter is based on the presentation of Hansen, Hurwitz, and Madow (1953; 1962). (For a more complete discussion on sampling theory consult these sources.)

As an aid to the reader, some basic terms are defined, which are used to describe the various sampling models illustrated in this chapter. The persons or units whose characteristics are to be measured are called the *elementary units*. Typical elementary units in health research are patients, nurses, doctors, hospitals, and like units. The aggregate of the elementary units constitute the *population* or *universe*. The sample of elementary units are selected from the population and are denoted by the N values, $[y_1, y_2, \ldots, y_N]$. The population of elementary units are denoted by the M values $[Y_1, Y_2, \ldots, Y_M]$. As indicated, in what follows N always refers to sample sizes and M always refers to population sizes. A sample of N elementary units is called a *simple random sample* if each combination of N elementary units has the same chance or probability of being selected as any other combination of N elementary units.

As an example, consider the data of Table 6–2. These data represent a universe of M = 8 nurses working in four different hospitals located in two different geographical areas. Also shown is the number of years each nurse has been employed as a professional. Suppose that a health researcher wanted to select a simple random sample of size N = 2 from the population of M = 8 nurses and then use the data to determine the mean length of employment, not for just the two nurses sampled, but for all M = 8 nurses that constitute the population. This can be done with simple random sampling if the researcher ignores all other information concerning the nurses when making the selection. Under this condition, no attention is paid to hospital of employment nor to the geographical region in which each nurse lives. In simple random sampling, such information is superfluous, unimportant, and extraneous.

The purpose of using this small population of nurses is strictly pedagogical; that is, it is used to describe and illustrate the many sampling models that are available for survey research. In practice, the populations may involve hundreds or even thousands of elementary units. In addition, the sample sizes will most likely be 200 to 2000 elementary units. Even so, the characteristics of the various models can be understood with a small number of 8 nurses. Remember that the goal is to provide understanding about various sampling schemes so that when a nurse plans a study, informed decisions can be made as to the best way to proceed.

6–6 PROPERTIES OF STATISTICAL ESTIMATORS AND METHODS USED TO EVALUATE DIFFERENT SAMPLING METHODS

One way to understand sampling theory is to consider the *universe of samples* that could be generated by a study. In practice the sample actually selected is only one of the large number of samples that could be selected. Consider simple random sampling as an example. The complete list of N = 2 sim-

TABLE 6–2 AN ARTIFICIAL POPULATION OF M = 8 NURSES EMPLOYED IN FOUR HOSPITALS IN TWO GEOGRAPHICAL REGIONS

Region	Hospital	Nurse	Years of Employment
Northern	One	Alice	6
		Bob	2
	Two	Carol	7
Southern	Three	Donald	9
		Elvira	4
	Four	Frank	12
		Grace	10
		Hilda	3

ple random samples that can be generated for the M = 8 nurses is shown in Table 6–3. There are 28 such samples. The first of the possible samples that could be selected consists of Alice and Bob, (A, B), and the last of the possible samples consists of Grace and Hilda, (G, H). Suppose that the sample consisting of Carol and Hilda, (C, H), had actually been selected. The mean years of employment for these two nurses is given as $\bar{Y} = 1/2(7 + 3) = 5$ years. This would be the estimate of the mean for the entire population. In this case, the estimate would be in error because the population mean defined as

$$\mu_Y = \frac{1}{M}(Y_1 + Y_2 + \ldots + Y_M)$$

is equal to

$$\mu_Y = 1/8(6 + 2 + 7 + 9 \\ + 4 + 12 + 10 + 3) = 6.625.$$

It should be noted that any sample of size N = 2 selected from the population is going to produce an estimate of μ_Y that is unquestionably in error. This is apparent in the mean values listed in Table 6–3. None is equal to 6.625. They range from a low of 2.5 years to a high of 11.0 years. Even so, note that 50% are in the narrow range of 5.0 years to 8.0 years, values close to 6.625. Thus, even though *none* is equal to the true population mean, *most* are fairly close to the true value, considering that each mean is based on only two observations.

To evaluate different sampling designs, a number of properties are examined that characterize estimators as good or bad. In particular, estimates are desired that give the correct answer on the average, are cost-efficient, and in large samples are very close to the population values. These three properties are termed unbiasedness, efficiency, and consistency.

Unbiased Estimators

The mean value of the 28 means reported in Table 6–3 is equal to 6.625 years. This mean is identical with the mean of the population. The example provides a demonstration of an important statistical concept useful in understanding survey research methodology. If a sampling scheme produces overall possible samples, a mean value that is equal to the numerical value being estimated in the original population, that is, the statistic that is used to estimate the population value, is said to be an *unbiased* estimate of the unknown true population value. Thus, we would conclude that the *mean* of a simple random sample of size N = 2 is an unbiased estimator of the population mean.

Now consider samples of size N = 3. The complete list is presented in Table 6–4. Note that the number of possible samples has increased from 28 to 56. This increase is very dramatic in large universes with large samples. As sample sizes increase, the number of possible samples can increase to the billions and trillions, but only one is ever selected. Hopefully, it is a true representative

TABLE 6–3 ALL POSSIBLE SIMPLE RANDOM SAMPLES OF SIZE N = 2 THAT CAN BE GENERATED FROM THE POPULATION OF TABLE 6–2

Sample	Years of Employment	$\bar{Y}$	Sample	Years of Employment	$\bar{Y}$
A, B	6, 2	4.0	C, E	7, 4	5.5
A, C	6, 7	6.5	C, F	7, 12	9.5
A, D	6, 9	7.5	C, G	7, 10	8.5
A, E	6, 4	5.0	C, H	7, 3	5.0
A, F	6, 12	9.0	D, E	9, 4	6.5
A, G	6, 10	8.0	D, F	9, 12	10.5
A, H	6, 3	4.5	D, G	9, 10	9.5
B, C	2, 7	4.5	D, H	9, 3	6.0
B, D	2, 9	5.5	E, F	4, 12	8.0
B, E	2, 4	3.0	E, G	4, 10	7.0
B, F	2, 12	7.0	E, H	4, 3	3.5
B, G	2, 10	6.0	F, G	12, 10	11.0
B, H	2, 3	2.5	F, H	12, 3	7.5
C, D	7, 9	8.0	G, H	10, 3	6.5

TABLE 6–4 SIMPLE RANDOM SAMPLES OF SIZE N = 3 GENERATED FROM THE POPULATION OF TABLE 6–2

Sample	Years of Employment	$\bar{Y}$	Sample	Years of Employment	$\bar{Y}$
A, B, C	6, 2, 7	5.00	B, D, G	2, 9, 10	7.00
A, B, D	6, 6, 7	5.67	B, D, H	2, 9, 3	4.67
A, B, E	6, 2, 4	4.00	B, E, F	2, 4, 12	6.00
A, B, F	6, 2, 12	6.67	B, E, G	2, 4, 10	5.33
A, B, G	6, 2, 10	6.00	B, E, H	2, 4, 3	3.00
A, B, H	6, 2, 3	3.67	B, F, G	2, 12, 10	8.00
A, C, D	6, 7, 9	7.33	B, F, H	2, 12, 3	5.67
A, C, E	6, 7, 4	5.00	B, G, H	2, 10, 3	5.00
A, C, F	6, 7, 12	8.33	C, D, E	7, 9, 4	6.33
A, C, G	6, 7, 10	7.67	C, D, F	7, 9, 12	9.33
A, C, H	6, 7, 3	5.33	C, D, G	7, 9, 10	8.67
A, D, E	6, 9, 4	6.67	C, D, H	7, 9, 3	6.33
A, D, F	6, 9, 12	9.00	C, E, F	7, 4, 12	7.67
A, D, G	6, 9, 10	8.33	C, E, G	7, 4, 10	7.00
A, D, H	6, 9, 3	6.00	C, E, H	7, 4, 3	4.67
A, E, F	6, 4, 12	7.33	C, F, G	7, 4, 10	7.00
A, E, G	6, 4, 10	6.67	C, F, H	7, 4, 3	4.67
A, E, H	6, 4, 3	4.33	C, G, H	7, 10, 3	6.67
A, F, G	6, 12, 10	9.33	D, E, F	9, 4, 12	8.33
A, F, H	6, 12, 3	7.00	D, E, G	9, 4, 10	7.67
A, G, H	6, 10, 3	6.33	D, E, H	9, 4, 3	5.33
B, C, D	2, 7, 9	6.00	D, F, G	9, 12, 10	10.33
B, C, E	2, 7, 4	4.33	D, F, H	9, 12, 3	8.00
B, C, F	2, 7, 12	7.00	D, G, H	9, 10, 3	7.33
B, C, G	2, 7, 10	6.33	E, F, G	4, 12, 10	8.67
B, C, H	2, 7, 3	4.00	E, F, H	4, 12, 3	6.33
B, D, E	2, 9, 4	5.00	E, G, H	4, 10, 3	5.67
B, D, F	2, 9, 12	7.67	F, G, H	12, 10, 3	8.33

of the population. For the 8-nurse universe, the mean value of the 56 means listed in Table 6–4 is equal to 6.625, the mean of the population. This shows that, at least for this example, the mean of a simple random sample of size N = 3 is also an unbiased estimator of the population mean. As might be expected, it can be shown that *any* simple random sample of *any* size provides an estimate of a population mean that is unbiased. This is one of the main characteristics and advantages gained in the use of simple random samples. The mean values generated from simple random samples are unbiased estimators of the population mean values.

Efficient Estimators

Consider the range in mean values for samples of size N = 3. In this example, it is seen that the smallest mean is 3.0 and the largest mean is 10.33. Both of these extreme values are closer to the population value of 6.625 than were the means provided by the extreme samples for N = 2. This is expected because when N = 3, 37.5% of the population is in the sample, whereas when N = 2, only 25% is included in the sample. The higher level of *precision* is also seen in the fact that 50% of the means are between 5.33 and 7.67 for samples of size N = 3. This range is smaller than that for N = 2. Thus, a sample of size N = 3 has a better chance of providing an estimate that is closer to the true value than is a sample of size N = 2. In practice, a large sample is more likely to be closer to the population value than is a small sample. This agrees with our intuitive notion that a large sample is better than a small sample.

Another way to assess the precision of a sampling scheme is to measure the variation in the complete set of possible estimates. A good measure of homogeneity is the population variance. For simple random sampling, it can be shown that the variance of the set of all possible means is given as

$$\sigma_{\bar{Y}}^2 = \frac{\sigma_Y^2}{N}\left(\frac{M - N}{M - 1}\right)$$

where σ_Y^2 is the variance of the original population. By definition the variance of a population of M values is given as

$$\sigma_Y^2 = \frac{1}{M} \sum_{m=1}^{M} (Y_m - \mu_Y)^2$$

For the eight nurses of Table 6–2, the population variance is equal to

$$\sigma_Y^2 = 1/8[(6 - 6.625)^2 + (2 - 6.625)^2 \\ + \ldots + (3 - 6.625)^2] \\ = 10.9844$$

Thus, for the samples of size N = 2 reported in Table 6–3, the variance is given as

$$\sigma_{\bar{Y}}^2 = \frac{10.9844}{2} \left(\frac{8 - 2}{8 - 1} \right) = 4.7076$$

whereas for the samples of size N = 3 reported in Table 6–4, the variance is given as

$$\sigma_{\bar{Y}}^2 = \frac{10.9844}{3} \left(\frac{8 - 3}{8 - 1} \right) = 2.6153$$

As shown, the means for samples of size N = 3 are more homogeneous than are the means for samples of size N = 2. This shows that samples of size N = 3 provide more precise estimates of μ_Y than do samples of size N = 2. In agreement with our intuition, large samples provide estimates that are more precise than small samples.

This example illustrates a second important statistical property of survey sampling. If one has two ways of estimating the same population characteristic, the estimator with the smaller variance computed across all possible samples is said to be the *efficient estimator* and is the preferred estimator. Sampling schemes are rated in terms of their efficiencies, E. The rating is done in terms of the following ratio:

$$E = \frac{\sigma_2^2}{\sigma_1^2}$$

where the denominator, σ_1^2, is the variance of the estimator with the smaller variance. For our example, $\sigma_1^2 = 2.6153$ and $\sigma_2^2 = 4.7076$. With these values,

$$E = 4.7076/2.6153 = 1.80$$

In this case, a sample mean based on three observations is more efficient as an estimator of the population mean than a sample of size N = 2 because E = 1.80 is a number greater than 1. On the basis of the efficiency ratio, it would be said that samples of size N = 3 are 1.8 times more efficient in providing estimates of the population mean than are samples of size N = 2.

This concept of efficiency is very useful when dealing with very large universes, not small ones as in our small universe of eight nurses. If the universe is large and if the efficiency ratio were to be computed for two different sampling schemes and if it were found that the ratio were equal to 1.80, then one could operationalize the meaning of the ratio as follows.

Suppose that the efficient estimator were based on a sample of 1000. The same precision could be attained with the less efficient sampling scheme if the number of elementary units were increased to 1800. Of course, no reasonable person would adopt the less efficient model because of the great increase in cost necessary to achieve the same level of precision offered by the smaller, more efficient sample. The point to be made is that efficiency is a highly desirable property, which translates easily into the saving of dollars and cents, a concept with which most researchers have an intimate acquaintance.

Operationally, the ratio of the two variances can be interpreted as a ratio of sample sizes that produces two sampling schemes of equal precision. Because of cost considerations, the sampling procedure that provides efficient estimators should always be chosen. Sometimes this means sacrificing the property of unbiasedness in favor of efficiency. In practice, the sacrifice is usually minimal because most surveys are based on large samples. Even if a sampling scheme produced biased estimators, the bias is usually negligible because in large samples, the bias is typically small.

Consistent Estimators

The last statement is based on a third important statistical property associated with large samples, the property of *consistency*. A statistic that converges upon an unknown population value as the sample size increases is said to be a *consistent estimator* of the pop-

TABLE 6–5 EXTREME SAMPLES AND VARIANCES FOR INCREASING SAMPLE SIZES

Sample Size	Sample With Smallest Mean	Mean	Sample With Largest Mean	Mean	Variance
1	2	2.00	12	12.00	10.9844
2	2, 3	2.50	10, 12	11.00	4.7076
3	2, 3, 4	3.00	9, 10, 12	10.33	2.6153
4	2, 3, 4, 6	3.75	7, 9, 10, 12	9.50	1.5692
5	2, 3, 4, 6, 7	4.40	6, 7, 9, 10, 12	8.80	0.9415
6	2, 3, 4, 6, 7, 9	5.17	4, 6, 7, 9, 10, 12	8.00	0.5231
7	2, 3, 4, 6, 7, 9, 10	5.86	3, 4, 6, 7, 9, 10, 12	7.29	0.2242
8	2, 3, 4, 6, 7, 9, 10, 12	6.625	2, 3, 4, 6, 7, 9, 10, 12	6.625	0.0000

ulation value. In essence, this implies that if an estimator has the property of consistency, the bias in large samples is very small and thus not large enough to be of any practical concern. In most cases, a large sample statistic is close to the population value even if the estimator is biased. In other words, given a first sample of size N, a second sample which is smaller and a sampling scheme producing biased estimators, the bias will be less for the large sample of size N. This further supports the intuitive feeling held by many researchers that a large sample is better than a small sample. Operationally this means that, for example, a sample of 200 is expected to be closer to the unknown population value than a sample of 100. In almost every case, this is true.

For completeness, a summary table showing the extreme samples, the extreme means, and the variances for increasing sample sizes from N = 1 to N = 8 is provided in Table 6–5. Note that when the sample size N equals the population size M, the mean of the sample is the mean of the population and the error in the estimate is zero. As indicated, the error in estimation decreases as sample size increases. The implication of this example is that, in practice, a researcher will want to choose a large sample whenever contemplating a field survey.

6–7 USING LISTS OF ELEMENTARY SAMPLING UNITS TO OBTAIN A SIMPLE RANDOM SAMPLING FOR A MAIL SURVEY

In order to select a simple random sample, a roster must be available. This is very limiting to the nurse researcher and can be a serious barrier to the use of probability sampling. In addition to the problem of acquiring an up-to-date roster or list of elementary sample units, strict guidelines on informed consent increase the difficulty of performing a scientifically valid survey sample investigation in a human population. Probability sampling schemes almost always require a listing by name and address of possible sample members. This information is highly protected, and access to a roster of names is restricted by many organizations. Some organizations have formal policies which deny the release of any lists of its members to a group wanting to conduct a field or sample survey. Other organizations insist on contacting their members directly and eliciting individual agreement to distribute a person's name to a research group. Other organizations insist on directly distributing the survey instruments or questionnaires. No information about any organization member is ever made available to the survey team. Consequently, the care, tact, and veracity demonstrated in the query letter and the informed consent materials to be sent to each sample member have a great effect on access to a desired list of names or sampling frame (Singer, 1978a; Singer, 1978b).

As an illustration requiring a current listing of possible sample members, consider a large-scale survey of nurses and their attitudes toward treating patients with AIDS in the state of California. Without a roster, sampling would be impossible. Fortunately, in a state like California, a registry of licensed nurses exists. Even so, it should be noted that merely the existence of a roster is not sufficient, because a registry may not be complete. Although it is not legal to be employed as a nurse in California without a license, there are nurses who are working without a legal license. Some may have intentionally allowed their license to lapse, and many more may have forgotten to renew their old license. Also, some addresses are certain to be in error. Some nurses will have moved after the last record updating took place, and some will have changed their names. Furthermore, licensed nurses in military health care agencies may not necessarily be licensed in California and therefore are not included in the registry. The records may also contain other errors. These kinds of inadequate record keeping are certain to create errors in sampling. As a consequence, the research nurse must be ready to deal with recording and registration errors before selecting the elementary units in a survey. Although very little can be done to correct these errors, except for spending great sums of money, it is important for the researcher to know that such potential errors may exist. Thus, results should be interpreted cautiously after the survey is completed.

Selecting a simple random sample is not easy. A code number must be established for each elementary unit. Some rosters are already coded and those numbers can be used for sample selection. Finally, the sample must be selected using a table of *random numbers*, or prepackaged computer programs can be used to identify the elementary units to sample. (A model based on random number tables is described in detail by Marascuilo and Serlin, 1988.)

6–8 SAMPLE SIZE FOR SIMPLE RANDOM SAMPLING

Before a sample can be selected, the investigator has to decide on the number of elementary units to include in the survey. At first it may seem that the bigger the sample, the better. In a sense that is true. However, limitations exist because, as sample sizes are allowed to increase, a *law of diminishing returns* sets in operation. To increase the precision of an estimator, a large amount of money may have to be spent. This is illustrated in the following example.

Consider sampling nurses in California to determine attitudes toward the treatment of AIDS patients. Suppose that the number of nurses in the registry is equal to M = 98,835 and suppose that the mean length of employment is given as $\mu_Y = 6.625$ years, with variance given as $\sigma_Y^2 = 10.9844$. As previously discussed, no random sample can produce a sample mean that is absolutely equal to the population mean. As a consequence, the re-

searcher must decide on the maximum error that can be tolerated in estimating the population values. This is not an easy problem to solve. One solution is to decide that the error should not exceed a certain percentage of the value to be estimated. Suppose that the maximum error, δ, is chosen so that the sample mean does not differ from the population mean by more than 10%. This means that an error that does not exceed

$$\delta = (0.10)(6.625) = 0.6625 \text{ years}$$

is acceptable. It can be shown that the relationship between δ and μ_Y and σ_Y^2 is given as

$$\delta = 3\sqrt{\frac{\sigma_Y^2}{N}\left(\frac{M-N}{M-1}\right)}$$

The number 3 appearing in the above equation can be changed to a larger or smaller value, depending on the risks in making a type I error that a researcher is willing to assume. We have set the risk at a very low value of about .0001. Although the selection of this low risk of error represents a very conservative position, it also represents one that will prove to be expensive in terms of dollars and cents. A conservative rule forces the sample size upward. The Gallup Poll actually uses a much less conservative rule in that the risk of a type I error is set at .05. With this rule, the number 3 is replaced by 1.96. Throughout this chapter, we use the value of 3 as the multiplier. As a consequence, we require large samples.

If we now substitute the known numbers into this equation, we have:

$$0.6625 = 3\sqrt{\frac{10.9844}{N}\left(\frac{98,835-N}{98,835-1}\right)}$$

an equation with one unknown. If this equation is solved for N, it is found that N = 225 elementary units are required.

Suppose that the researcher wished to double the precision so that the maximum error did not exceed 5% of the unknown population value. To do this, a sample of size N = 892 elementary units would be required. In other words, to *double* the precision, one would have to *quadruple* the costs of conducting the survey. If the budget permits, this is the appropriate thing to do. Even so, note that it takes money to achieve a high level of precision. A word of advice is offered to the nurse researcher. Surveys based on N = 1000 elementary units are generally more than sufficient. Surveys based on more elementary units are certain to be more precise, but the precision obtained is frequently more than is necessary. The Gallup polls reported in the daily newspapers are usually based on about N = 1400 interviews. With this size sample, the maximum errors in the Gallup poll are about 3.5%. For most studies, this level of precision is more than adequate.

Before closing this section, we would like to dismiss a common myth. It was seen that for M = 98,835 nurses a sample of size N = 225 would suffice. Suppose, however, that the universe size was actually M = 197,760, or twice what was used earlier. It is easy to conclude that this universe requires a sample of N = 450 or twice the size of the previous sample to obtain the same degree of precision. In this case, the conclusion is false. The correct sample size is still given as N = 225. This can be shown by replacing M with 197,670 in the equation defining δ. The population size is of no consequence when determining sample size. *Population size has no relationship to sample size in large samples.*

In sampling theory, large population size is defined relative to sample size. Thus, a large population is one in which N/M is less than .05. Consider the factor

$$f = \left(\frac{M - N}{M - 1}\right)$$

used as a multiplier to σ_Y^2/N. If M is large, this factor is very close to 1.0 in numerical value. As we see,

$$f = 1 - N/(M - 1).$$

If M is large, f is nearly equal to $1 - N/M$. As long as f is greater than $1 - .05 = .95$, population size is irrelevant to sample size determination. For our example, f is equal to 0.9977. Because it is so close to one, a highly effective approximation equation for sample size determination is given as

$$\delta = 3\frac{\sigma_Y}{\sqrt{N}}$$

From this equation, the sample size can be determined with

$$N = \frac{9\,\sigma_Y^2}{\delta^2}$$

For our example,

$$N = \frac{9(10.9844)}{(0.6625)^2} = 225$$

Finally, it must be noted that all surveys have nonresponse rates, and so the sample sizes determined from these equations must be adjusted upward. Suppose it is assumed that 40% of the questionnaires will not be returned. To maintain the degree of precision desired, it is advisable to increase the sample size to $(1/0.60)(225) = (1.67)(225) = 375$ subjects, or to the nice round figure of 400 elementary units. With this increase in sample size, the expected return is about N = 240.

6–9 SIMPLE RANDOM SAMPLING FOR ESTIMATING A POPULATION PROPORTION

In survey research, it is common to ask questions that have a yes or no type of response. The variance for such estimators is given as

$$\sigma_{\hat{p}}^2 = \frac{pq}{N}\left(\frac{M - N}{M - 1}\right)$$

where $\hat{p}$ equals the proportion who say yes. If N/M is less than .05, sample size can be determined from

$$N = \frac{9}{4\delta^2}$$

As an example, suppose one wanted to ask the question:

Are you willing to work with persons with AIDS?
Yes ___ No ___

If the maximum error is set equal to δ = 0.035, the sample size is given as

$$N = \frac{9}{4(0.035)^2} = 1836$$

To cover a 40% nonresponse, it would be wise to increase N to 1836/0.6 = 3060, or 3000 nurses.

Most investigators would find a sample

size of this magnitude too large to handle from both an economic point of view and from a logistical viewpoint. For this reason, some compromises are in order. One compromise that is always possible is to lower the level of acceptable precision. Suppose that it is decided to increase the maximum error from $\delta = 0.035$ to $\delta = 0.04$. With this adjustment, $N = 9/4(0.04)^2 = 1,406$. Although this provides a reduction in sample size, the reduction may not be sufficient for most budgets. With $\delta = 0.05$, $N = 900$. As illustrated, smaller, more manageable samples can be obtained by increasing δ. Unfortunately, increasing δ can make the study so imprecise that it might be wise to forget the whole thing.

To overcome the decline in precision with smaller sample sizes, another compromise can be made when choosing the sample size for a study. The derivation of the equation for N is based on the assumption that a risk of a type I error is set at the exceedingly low level of $\alpha = 0.001$. Social science research rarely uses such small type I error rates. The more typical value is $\alpha = 0.05$. With this value, the equation for N is exceedingly simple and is given for a dichotomous variable like {yes, no} by $N = 1/\delta^2$. Thus, for $\delta = 0.04$,

$$N = 1/(0.04)^2 = 625$$

Assuming a response rate of 60%, the sample size should be increased to $625/(0.60) = 1042$, which we round to the easy-to-remember number of 1000.

The procedure just illustrated may appear to be arbitrary. It may appear to be based on subjective decisions concerning the maximum error to be tolerated, a wild guess about a response rate, and a rounding down to an easy-to-remember sample size. In a certain sense the decisions are subjective, but survey after survey shows that the method works well. In social science surveys, a response rate of about 60% is not unreasonable, and a 0.04 maximum error from the true value is not going to lead to many false decisions. In practice, the errors are generally *smaller* than that tolerable for the maximum error used in the planning stage.

For a quantitative variable and type I error control of $\alpha = 0.05$, the equation for N reduces to

$$N = 4\,\sigma_Y^2/\delta^2$$

For our example,

$$N = 4(10.9844)/(0.6625)^2 = 100$$

With a response rate of 60%, the final sample size to select is given as $N = 167$. Note that the mean of a quantitative variable can be estimated with a sample that is considerably smaller than that required to estimate a proportion for a dichotomous variable.

6–10 STRATIFIED PROBABILITY SAMPLING

Note that in the previous $N = 8$ nurse example, the nurses of Table 6–2 are located in two different geographical regions. This knowledge can be put to good use in many surveys. We will use this knowledge in designing our AIDS survey to be discussed later. One of the problems in simple random sampling is that an unusual sample might be generated that does not reflect the nature of the universe. For example, if sample (A, B) had been selected, one might be a little disturbed because both nurses live in the same geographical region and work in the same hospital. Fortunately, in large universes with large samples such extreme cases are rare or almost nonexistent in practice. Even so, the possibility of obtaining a strange or unusual sample can be reduced by *stratification* of the universe before selecting the sample.

Suppose that it is desired to stratify on the basis of geographical region and use $N_1 = 1$ and $N_2 = 1$ nurses from each geographical region. The samples that could be selected which satisfy this external requirement are reported in Table 6–6. Note that the number of possible samples is reduced from 28 to 15. The smallest mean in this restricted set of samples is 2.5 and the largest is 9.5. The range in sample means is less than that of simple random sampling because some of the extreme samples have been eliminated. Suppose that the mean of the 15 sample means is computed. In this case, $\mu_{\bar{Y}} = 6.3$. This is not equal to the population mean of 6.625, as found for simple random sampling. Clearly, this procedure generates a biased estimator and the amount of the bias is given as

$$B = 6.3 - 6.625 = -0.325 \text{ years.}$$

TABLE 6-6 ALL POSSIBLE STRATIFIED SAMPLES FOR THE DATA OF TABLE 6-2*

Sample	Years of Employment	Simple Average	Stratified Mean
A, D	6, 9	7.5	7.875
A, E	6, 4	5.0	4.750
A, F	6, 12	9.0	9.750
A, G	6, 10	8.0	8.500
A, H	6, 3	4.5	4.125
B, D	2, 9	5.5	6.375
B, E	2, 4	3.0	3.250
B, F	2, 12	7.0	8.250
B, G	2, 10	6.0	7.000
B, H	2, 3	2.5	2.625
C, D	7, 9	8.0	8.250
C, E	7, 4	5.5	5.125
C, F	7, 12	9.5	10.125
C, G	7, 10	8.5	8.875
C, H	7, 3	5.0	4.500

*$N_1 = 1$ and $N_2 = 1$

This is not acceptable because most of the samples that could be generated tend to underestimate the true number of years that the nurses were employed. A correction is called for.

Note that the two strata are of different sizes. The northern stratum contains $M_1 = 3$ nurses, whereas the southern stratum contains $M_2 = 5$ nurses. This information can be used to generate an unbiased estimator, by simply weighting each of the stratum means by the number of nurses in the stratum. Thus, an unbiased estimator is given as

$$\overline{Y} = \frac{M_1}{M} \overline{Y}_1 + \frac{M_2}{M} \overline{Y}_2$$

where $\overline{Y}_1$ and $\overline{Y}_2$ are the mean values in the two strata samples.

For our example, the sample means are equal to the individual values because $N_1 = N_2 = 1$. For the possible 15 stratified samples, the set of unbiased estimates are reported in Table 6-6. As can be seen, the lowest possible mean value is now 2.625, with the highest possible mean given as 10.125. The mean of these means is equal to 6.625, the mean of the original eight nurses. This shows that weighting each stratum by its size produces an estimator for the population mean that is unbiased, because across all 15 potential samples the mean is equal to 6.625, the population value.

Means that are computed by weighting according to strata characteristics are called stratified means. If, in particular, the weights are the ratios of the strata sizes to the population size, the mean is called the proportional stratified mean. In practice, proportional stratified means are preferred. Another way to obtain an unbiased mean is to sample each stratum proportionally to sample size and thereby have a self-weighting estimator. With a self-weighting mean, the formula for a simple random sample is to determine $\overline{Y}$. Weighting is not required. This property of proportional sampling is illustrated in Section 6-11.

In our example, to obtain a stratified proportional sample of size N = 2, we would have to choose $N_1 = (3/8)2 = .75$ and $N_2 = (5/8)2 = 1.25$ nurses from the northern and southern strata respectively. Of course, for M = 8, this is not possible, but in a large universe with large samples no problem exists in determining the appropriate sample sizes. For example, in a real survey 75 nurses from the northern strata and 125 nurses from the southern strata could be sampled. In fact, most surveys today use this strategy. It is used here in the survey of nurses' attitude toward persons with AIDS. Stratified proportional sampling is a good strategy and is easy to apply. It avoids the bias problem illustrated in Table 6-6. It provides self-weighting samples, so that weighting as illustrated in Table 6-6 is not necessary. This is a real advantage because by selecting samples proportional to strata size the adoption of all of the statistical models described in subsequent chapters is possible and defensible. In the end, these statistical models are used to analyze sample data. Thus, the prudent nurse researcher is advised to use proportional allocation whenever possible. It is not always the most efficient model but is the most useful model when it comes to data analysis. It is recommended highly.

We close this section by comparing the efficiency of the weighted stratified mean to that of simple random sampling. In this case the variance of the mean is given in the equation at the top of page 127.

As we see, simple random sampling is preferred because when it is compared with the stratified mean weighted by strata sizes the efficiency ratio is given as

$$E = (5.4375)/(4.7076) = 1.16$$

Because the stratified mean was less efficient than the simple random sampling mean in this example, it should not be con-

$$\sigma_{\bar{Y}_S}^2 = 1/15[(7.875 - 6.625)^2 + (4.750 - 6.625)^2 + \ldots + (4.500 - 6.625)^2] = 5.4375$$

cluded that this is usually the case. In fact, the stratified mean is usually the more efficient of the two. It is always more efficient if the variation between the strata is large and the variation within the strata is small. These same conditions make a multifactor analysis of variance, randomized block, and repeated measure analysis more efficient. If the northern stratum consisted of Bob, Hilda, and Elvira with years of employment of 2, 3, and 4 years, it would be seen that stratification is highly efficient. Stratification is always preferred if there is homogeneity of values within the strata and heterogeneity of values between the strata.

This high efficiency of stratification suggests that attempts should be made to increase the efficiency of a survey by finding stratification variables that can be used to capitalize on the correlation that exists between a response variable and some other confounding variable. In the AIDS survey, it is certain that attitudes toward treating persons with AIDS (PWAs) are influenced, for example, by religious background and affiliation, political party and social group membership or reference group orientation, and marital status. If information were available on marital status and if it were believed that attitude is related to marital status, the nurses could be divided into four groups consisting of single nurses, married nurses, divorced nurses, and widowed nurses. Each group could be sampled individually, and the information could be pooled using the formulas for stratified sampling.

Problems almost always exist in stratification of a population on these types of variables. A good stratification variable for one set of questions may not be a good stratification variable for another set of questions. The other problem encountered in attempting to stratify psychological constructs like self-esteem, locus of control, intelligence, knowledge about harmful effects of drugs, attitudes toward alternative life-styles, and like dispositional states is that the data are usually not available. Although stratification of variables correlated with the dependent variable may be an ideal goal or desirable attribute of a survey, most surveys rely on demographic variables for stratification. Variables may include such characteristics as

gender, religious affiliation, census tracts, cities, counties, hospitals, voting registration sites, schools, and health facilities. Because of unavailability, psychological constructs rarely can be used. In experimental design literature, stratification is referred to as *blocking*. The principles that apply to stratification also apply to blocking. (For a further discussion on this topic see Section 10–12.)

Often, researchers oversample one or two strata so as to have a sufficient number of subjects in the sample to provide sample estimates that are efficient. For example, consider strata defined by nurses with hospital diplomas, bachelor of science degrees, master of science degrees, and doctor of philosophy degrees. Suppose the numbers in the four groups are given as 700, 200, 80, and 20, respectively. Sample determination computation may have shown that 36 nurses should be sampled from each category. Such a large number cannot be obtained in the class of nurses with doctoral degrees. For this category, one would oversample and take all 20 into the sample. Oversampling is sometimes the only option available to fill all the strata of a survey.

6–11 SAMPLE SIZES FOR STRATIFIED SAMPLING

Sample sizes to be selected from each subpopulation or stratum can be determined in many ways. All require advanced knowledge about the strata such as strata size and the variance of the characteristic to be measured on the elementary units. In most cases, this information is not available. In addition, most surveys contain many different questions so that what is the best sampling scheme for one variable may be of little value for another variable. One solution is to arbitrarily decide on a sample size that can be handled by the staff and supported by the budget and then use this sample size for the *proportional* allocation of sample sizes to the individual strata. Proportional allocation generates self-weighting samples. (Other allocation models can be found in Hansen,

TABLE 6–7 UNIVERSE SIZE, SAMPLE SIZE, AND RETURNS FOR THE SURVEY ON NURSES' ATTITUDES IN CALIFORNIA CONCERNING THE TREATMENT OF AIDS PATIENTS

County	Number of Nurses		
	Universe	Sample	Return
Los Angeles	49,708	503	377
San Diego	14,467	146	129
Santa Clara (San José)	9,780	99	69
San Francisco	6,643	67	42
Sacramento	5,933	60	40
Alameda (Oakland)	5,580	56	40
Sonoma (Santa Rosa)	2,534	26	18
San Joaquin (Stockton)	2,125	22	21
Kern (Bakersfield)	2,065	21	10
Total	98,835	1,000	748

Hurwitz, and Madow, 1962; Cochran, 1977; and Kish, 1965.)

As an example of proportional stratification, consider the sampling of nurses in the state of California and the assessment of the nurses' attitudes toward PWAs. In order to sample a representative population, we use the roster of the State Board of Registered Nursing, which contains 210,000 licensed nurses, as of December 1985. Because AIDS is not uniformly distributed throughout the state, cost-effectiveness principles suggested that only counties with a known incidence of the illness should be sampled. Because the State Board of Registered Nursing maintains statistics only by counties, cities cannot be selected as the primary strata. Let the specific counties chosen for this survey be Los Angeles, San Diego, Santa Clara (San José), San Francisco, Sacramento, Alameda (Oakland), Sonoma (Santa Rosa), San Joaquin (Stockton), and Kern (Bakersfield). The number of registered nurses in each of these counties is reported in Table 6–7. As can be seen, Los Angeles County contains about 50% of the registered nurses in the nine-county sampling universe and, as such, it will receive the largest sampling and weighting. At the same time, Kern County will receive the smallest sampling and weighting.

The main research question in this proposed study is: Are you willing to work with persons with AIDS? As seen in Section 6–9, we plan to sample 1000 registered nurses. To obtain a self-weighting sample, these 1000 elementary units should be distributed across the nine strata, proportional to the number of nurses in each stratum. Thus, for Los Angeles, we would allocate

$N_1 = (49,708/98,835)(1000) = (0.5029)(1000)$
$= 503$ nurses.

The allocation of nurses to the remaining strata would be as shown in Table 6–7. As we see, Kern County is sampled with

$N_9 = (2,065/98,835)(1000) = (0.0209)(1000)$
$= 21$ nurses.

With these numbers a simple random sample would now be selected within each stratum.

6–12 CLUSTER PROBABILITY SAMPLING

In addition to seeking precise estimates, the survey researcher also wishes to save money and maximize the amount of information collected for a fixed budget. Simple random sampling is the most expensive sampling model to adopt. Stratified sampling is a good model with respect to increased efficiency and reduced costs, provided that the variation between the strata is large and the variation within the strata is small. But if the variation between the strata is small and if the variation within strata is large, it is not an effective sampling model to apply. What can be done is to adopt a *cluster* sampling procedure because whenever stratified sampling is a poor choice, cluster sampling works fine.

A cluster sampling scheme is one in which elementary sampling units are selected as a group and analyzed as a group. It is used when a roster of individual subjects is not available and when there is a roster of cluster units consisting of elementary sampling units. An example is provided in a study in which the goal is to sample hospital patients with cardiovascular illness with only a listing of hospitals with cardiovascular patient care units. Here, a roster of hospitals can be generated from which a sample of patient care units can be selected with known probabilities. After the units are selected, a target date for the study can be specified and a roster of the patients in the unit on that specific date can be constructed. Patients are then sampled from the newly prepared rosters with known probabilities. Thus, in general, first a sampling of the patient care units with known probabilities can be made, and then a second sampling performed of the patients being treated at a specific date based on the probabilities in operation at the time of the sampling.

Another case in which cluster sampling is preferred to stratified sampling is when the sample covers a large geographical area. Transportation costs can absorb a large share of a survey budget if the elementary units selected are far apart in travel or time. As an example, consider a study in which the roster of nurses living in the greater New York City area is available for sampling. One-hundred names can be sampled for this roster and an interviewer can be sent to each nurse to assess their attitudes toward treating PWAs. If the nurses are spread across the five boroughs of New York, much of the cost of the survey could be spent in traveling to the homes of each nurse. With the problems in scheduling and not finding people at home, the costs could skyrocket and prevent the completion of the survey. If the roster can be matched to census tract boundaries, a solution would be to divide the city into census tracts and then to choose a random 10 census tracts to poll. Within each census tract, 10 nurses could be sampled to be interviewed. At this point, the interviewer could travel to a census tract and interview all 10 nurses in a very short period of time.

Another option for sampling nurses in the New York City area is to use a multistage cluster sampling strategy. For example, the five boroughs could be treated as stratification units. Within each borough, a roster of census tracts can be generated and two can be selected as primary sampling units. Within each primary sampling unit, a secondary unit could be sampled. Thus, in the 10 sampled census tracts, a second set of rosters could be generated in which hospitals, health departments, nursing homes, and other health facilities are listed. A sampling can be made of five of these units in each sampled census tract. Finally, a roster can be made of the nurses in each of the five health facilities sampled, and from each, 10 nurses can be selected and interviewed.

There are no limits to the kinds of sampling schemes that an investigator can produce. The main problems to be encountered in designing any survey are those of obtaining a roster to sample from and cost constraints that are always limiting.

In our proposed study on AIDS, we are not adopting cluster sampling, even though it would be more precise than stratified sampling. A great deal more information on sampling units is needed in cluster sampling than is necessary in stratified sampling. Later it will be illustrated why cluster sampling would not be appropriate for the AIDS study.

At this point, let us again consider the eight nurses described in Table 6–2 to illustrate the statistical properties of cluster sampling. Cluster sampling may actually be the most efficient and the least expensive. Here, a hospital could be selected as a cluster, all the questionnaires could be placed in a single mailing packet and sent to the hospital or nurse administrator, who would then distribute, collect, and mail the questionnaires back to the research team in a single packet. In addition to the reduced costs, such a sampling scheme tends to lower the nonresponse rate because the responsibility for collecting the distributed questionnaire falls on the person to whom the original packet is addressed. Of course, if the administrator does not want to cooperate, the entire packet could wind up in the wastebasket or in the return mail to the research team.

For our example, suppose that it is decided to sample one hospital and use the nurses in that hospital as a single cluster. There are four such samples. They are listed in Table 6–8. Note how small the range in mean values is for this version of cluster sampling. This is expected because we know that stratified sampling is not efficient with these data. The mean of the means is equal to

$$\overline{Y} = 1/4(4.00 + 7.00 + 6.50 + 8.33)$$
$$= 6.4575$$

TABLE 6-8 ALL POSSIBLE CLUSTER SAMPLES OF HOSPITALS THAT CAN BE GENERATED FROM THE POPULATION OF TABLE 6-2

Cluster	Nurses	Years of Employment	Mean
One	A, B	6, 2	4.00
Two	C	7	7.00
Three	D, E	9, 4	6.50
Four	F, G, H	12, 10, 3	8.33

showing that the estimates are biased, with the bias being equal to

$$B = 6.4575 - 6.625 = -0.1675 \text{ years}$$

To most, this small amount of bias is not important. The variance of the means is very small and equal to 2.4604 so that the efficiency of cluster sampling relative to simple stratified sampling is given as

$$E = (4.7076)/(2.4604) = 1.91$$

Without doubt, cluster sampling is a highly viable sampling scheme for these data.

Cluster sampling can be very effective when used in conjunction with stratified sampling. As an example, suppose it were decided to choose one hospital per geographical region. The results of this sampling are shown in Table 6-9. As can be seen, the range in the means is very small. In addition, the means cluster about the

mean value of 6.86 with a variance of 1.1267. As before, the estimate is biased with the amount of the bias equal to

$$B = 6.86 - 6.625 = -0.235 \text{ years}$$

From a practical point of view, this sampling scheme looks very good. But for the proposed AIDS survey, this sampling scheme is poor.

Note that the bias can be reduced by using weights proportional to strata size. In this case,

$$\overline{Y}_{S(C)} = \frac{N_1}{N} \overline{Y}_{1(C)} + \frac{N_2}{N} \overline{Y}_{2(C)}$$
$$= \frac{3}{8} \overline{Y}_{1(C)} + \frac{5}{8} \overline{Y}_{2(C)}$$

For the example, $\overline{Y}_{S(C)} = 6.70$, so that the bias is reduced to

$$B = 6.70 - 6.625 = .075$$

TABLE 6-9 ALL POSSIBLE STRATIFIED CLUSTER SAMPLES THAT CAN BE GENERATED FROM THE POPULATION OF TABLE 6-2

Cluster	Nurses	Years of Employment	Mean Value	
			Unweighted	Weighted
One	A, B	6, 2		
Three	D, E	9, 4	5.25	5.56
One	A, B	6, 2		
Four	F, G, H	12, 10, 3	6.60	6.71
Two	C	7		
Three	D, E	9, 4	6.67	6.69
Two	C	7		
Four	F, G, H	12, 10, 3	8.00	7.83

For our AIDS study, this would be a poor sampling technique, as is easily illustrated by considering the population distribution of a city such as San Francisco.

Suppose that a specific hospital is located in a community such as San Francisco, with a sizable homosexual population, and suppose that the nurses working at the hospital live in that same community. Under these circumstances, it could be reasonably expected to find at this hospital a high proportion of nurses who would be willing to work with AIDS patients. Because the proportion would be higher than the San Francisco community at large, an invalid estimate would be obtained for the entire city. At the other extreme, when a hospital is selected that is located in an area of San Francisco with few homosexual residents and with nurses living in the same area, it may be possible that a considerable amount of fear may be expressed toward working with AIDS patients. Again, the estimate generated from this hospital would be invalid because it would provide a low estimate for the entire city of San Francisco. When the clusters are homogenous, cluster sampling is not recommended.

6–13 SAMPLE SIZES FOR CLUSTER SAMPLING

Sample allocation for cluster sampling depends on having a roster of potential clusters. Without it the model cannot be adopted. If the listing is available, it operates as follows. It has already been seen that for simple random sampling N = 225 nurses are required to estimate the mean length of employment. With a table of random numbers, hospitals are selected at random. Suppose that the first hospital selected has 37 nurses that meet the criteria of the survey. These 37 nurses are included in the sample, leaving 225 − 37 = 188 nurses to be included. If the second hospital has 16 nurses, they are admitted to the sample leaving 188 − 16 = 172 for the remaining clusters. The process continues until the sample size of 225 is reached.

If cluster sampling is to be used in conjunction with stratified sampling, the above sample construction procedure is followed with each stratum. To obtain self-weighting samples, it would be necessary to sample hospitals proportional to the number of nurses eligible to be included in the survey. With this model costs are reduced and the statistical models of later chapters can be applied directly without having to weight the observations because of the difference in probabilities of being selected into the sample.

6–14 SYSTEMATIC PROBABILITY SAMPLING

A very simple model that can be employed if a complete register is available is *systematic sampling*. For this model, a decision is made about the size of the sample to be selected. After this, the roster is divided systematically into samples, and one sample is selected by using a table of random numbers.

As an example, suppose that we select a systematic sample for the M = 8 nurses of Table 6–2 with N = 2. All such samples are listed in Table 6–10. As indicated, the mean values are tightly clustered about the mean value of 6.625, the mean of the population. In addition, the small variance of 1.6719 suggests high efficiency. The efficiency of this model when compared with simple random sampling shows that it is a good model for

$$E = (4.7076)(1.6719) = 2.91$$

Of the models discussed in this chapter, systematic sampling appears to be the best for the data of Table 6–2.

For the study on AIDS, consider the universe of M = 98,835 nurses and, of those, the N = 1000 who would be included in the sample. Begin by identifying S = M/N = (98,835)/(1000) = 98 unique samples. Sample number one consists of the nurses who have been coded [00001, 00099, 00197,

TABLE 6–10 ALL POSSIBLE SYSTEMATIC SAMPLES OF SIZE N = 2 THAT CAN BE GENERATED FROM THE POPULATION OF TABLE 6–2

Sample	Years of Employment	Mean
A, E	6, 4	5.00
B, F	2, 12	7.00
C, G	7, 10	8.50
D, H	9, 3	6.00

00295, . . . , 97903]. Sample number two consists of the nurses who have been coded [00002, 00100, 00198, 00296, . . . , 97904]. Proceeding in this manner sample number 98 consists of the nurses who have been coded [00098, 00196, 00294, . . . , 98002]. As indicated, all nurses except those with code numbers 98003 to 98835 are systematically assigned to only one possible sample. The sample selected is based on choosing a number at random between 01 and 98 from a random number table. In most cases, systematic sampling reproduces the properties of simple random sampling.

Note that 832 nurses have been eliminated from the study because nurses with code numbers 98003 to 98835 are not included. With systematic sampling this elimination of subjects is of no consequence because if it were, systematic sampling could not be performed. The only instance in which a researcher can justify a systematic sampling procedure is when the responses are unrelated to the order on the roster. If a correlation exists between the order on the list and the responses, systematic sampling is invalid.

In this particular case for the study on AIDS, systematic sampling would not be recommended. Differences in attitude would be expected to exist across the strata. The smallest degree of fear could be anticipated in counties such as San Francisco because of the long-term tradition of community tolerance of life-style differences and the extensive community education programs pioneered by the city government and gay activist community agencies and support groups. In essence, systematic sampling should be considered only when the estimates across the strata can be expected to be equal.

6–15 THE QUESTIONNAIRE FOR THE STUDY ON AIDS

Most surveys are conducted only to obtain information that can be used for planning and administrative decision making; however, surveys can be used to provide information and understanding about some population characteristics. In the survey about AIDS, survey methodology is being used to answer research questions related to nurses' attitudes toward treating PWAs. This information can be used for administrative or educational purposes, and it also can be used to make a scientific inquiry about attitudes and behavior.

As indicated earlier, before formulating the questions that are to appear on the questionnaire, the researcher needs to clearly define goals and objectives. In this case, the goals and objectives are built around a theoretical framework proposed by Herek (1984; 1986a; 1986b) and research conducted by Crosby and Herek (1986). According to Herek's model, attitudes toward homosexuality can be viewed from a three-dimensional perspective based on:

1. past experience with homosexual persons,
2. coping responses with inner conflicts or anxieties,
3. expressions of self-identity through social networks and reference groups.

These dimensions have been used to focus on three interrelated research questions. Items for the survey were devised to obtain information about the following research objectives:

1. Is the willingness to work with PWAs a function of a nurse's homophobia?
2. Is the willingness to work with PWAs a function of prior experience of having cared for dying persons?
3. Is the willingness to work with PWAs a function of a nurse's knowledge about AIDS?

It is tempting to test all three questions using a single questionnaire. In many situations, one questionnaire is sufficient. However, in this case, it would not be advisable because, as will be seen, the set of proposed questions is extensive. It is well known by survey analysts that the use of a long questionnaire is defeating. The response rate to a long questionnaire is almost always low. In fact, there appears to be an inverse relationship between the length of the instrument and the response rate. Short questionnaires have a higher probability of being completed and returned than long questionnaires. To ensure a high response rate in the proposed survey, it was decided to use three questionnaires—one for each objective. Questions 1 through 12 are common to each questionnaire. These items define the independent variables of the study. The response categories associated with each of these items generate what are called *domains of study*. For instance, the domains of study defined by item 10 are:

1. nurses who will work with PWAs,
2. nurse who will not work with PWAs

The three questionnaires for this survey are as follows:

Questionnaire 1. Nurses' Attitudes Toward Homosexuality

1. How old were you on your last birthday? ___ (in Years).
2. Are you Male___ Female___?
3. What is your present marital status? Are you Married___ Single___ Divorced___ Widowed___ (check one)
4. Are you a member of an organized religion? Yes___ No___
5. How many years have you been employed or worked as a registered nurse?
___
6. For the years worked as an RN, how many were spent in direct patient care?
___
7. In your present work setting are there patients diagnosed as having AIDS? Yes___ No___
8. How would you describe attitude of your work setting toward admitting and caring for PWAs? Very positive___ Positive___ Somewhat positive___ Not positive at all___
9. Have you in the past or are you presently working with patients with a diagnosis of AIDS? Yes___ No___
10. Are you willing to work with PWAs? Yes___ No___
11. Do you have friends, coworkers, or family members who are gay/lesbian? Yes___ No___
12. How would you describe your sexual orientation? Heterosexual___ Bisexual___ Gay/lesbian___

Please circle the following questions as either true or false.

13. Homosexual couples should be allowed to adopt children the same as heterosexual couples.
        True   False
14. I would not be upset if I learned that my child was gay/lesbian.
        True   False
15. I would be nervous if a gay/lesbian sat next to me on a bus.
        True   False
16. Homosexuality is merely a different kind of life-style that should not be condemned.
        True   False

17. There is an element of homosexuality in all men and women.
        True   False
18. I think lesbians/gays are disgusting.
        True   False
19. Homosexuals should not be allowed to teach school.
        True   False
20. If my best friends told me that they were gay/lesbian, it would distress me greatly.
        True   False
21. Homosexuality is detrimental to society because it breaks down the natural divisions between the sexes.
        True   False
22. Gays/lesbians just don't fit into our society.
        True   False
23. A man's or a woman's homosexuality should not be a cause for job discrimination in any situation.
        True   False
24. Homosexuality is a threat to many of our social institutions.
        True   False
25. I would not be upset if a family member told me that he or she was gay/lesbian.
        True   False

Questionnaire 2. Nurses' Attitudes Toward Working with Dying Patients

1. How old were you on your last birthday?
___
2. Are you Male___ or Female___?
3. What is your present marital status? Married___ Single___ Divorced___ Widowed___ (check one)
4. Are you a member of an organized religion? Yes___ No___
5. How many years have you been employed or worked as a registered nurse?
___
6. For the years worked as an RN, how many were spent in direct patient care?
___
7. In your present work setting, are there patients diagnosed as having AIDS? Yes___ No___
8. How would you describe the attitude in your work setting toward admitting and caring for patients with AIDS (PWAs)? Very positive___ Positive___ Somewhat positive___ Not positive at all___
9. Have you in the past or are you presently working with patients with a diagnosis of AIDS? Yes___ No___
10. Are you willing to work with PWAs? Yes___ No___
11. Do you have friends, coworkers, or family members who are gay/lesbian? Yes___ No___

12. How would you describe your sexual orientation? Heterosexual___ Bisexual___ Gay/lesbian___
13. During the past five years, have you worked with terminally ill patients? Yes___ No___
14. How many patients died in the setting(s) where you worked during the past five years? None___ A few___ Many___ A great many___
15. How difficult has it been for you to work with dying patients? Very difficult___ Difficult___ Somewhat difficult___ Not difficult at all___
16. How difficult do you find it to work with terminally ill children and adolescents? Very difficult___ Difficult___ Somewhat difficult___ Not difficult at all___
17. How difficult do you find it to work with terminally ill patients who are age 21 through 45? Very difficult___ Difficult___ Somewhat difficult___ Not difficult at all___
18. How difficult do you find it to work with terminally ill patients who are elderly? Very difficult___ Difficult___ Somewhat difficult___ Not difficult at all___
19. Are you presently willing to work with terminally ill patients? Yes___ No___
20. Do you have anything to add about working with terminally ill patients and PWAs in particular?

Questionnaire 3. Nurses' Knowledge About AIDS

1. How old were you on your last birthday?
___
2. Are you Male___ Female___?
3. What is your present marital status? Are you Married___ Single___ Divorced___ Widowed___ (check one)
4. Are you a member of an organized religion? Yes___ No___
5. How many years have you been employed or worked as a registered nurse?
___
6. For the years worked as an RN, how many were spent in direct patient care?
___
7. In your present work setting, are there patients diagnosed as having AIDS? Yes___ No___
8. How would you describe the attitude in your work setting toward admitting and caring for PWAs? Very positive___ Positive___ Somewhat positive___ Not positive at all___
9. Have you in the past or are you presently working with patients with a diagnosis of AIDS? Yes___ No___
10. Are you willing to work with PWAs? Yes___ No___
11. Do you have friends, coworkers, or family members who are gay/lesbian? Yes___ No___

12. How would you describe your sexual orientation? Heterosexual___ Bisexual___ Gay/lesbian___

For the following questions, please circle whether they are True or False.
13. Gay or bisexual men and intravenous drug users are most at risk for AIDS.
    True   False
14. The AIDS virus is very virulent and is easily transmitted.
    True   False
15. The most effective control precaution that health care workers can use in caring for persons with AIDS is good handwashing.
    True   False
16. A positive result from the HIV antibody test means that a person will get AIDS.
    True   False
17. Because of the complex issues associated with AIDS, the multidisciplinary team approach has proven to be the most effective.
    True   False
18. AIDS is spread through saliva and tears.
    True   False
19. It is important for nurses to be aware of the psychosocial issues of AIDS to be able to offer emotional support to patients, to significant others, and to other nurses.
    True   False
20. Most people with AIDS die from opportunistic infections.
    True   False
21. Health care workers should always wear masks when working with AIDS patients.
    True   False
22. Health care workers are not at risk for AIDS.
    True   False
23. Family members living with patients with AIDS are at high risk of contracting AIDS.
    True   False
24. AIDS patients must be isolated.
    True   False
25. Incubation period for AIDS is short.
    True   False

For an example of a survey, which was not based on a theoretical model and was conducted with nurses about their knowledge of AIDS and attitudes and fears toward persons with AIDS, see van Servellen, Lewis, and Leake (1988).

6–16 STATISTICAL METHODS FOR QUANTITATIVE VARIABLES

As an illustration on how to estimate the parameters and test hypotheses for survey data based on stratified sampling, consider the homophobic items of Questionnaire 1. In it, 13 homophobic items are present, which, when summed up, produce a homophobic scale ranging from a low of zero to a high of 13, with the high scores representing high homophobia. Hypothetical data for this scale are reported in Table 6−11 where nurses' responses are classified on the basis of county and how they responded to item 10 given as

10. Are you willing to work with PWAs?
Yes___ No___

Note that the response rate is given as $r = 748/1000 = 74.8\%$. As indicated, the mean homophobic score for the nurses who said yes in Los Angeles County is 7.51. Their standard deviation is 2.61 and the number of nurses who provided information is 103. For the 274 nurses of Los Angeles County who said no, the mean value on the homophobic scale is 10.31, with a standard deviation of 3.64. These numbers are used to estimate the mean scores and standard errors for the two types of nurses. With the mean scores and the standard errors, confidence intervals can be set up for the mean homophobic scores for the two groups of nurses, and the statistics can be used to test the hypothesis that the mean homophobic scores for the two groups are identical.

By definition the stratified mean is given as

$$\overline{Y}_S = \frac{N_1}{N} \overline{Y}_1 + \frac{N_2}{N} \overline{Y}_2 + \ldots + \frac{N_K}{N} \overline{Y}_K$$

where N_1 = number in stratum number one, N_2 = number in stratum number two, and so on. Also, $N = N_1 + N_2 + \ldots + N_K$. Because we have used proportional sampling, we can replace each N_k/N by n_k/n to give the following formula for computing the mean values:

$$\overline{Y}_S = \frac{n_1}{n} \overline{Y}_1 + \frac{n_2}{n} \overline{Y}_2 + \ldots + \frac{n_K}{n} \overline{Y}_K$$

These weights definitely apply to the total sample and can be applied to the marginal means; however, because we are illustrating a research investigation, we wish to apply the weights to interesting domains of study. At this point, proportional sampling takes on importance. We did not sample nurses who said yes or no to treating PWAs, but under proportional sampling, it is reasonable to assume that the sampling weights are applicable to all variables on the questionnaire and the domain of study defined by item categories.

For the nurses who said that they would treat PWAs,

$$\begin{aligned}\overline{Y}_{yes} &= (0.503)(7.51) + (0.146)(7.91) \\ &\quad + \ldots + (0.021)(6.32) \\ &= 6.89\end{aligned}$$

and for the nurses who said that they would not treat PWAs, the corresponding mean homophobic value is given as

$$\begin{aligned}\overline{Y}_{no} &= (0.503)(10.31) + (0.146)(11.36) \\ &\quad + \ldots + (0.021)(12.16) \\ &= 10.22\end{aligned}$$

These values are used to characterize the population of 98,835 nurses on the original registry. Among those who are willing to treat AIDS patients, the mean homophobic scale is about 7, whereas for those nurses who are not willing to treat AIDS patients, the mean value is about 10.

TABLE 6−11 SAMPLE STATISTICS FOR THE HOMOPHOBIC SCALE FOR THE NINE STRATA ACCORDING TO NURSES' WILLINGNESS TO TREAT PWAS

County	Statistics							
	$\overline{Y}_s$	n_s	S_y	S_y^2/n_s	$\overline{Y}_s$	n_s	S_y	S_Y^2/n_s
Los Angeles	7.51	103	2.61	0.0661	10.31	274	3.64	0.0484
San Diego	7.91	51	2.81	0.1548	11.36	78	4.21	0.2272
Santa Clara	7.10	15	3.41	0.7752	9.37	54	4.00	0.2963
San Francisco	4.20	13	2.91	0.6514	9.36	29	3.98	0.5462
Sacramento	5.21	16	2.10	0.2756	10.39	24	3.46	0.4988
Alameda	5.10	12	2.01	0.3367	9.22	30	2.41	0.1936
Sonoma	5.03	6	2.98	1.4801	8.22	12	2.71	0.6120
San Joaquin	5.29	7	1.42	0.2881	9.36	14	1.98	0.2800
Kern	6.32	3	1.91	1.2160	12.26	7	1.36	0.2642
Total	6.94	226			10.21	52		

① $$SE^2(\overline{Y}_S) = \frac{S_1^2}{n_1}\left(\frac{N_1 - n_1}{N_1 - 1}\right)\left(\frac{N_1}{N}\right)^2 + \frac{S_2^2}{n_2}\left(\frac{N_2 - n_2}{N_2 - 1}\right)\left(\frac{N_2}{N}\right)^2 + \ldots + \frac{S_K^2}{n_K}\left(\frac{N_K - n_K}{N_K - 1}\right)\left(\frac{N_K}{N}\right)^2$$

② $$SE^2(\overline{Y}_S) = \frac{S_1^2}{n_1}\left(\frac{n_1}{n}\right)^2 + \frac{S_2^2}{n_2}\left(\frac{n_2}{n}\right)^2 + \ldots + \frac{S_K^2}{n_K}\left(\frac{n_K}{n}\right)^2$$

By definition, the squared standard error of the stratified mean is given in equation 1 at the top of this page.

With large universes, the $(N_k - n_k)/(N_k - 1)$ tend to be close to 1 in value and are ignored whenever $n_k/N_k < 0.05$. Because this is the situation for this study and because proportional sampling has been used, the formula reduces to equation 2, at the top of this page.

For the nurses who said yes to treating PWAs,

$$SE^2(\overline{Y}_{yes}) = (0.0661)(0.503)^2 + (0.1548)(0.146)^2$$
$$+ \ldots + (1.2160)(0.021)^2$$
$$= 0.0343 = (0.185)^2$$

and for the nurses who said no to treating PWAs,

$$SE^2(\overline{Y}_{no}) = (0.0484)(0.503)^2 + (0.2272)(0.146)^2$$
$$+ \ldots + (0.2642)(0.021)^2$$
$$= 0.255 = (0.1597)^2$$

The 95% confidence intervals for the two groups of nurses are given as

$$\mu_{Yes} = \overline{Y}_{yes} \pm Z\,SE_{\overline{Y}_{yes}}$$
$$= 6.89 \pm 1.96(0.1851) = 6.89 \pm 0.34$$

and

$$\mu_{No} = \overline{Y}_{no} \pm Z\,SE_{\overline{Y}_{no}}$$
$$= 10.22 \pm 1.96(0.1597) = 10.22 \pm 0.31$$

As we see, there is no overlap in the two intervals,

$$6.55 \le \mu_{Yes} \le 7.23 \quad \text{and} \quad 9.91 \le \mu_{No} \le 10.53.$$

To test the hypothesis H_0: $\mu_{Yes} = \mu_{No}$, the test statistic is given as

$$Z = \frac{\overline{Y}_{yes} - \overline{Y}_{no}}{\sqrt{SE^2(\overline{Y}_{yes}) + SE^2(\overline{Y}_{no})}}$$

$$= \frac{6.89 - 10.22}{\sqrt{0.0343 + 0.0255}} = \frac{-3.33}{0.2455} = -13.56$$

Because Z is in the critical region defined by $Z < -1.96$ or $Z > +1.96$, the hypothesis of equal mean homophobic scores is rejected. The nurses who said no to working with PWAs have higher homophobic scores than do the nurses who said yes. The 95% confidence interval for the difference in the means is given as

$$\mu_{Yes} - \mu_{No} = -3.33 \pm 1.96(0.2455)$$
$$= -3.33 \pm 0.48$$

As we see, the population difference might be as large as 4.05 units or as low as 3.11 units on the homophobic scale.

6–17 STATISTICAL METHODS FOR DICHOTOMOUS VARIABLES

As an illustration on how to estimate the parameters and test hypothesis for survey data based on dichotomous variables in stratified sampling consider item number 11 of Questionnaire 1. this item is as follows:

11. Do you have friends, coworkers, or family members who are gay/lesbian?
Yes___ No___

Responses to this item are reported in Table 6–12 for nurses classified on the basis of county and how they responded to item 10:

10. Are you willing to work with PWAs?
Yes___ No___

As indicated, the proportion of nurses in Los Angeles who said yes to working with AIDS patients and who know gay/lesbian people is given by 0.5340. For the 274 nurses of Los Angeles County who said no to working with

TABLE 6–12 PROPORTION OF NURSES WITH GAY/LESBIAN ACQUAINTANCES ACCORDING TO COUNTY AND WILLINGNESS TO WORK WITH PWAS

County	$\hat{p}_k$	n_k	$\dfrac{\hat{p}\hat{q}}{n_k}$	$\hat{P}_k$	n_k	$\dfrac{\hat{p}\hat{q}}{n_k}$
					Statistic	
Los Angeles	0.5340	103	0.002416	0.0438	274	0.000153
San Diego	0.4314	51	0.004810	0.0512	78	0.000623
Santa Clara	0.5333	15	0.016593	0.0741	54	0.001271
San Francisco	0.8462	13	0.010011	0.1379	29	0.004099
Sacramento	0.6250	16	0.014648	0.1667	24	0.005788
Alameda	0.8333	12	0.011574	0.1333	30	0.003851
Sonoma	0.6667	6	0.037035	0.0833	12	0.006363
San Joaquin	0.5714	7	0.034986	0.0714	14	0.004736
Kern	0.3333	3	0.074070	0.0000	7	0.000000

AIDS patients, the proportion of nurses who said that they know gay/lesbian people is 0.0438. For nurses willing or not willing to work with AIDS patients, these numbers are used to estimate the proportions and standard errors for nurses who know gay/lesbian people in the state of California. For the two types of nurses, the estimated proportions and the standard errors can be used to set up confidence intervals for the proportions of nurses who know gay/lesbian people. These same statistics can be used to test the hypothesis that the proportions of nurses who know gay/lesbian people are equal.

By definition, the stratified proportion is given as

$$\hat{P}_S = \frac{N_1}{N}\hat{p}_1 + \frac{N_2}{N}\hat{p}_2 + \ldots + \frac{N_K}{N}\hat{p}_K$$

Because we have used proportional sampling, we can replace each N_k/N by n_k/n to give the following formula for computing the proportions for each group:

$$\hat{P}_S = \frac{n_1}{n}\hat{p}_1 + \frac{n_2}{n}\hat{p}_2 + \ldots + \frac{n_K}{n}\hat{p}_K$$

For the nurses who said yes to treating AIDS patients,

$$\begin{aligned}\hat{p}_{yes} &= (0.5340)(0.503) + (0.4314)(0.146) \\ &\quad + \ldots + (0.3333)(0.021) \\ &= 0.5621\end{aligned}$$

and for the nurses who said no,

$$\begin{aligned}\hat{p}_{yes} &= (0.0438)(0.503) + (0.0512)(0.146) \\ &\quad + \ldots + (0.0000)(0.021) \\ &= 0.0673\end{aligned}$$

By definition the squared standard error of the stratified proportion is given in equation 1 at the bottom of the page.

Because we have used proportional sampling and because each $N_k/N < 0.05$, the formula reduces to equation 2 at the bottom of this page.

For the nurses who said yes to treating AIDS patients,

① $$SE^2(\hat{P}_S) = \frac{\hat{p}_1\hat{q}_1}{n_1}\left(\frac{N_1 - n_1}{N_1 - 1}\right)\left(\frac{N_1}{N}\right)^2 + \frac{\hat{p}_2\hat{q}_2}{n_2}\left(\frac{N_2 - n_2}{N_2 - 1}\right)\left(\frac{N_2}{N}\right)^2 + \ldots + \frac{\hat{p}_K\hat{q}_K}{n_K}\left(\frac{N_K - n_K}{N_K - 1}\right)\left(\frac{N_K}{N}\right)^2$$

② $$SE^2(\hat{P}_S) = \frac{\hat{p}_1\hat{q}_1}{n_1}\left(\frac{n_1}{n}\right)^2 + \frac{\hat{p}_2\hat{q}_2}{n_2}\left(\frac{n_2}{n}\right)^2 + \ldots + \frac{\hat{p}_K\hat{q}_K}{n_K}\left(\frac{n_K}{n}\right)^2$$

$$Z = \frac{\hat{P}_{yes} - \hat{P}_{no}}{\sqrt{SE^2(\hat{P}_{yes}) + SE^2(\hat{P}_{no})}} = \frac{0.5621 - 0.0673}{\sqrt{0.001085 + 0.000122}} = \frac{0.4948}{0.0347} = 14.26$$

$$\begin{aligned}
SE^2(\hat{P}_{yes}) &= (0.002416)(0.503)^2 \\
&\quad + (0.004810)(0.146)^2 \\
&\quad + \ldots + (0.074070)(0.021)^2 \\
&= 0.001085 = (0.0329)^2
\end{aligned}$$

and for the nurses who said no,

$$\begin{aligned}
SE^2(\hat{P}_{no}) &= (0.000153)(0.503)^2 \\
&\quad + (0.000623)(0.146)^2 \\
&\quad + \ldots + (0.000000)(0.021)^2 \\
&= 0.000122 = (0.0110)^2
\end{aligned}$$

The 95% confidence intervals for the two groups of nurses are given as

$$\begin{aligned}
P_{Yes} &= \hat{P}_{yes} \pm Z\, SE(\hat{P}_{yes}) \\
&= 0.5621 \pm 1.96(0.0329) \\
&= 0.562 \pm 0.064
\end{aligned}$$

and

$$\begin{aligned}
P_{No} &= \hat{P}_{no} \pm Z\, SE(\hat{P}_{no}) \\
&= 0.0673 \pm 1.96(0.0110) \\
&= 0.067 \pm 0.022
\end{aligned}$$

As we see, there is no overlap in the two intervals,

$$0.50 < P_{Yes} < 0.63 \quad \text{and}$$
$$0.04 < P_{No} < 0.09$$

To test the hypothesis $H_0: P_{Yes} = P_{No}$, the test statistic is given in the equation at the top of this page.

Because Z is in the critical region defined by $Z < -1.96$ or $Z > +1.96$, the hypothesis of equal proportions in the two sets of nurses' scores is rejected. Among the nurses who said no to working with PWAs, fewer are acquainted with gay/lesbian persons than nurses who said they were willing to work with PWAs. The 95% confidence interval for the difference in the proportions is given as

$$\begin{aligned}
P_{Yes} - P_{No} &= 0.4948 \pm 1.96(0.0347) \\
&= 0.495 \pm 0.068
\end{aligned}$$

As we see, the population difference can be as low as 0.34 or as high as 0.56.

Recall that to obtain population estimates that were within 4% of the true value, a sample of 625 nurses was needed, which was increased to 1000 to account for an expected response rate of about 60%. Note that the estimate for P_{Yes} is within 11% of the correct value and the estimate for P_{No} is within 2% of the correct value. In general, errors in estimation for the domain estimates are usually larger than for the total sample. Statistics for the total sample are provided in Table 6–13. With these figures,

$$\begin{aligned}
P_{yes} &= (0.177)(0.503) + (0.2016)(0.146) \\
&\quad + \ldots + (0.1000)(0.021) \\
&= 0.2142
\end{aligned}$$

and

$$\begin{aligned}
SE^2(\hat{P}_{yes}) &= (0.000388)(0.503)^2 \\
&\quad + (0.001248)(0.146)^2 \\
&\quad + \ldots + (0.009000)(0.021)^2 \\
&= 0.000222 = (0.0149)^2.
\end{aligned}$$

The 95% confidence interval for P_{Yes} is given as

$$\begin{aligned}
P_{Yes} &= \hat{P}_{yes} \pm Z\, SE(\hat{P}_{yes}) \\
&= 0.2142 \pm 1.96(0.0149) \\
&= 0.21 \pm 0.03.
\end{aligned}$$

As we see, the error in the estimate is less than 4%.

Many researchers are tempted to collapse the frequencies of Table 6–13 and to use simple random sampling theory on the single sample. Under this model, $\hat{P}_{yes} = 159/748 = 0.2126$. In addition, the squared standard error for $\hat{P}_{yes}$ is given as

$$\begin{aligned}
SE^2(\hat{P}_{yes}) &= \frac{\hat{P}_{yes}\hat{q}_{yes}}{n} = \frac{(0.2126)(0.7874)}{748} \\
&= 0.000224 = (0.0150)^2
\end{aligned}$$

Note the closeness in numerical value of the simple random sample squared standard error and the standard error obtained under stratified sampling. The reason why the values are so close is that proportional sampling was used. Under proportional sampling, collapsing across strata is justified, provided that the response ratios in all strata are equal

TABLE 6-13 RESPONSES ACCORDING TO COUNTY TO ITEM 10*

County	Yes	No	n_k	p_k	$\dfrac{\hat{p}_k \hat{q}_k}{n_k}$
Los Angeles	67	310	377	0.1777	0.000388
San Diego	26	103	129	0.2016	0.001248
Santa Clara	12	57	69	0.1739	0.002082
San Francisco	15	27	42	0.3571	0.005466
Sacramento	14	26	40	0.3500	0.005688
Alameda	14	28	42	0.3333	0.005291
Sonoma	5	13	18	0.2778	0.011146
San Joaquin	5	16	21	0.2381	0.008638
Kern	1	9	10	0.1000	0.009000
Total	159	589	748		

*10. Are you willing to work with PWAs?

___ Yes ___ No

or very similar. If proportional sampling is not used and if the response rates differ across strata, collapsing sample data into one single sample cannot be justified. For this reason, researchers are advised to sample proportional to stratum size. Under such a sampling scheme, *all* the advanced statistical models described in this text can be used without fear of violation of weighting principles, provided that response rates across strata are similar. Although proportional sampling is not always the most efficient method, it is the most convenient and the easiest to use from a statistical point of view.

6-18 RANDOMIZED RESPONSE TECHNIQUE FOR STUDYING SENSITIVE AND EMBARRASSING BEHAVIOR

In many studies, researchers are interested in asking subjects about very sensitive issues related to sexual practices, drug and alcohol usage, abortion, child abuse, gambling behavior, cheating and lying, over eating and other perceived socially deviant and unacceptable behaviors. The three major problems that can be encountered in these types of investigations are:

1. the lack of willingness of the informants to answer questions dealing with topics that are assumed to be personal and private,

2. the truthfulness of the responses that people give to an interviewer or provide as answers to a questionnaire,

3. the emotional turmoil that some subjects may experience in an interview or in responding to a questionnaire in which they are asked to consider their own behavior in very threatening social areas.

The first problem occurs when some subjects are unwilling to talk about who makes the decision to use condoms or other contraceptive measures to prevent pregnancy or socially transmitted diseases. The second problem occurs when, for instance, a drug user tells an interviewer that he or she has never smoked marijuana when, in fact, the person has been doing it for years. The third problem may be encountered when a woman goes to an abortion clinic and is asked to review with a health practitioner any prior experiences with abortion procedures.

One way to help solve the three problems associated with inquiries related to sensitive issues is to use the *randomized response technique* presented by Warner (1965) and expanded on by Warner (1971) and developed by many writers including Liu, Chow, and Mosley (1975), Goodstadt and Gruson (1975), Dowling and Shachtman (1975), and Carr, Marascuilo, and Busk (1982).

As an example of the technique, consider a study of safe sex practices in bisexual men. The randomized response technique can be used in the following way to estimate the prevalence of safe sex behavior in the population of bisexual men.

Each respondent is given a card containing two questions. A typical example follows:

A. George Washington was the King of England.
   Yes ___ No___
B. I practice safe sex with all of my partners.
   Yes ___ No___

The subject is also given a random number generator. As an illustration, a die or a pair of dice to roll. Warner (1965) describes the method in terms of an arrow spinning around a circle with two colored sections— red or blue. Suppose that a pair of dice is used. The subject is told to:

1. roll the dice and add up the sum on the two upper faces,
2. answer Question A if the total is 2, 3, 4, or 5,
3. answer Question B if the total is 6, 7, 8, 9, 10, 11, or 12 and,
4. keep the identification of the question answered secret and unknown to the investigator.

A number of important features in this example are the following:

1. The answer to Question A has only one answer and is an answer known to everyone who would ever be included in the sample.
2. The probabilities associated with the two questions are different.
3. The investigator never knows which response is made with respect to the sensitive issue.

The question about George Washington could be replaced by a declarative statement. For example: "If a 2, 3, 4, or 5 appears, say no." If the probabilities for the two questions are equal, the method fails. Thus, the probabilities must be different but not too far from equal. If one question has a high probability of occurrence, large samples are required and subjects become suspicious. The fact that the interviewer does not know which question is being answered places the informant in a less threatening position and helps to overcome the fear of providing an answer to a question that asks about socially compromising or embarrassing behavior.

For example, suppose 180 men are interviewed and 70 say no. It is immediately known that

$$\begin{aligned}\text{(Number who say no)} &= \text{(Number who say}\\ &\quad \text{no to A)}\\ &\quad + \text{(Number who say}\\ &\quad \text{no to B)}.\end{aligned}$$

Although the *exact* number who say no to A is unknown, an accurate estimate can be made with a large sample. The probability of being told to answer question A is given as

$$P \text{ (total is 2, 3, 4, or 5)} = 10/36.$$

Thus, the estimated number of no responses to question A is given as

$$\begin{aligned}&\text{(Estimated number who say no to A)}\\ &\quad = 180(10/36) = 50.\end{aligned}$$

An estimate of the number who say no to question B is

$$\begin{aligned}&\text{(Estimated number who say no to B)}\\ &\quad = 70 - 50 = 20.\end{aligned}$$

Thus, our estimate of the percentage of bisexual men who do not practice safe sex is $(20/180)100 = 11.1\%$.

Originally the method was designed to obtain information to only one socially sensitive question. Of course, the method can be expanded to cover a battery of items all related to a single or multiple topics. In addition, the technique has been extended in a number of different directions. Questions can be asked with polychotomous responses and responses made on a quantitative scale. For example, questions like the following can be asked:

1. Safe sex practices will stop the spread of AIDS.
   a. Strongly agree
   b. Agree
   c. Undecided
   d. Disagree
   e. Strongly disagree
2. How many times during the past week have you gone off your diet and eaten desserts and sweets?___

Many such questions can be asked using the random response technique.

To reduce costs, the model can be transferred from a personal interview format to a mail questionnaire. The flexibility of the questionnaire makes the technique ideal for computer data collection methods and analysis. Standard errors are available for all the extensions. Thus, the method can be used to obtain data to compare men with women, control subjects with experimental subjects, and other independent variables defined by mutually exclusive and exhaustive classes. In the previous example, the negative response was used as the dependent measure. In other situations, the positive response may be preferred. The choice depends on the issue and the way in which the questions are worded.

6-19 BUDGET PREPARATION FOR SURVEY SAMPLING RESEARCH

An important part of any survey is adequate money to carry it out successfully. Survey research is not an inexpensive model for nursing research. To contact subjects, to induce them to respond, to transfer responses to a computer system, to process the data, and to write the results for general consumption by a lay and professional audience is time-consuming and requires a sufficient amount of money. It is very easy to lose sight of this important component of a survey. Many researchers discover too late that they do not have enough money to complete the survey satisfactorily.

We will use the hypothetical survey on nurses' attitudes toward the treatment of PWAs to illustrate the kinds of expenses that must be considered when planning a mail survey. The basic costs are summarized in Table 6-14.

Item 1 is an estimate of the mailing expenses for three separate mailings based on the assumption that the response rate will be about 60%. For the example, the survey is based on three separate questionnaires and a sample of 1000 nurses per questionnaire. On the first mailing, 3000 questionnaires will be distributed with return envelopes. The total costs for this initial mailing is 3000 × $0.50 = $1500. Across three mailings, the total cost is $2500.

Item 2 covers the costs of preparing and printing the questionnaires. The labels can be purchased from the Board of Registered Nursing in Sacramento for $.10 per name. To reproduce one page of the mailed material, the cost should be about $.10, and with two pages for each questionnaire and one page for the cover letter the total cost will be about $550.

Item 3 provides an estimate of the costs to hire a secretary/clerk to address, stuff and mail the envelopes, keep a record of the returns, and type the reports and research articles to come out of the survey.

Item 4 describes the salary of the research assistant employed for 20 hours per week for 3 months to do the library research, run the computer programs, and perform other research duties.

Item 5 provides an estimate of mainframe computer time at $400 per hour for 4 hours.

Item 6 provides an estimate of reproduction costs for survey material and research reports.

Item 7 describes the costs of preparing the final reports and disseminating the findings to professional readers, as well as other related costs.

The projected costs are underestimates and do not recognize yearly inflational costs. In addition, these figures are based on the assumption that everything about the survey progresses smoothly and on time. This may be a dangerous assumption.

6-20 SUMMARY

Typical surveys are used to obtain information on a large series of questionnaire items. What may be an acceptable allocation of sample sizes to strata for one question may

TABLE 6-14 MINIMAL BUDGET FOR A SURVEY SAMPLING OF 3000 NURSES

Item		Cost
1. Mailing		
First wave	3000 @ $0.50	$1,500.00
Second wave	1200 @ $0.50	600.00
Third wave	600 @ $0.50	300.00
	Total	$2,500.00
2. Preparation of questionnaire		
Printing	5000 @ $0.10 per page	$450.00
Materials	5000 @ $0.10 mail & return	100.00
	Total	$550.00
3. Secretary/clerk	120 hours @ $15.00 per hour	1,800.00
4. Research assistant	@ $1000/month for 3 months	3,000.00
5. Computer	@ $400/hour for 4 hours	1,600.00
6. Xeroxing		2,000.00
7. Preparation and dissemination of report		1,938.00
Grand total		$13,388.00

not be an acceptable allocation for another question. Thus, the research nurse is advised to choose the sampling plan that is optimum for the most important questions. Often the best allocation cannot be achieved because it almost always requires specific knowledge about the strata and the clusters; such information may not be available. Cluster sampling can still be achieved even if the size of the clusters is not known. For example, the first hospital selected can be reached by a telephone call to the administrator to determine the number of nurses that are eligible for the survey. The phone call also provides a good chance to do some public relations work to obtain cooperation and explain the purposes of the survey. These presurvey contacts can help reduce the nonresponse rate and actually improve the kind of information obtained from the individual nurses because a resource person is immediately available to answer questions. Systematic sampling is also useful and in many cases may prove to be more efficient than simple random sampling, although in most cases it mimics the findings that could be obtained from the most basic sampling model.

Most questionnaires contain items that can be treated as independent variables. Examples are sex, age, type of job, years of education, type of nursing degree. These variables can be used as domains of study to make comparisons with respect to dependent variables of interest. For example, a researcher may want to know the following:

1. Do male nurses show a lesser aversion to working with persons with AIDS than female nurses do?

2. Do younger nurses show less aversion to working with persons with AIDS than older, more experienced nurses do?

3. Is there more burnout among nurses who have worked with AIDS patients when compared with nurses who have not worked with AIDS patients?

4. Do nurses who are members of fundamentalist religions demonstrate a higher level of aversion to working with persons with AIDS than nurses who are not members of fundamentalist religions?

5. Do nurses who have gay/lesbian acquaintances show less aversion to working with AIDS patients than nurses do who have no gay/lesbian acquaintances?

Except for subject matter, these types of questions are not unusual in survey research. Unfortunately, they are not easy to analyze in an unbiased fashion using the procedures described in later chapters. Familiar statistical procedures such as chi-square, ANOVA, and regression can be used *if* the elementary units are selected with equal probabilities. Thus, they are valid directly for simple random sampling and systematic sampling. These procedures are also valid for stratified sampling but only if the analyses are carried out between and within samples. In other words, collapsing across strata is not permissible. An important exception to this general rule exists if proportional allocation has been adopted. With proportional allocation self-weighting samples are generated. The models can be adopted with cluster sampling combined with proportional allocation, but if proportional allocation is not used and if the models of subsequent chapters are adopted, the estimates are almost certain to be biased.

Finally, sample sizes may be dictated not by sampling requirements but by analytical requirements. This is especially true if frequency data are to be analyzed using cross-tabulations and chi-square methodology. For example, a researcher may wish to compare males with females with respect to 5 different job classifications. For a chi-square test these 2 variables define 10 unique cells. If these variables are now crossed with an attitude scale containing 5 categories, the resulting 3-dimensional contingency table has 50 cells. One assumption of the chi-square test is that none of the expected frequencies can be below 5. Thus, the test requires a minimum of 250 subjects and actually many more because some cells contain 20 to 30 subjects, thereby producing a contingency table with cells whose frequencies are below 5. In this case, it may be wise to increase the sample size to 500 to ensure that the statistical analysis can be carried out.

Frequently survey data are submitted to multivariate analysis models in which correlation coefficients play an important role. Correlation coefficients are exceedingly unstable and require large samples, especially for regression analysis, multivariate analysis of variance, and factor analysis. Many rules are provided by various authors concerning sample sizes for such studies. The proper approach is to consider power computations and to use specialized tables for determining sample size. Marascuilo and Serlin (1988) provide specific directions for many designs and for multiple regression. (For the exact procedure, see their Chapter 50.)

Here, we recommend a conservative rule of thumb which approximates the exact procedures adequately, that is, to use N = 20 subjects for each variable. For example, to regress P = 10 variables onto a dependent variable and make comparisons across the two sexes, S = 2, and the five job classifications position, J = 5, it would be necessary to have $T = S \times J \times P \times N = 2 \times 5 \times 10 \times 20 = 2000$ observations just to satisfy the statistical requirements of having at least 20 observations per variable for each of the regressions. Thus, when choosing sample sizes consideration must also be given to the kinds of statistical analyses that are planned for the data. They too contribute to the decisions of how large a sample to take to make the survey a success.

REFERENCES

American Nurses' Association: Human Rights Guidelines for Nurses in Clinical and Other Research. Kansas City, MO, American Nurses' Association, 1975.

Carr, J., Marascuilo, L., and Busk, P.: Optimal randomized models and methods for hypothesis testing, J. Ed. Stat., 7: 295–310, 1982.

Cochran, W. G.: Sampling Techniques, ed. 3. New York, John Wiley & Sons, 1977.

Code of Federal Regulations, Title 45, Part 46, Washington, DC, January 26, 1981.

Crosby, F., and Herek, G.M.: Male sympathy with the situation of women: does personal experience make a difference, J. Soc. Issues, 42: 55–66, 1986.

Dowling, T.A., and Shachtman, R.H.: On the relative efficiency of randomized response models, J. Am. Stat. Assoc., 70: 84–87, 1975.

Goodstadt, M.S., and Gruson, V.: The randomized response technique: a test on drug use, J. Am. Stat. Assoc., 70: 814–818, 1975.

Gortner, S.R., et al.: The institutional review board: a case study of no-risk decisions on health-related research, Nurs. Res., 30: 21–24, 1981.

Hansen, M., Hurwitz, W., and Madow, W.: Sample Survey Methods and Theory, vol. 1. New York, John Wiley & Sons, 1953.

Hansen, M., Hurwitz, W., and Madow, W.: Sample Survey Methods and Theory, vol. 2. New York, John Wiley & Sons, 1962.

Herek, G.M.: Beyond "homophobia": a social psychological perspective on attitudes toward lesbian and gay men, J. Homosex., 10: 1–21, 1984.

Herek, G. M.: On heterosexual masculinity: some psychical consequences of the social construction of gender and sexuality, Am. Behav. Sci., 29: 563–577, 1986a.

Herek, G.M.: The instrumentality of attitudes: toward a neofunctional theory, J. Soc. Issues, 42: 99–114, 1986b.

Katz, J.: Experimentation with Human Beings: The Authority of the Investigator, Subject, Professions and State in the Human Experimentation Process. New York, Russell Sage Foundation, 1972.

Kish, L.: Survey Sampling. New York, John Wiley & Sons, 1965.

Kruskal, W., and Mosteller, F.: Representative sampling II: scientific literature, excluding statistics, Internat. Stat. Rev., 47: 111–127, 1979.

Liu, P.T., Chow, L.P., and Mosley, W.H.: Use of randomized response technique with a new randomizing device, J. Am. Stat. Assoc., 70: 329–332, 1975.

Marascuilo, A., and Serlin, R.C.: Statistical Methods for the Behavioral Sciences. New York, Freeman, 1988.

Serlin, R.C.: Hypothesis testing, theory building, and the philosophy of science, J. Counseling Psychol., 34: 365–371, 1987.

Serlin, R.C., and Lapsley, D.K.: Rationality in psychological research: the good-enough principle, Am. Psychol., 40: 73–83, 1985.

Singer, E.: Informed consent: consequences for response rate and response quality in social surveys, Am. Sociol. Rev., 43: 144–162, 1978a.

Singer, E.: The effects of informed consent procedures on respondents' reactions to surveys, J. Consumer Res., 5: 49–57, 1978b.

Smith, R.J.: Electroshock experiment at Albany violates ethics guidelines, Science, 198: 383–386, 1977.

US Department of Health, Education, and Welfare: The Institutional Guide to DHEW Policy on Protection of Human Subjects. Washington, DC, US Government Printing Office, 1971.

US National Commission for the Protection of Human Subjects of Biomedical and Behavioral Research: The Belmont Report: Ethical Principles and Guidelines for the Protection of Human Subjects of Research. DHEW Publication No. (05) 78-0012. Washington, DC, US Government Printing Office, 1978.

van Servellen, G.M., Lewis, C.E., and Leake, B.: Nurses' knowledge, attitudes, and fears about AIDS, J. Nurs. Sci. Pract., 3: 1–7, 1988.

Warner, S.L.: Randomized responses: A survey technique for eliminating evasive answer bias, J. Am. Stat. Assoc., 60: 63–69, 1965.

Warner, S.L.: Linear randomized response model, J. Am. Stat. Assoc., 66: 884–888, 1971.

Chapter 7

INTRODUCTION TO EXPLORATORY DESCRIPTIVE RESEARCH APPROACHES TO INVESTIGATE NURSING PHENOMENA

7–1 ROLE OF QUALITATIVE STUDIES IN NURSING RESEARCH

In the previous chapters we have laid the groundwork for studies in nursing that are variants of experimental, quasi-experimental, and survey designs and are basically quantitative in nature. The basic premise underlying this text is an emphasis on hypothesis testing and the quantification of research data to support or refute nursing conjectures. It is important to note that a number of research strategies actively employed by nurse researchers could be characterized as hypothesis generating. Although necessary in the development of knowledge, these particular research styles and strategies are not treated in the following discussion systematically or with the in-depth presentation required to execute them properly. In this chapter, we are interested in providing an overview and flavor of a few qualitative investigational approaches used by nurse researchers. The basic point of this chapter is to suggest models by which qualitative data can be subjected to selected quantitative analyses. The reader is forewarned that he or she cannot successfully engage in the sophisticated investigational techniques subsumed under the broad category of qualitative research through only the perusal of this very brief chapter. We have tried to indicate and name some of the major references and authors in several qualitative research traditions. The reader should consult these references to gain a preliminary insight and appreciation of qualitative research methods.

The studies that play a major role in nursing research are studies that are termed *exploratory descriptive* investigations or *qual-*

itative studies. According to Knafl and Howard (1984), ". . . qualitative methods include ethnography, case studies, in depth interviews, and participant observation." To these specific types of qualitative research can be added content analysis, descriptive statistics, grounded theory, field method research, historiography, hypothesis generating studies, phenomenological research methods, and related methodologies.

In this chapter, a selective examination is made of some of these methodologies and their use in nursing research. The relative advantages and disadvantages of these methods are assessed, and illustrations of their use are provided. Following this exposition, qualitative research strategies that serve as an adjunct to quantitative methods are examined. Next, an example of a qualitative research inquiry is provided. In the process of data analysis and synthesis, variables are identified, dimensions and categories emerge, and tentative propositions are generated which can be treated statistically, if desired.

7-2 STRENGTHS AND WEAKNESSES OF QUALITATIVE RESEARCH METHODS

Strengths

The following strengths are integral to qualitative research methods.

1. Qualitative research methods bring to light important variables, processes, and interactions that deserve more extensive attention. Chenitz and Swanson (1986) describe a study that takes place in a methadone clinic. Using a series of repeated observations of nurse–drug addict interactions, they conceptualized a new set of variables. One variable that they identified is termed *selectively attending or specifically focusing in* and is used to describe confrontational activities engaged in by nurses when dealing with drug addicts about current drug use. This new variable can be treated as the basis for new studies in which these types of interactions are studied in other qualitative designs, correlational studies, and quasi-experimental designs.

2. They pioneer new ground and offer new sources for fruitful hypotheses to be studied in another planned study. Bailey (1985) describes an ethnographic study that takes place in two different residences for the elderly. She discovered that there was a difference in the levels of energy and activity between the elderly in one site and those in the other study site. Residents in a private-paying setting appeared passive and less involved in ongoing community and in-house activities. The residents of a federally subsidized housing area were essentially the opposite. This finding could be put to a test of a hypothesis in a carefully planned second investigation. Factors that might be important in explaining this finding is that the two different sites attract different kinds of residents. Elderly with limited financial resources may have no alternative but to choose the federally subsidized housing area. The more physically unstable patients may have the resources to choose the private-paying resident program.

3. They provide anecdotal or illustrative examples to illustrate quantification findings. McLaughlin and colleagues (1978a; 1979a; 1979b) in a quasi-experimental study compared physicians' and nurses' performances on two patient problem exercises. Participants were interviewed after the administration of a paper and pencil test to elicit their reactions to and understanding of the problem situations of the study. It was discovered that in spite of hypothesized predictions, a number of public health nurses performed as well as physicians and nurse practitioners on the clinical test. From anecdotal materials, it was learned that a number of public health nurses had recently worked in an acute care setting or had taken a refresher course on the clinical topic. This provided a reason for the finding. Without the anecdotal information, this finding would not have been discovered.

4. They provide a useful opportunity to develop nursing concepts derived from systematic observations of nursing practices. Hutchinson (1984) describes responses of nurses working in a neonatal intensive critical care unit with very sick babies. This investigator describes the visual, aural, tactile, and emotional stimuli that elicit feelings of horror among many nurses at some time during their nursing unit experience. With the acknowledgment of this horror, the question emerged, "What enables nurses to survive and choose to work day after day in this environment?" A concept that emerged is what

the author called *creating meaning*. This refers to the cognitive emotional process of attributing psychological meaning or value to the babies whom a nurse cares for. This variable can be used for future investigation in other settings that might involve surveys, field studies, and quasi-experimental and experimental designs.

5. They can be used to generate propositions that can be tested in new settings. Mishel (1981) did a qualitative study in which she interviewed hospitalized patients to develop statements of uncertainty associated with illness or hospitalization. The qualitative data were categorized according to sources and types of uncertainty and transformed to a 54-item Likert scale. The resulting scale was administered to a larger sample of hospitalized patients and then factor analyzed. In numerous subsequent studies, Mishel and other investigators (Christman et al., 1988) have continued to use the factors to test propositions about uncertainty and patients' responses to hospitalization (1983a; 1983b; 1984a; 1984b; 1988).

6. They are easier to interpret because they generally relate more directly to the everyday experiences of practitioners and consumers. Fagerhaugh (1973) did a series of studies concerning how patients with advanced emphysema get around physically in their environment because of their extreme oxygen shortage. She categorized the resources of emphysema patients into time, energy, and money. She identified the variables that assisted patients to get around in terms of these three basic resources. Her research is extremely easy to describe to emphysema patients, their families, and their caretakers.

7. They can be performed in naturalistic and nonartificial environments. All the studies described in this section were performed in naturalistic settings. A review of the literature will uncover many more.

Weaknesses

The following weaknesses have been identified in qualitative research methods.

1. Qualitative research methods are used too often to study atypical environments and atypical events (Fielding and Fielding, 1986). Qualitative researchers are like all human beings—fascinated by the unusual, the bizarre, the extreme, and the idiosyncratic. Although these groups are interesting, their numbers are few and findings for these types of specialized research topics probably possess limited usefulness for the advancement of nursing research and practice. Nursing research will advance more rapidly if the *typical patient* and the *typical event* are studied, described, and understood better.

2. They are difficult to repeat or replicate in other settings by different investigators (Chenitz and Swanson, 1986). With the information frequently provided in the resulting reports, replication is very difficult to achieve because the events, personalities, situations, and encounters seem to be time-bound and specific to a special set of circumstances and to particular places. Furthermore, the distinct theoretical perspectives and personality of the investigator are often difficult to separate from the body of the report. It is in essence an art form representative of a highly artistic, creative, and imaginative portrayal of special occurrences and particular personalities.

3. They are inordinately inefficient because of the high labor-intensive cost. Entering a naturalistic setting for long periods requires considerable commitment and investment of the investigator's time and energy. Long periods of sustained observation over varying 24-hour cycles lasting for months or years are frequently reported by qualitative researchers. Extensive time intervals are generally required for these types of studies. After permission is obtained to enter the environment, gaining credibility, trust, and acceptance is also a long-term process. In addition, it takes a long time to become familiar with the scene, know the key players, understand the themes and behaviors of the participants, and gain critical insights into variables affecting the phenomena of interest.

Other factors to consider are that qualitative researchers frequently study questions that are highly volatile, interpersonally sensitive, politically threatening, emotionally charged, and culturally controversial. As a consequence, the time periods for data collection must, of necessity, be extensive in order to gain acceptance and familiarity with very threatening or uncomfortable sources of interpersonal transactions and social behaviors.

4. They are highly dependent and rely on data that are for the most part hand- or type-

written and that are essentially long, written narratives. The qualitative researcher in the conduct of a project records voluminous notes, which are coded periodically and placed in logs. At the end of a project, it is not unusual to be faced with hundreds or thousands of pages of narration. It is, indeed, a formidable exercise to extract meaning and summarize salient concepts from the morass of copious records kept by the researcher (Leininger, 1985). Here the term *immersed in the data* has true meaning.

In the hand of a creative writer, unimportant, poorly documented studies can be very persuasive in affecting a reader's point of view on any topic, whether it is nursing research or whether it is a study regarding which opera singer is the best in the world. Many qualitative studies are free of investigator bias and preconceived notions. Two excellent examples of a collection of qualitative research reports are to be found in Chenitz and Swanson (1986) and in Leininger (1985).

5. They are easily open to bias if an investigator cannot remain detached and objective about the environments, settings, and people studied (Fielding and Fielding, 1986). This is a problem that all researchers must face. It is not a problem exclusive to any one research method or theoretical perspective. It is necessary to use rules for both qualitative and quantitative research to counteract the possibilities of bias or subjectivity in the collection or analysis of data. Qualitative guidelines are found in Chenitz and Swanson (1986) and in Leininger (1985). Rules for quantitative studies can be found in Campbell and Stanley (1963), Cook and Campbell (1979), and Trochim (1986).

6. They are subject to generating hypotheses that cannot be tested using other research methods or designs. A dispassionate review of nursing literature on a specific topic does not provide strong evidence that many hypothesis-generating studies have led to hypothesis-testing investigations. This may be partly a function of the newly developing body of nursing science because the bulk of extant research reports are in the descriptive exploratory mode.

7. They fail to produce findings that can be incorporated into an already existing body of knowledge about a general topic. Not enough qualitative studies represent a sequential development of knowledge in a specific substantive area. Too often, highly creative and conceptually exciting qualitative studies are reported, and the investigator moves on to different areas of research interest. At times, the connections—both theoretical and empirical—between a piece of qualitative research and the subsequent work of the same investigator are difficult to identify or cannot be easily connected.

7–3 QUALITATIVE METHODOLOGY FOR NURSING RESEARCH

Considerable diversity in views seems to exist among researchers in the behavioral science and nursing fields regarding the definition of qualitative methodology. Each author appears to use a definition that is specific to the interest and philosophical position held by the person doing the qualitative research. The following set of proposed definitions should point out the problems involved in specifying the nature of this type of research, and yet the definitions collectively describe the general notions and themes involved in qualitative research. It should be noted that the 10 definitions do not represent a random sample of definitions from a universe of definitions. They represent a convenience sample that was readily available.

1. According to Chenitz and Swanson (1986), "Qualitative research . . . is viewed within a symbolic interactionist framework . . . (that) is both a philosophy of human life and social experience and a distinctive approach to the study of human life."

2. According to Chinn and Jacobs (1987), "[qualitative research] . . . is theory generating . . . [and] includes field observations as used in anthropology and participant observation as used in sociology. The investigator attempts to minimize any intrusion or effect on events observed and seeks to view and describe things occurring as they would if the observer were not present."

3. According to Fawcett and Downs (1985), "Descriptive [Qualitative] studies [employ] the empirical method [involving] observation of a phenomena in its natural setting. Data are gathered by participant or nonparticipant observation, as well as by open-ended or structured interview schedules or questionnaires. Qualitative data may be analyzed by means of content analysis . . . which sort data into a priori categories

or into categories that emerge during the analysis."

4. According to Jacob (1987), "Qualitative research [emanates] from five contemporary American qualitative research traditions [representing] ecological psychology, holistic ethnography, cognitive anthropology, ethnography of communication, and symbolic interactionism. . . . Methodologies developed in qualitative traditions are the product of assumptions and particular foci of study."

5. According to Johnson (1975), [Qualitative researchers] go directly to [nursing] phenomena. . . . [Such research] is based upon the following features: a philosophy of human freedom, choice, responsibility; a belief in human and cultural spirituality; a biology and psychology of wholism [a nonreducible, nondivisible, person interconnected with others and nature, a mind, a body, a spirit, gestalt]; ontology of time and space; a context of interhuman events, processes, and relationships; a scientific world view that is open; and a method that allows for esthetics, empirics, human values, and process discovery."

6. According to Knafl and Howard (1984), "Qualitative research is equated with those methods or data gathering techniques which generate narrative as opposed to numerical data. Qualitative data takes the form of verbatim interview or field note transcripts."

7. According to Leininger (1985), "Qualitative . . . research refers to the mehods and techniques of observing, documenting, analyzing, and interpreting attributes, patterns, characteristics, and meanings of specific contextual or gestaltic features of phenomena under study."

8. According to Oiler (1986), qualitative research methods ". . . [pay] attention to subjects' realities in formulating the research question . . . attention to such realities requires that the researcher approach the study with a holistic perspective . . . the researcher must recognize that she is herself immersed in the phenomenon of study by virtue of studying it. . . . [Qualitative research] aims to describe experience rather than to define, categorize, explain, or interpret it."

9. According to Reinharz (1979), "Qualitative research includes the creation of gestalts and meaningful patterns. It also includes viewing natural events in their ongoing contexts with theory emerging from research facts or findings."

10. According to Tripp-Reimer (1985), "Qualitative studies tend to be exploratory providing rich descriptive and documentary information and . . . tend to be hypothesis generating. [It] is used appropriately when an investigator does not have a comprehensive understanding of the topic . . . or when investigators do not know the way important questions should be asked or the range of responses likely to be elicited . . . [It] facilitate(s) serendipitous findings, raise(s) unexpected questions, and identify(ies) topics the investigator might not otherwise have considered."

As is evident in reviewing the diverse perspectives enunciated in the preceding quotations, qualitative methods encompass a wide array of theoretical viewpoints, philosophical assumptions, empirical methods, investigative strategies, data analytical procedures, interpretative rules, cultural references, and humanistic frameworks. That it is difficult, if not impossible, to provide a unifying definition of qualitative methods should be obvious from a review of these 10 definitions selected from a whole population of definitions of qualitative methods. The remainder of this chapter contains descriptions of what we view to be qualitative methods. Because the presentation represents our views, it is suggested that other sources be examined to learn what qualitative methods mean to other authors.

7-4 GROUNDED THEORY: A MODEL FOR NURSING RESEARCH

According to Chenitz and Swanson (1986), "grounded theory is a highly systematic research approach for the collection and analysis of qualitative data for the purpose of generating explanatory theory that furthers the understanding of social and psychological phenomena." From a historical point of view, grounded theory is nested in the ideas of *symbolic interactionism*. Symbolic interactionists assume that meanings about human behavior arise through social encounters and interactions with other persons. A person's interpretation of the meaning of an interaction is not an automatic application of socially acceptable or sanctioned meanings.

The interpretative process that a person goes through to arrive at meaning is the focus of the research conducted by symbolic interactionists. Whereas, on the one hand, a number of schools of psychology believe that human behavior is a reaction or response to instincts, conscious and unconscious drives, and motivational factors, symbolic interactionists do not see human behavior as being caused by such deterministic forces. Symbolic interactionists, on the other hand, see group life as a process in which, in their various interpersonal transactions, people indicate individual lines or modes of behavior and action, and each person interprets the indicated behaviors of others in light of their own behaviors and understandings. Symbolic interaction theorists want to understand the process by which the point of view of each person is developed knowing that each viewpoint is shaped and bounded by the social groups to which each individual is a member.

Grounded theorists are not interested in testing or proving theory. Their goal is to identify themes and to construct hypotheses as they are extracted from the research data. Data analysis and data collection are done simultaneously, with preliminary data analysis informing future data collection. Participant observation and informal interviews are the principle means by which data are collected. Earlier in the data collection, theoretical notes are generated, which are self-conscious, controlled attempts to *derive meaning* from the notes made during the interviews or participant observation sessions. These short notes are linked together and expanded into longer analytical memos with the goal to increase conceptual development (Glaser and Strauss, 1965; 1968).

Symbolic interactions do not operationalize a concept until after they have been in the field. From one perspective, the grounded theory investigator plays with data, relating different observations to one another in the hope that new concepts will emerge and that those new concepts will be linked to concepts in the extant literature. In following these phases, the grounded theory researcher aims to identify and discover important classes of things, persons, and events and the properties that characterize them.

The way in which a grounded theory investigation can be conducted is summarized here. It might be assumed that the last step in a grounded theory study consists of an analysis of the data and generation of the theory and hypotheses. Unfortunately, that is not how a grounded theory study operates. Instead the theoretical linkages and conceptual development emerge throughout the entire operation of the study. The last step is truly a production of a written narrative based on the ever-constant analysis and reanalysis. The steps in a grounded theory study are as follows:

1. The place in which the study is performed must be identified. To assist a reader, reasons for choosing the site should be indicated.

2. Gaining access to the setting or site to do the study must be negotiated with participants and agencies. This means that informed consent procedures must be followed. For a review of informed consent procedures see Section 6–2.

3. Establishing a role as either a complete participant or a complete observer must be completed before any data can be collected. Depending upon which role is selected, different notes are taken and different hypotheses can result. This suggests that two different, grounded theorists could conceivably produce dissimilar and perhaps contradictory final narratives.

4. Collecting and recording field notes and interview data must be done on site when people are in interactions in social settings. Protocols should be so defined that, in theory, another grounded theorist would collect the same data.

5. Exiting or leaving the field where the study was conducted must be carefully managed and performed only when *all* pertinent data have been collected. To some researchers this process could be viewed as never ending. To some a grounded theory study must be viewed as written narrative based on the ever-constant analysis and reanalysis and tentative in its interpretation of human behavior.

6. The last step is writing the report from which tentative theory and hypotheses are generated.

When a researcher begins a grounded theory research study, he or she goes into the environment in which events, interactions, and situations occur that have theoretical interest to a particular research issue. The investigator generally has a preliminary idea of some of the key forces at work in the environment, but a formal set of hypotheses are not set up before entrance into the environment of the study. The principle research tool employed by a researcher is the person who observes and records selective events.

The data used for the study are primarily based on informal interviews, direct observations, papers and official documents, letters, newspapers, official organization memos and handouts, and any other typical communication used by persons in the environment. Field work is highly dependent on disciplined note taking. Notes may be taken directly in front of the key players or actors, but more often after a significant observation or interview has taken place. Some researchers use a code book in which notations are made in the margins of each field note or interview. Theoretical notes are then made and the individual researcher reenters the environment to establish the veracity or soundness of the theoretical linkages. A cyclical process is enacted through subsequent analysis of notes with a theoretical proposition. When the researcher has concluded that the environment is saturated or has exhausted all possible instances of the phenomena under study, the study is halted. To some this is a difficult decision to make.

7–5 PHENOMENOLOGICAL NURSING RESEARCH METHODS

According to Chinn and Jacobs (1987), ". . . phenomenology is a research method which explicitly seeks to describe the subjective lived experience of people and comprehend the meanings that people place on their experience." Phenomenological methods in nursing research adhere to certain principles consistent with primary phenomenological themes (Oiler, 1986).

First, the attention paid by researchers to each subject's definition of reality in posing a research question is a preeminent consideration. At this stage it is important to the phenomenologist to capture and disclose human experience in *all* its magnificent and variegated complexities.

Second, the researcher must approach the study with a holistic perspective. The selection of data collection procedures at this stage is guided by the intent to preserve the natural spontaneity of each person's lived experiences. Repeated contacts with study subjects are necessary to gain an understanding of the range of each person's expression in order to exhaust all possible instances of the phenomena under study. At this point, a phenomenologist must be careful not to fall into the trap of homing in on certain behaviors and events nor to consciously or unconsciously pay attention to only particular or specialized events, processes, or persons in the environment. Selective observations at this stage must be guarded against, and premature closure must not occur.

Third, the researcher becomes an integral part of the research process because of total immersion in the phenomena. A full range of interpersonal modes of awareness on the part of the researcher are used in data collection. Empathetic and intuitive awareness are included in research design choices. Information is gathered about the broad scope in which people depict their life experiences to others. Here, researchers must control their involvement in the phenomena in order to avoid idiosyncratic bias. This bias can be avoided by explicating the researcher's perspective, bracketing prior explanations about the phenomena, selecting unfamiliar settings, people, and circumstances, assuming an unobtrusive presence, and using a coinvestigator as a check on personal biases. To some investigators the immersion of the observer into an environment is a stimulus that changes the contexts of the events to be observed. The environment is different when the observer is not there. Thus, the applicability of the researcher's findings may be called into question.

Fourth, the enlargement of the qualitative expression of the findings can be achieved by methods other than the specification of dimensions and categories. A successful description directs the consumer of research to his or her own experiences and conclusions. The test for validating a phenomenological research study resides in the consumer. The study is valid if the consumer recognizes the descriptions as true. This means that a reader of the phenomenological narrative can deny or reject the findings if the report does not agree with the reader's own experiences and perceptions.

Fifth, the results of phenomenological studies can be reported through such media as photographs, poems, and narrative descriptions (Lynch-Sauer, 1985). These alternative methods of data presentation must be used with care if the results are to have meaning for nursing research.

7–6 ETHNOGRAPHY AS A RESEARCH MODEL FOR NURSING RESEARCH

According to Leininger (1985), "ethnography . . . can be defined as the systematic process of observing, detailing, describing, documenting, and analyzing the lifeways or particular patterns of a culture [or subculture] in order to grasp the lifeways or patterns of the people in their familiar environment. An ethnographer documents, describes, and analyzes physical, cultural, social, and environmental features as these factors influence people's patterns of living." Ethnographers generate both real life (grounded) and abstract theories about people and in general phenomena. The data can be used to gain fresh insights or interpret behavior. Ethnographic methods in nursing have been used by nurse anthropologists.

The ethnographic nursing research process, according to Leininger (1985), encompasses a series of steps, summarized here.

1. The first step is to identify a domain of inquiry.
2. After the domain of study has been made, a literature search of the domain should be made to see what others have done and learned about the domain.
3. The research tool and instruments should be established and approvals to perform the study should be obtained.
4. The study subjects should be identified and chosen for study.
5. The study is performed by observing, participating, interviewing, and validating data.
6. The analytic strategies must be formulated and the data must be analyzed.
7. The research findings are reported.

Much of what was stated for grounded theory and phenomenological research can be repeated here.

7–7 CONTENT ANALYSIS IN NURSING RESEARCH

Content analysis is a method for categorizing verbal, behavioral, and pictorial information which represents unstructured qualitative data. The goal of content analysis is to identify the structure of the collected information. All qualitative research involves content analytic procedures and techniques in one form or another. Each behavioral science discipline such as sociology, anthropology, and psychology among others has developed specific rules and procedures for conducting a content analysis. The content analysis models used in grounded theory, ethnography, and phenomenological research are based on the theoretical perspectives and specific techniques developed from each of the respective three behavioral sciences. These are not described here. Instead a generic content analytic process applicable to both qualitative and quantitative nursing research studies is illustrated.

There are three overall phases to a typical content analysis. They are as follows:

1. Deciding on the unit of analysis
2. Creating or using existing set of mutually exclusive and exhaustive categories for classification of information of each identified dimension
3. Developing rules for coding data into appropriate categories for each dimension associated with the entire set of data

At the outset the investigator must make a decision on how the verbal, behavioral, or pictorial information is to be examined. For instance, in examining verbal data, are individual words or terms to be the particular unit, or are themes abstracted from collections of words to be the unit? Verbal behavioral or pictorial information can be broken down into highly refined or micro units or one can use a macro-analytical system such as themes, patterns, and trends.

After selecting a micro or macro unit of analysis, the investigator must decide whether existing classification systems are appropriate to the particular study. It is inherently more desirable to use an existing classification system which is tried and true than to establish a new system. Most investigators, however, in qualitative research, tend to create their own dimensions and category systems. This is true because most qualitative researchers are pioneering unexplored or poorly defined substantive research areas. If the latter is the case, then the task is a much more complex and involved process. The problem facing most researchers at this point is to identify enough theoretically relevant variables with categories to assign the appropriate data. The problem becomes one of identifying either too many classes or too few.

After a satisfactory listing and division of

dimensions and categories have been established, specific rules should be stated so that instances defined by one category are always placed in that category and not in any other. At this point, qualitative researchers have a tendency to falter. Generally the qualitative researcher develops the dimensions and their categories, establishes the rules for assigning the appropriate information to a specific dimension and category, and then notes or counts instances of where the information appears and does not appear in the different categories. It is unusual to read in a qualitative study that, prior to publication, someone other than the researcher independently examined the same verbal, behavioral, or pictorial data. At this stage, it would be advisable to perform a test of reliability.

A test of reliability can be done by using a second researcher. This second reader would follow the stated rules and match the verbal, behavioral, or pictorial information to the categories used by the original researcher. The original researcher would then check to see how well they agreed in their classifications. In quantitative research, it is the rule rather than the exception for different researchers to separately examine the identical data and independently assign the information to mutually exclusive and exhaustive categories. In this instance, particular rules for the development of interrater reliability or agreement have been described and illustrated in Chapter 3. Here, we present an example.

In a health care agency, a nursing union has proposed a strike resulting from unsatisfactory contract renegotiations. To determine how the typical nurse feels about joining the strike, an informal interview was conducted with five staff nurses. Here are the responses of these five nurses to the question:

Question: What is your view about the success of the proposed strike?

Response A. I really don't know how I feel about the strike at this time. I have never had an experience in joining a strike. Things are pretty bad here and most of the staff want some definite changes made. So far we have not been too successful. It would be a financial hardship for me to leave my job for weeks or months.

Response B. I think I am now 150% in favor of the strike. Two weeks ago I was not, but now the administration has really become awful. I have to tell you that I am fed up to my neck with their attitude. I know the strike will be 150% successful because we are determined to win and get our raise. I have to tell you I am in favor.

Response C. I don't support a strike. I've worked here over 20 years and I have too much invested in this place to walk out. I'm concerned about my pension, my seniority, and my day shift work schedule. I have a pretty good deal here and, at age 50, I'm not about to throw everything away. The younger ones have nothing to lose and I say, more power to them, but I'm not walking out.

Response D. Gosh, I don't know what I think. I don't want to go on strike, but I don't know how to make things better here. I know some of my friends want the strike but I'm not so sure. I don't know what good it will do. If we go on strike, who will take care of these poor patients? I just can't leave them alone to suffer.

Response E. I come from a labor family. Everyone has belonged to a union and we are used to having some member of the family being on strike. We all put away three months' salary in case we are out on strike and need money to pay our bills and eat. I'll be out there on the picket line and I've already agreed to appear on our local TV station to present the nurses's side.

These data can be categorized in a number of ways. The unit of analysis can be words, terms, themes, ideas, feeling tone, latent content, and so on. More on this topic appears in Section 7–9. The researcher must decide which of these units is best for the particular item to be analyzed. In a single interview, it would not be unusual to use different units for different items. Here we use themes as the unit of analysis. We begin by listing the themes for each response. These are summarized in Table 7–1. In practice, it is advisable to use about 20 to 30 interviews that are randomly or systematically selected from the full pool of completed interviews.

For these five nurses, the number of identifiable themes is 27, of which 18 are unique. A number of overlaps occur in the themes across these five nurses, which can be combined into a smaller set of dimensions. Let us consider the dimension *degree of support for the strike*. Each of the five nurses can be placed on this dimension. Their responses follow:

Nurse A. Indecisive or ambivalent about the strike: "I really don't know how I feel about the strike at this time."

TABLE 7–1 THEMES ASSOCIATED WITH THE FIVE INTERVIEWS OF NURSES GOING ON A PROPOSED STRIKE

Nurse A.
Indecisiveness or ambivalence about the strike
Previous history with a strike
Satisfaction with current work environment
Desire for changes in work environment
Ability to make changes in work situation
Financial hardship of a strike

Nurse B.
Degree of support of a strike
Changes by administration that shift opinions
Satisfaction with administration policies
Perceived success of the strike

Nurse C.
Degree of support of a strike
Longevity in work situation
Investment in work situation
Perceived negative consequences of a strike
Satisfaction with current work environment
Perceived consequences to others' participating in strike

Nurse D.
Indecisiveness or ambivalence about the strike
Degree of support of a strike
Perceived inability to effect change in work situation
Perceived peer group support of the strike
Indecisiveness or ambivalence about the strike
Perceived consequences of the strike
Empathy and concern for patient welfare during the strike

Nurse E.
Existence of a primary support system that favors strikes
Previous history with a strike
Financial planning for a strike
Prepared to actively participate in strike

Nurse B. Support of a strike: "I think I am now 150% in favor of the strike."

Nurse C. Nonsupport of a strike: "I don't support a strike. . . . I'm not walking out."

Nurse D. Indecisive or ambivalent about the strike: "Gosh, I don't know what I think." Nonsupport of the strike: "I don't want to go on strike. . . ."

Nurse E. Support of a strike: "I'll be out there on the picket line and I've already agreed to appear on our local TV station to present the nurses's side."

If we define this dimension in terms of the following three categories (Nonsupport, Indecisive, Support), the five nurses would be classified as shown in Table 7–2.

If each nurse could have been placed into only one category, a Likert type scale could be assigned to the categories and the resulting numbers could be used for statistical analysis. But the problem here is that Nurse D is assigned to two categories.

One option is to place Nurse D into one of the two categories, based on a reading of the entire interview to determine the general feeling tone to the response. The general tone is that of nonsupport, and that is where

we would place this nurse. If we wanted to draw an inference about this individual nurse, the prediction would be that Nurse D would cross the picket line. The statement, "I just can't leave them alone to suffer," suggests that the nurse will continue to care for patients while other nurses are out on strike.

The second option is to increase the number of categories on the dimension. In this case, the categories could be increased to strong nonsupport, nonsupport, indifferent, support, strong support. After reading the total interview of Nurse E and assessing the total feeling tone, it can be readily seen that this nurse will completely and totally support a strike. This particular nurse comes

TABLE 7–2 CODING USING THREE POINT SCALE

	Nonsupport	Indecisive	Support
Nurse A		X	
Nurse B			X
Nurse C	X		
Nurse D	X	X	
Nurse E			X

from a family of union members, all of whom have participated in strikes and have saved money to ensure their ability to override the financial losses resulting from their participation in a strike. When a strike is called, this nurse will be marching in the picket line around the hospital. In addition, the nurse has agreed in advance to appear on a local TV station to voice the union's position about why they are on strike. The inference for a future course of action based on this transcript is a nurse completely involved and committed to ensure the success of the strike. Because of this position, Nurse E would be coded in the strong support category. The coding of all five nurses with this five point Likert scale is shown in Table 7–3.

Not all dimensions can be defined by ordered categories. Sometimes a dichotomy is all that can be achieved so that some dimensions can be classified only as yes or no, or positive or negative. An example is associated with the theme *previous history with a strike*. A nurse has or has not participated in a strike prior to that being considered in this study.

One other problem needs to be addressed when a researcher is setting up dimensions and associated categories. Sometimes no mention is made of a dimension by an interviewee. For example, among the five nurses, previous history with a strike was mentioned by only two nurses. Thus, the categories for this dimension would have to be defined by (Yes, No, Not mentioned).

The process of combining categories and defining dimensions would have to be done with the remaining themes identified in the sample of interviews. In addition, coding rules would have to be specified so that coders can classify each subject with as much ease as can possibly be generated. It is a good idea to use two coders who code responses

independently of one another. With two coders, checks on interrater reliability and agreement can be made as described in Chapter 3.

7–8 USE OF QUALITATIVE METHODS IN QUANTITATIVE RESEARCH STUDIES

As already discussed in Chapter 2, the development of nursing research is relatively recent. Many questions and concerns of nurses have been addressed through systematic research only recently. A close study of the types of articles that appear in nursing research journals would reveal that many articles are not theoretically based and even fewer make use of traditional experimental paradigms as found in many other empirically based disciplines. The studies that dominate the nursing research literature are exploratory or descriptive in their approaches.

There are good reasons why exploratory and descriptive studies are so common in the newly emerging clinical and research interests of the nursing profession. Probably the main reason is that in the past nursing was not viewed as a scientifically based profession. Decisions on how to best treat patients were based on experience and intuition. Nursing practices that worked in the past were kept and by repetition became reinforced through hospital procedures and nursing textbooks. Practices that failed to help patients recover quickly and to bring about favorable results were discarded. Today, the nursing profession is caught in the rapidly changing world being produced by scientists who are at the cutting edge of research and technology. With the rapid growth in public health problems, the expansion of knowledge in the biological and behavioral sciences, the accelerated fine tuning in medical practice, and the expanding technology associated with these fields of study and inquiry, it follows that the nursing profession also must change and develop methods that are appropriate and timely for the new world of health care. The ad hoc patient care procedures that were useful just a few years ago are not necessarily very useful today. In fact, many standard patient care protocols may be obsolete in the care of patients in the newly adopted cost-effective-

TABLE 7–3 CODING USING FIVE POINT SCALE

	Strong Non-support	Non-support	Inde-cisive	Sup-port	Strong Support
Nurse A			X		
Nurse B					X
Nurse C	X				
Nurse D			X		
Nurse E					X

ness approaches to health care in the 1980s and 1990s.

In any emerging discipline, observations and descriptions are the precursors of theory generation. Clear descriptions of the attributes of a set of events related to some aspect of health status, nursing behaviors, client characteristics, and environmental factors are needed. Theories supporting nursing practices that permit the generation of hypotheses for testing and theory refinement are dependent on precise descriptions of nursing processes and events. For a long time, nursing research has stagnated at the observation and description phase. Although movement to another form of investigation is necessary for growth, there is no reason to believe that observation will not continue to be the dominant mode of the nurse scientist. Much can be learned by systematic observation and rigorous description. Before sound theories can be formulated which accurately reflect domains of nursing practice and health care, reliable and valid reports on observed events are required and needed.

Careful observation leads to a better understanding and appreciation of the forces at work in a research context. For example, in terms of the preoperative teaching program described in Chapter 1, three different teaching strategies were used. One component in the evaluation of the three teaching strategies that should concern practitioners is the nature of the typical or standard level of nursing care provided to patients before surgery. In other similar studies, nurse investigators testing different intervention programs have frequently assumed that the level of care given to patients was poor, haphazard, unplanned, and inconsistent. In a number of studies, the presumption that the typical level of preoperative preparation was less than adequate was not supported.

No differences could be established between a new intervention program and the typical or standard nursing program used with patients. Two possible explanations for this finding exist. One explanation is that both the intervention program and the standard program were equally effective in terms of the dependent measures used in the study. If both programs are equally effective, chances for showing that an innovative program is better can hardly be demonstrated. The second explanation is that both programs were equally ineffective and are not statistically different from one another on the dependent measurements used in the comparisons. Again, demonstration of a difference is not to be expected.

Before instituting a new nursing intervention program, a discerning investigator should spend a considerable amount of time observing and describing the behaviors of nurses with patients of different health statuses on the patient care unit where a research program is to be inaugurated. Descriptions and observations, over a period before a new program is started, could and should provide an accurate portrayal of the quality of nursing care provided to all patients. In some instances, it would be prudent for investigators to forego an investigation until information about the existing program is documented, analyzed and understood, especially when comparisons are to be made between a new intervention program and an existing nursing care program. If the old nursing care program is a model of nursing excellence or exceptional practice, there is no need for change. In addition, the probability of finding meaningful differences between the old program and the new program would seem less than likely. If the old program is performing well, it will be very difficult to prove that a new nursing care program is more effective. New nursing care programs should be contemplated only when the old nursing care programs are not living up to expectations.

In the case of the hypothetical preoperative teaching study, a careful researcher must make many observations about the quality of nursing care provided in the three different teaching programs. These observations are important because a researcher may believe that one program already exemplifies the optimum or model teaching practice. Information on all three programs is required to guard against this bias.

In addition, observations and descriptions are required throughout the course of the study to ensure that the interventions are being put into practice. Another reason for consistent observations of both nurses and patients is to describe and identify possible intervening or confounding factors that may influence the outcome of the study. For example, an investigator must know with certainty that nurses participating in less desirable treatment programs are in fact consistently performing the requisite teaching practice designed for that particular experimental condition. At the same time, observations should be made and records kept on the behaviors of the patients in each of the treatments. Just because patients were given preoperative training, it does not follow that they will necessarily put their training into practice. Some will; some will not! Careful surveillance of patients is always required in this type of study. If the patient does not do what is expected, no treatment has been put into practice.

In addition to the knowledge gained by observing nurses and patients, a researcher can begin to learn about other patterns of behavior developing among some patients in a specific experimental teaching program. Careful detailed narrative descriptions of particular patients and subsets of patients may provide insights into whether or not their recovery is faster or slower than other patients in other subsets of patients. Observation may show that other factors may help explain why one treatment was more successful than another for various subgroups of patients.

On-site observation permits close connections to develop among the researcher, nurses, staff, practices, patients, and study setting. Clusters of behavior patterns can be identified, which may help to explain the findings or which can be used to modify the treatment for a further investigation. For instance, it may become apparent that particular patients, though having agreed to participate in a study, are tuning out or selectively attending to the preoperative teaching materials in one of the preoperative preparation programs. It is also possible that some patients would like to be dropped from their assigned program, even though no formal requests to be dropped are made. With on-site observations, an investigator has a better chance of noting that the teaching program is not reaching or having the desired effect on all patients. It would be important for the investigator to keep a record of the times in the preoperative recovery period that nurses first notice an adverse response in patients. Systematic notations of adverse responses may assist in the description and identification of similarities among groups of patients. A record of these events may help to generate hypotheses and to design future studies that assess a person's readiness to participate in other preoperative teaching programs.

Some of the early research on preoperative preparation of patients was based on explor-atory investigations. For instance, the research on the preoperative preparation of patients for stressful hospital events such as surgery had, as precursors, a number of descriptive and anecdotal reports in the late 1950s and early 1960s. These reports detailed specific approaches thought to be useful with surgery patients. In these early studies, the main focus was on describing the typical surgical patient's experiences before and after surgery. Fears and anxieties expressed by patients were reported. Also described were typical questions asked by patients, such as:

1. What will happen to me in the operating room?
2. What will happen to me during recovery from anesthesia?
3. What will my body look like upon recovery?
4. How much pain will I have?
5. How will the pain be treated?
6. How soon will I be able to resume normal activities?

In addition to the various descriptions about the surgical patient's concerns, detailed reports appeared in the literature about individual efforts by nurses to intervene with patients about their fears and questions. Several exploratory projects depicted individual efforts to teach patients about the surgical experience. Such projects were organized around information that the nurse researcher felt must be imparted to every patient before undergoing surgery. Several articles discuss the advantages of various physical exercise programs such as deep breathing, coughing, and passive range of motion exercises.

Johnson (1965; 1966) consulted the literature and derived significant benefits from these descriptive and exploratory reports of individual nurse studies on preoperative teaching. However, Johnson, through her own observations and explorations, speculated on why preoperative teaching programs might be effective with surgical patients. It was not until the mid-1960s that Johnson collected quantitative data to test propositions concerned with various preoperative preparation strategies.

A number of recently proposed programs by nurses follow the sequence seen in the preoperative preparation research literature. In a typical case, an investigator may examine a particular clinical issue by observing naturalistic occurrences in the patient care arena. Through detailed observations over the course of time, certain hunches or enlightened guesses of what seem to be important variables should emerge. In Johnson and associates' research program, the critical variables seemed to be, from her perspective, the types and kinds of information given about the particular physical sensations that a patient would experience through the preoperative and postoperative period (1978a; 1978b). Johnson linked her observations to a theoretical perspective formulated by Janis (1958) and Leventhal (1970). This perspective about the cognitive structuring or emotional inoculation programs eventually produced ideas on how to help persons develop or strengthen coping abilities when undergoing a stressful experience. The time frame for making these connections followed from the early observations made by Johnson when working with surgical patients. The theoretical connections were begun in her masters' thesis and later systematized in her doctoral program.

An alternative approach concerned with the same issue of preparing patients for surgery was undertaken by Lindeman and associates (1971; 1973), who essentially took an inductive approach to the whole issue of preoperative preparation. Lindeman and associates reasoned from their own professional experiences that patients seemed to do better after surgery, provided that they were given sufficient and accurate information about the typical experiences a patient would have during the time in the hospital. Little substantive theoretical propositions or explanations were offered by Lindeman as to why the patients who received information did better than those who did not. Lindeman stopped at observations. The scientific question of *why* was not answered.

Much of the literature on the preoperative preparation of patients from studies conducted by nurses, physicians, anesthesiologists, and psychologists are more like Lindeman's than Johnson's approach (Hathaway, 1986). Strong compelling theoretical arguments do not seem to exist in the literature about why preoperative preparation programs work. Most of the reports simply note that a variety of different psycho-educational approaches work with patients undergoing surgery (Devine and Cook, 1983; 1986). Obviously, the research in preoperative teaching is an area of inquiry that has clearly led to improved patient outcomes. In defense of this finding, the pragmatist would argue, "Is it better to test theory but not impact patient care?" Alternatively the scientist would ask, "Why did the improvement occur?"

Lindeman has challenged Johnson's theoretical perspective about the underlying reasons why patients do well when exposed to a systematic preoperative preparations protocol (Meleis, 1985). Offering an explanation, Lindeman states that persons with a strong self-care capacity or perspective benefit from preoperative preparation instructions. From this researcher's viewpoint, a strong self-care capacity suggests that a person has a vital sense of mastery and assertion about his or her own lifestyle and a concomitant ability to control and influence events such as illness or physical incapacities. Using observations only, Lindeman reasons that an informed educational program conducted by registered nurses with these persons further reinforces their self-care capabilities and personal sense of mastery.

Recently, a third perspective on the effectiveness of preoperative teaching emerged in the work of Ziemer (1983). Ziemer used Neuman's system model (1982) for her study of the effects of preoperative information on clients' postoperative coping behavior. Neuman's model offers propositions concerned with nursing interventions that strengthen a patient's line of defense prior to the impact of potential stressors. These primary prevention nurse intervention behaviors are demonstrated with patients prior to the stress event. The propositions predict that primary prevention actions avoid stressors or reduce their intensity as a function of appropriate nurse preparation or educational activities engaged with patients. Ziemer linked Johnson and associates' (1978a; 1978b) theory of cognitive preparation, sensory imagery, and emotional inoculation to Neuman's conceptual framework. Ziemer found that preoperative information did not result in the expected coping behaviors nor did the use of coping behaviors result in the anticipated reduction of postoperative symptoms. Therefore, a researcher in the preoperative preparation area is now faced with at least three different theoretical rationales for why a preoperative teaching program may or may not work.

The main point established in the preceding discussion is that few research areas have progressed from the exploratory to the experimental hypothesis-testing models traditional to scientific practice. Ideas and premises about nursing phenomena logically proceed from research reports rich in descriptions about patient events, nursing situations, health factors, and environmental circumstances in which nurses are involved. Highly detailed narration and intricate weaving of forces at work in the health care arena, with the corollary indication of themes, patterns, and subtle factors at play, allow hunches and tentative hypotheses to come to the forefront for further investigation.

Exploratory studies may pursue a variety of factors based on collected descriptions of nursing phenomena. Possible approaches in an exploratory design might be:

1. to immerse oneself in a situation to gain familiarity or to achieve new insights into it,

2. to portray accurately the characteristics of a particular person, situation, or group,

3. to determine the frequency with which something occurs or with which it is associated with something else, and

4. to pilot test hunches or hypotheses about possible relationships between variables.

All research should be guided by a statement of purpose. Most investigators have particular notions about key factors or variables at work in the substantive areas that they choose to examine. Therefore, it is important to state at the outset what one anticipates finding in an exploratory study. Rarely does a nurse researcher *not* have some preliminary estimate of what are important variables in a particular nursing domain. Stating initial predictions at the beginning of the study does not preclude identifying other crucial components of the area of interest. It simply gives an initial focus to an exploration of what can be, to both novice and experienced researcher, a somewhat overwhelming plethora of situational and interpersonal variables.

7–9 EXAMPLE OF AN EXPLORATORY STUDY INVOLVING A NURSING STRIKE

A number of exploratory studies have the purpose of formulating a problem for more precise definition, for further investigation,

or for the development or refinement of hypotheses. Other functions to be served by exploratory designs might be:

1. to serve as a pilot study to test nonparticipant observational or participant observation techniques before launching a more extensive study,

2. to establish the feasibility of studying a particular setting with unpredictable or unusual set of persons, patients, procedures, or locales,

3. to identify, clarify, or prioritize concepts for further investigation,

4. to gather information about the practicalities for doing a project in a particular health care setting, and

5. to gather an estimate or tentative appraisal of what practitioners in a particular nursing specialty or practice domain regard as worthwhile or vital nursing problems or central variables to be examined.

Of concern in discussing exploratory studies are the identification or refinement of researchable problems and the generating and testing of hypotheses. It goes without saying that in order to gain insight and appreciation into the issues contained in a specific health care arena, the nurse investigator must locate the pertinent literature that treats the issue and related topics. This is a task easier said than done. Not infrequently, novice investigators believe that it is a formidable assignment to locate pertinent literature that can provide critical insights into a topic deemed to be too novel even to have been mentioned in a professional journal or research publication. To illustrate, consider the following hypothetical scenario. A staff nurse employed in a health care facility soon to undergo renegotiation of a collective bargaining agreement redirected his interest in the perceptions of nurses about the effectiveness of such agreements on improving the salaries, benefits, and working conditions of nurses into a qualitative study of the issues surrounding the strike.

Before presenting the results of the study, it would be helpful for the reader to know about the events that transpired throughout the history of the study. The study was initiated on 15 June of last year and was terminated on 31 December of the same year. This termination date was forced upon the study because the funding institution failed to support a second year of investigation. The report had to be completed by 15 June of this year.

As a first step, a computer bibliographic

Medline retrieval search for nursing studies concerned with this topic was initiated. It was disappointing to learn that appropriate nursing research studies were not available on nurses' perceptions toward the relative value of collective bargaining agreements in improving the professional life of staff nurses. A number of descriptive and anecdotal reports were located which supported the idea that this topic of investigation was important to examine. Also found in the literature were numerous controversies and diverse views held by different groups of nurses about the merits of this labor-management contractual procedure. It was disappointing to learn that definitive nursing research reports did not exist which clearly and unambiguously address the issue of nurses' perceptions about strikes and associated work stoppage procedures.

As a consequence of a consultation session with the director of nursing research, it was suggested that the search statement be recast. A new computer bibliographic retrieval search was initiated that had, as a data base, business, labor relations, organizational and corporate management, public administration, and union literature in its system. The reworked search statement identified numerous studies detailing worker and management attitudes about the collective bargaining process and its contemporary status in meeting the needs of workers in different industries. It became obvious that the industrial model of establishing worker benefits and job security measures had been essentially incorporated into the current hospital industry. Strong parallels existed between nurses and workers in many fields. It was also learned that conceptual models such as Herzberg's Dual Factor Job Satisfaction Theory (1966) and Vroom's Expectancy Model (1967) among others served to identify pertinent concepts on which to base a nursing research study concerned with collective bargaining.

Let us describe how he would continue to investigate his research question in practice. A number of crucial questions must be asked and decisions must be made at the outset. Here are some of the questions.

1. Does the background literature provide enough support for identifying key variables about the individual nurse's views about collective bargaining?

2. Is there sufficient theoretical support for framing specific research questions?

3. Is the research on industrial workers directly related to what could logically be connected to forces which would affect the nurse's viewpoint about collective bargaining?

4. Are there data that addresses the problems of worker groups composed predominantly of women?

5. Are there clear indications where the industrial model does not work or poorly fits the area of 24-hour round-the-clock, 365 days a year health care provision?

6. Does reported research adequately address the changing relationships between management and labor under the revolutionary changes created by the prospective payment schedules of the federal government and third party insurance?

These are but a few of the salient questions that must be answered in the affirmative before an extensive formal investigation can be launched. Even if all these questions could be answered from a research base found in the contemporary literature with a positive "Yes," other pertinent considerations must be weighed.

The consultant and the investigator pondered over the following issue. Would the targeted health care institution or labor union representing registered nurses support or allow the distribution of a formal questionnaire about the issue of collective bargaining? Both the investigator and the consultant were aware that collective bargaining is a very hot issue in today's volatile health care scene. Extremely strong views are held by both management and labor unions about what is contained in a collective bargaining agreement and the changes required in each new round of extensive and exhaustive negotiations. Strong emotions, suspicion, distrust, and frank hostility pervade a number of health care institutions and the unions representing large groups of health workers, including registered nurses. It was all too apparent to the investigator and the consultant that, even in those labor-management situations in which there appears to be a relatively stable set of relationships and mutually satisfied expectations, the equilibrium was and continues to be fragile.

At this point a well-constructed questionnaire was developed with clear research objectives, but it was never distributed. The introduction of a survey instrument was seen as a threat to both sides of the labor-management relationship. Both could be supported or challenged by the study's findings.

Given the considerations of unsubstantial research literature and an unsympathetic or volatile health care environment, it was decided to adopt a different research strategy using the investigator as the major research instrument. At this point, conversations were held with fellow nurses about their expectations concerning the new collective bargaining agreement. The following questions were entertained.

1. What do they like and dislike about the present work contract?

2. What do they want in a new contract?

3. What do they think they will have to settle for?

4. What is their perception of management's position?

5. What role will the union take?

6. Are they prepared for any work stoppage action to back up their demands?

7. Have they put away money to support themselves if a strike is called?

A log was kept of the interviews conducted with individual nurses or groups of nurses on how they responded to these questions. Also noted were additional comments or associated thoughts generated by these open-ended questions. As new issues and questions arose, they were added to the list of open-ended questions or probes asked by the investigator.

The director of nursing research at the hospital, serving as the nurse researcher's consultant and advisor, provided external checks and monitored the procedures and information established in the study. A research data book was kept for recording separate consecutively dated sections for observations, informal interviews, copies of management and labor union memoranda, and newsletters detailing the various stages of progress in the new collective bargaining agreement. In addition, copies of newspaper articles, published reports in national magazines or professional journals, and television stories were also entered into this record book. A chronology of both the individual nurse's views and the institution's responses to labor union proposals were determined from periodic examination of the record book.

When the investigator was observing groups of nurses, he was faced with decisions about what was to be noted and recorded about certain aspects of each situation or encounter. For instance, the number and types of participants, the characteristics of the setting, the purpose of the activity, the social behavior of participants in the setting, and the frequency and duration of the activity engaged in by participants were noteworthy elements to record. Specific questions about these aspects were observed and documented. Some are listed here.

1. Questions about the participants.
   (a) Who were the participants?
   (b) What were their ages and gender?
   (c) What were their roles and functions in the strike and in the collective bargaining procedures?
   (d) How were they related to each other? Were they strangers, family members, colleagues, or members of the same work group?
   (e) What was their position in the hierarchy of the organization?
   (f) How many persons were in attendance?

(g) Was membership in the group consistent?
   (h) Who were the leaders?
2. Questions about the setting.
   (a) Where did the interaction of participants occur?
   (b) What was the apperance of the places where the interaction happened?
   (c) What kinds of behavior did the location encourage, discourage, or prevent?
3. Questions about the purpose.
   (a) What purpose brought the participants together?
   (b) Was the gathering of participants a planned event, or did the collection of persons occur by chance?
   (c) Was the group an ongoing one?
   (d) Was there a history to the group's membership and reason for being?
4. Questions about the social behavior.
   (a) What actually happened?
   (b) What did the participants do?
   (c) How did they do it?
   (d) With whom did they do it?
5. Questions about frequency and duration of the activity.
   (a) How long did it last?
   (b) If it reoccurred, how frequently did it recur?

After several weeks of recordings, the nurse investigator began to look for themes and patterns in the observational data. In addition to the observational data, interview data were collected from 20 nurses. Preliminary analyses showed that certain similarities emerged from the data. In trying to extract meaningful dimensions and categories from these interviews, the researcher used content analysis. In thinking about the range of social phenomena that could be classified in the interview data the nurse investigator could arrange them along a continuum from the most microscopic to the most macroscopic social events or occurrences. According to Lofland (1971), they are

(1) Acts: Acts are action in a situation that is temporally brief, consuming only a few seconds, minutes, or hours.
(2) Activities: Activities are action in a setting of a more major duration involving days, weeks, months. They constitute significant elements or involvement of a person or numerous persons.
(3) Meanings: Meanings are the verbal productions of participants that define and direct action.
(4) Participation: Participation involves a person's or multiple persons' holistic involvement or adaptation to a situation or setting under study.
(5) Relationships: Relationships are the interrela-

tionships that occur among several persons considered simultaneously.

(6) Settings: The setting refers to the entire milieu under study conceived as the unit of investigation.

In looking at the meaning of the verbal productions of the 20 interviews, a number of classification schemes were suggested by the consultant to the nurse researcher. One suggested scheme described by Kerlinger (1964) involved five possible units of analyses. They are words, themes, characters, items, and time and space measurements.

The nurse investigator could use specific value *words* employed by staff nurses to characterize their perceptions of the present collective bargaining contract. This would involve counting the number of times that negative words like poor, inadequate, demeaning, and so on, are used. Likewise, the frequency of positive words like good, satisfactory, adequate, and so on, could be counted. A summary of the use of both negative and positive terms can provide an indication of the views about the contract.

Similarly the nurse researcher could count the number of times that certain themes appear in the interview data. A *theme* is a very useful though a somewhat more complex unit to extract from the verbal reports of the nursing staff. A theme is often a sentence or sequence of sentences which represent a belief, perception, feeling, attitude, or opinion about a particular proposition. For example, the perceptions of the nursing staff about how successful the renegotiated labor-management contract will be in meeting their increased expectations for greater benefits and promotional opportunities can be derived from themes in the interview data for the nurse respondents. Themes are an important and useful unit because they are ordinarily realistic and close to the original content.

In addition to the use of words and themes as content analysis units, *character* can be used to indicate the perception of who the key players are and what the likely course of action might be if an impasse is reached in the contract negotiation process. The realm of fantasy and imagination can be captured in the verbal comments of staff concerning their highest and lowest expectations as to contract negotiations outcomes. For instance, how often were strike-breaking mechanisms mentioned? Did the hospital management fly in nurses from other parts of the country to replace nurses who went out on strike? How often was it mentioned that the institution would close or disband many present health care programs if a strike action took place?

Time and space measurements can be used as actual physical measurements of both the verbal interview content and as a means to classify the many written reports found in the hospital and union publications concerned with collective bargaining. The number of inches of space, number of pages, number of paragraphs, number of minutes of discussion and similar quantifications can provide yet another index of meaning to the nurse researcher's efforts to categorize observational and interview data. For example, the amount of space in the local community newspaper devoted to either the union's position or the management's position regarding a contract impasse could be a gauge of the success of either group's position in the new contract. Or, the nurse investigator, by counting the number of paragraphs in the hospital newsletter prior to and after a new contract was signed, could discern a pattern that suggests the likely outcome of the negotiation.

Like the theme, the *item* unit is a crucial categorization procedure to the nurse investigator's efforts to construct meaning from observational and interview data. The item refers to a whole production such as an article, a news story, a television program, a union meeting, a nursing staff conference, and a complete interview. For instance, each article, news story, or television program concerning the contract negotiation process could be classified as either pro-union, pro-management, or neutral. This classification scheme could be used throughout the study and positive, negative, or neutral news coverage could be connected to the final results.

Using the theme classification procedure, it was learned that the interviews revealed that nurses wanted a new promotion program. The instituted program must reward them for clinical excellence demonstrated in direct patient care functions. In particular, these nurses wanted a five-step clinical or career ladder program with increased pay differentials instituted in the new collective bargaining agreement. In examining the interviews, it also became apparent that the bulk of the data was collected or observed on critical care nurses. As a consequence, to broaden the base of data, the consultant encouraged the investigator to seek nurses from other specialty areas to observe or informally query. This strategy was adopted to see which other patterns or themes would come to the forefront for noncritical care nurses. After a period, a different pattern emerged when general medical-surgical unit nurses were observed or interviewed. Interest seemed to be stronger in increasing the number of paid leave days for professional education programs among that group of nurses. Furthermore, they wanted to expand the child care provisions paid for by the hospital so that weekend workers would be covered. In this case, the analysis of early collected data led to a search in another area with different outcomes.

A predominant theme elicited from the interviewed nurses who worked in the outpatient program and home health care program revealed that they were more concerned about adequate staffing of their programs. Several reductions had been implemented over the course of the present collective bargaining agreement, and a consistent theme from their data suggested that staff reduction would be the priority issue to be addressed in a new agreement. All three sets of nurses expected an across-the-board pay raise of 12% to 14% and maintenance of current fringe benefits. Few anticipated that a strike would be called, and even fewer had put money aside to cover that contingency. Most of the nurses seemed moderately comfortable in expecting that their proposals would be vigorously pursued by their elected union representatives. Most believed that hospital management would put up a strong counterproposal, meeting some but not all of their conditions.

The descriptive data which covered the six weeks prior to contract renegotiations, however, revealed a dramatic change in events. An article in the hospital newsletter reported extensive financial losses primarily due to the federal government's disallowance of charges for several of the hospital's principal DRG (diagnostic related groups), big money-earning patient services. Other disturbing events in the organization were noted and recorded. Rumors circulated about staff layoffs and programs being closed. Although there were three months remaining in the hospital's fiscal year, all nurse unit managers were directed to submit plans to reduce each unit's budget by 10%. The request for a budget reduction proposal was sent one week prior to the institution of formal collective bargaining renegotiations. The investigating nurse attended nursing staff meetings of several units. The tenor of these meetings was much changed from that of meetings previously observed. Considerable apprehension was voiced about whether the hospital would remain open, considering its poor financial picture. Concern was expressed about keeping one's job and the benefits associated with it, including a vested retirement system. Few comments were offered about the new proposals offered by the union on its members' behalf. Survival issue themes dominated the meetings attended by the staff nurse investigator.

A strike was averted when management agreed to keep present contract provisions in force but gave nurses only a 6% raise in pay for the subsequent three-year contract period. The renegotiated contract was reluctantly ratified by nurses. Much unhappiness prevailed. The work atmosphere for the first few months under the new contract was tense and brittle. Suddenly, an announcement in the hospital newsletter appeared, stating that the formal appeals made by the hospital to the federal government's disallowance of payment were supported. Several million dollars were paid. The hospital census took a dramatic upswing. The home health service was being inundated with patients. The financial picture changed overnight. But the nursing staff was locked into a new three-year contract.

As one might surmise, a great deal of data had been collected by the investigating staff nurse which covered the three months prior to the contract negotiations and the three months after the new contract was in place. This brief narrative of the six-month period does not do justice to a very complex set of events, persons, and forces affecting the individual nurse's perceptions about the effectiveness of the collective bargaining process in one health agency. In any case, several points need to be emphasized before a discussion can take place about possible analytic approaches to the data collected in this exploratory study.

It was assumed that the director of research at the institution had received the necessary administrative approval for the study prior to its initiation. It was also assumed that the staff nurse was able to maintain a consistently neutral viewpoint throughout the course of his investigation. The maintenance of an objective stance could be constantly challenged in the face of events that could have, at one point or another, threatened his own job security. Also, before data analysis began, the nurse investigator had to consciously recognize that the bulk of collected observational and interview data were heavily weighted toward staff nurses and union representation perspectives. On two occasions the nurse investigator attempted to interview hospital management after the new contract was in place and was rebuffed.

A number of micro- and macro-analytical approaches could be effectively used in this hypothetical investigation. Because the study was not based on a priori theoretical propositions, the investigator was free to examine the data from a number of qualitative perspectives. Inductively, the daily set of notes and interviews could have been examined for words, themes, and items. This search for recurring regularities or patterns is a continuous process. The search for patterns not only involves the discovery of commonalities across data but also a search for natural variation in observational and interview recordings. Patterns that emerge from unstructured observations and interviews are never universal. The researcher must not only attend to what words, themes, and items arise but also to how they are patterned. Do the themes or patterns apply only to certain subgroups of nurses, certain divisions of the hospital or organization, specific phases of the period studied, or certain social contexts? Again, in looking through the data the nurse investigator must infer what conditions preceded the observed phenomena and what are the apparent consequences. In other words, the researcher must be sensitive to relationships within the data.

At one point in the study, it was thought that Maslow's Hierarchy of Human Motivation Model directly pertained to the interview and observational data (1954). For instance, the generalized expectation by staff nurses for expanded educational and promotional options in the new contract suggested that nurses' primary survival needs had been met. Higher order needs for self-development and self-actualization predominated in the period preceding management's announcements about the dire financial condition of the organization. As the projected budget cuts were announced and the anticipated dismantling of programs was discussed in terms of the nursing department's assumption of additional responsibilities, the whole tenor of interview and observation data changed. Individual nurses were, at that juncture, talking about the possibilities of keeping their present positions, having to transfer to other services, or reducing the number of hours worked in light of anticipated staff reductions. Individual survival needs predominated up to and including the time when a strike was a possibility. A discussion of higher order needs by nurses did not reappear in any great number until the dramatic improvement in the hospital's economic status was revealed a month after the new contract had been in force.

In looking at the data from the home health nursing staff of the parent institution, it was noted that different words, themes, and items categories were used before a new contract was signed. In contrast to the inpatient nursing staff, the home health nursing staff were relatively low-keyed, voiced few, if any, expectations for the new contract, and remained uninvolved even when a strike was a possibility.

In reviewing the research and record book, it was discovered that the nurses in home health were considerably older, had postbaccalaureate educational preparation, possessed both inpatient and community health nursing work experience, and all were relatively new employees in the organization. Their major concern, throughout the six-month period covered in the study, was the inadequate ratio of the number of nurses to the acutely ill patients who received direct nursing care at home. The home health nurses were not discomforted by the possibility of a strike action. They viewed themselves as very marketable. None would have difficulty in finding employment in the rapidly expanding home health care economic marketplace.

There was no readily handy theoretical formulation to describe and interpret the particular behavior of the home health nursing group, regarding the collective bargaining process. The home health nursing group had, from the investigator's view, an entrepreneurial approach to professional nursing. The behavior of inpatient nurses reflected an industrial approach. The descriptor *entrepreneurial* was formulated to capture a set of behaviors that depict a nurse who is self-confident and assertive, proactive and futuristic in thinking, constantly assessing the health care marketplace, and a pioneer. The descriptor *industrial* was coined to describe a set of nurse behaviors in which the nurse is concerned with the performance of an employee role in a bureaucratic, hierarchical administrative structure, conforms well to rules and regulations, and is reactive to problems and retrospective in viewpoint. These descriptors are short-hand expressions for complex types of nurse behaviors. There was concern about the validation of the thematic explorations derived from the home health nurses' data. The researcher was concerned whether the inferred themes are an accurate representation of the perspective of the observed or interviewed nurses. In this case, the preliminary thematic analysis was presented to some of the home health nurses and inpatient nurses for review and evaluation. They were encouraged to offer suggestions that might support or contradict this analysis.

The investigator was advised to view these labels as tentative descriptions of attributes of a set of professional nurse workers in one health care organization. In subsequent studies, the descriptive labels may be refined, discarded, or expanded to depict a set of nurses and their expected responses to collective bargaining.

Before leaving this hypothetical, exploratory descriptive study on a staff nurse's perceptions of the effectiveness of the collective bargaining process, it is well to point out that all the various material used to build categories or classification schemes lend themselves to quantification. There are three potential ways to assign numbers to the outcomes of a content analysis of interview or observational data.

The first method of quantification is to use a *normal classification technique*. That is, count the number of each category after assigning each object to its proper category. In reviewing the observation or interview notes, the nurse investigator assigned words, themes, or items to categories. When the investigator counted the number of words reflective of Maslow's survival needs, he summarized the frequency with which these terms were used by each group of nurses. The increased or decreased use of these words also were counted in the contract negotiation process.

A second form of quantification is using *ranks* or *ordinal measurement*. Using interview data, groups of nurses or clinical units were rank ordered according to their preferences of employing various work stoppage strategies including work slowdowns, sickouts, and strikes. When such a rank ordering was performed, interviews were reexamined for different items or themes that were related to the willingness to use work stoppage techniques to gain a favorable contract.

A third form of quantification is *rating*. A rating scale is a measuring instrument that requires a rater or observer to assign the rated object to the ordered categories of a dimension. For instance, the investigator rated each interview as an item on a five-point scale as to the favorableness of the work of the union in the renegotiation of an effective contract. The scale is represented as follows:

Highly Favorable	Favorable	Undecided	Unfavorable	Highly Unfavorable
1	2	3	4	5

Themes from each inteview were rated on a four-point scale as to the strength of each nurse's willingness to participate in a strike. This scale is as follows:

Very Strong	Strong	Weak	Very Weak
1	2	3	4

Certain conditions must be met before standard statistical procedures can be justified. Category counts must be done carefully. If the materials are not representative or if the categories appear with relatively low frequency, generalization from inferential statistical comparisons are unwarranted. The researcher should consult Chapter 3 for the various procedures for determining reliability and validity when enumeration, rankings, and ratings are used by two or more raters: Reliability and validity psychometric procedures are highly recommended with data such as that contained in this exploratory-descriptive study.

At the conclusion of this preliminary research, a brief report of the study was submitted to a professional journal. The report, based on an exploratory descriptive design, emphasized the tentativeness and incompleteness of the conclusions. The investigator clearly indicated the exploratory aims of the research and pointed out the specific limitations of the particular project. The report carefully pinpointed those descriptions that apply only to the samples of nurses used and thus constrained the reader from inferring that the results came from a population of working nurses at large. For instance, the description accorded to the behavior of home health nurses and the inpatient hospital nurses were tentative hypotheses. Others were encouraged to test the generated hypotheses in subsequent research on this topic. Highlighted in the study findings were the phases through which the nurses progressed in the collective bargaining process.

Excerpts of descriptive dialogue and key words and themes were presented to help understand the phases identified in the six-month period studied. The investigator presented the rationale for using a particular word, theme, or item analysis. Next, the data for a particular analysis were described, the results were interpreted, and the use of the findings and conclusions was stated. Because of the preliminary nature of the report, the ability of the research and professional community to weigh the possible merits and application of findings was heavily dependent on the logic, the clarity, the honesty, and the particular narrative ability of the investigator. The investigator was in the best position to know the shortcomings and tentativeness of offered conclusions and was encouraged by the research consultant to give the reader the advantage of that knowledge.

7–10 SUMMARIZING EXPLORATORY-DESCRIPTIVE DATA FOR DISSEMINATION AND PUBLICATION

At this juncture it is well to reiterate that the purpose of exploratory-descriptive research is to provide a way to formulate hypotheses that can be tested to establish cause and effect relationships. Through the systematic study of a dynamic set of events, such as the collective bargaining process described in Section 7–9, a number of possible explanatory variables can be related to the origins of the nurses' perceptions, the exact nature of the perceptions, and the generated behaviors concerning the effectiveness of collective bargaining. Through analysis and interpretation of the interview and observational data, hypotheses should emerge. The meaningfulness of the study can be established only when the researcher offers the reader a set of generalizations. The generalized statements identify the possible causes and consequences of events which led to the perceived failure of the contract renegotiation process to achieve both the economic and professional goals of the nurses.

In writing a report of an exploratory-description research project, a definite sequence of specific subject matter would be expected. These elements are briefly indicated here. In preparing written materials it is wise to introduce the topic by selecting a title that vividly and accurately highlights the central thrust of the study. A suggested title for the report is: "Why Collective Bargaining Failed: A Case Study of Nurses at a Northern California Hospital." Next, the introduction of the report should identify the purpose(s) of the study and provide an overview of the general sections which are included. In essence advanced organizers provide information to the reader about what to expect and why it is important. Having presented the general purpose of the study, the researcher would be expected to bring the reader up to date on the previous research in the area of collective bargaining and its effects on nurses. Because there seemed to be a paucity of such research, the researcher would briefly present the related literature and thus indicate the need for the present study based on the lack of substantive work in this crucial area. Following this exposition, the methodological design and execution of the study would be depicted. Here, the reader would be acquainted with the rationale and choice of a participant observational research strategy. It would be important for the reader to have a clear grasp of how this technique was used, under what conditions it was used, and the ways in which information was gathered and re-

corded. Furthermore, the sequence and timing of observations and the understanding of nurses about the role of the investigator would be delineated.

Having set the study in the perspective of previous research and having described its design and execution, the researcher must then present the data. Here, the reader would find summarized descriptions of both qualitative and quantitative material and the procedures used to achieve such summarized information. The findings would be presented so as to marshal an argument regarding why the collective bargaining process failed. The principle mode of presentation would be classical expository writing. For this, the researcher would take a chronological perspective through the description of distinct phases over the six-month period. In this section it would be important to identify the explanatory variables and show how they functioned in the context of the origin, status, and later behaviors of nurses' perceptions.

For example, one of the explanatory variables is *previous history* of success in contract negotiations. In this study, this variable was expressed by a number of nurses during the interview phase. Some had lowered expectations based on similar experiences at other hospitals. Because of these low expectations, they were not motivated nor prepared to push for success in the present negotiations. In addition, a greater number of nurses who worked at this hospital had experienced a successful conclusion to previous contract negotiations. As a consequence, they expected their additional demands to be met and they were lulled into a false sense of security. They anticipated little difficulty and did not prepare for the final contingency. Consequently, the nursing union and staff nurses failed to mobilize their personal, organizational, and economic resources in order to achieve their aims. When the hospital management refused all new requests, nurses new to the hospital were not surprised, whereas nurses with prior work experiences in the hospital were completely taken off-guard.

To support the premise that history is a possible explanation for failure of the negotiations, it is a good idea to present other data. For example, as further defense of previous history as a variable to explain *negotiation failure*, other sources of evidence can be found in minutes of previous union meetings, prior hospital newsletters, and earlier newspaper articles chronicling other negotiations at this and other hospitals in the same locale. It is possible that if the investigator had observed another institution undergoing contract negotiations, he might have noted similar or different previous history factors in operation. This added source of information can be documented and used to support the argument. All these sources of information can be mustered together and used to support the argument as to how previous history has an effect on negotiation failure. Note that three independent sources are collected to identify a single variable and concordant set of explanations. Such cross-validation of information is often referred to as *triangulation* (Denzin, 1973; Sohier, 1988). It is a useful model to adopt in qualitative research endeavors.

The final section of the manuscript should be an integration of all previous sections. A summary is called for and conclusions should be specified in detail. A particularly important part of the section should be a review of particular shortcomings and limitations of the study. Here, suggestions can be offered about possible ways to improve or expand the study to cover other settings and similar situations. One final part of this section should include a set of statements or hypotheses that should be subjects of other research based on the theory that the report has generated.

ysis and interpretation of observational, interview, and pictorial data. Next, an illustration of a hypothetical nursing research qualitative project was presented. The various phases and stages through which a qualitative researcher progresses were highlighted. Emphasis was placed on detailed, systematic, written recordings, observational notes, and pictorial data, which are organized in books and manuals for ease of access for the necessary analysis and interpretation of data.

The dynamic flow of historical, political, and social events affecting qualitative research also was noted. Particular attention was directed toward the need to cross-validate tentative analytical categories and interpretative strategies with a second independent researcher. Another suggested validation strategy was offered in the form of presenting preliminary or tentative findings to the research subjects or the groups studied. Furthermore, direction was offered regarding the appropriate quantification and statistical strategies and techniques to be employed with dimensions and categories of qualitative data.

Finally, the steps to be used in the reporting and dissemination of qualitative research were described. This chapter highlighted the important value of qualitative research for generating tentative propositions and hypotheses to be tested, if desired, in other research designs and settings.

7–11 SUMMARY

This exposition has explored the creative and exciting world of qualitative research. The historical debt that nursing researchers owe to the fields of anthropology, sociology, and psychology were noted in terms of the development of ethnography, grounded theory, and phenomenology. The advantages and disadvantages of qualitative research were enumerated. The unifying theoretical and empirical approaches among these distinct qualitative research traditions is to be found in the emphasis placed on naturalistic observations and interviews of persons about their perceptions of the world in general and health care in particular.

A methodological approach called *content analysis* was depicted in terms of procedures and techniques applicable to the anal-

REFERENCES

Bailey, M.: A qualitative research method to study the elderly in two residences. In Leininger, M., ed., Qualitative Research Methods in Nursing. Orlando, Grune and Stratton, 1985.

Campbell, D.T., and Stanley, J.C.: Experimental and quasi-experimental designs for research on teaching. In Gage, N.L., ed., Handbook of Research on Teaching. Chicago, Rand McNally, 1963.

Chenitz, W.C., and Swanson, J.A.: From Practice to Grounded Theory: Qualitative Research in Nursing. Menlo Park, Addison-Wesley, 1986.

Chinn, P.L., and Jacobs, M.K.: Theory and Nursing, ed. 2. St. Louis, The C.V. Mosby Co., 1987.

Christman, N.J., McConnell, E.A., Pfeiffer, C., et al.: Uncertainty, coping, and distress following myocardial infarction: transition from hospital to home, Res. Nurs. Health, 11: 71–82, 1988.

Cook, T.D., and Campbell, D.T.: Quasi-experimentation: Design and Analysis Issues for Field Settings. Chicago, Rand McNally, 1979.

Denzin, N.: The Research Act. Chicago, Aldine, 1973.

Devine, E., and Cook, T.: A meta-analytic analysis of effects of psychoeducational interventions on length of postsurgical hospital stay, Nurs. Res., 32: 267–274, 1983.

Devine, E., and Cook, T.: Clinical and cost-saving effects of psychoeducational interventions with surgical patients: A meta-analysis, Res. Nurs. Health, 9: 89–105, 1986.

Fagerhaugh, S.: Getting around with emphysema, Am. J. Nurs., 73: 94–99, 1973.

Fawcett, J., and Downs, F.S.: The Relationships of Theory and Research. East Norwalk, CT, Appleton-Century-Crofts, 1985.

Fielding, N.G., and Fielding, J.L.: Linking Data: Qualitative Research Methods, ed. 4. Beverly Hills, Sage, 1986.

Glaser, B., and Strauss, A.: Awareness of Dying. Chicago, Aldine, 1965.

Glaser, B., and Strauss, A.: A Time for Dying. Chicago, Aldine, 1968.

Hathaway, D.: Effects of preoperative instruction on postoperative outcomes: a meta-analysis, Nurs. Res., 35: 269–276, 1986.

Herzberg, F.: Work and the Nature of Man. Cleveland, World Publishing Co, 1966.

Hutchinson, S.A.: Creating meaning: a grounded theory of NICU nurses, Nurs. Outlook, 32: 86–90, 1984.

Jacob, E.: Qualitative research traditions: a review, Rev. Ed. Res., 57: 1–50, 1987.

Janis, I.J.: Psychological Stress. New York, John Wiley & Sons, 1958.

Johnson, J.E.: Effects of nurse-patient interaction on the patient's postoperative discomforts. Unpublished masters' thesis, New Haven, CT, Yale University, 1965.

Johnson, J.E.: The influence of purposeful nurse-patient interaction on the patient's postoperative course. In Exploring Progress in Medical-Surgical Nursing Practice ANA: 1965 Regional Clinical Conferences, 16–22. New York, American Nurses' Association, 1966.

Johnson, J.E., Rice, V.H., Fuller, S.S., et al.: Sensory information, instruction in a coping strategy, and recovery from surgery, Res. Nurs. Health, 1: 4–17, 1978a.

Johnson, J.E., Fuller, S.S., Endress, M.P., et al.: Altering patients' responses to surgery: an extension and replication, Res. Nurs. Health, 1: 111–121, 1978b.

Johnson, R.; In Quest of a New Psychology. New York, Human Science Press, 1975.

Kerlinger, F.: Foundations of Behavioral Research. New York, Holt, Rinehart, & Winston, 1964.

Knafl, K.A., and Howard, M.J.: Interpreting and reporting qualitative research, Res. Nurs. Health, 7: 17–24, 1984.

Leininger, M.M.: Nature, rationale, and importance of qualitative research methods. In Leininger, M.M., ed., Qualitative Research Methods in Nursing. Orlando, Grune & Stratton, 1985.

Leventhal, H.: Findings and theory in the study of fear communication. In Berkowitz, L., ed., Advances in Experimental Social Psychology, vol. 5. New York, Academic Press, 1970.

Lindeman, C.A., and Van Aernamn, B.: Nursing intervention with the presurgical patient—the effects of structured and unstructured preoperative teaching, Nurs. Res., 20: 319–332, 1971.

Lindeman, C.A., and Stetzer, S.L.: Effect of preoperative visits by operating room nurses, Nurs. Res., 22: 4–16, 1973.

Lofland, J.F.: Analyzing Social Settings. New York, Wadsworths, 1971.

Lynch-Sauer, J.: Using a phenomenological research method to study nursing phenomena. In Leininger, M.M., ed., Qualitative Research Methods in Nursing. Orlando, Grune & Stratton, 1985.

Maslow, A.H.: Motivation and Personality. New York, Harper & Row, 1954.

McLaughlin, F.E., et al.: Primary Care Judgments of Nurses and Physicians, vol. 1. Veteran's Administration Hospital, San Francisco, CA (NTIS No. HRP-0900605), 1978.

McLaughlin, F.E., et al.: Nurse practitioners', public health nurses', and physicians' performance on clinical simulation test: COPD, West. J. Nurs. Res., 1: 273–295, 1979a.

McLaughlin, F.E., et al.: Nurses' and physicians' performance on clinical simulation test: hypertension, Res. Nurs. Health, 2: 61–72, 1979b.

Meleis, A.I.: Theoretical Nursing: Development and Progress. Philadelphia, J.B. Lippincott Co., 1985.

Mishel, M.H.: The measurement of uncertainty in illness, Nurs. Res., 30: 258–263, 1981.

Mishel, M.H.: Adjusting the fit: development of uncertainty scales for specific populations, West. J. Nurs. Res., 5: 355–370, 1983a.

Mishel, M.H.: Parents' perception of uncertainty of their hospitalized child, Nurs. Res., 32: 324–330, 1983b.

Mishel, M.H.: Perceived uncertainty and stress in illness, Res. Nurs. Health, 7:163–171, 1984a.

Mishel, M.H., Hostetter, T., King, B., et al.: Predictors of psychosocial adjustment in patients newly diagnosed with gynecological cancer, Cancer Nurs., 7: 291–299, 1984b.

Mishel, M.H., and Broden, C.S.; Finding meaning: antecedents of uncertainty in illness, Nurs. Res., 37: 98–103, 1988.

Neuman, B.: The Neuman Systems Model: Application to Nursing Education and Practice. New York, Appleton-Century-Crofts, 1982.

Oiler, C.J.: Qualitative methods: phenomenology. In Moccia, P., ed., New Approaches to Theory Development. New York, National League for Nursing, 1986.

Reinharz, S.: On Becoming a Social Scientist. San Francisco, Jossey-Bass, 1979.

Sohier, R.: Multiple triangulation and contemporary nursing research, West. J. Nurs. Res, 10: 732–742, 1988.

Tripp-Reimer, T.: Combining qualitative and quantitative methodologies. In Leininger, M.M., ed., Qualitative Research Methods in Nursing. Orlando, Grune & Stratton, 1985.

Trochim. W.M., ed: Advances in Quasi-experimental Design and Analysis. San Francisco, Jossey-Bass, 1986.

Vroom, V.H.: Work and Motivation. New York, John Wiley & Sons, 1967.

Ziemer, M.M.: Effects of information on postsurgical coping, Nurs. Res., 32: 282–287, 1983.

Chapter 8

GRAPHIC AND TABULAR METHODS FOR DISPLAYING DATA

8–1 GRAPHIC AND TABULAR METHODS

In the previous chapters, descriptions of experimental, quasi-experimental, sample surveys, and qualitative research methods were provided. All investigations generate data that can be used for analysis and understanding about relationships among variables. Investigations always generate information that can be used to illustrate and display research findings to discerning colleagues who attend meetings and conferences or who read and make use of reports and journal articles.

Well-thought out and well-executed graphical displays and tables provide a very effective medium that can be used to inform readers about the relationships that may exist among the constructs, propositions, and variables of research interest. If graphs and tables are made with care, they are easy to understand and interpret. Sometimes a picture is much better than a thousand words. An example provided in Chapter 7 involved the reported degree of positive or negative support of strikes by nurses. To aid in communicating the findings to others, the distribution of responses may be summarized for presentation in the form of a frequency table or a bar graph.

The construction of helpful visual aids and pictorial displays for written reports and oral presentations are described in this chapter. Guidelines for the construction of histograms, scatter plots, and other statistical graphs are provided. Directions are offered for assessing randomness in quantitative and qualitative data. Methods for estimating medians, percentiles, and related summary measurements about frequency distributions are illustrated.

After the data have been collected and prepared for processing, the next step is to inspect the data set to gather preliminary impressions concerning the interrelationships that exist among the major variables of research interest. This can be done by viewing the data graphically and by studying of summary tables. By using these visual aids, a researcher can get an intuitive or heuristic sense concerning the relationships that exist among the constructs, propositions, and variables. The information that is obtained at this point has multiple uses. In particular, tables and graphs can be used to

1. provide information that aids in the understanding of the relationships that exist among independent and dependent variables and among constructs and propositions,
2. present the basic and important findings by means of tables and graphs to readers and attendants at conferences and meetings,
3. generate strategies for analyzing the data,
4. detect and correct errors that were missed in the initial inspection of the data,
5. generate research questions that were not considered at the initial planning and development stage of the study,
6. provide visual inspection of the data, and
7. detect study flaws and possible hidden biases in the data that have been collected.

Demonstrations of how graphs and tables can be used are provided throughout this chapter.

8–2 FREQUENCY TABLES FOR QUALITATIVE AND QUANTITATIVE DATA

One of the most useful tables available to the nurse investigator is the *frequency table*. A frequency table is a two-dimensional display of a set of categories with the number or percentage of instances observed in each category. Frequency tables can be used to detect data entry and data processing errors. Potential sources of experimental bias also can be detected. Frequency data can provide information to readers of reports and journal articles in easily understood or intuitively appealing form. When set up properly, frequency tables offer a highly effective form to help both researchers and readers of research material to understand and evaluate the outcomes of surveys, qualitative investigations, and quantitative studies that are experimental or observational in design and emphasis.

Frequency tables are very easy to construct, even though the initial tabulation of the data may be time-consuming and fraught with errors. Before the days of the personal and main frame computers and the introduction of key-punched data cards, the typical method for making a frequency table was to take a paper and pencil in hand and simply tabulate the data, piece by piece.

For example, to obtain the distribution of severity for the patients admitted to surgery in Hospital One of the preoperative teaching study of Chapter 1, a researcher would have to tabulate the severity scores of each subject, one by one. For this a frequency table of severity levels would have to be drawn up. To fill in the body of the table, a tally mark would be made for each subject in the appropriate severity level. As soon as five subjects are found that fit a specific severity level, a straight line is cut across the four existing tally marks which produces a grouping or bundle of five tally marks to represent the five subjects. Such a tedious task would provide a table such as that shown in Table 8–1. Of course, no one would want to do that today. The opportunities for error are legion. The chances that the tabulation would be repeated four or five times before two tabulations were found to agree is high. Certainly, the method is not recommended, even though the concept is still pertinent.

The display, consisting simply of the tally marks and the frequencies of Table 8–1, provides information about the severity levels and the number of patients experiencing each level of severity. As will be shown later, this type of tabulation provides the basis for a numerical presentation of frequency data and acceptable visual presentations commonly encountered in standard statistical graphs. These graphs are the *bar graph* and the *histogram*. They are described in Sections 8–11 and 8–12, respectively.

The tally marks of Table 8–1 provide a visual impression of the distribution of severity of the 39 patients undergoing surgery in Hospital One located in a rural environment. A visual inspection of the tabulation clearly reveals that most of the patients have been classified as having a mild (less fragile preoperative physiological status) form of severity. An examination of the number of bundles of tally marks shows that about half the patients have a mild level of severity. A possible reason for the large number of mild severity cases is that doctors may have advised these patients to undergo treatment before the condition became serious. These impressions are further reinforced by examining the numbers in the right two columns of Table 8–1, which summarize the number and percentage of patients belonging in each category. These two columns provide a quantitative *picture* of the distribution. The column of least interest is the column headed *frequency*. In most investigations, frequencies defy scientific interpretation.

Often, researchers provide only the column of frequencies to their readers. Although the frequency column contains some information, it does not provide the information that a reader needs for understanding and interpretation. To omit the last column of *percentages* is a mistake. A researcher wants to know what percentage of the patients are classified as severe, moderate, and mild, because percentages provide a stable estimate of the proportion of cases that belong to each category that is independent of sample size. As a researcher adds more subjects to a sample, frequencies assigned to a category naturally increase. But, as the sample size increases, percentages for a category remain essentially constant, fluctuating

slightly about a fixed value with the addition of each subject. The convergence to a fixed value or constant is a function of the *law of large numbers*, which is a basic principle of statistical theory (Hays, 1981). Operationally, the law of large numbers states,

There is a convergence upon an unknown population parameter of a statistical measurement made serially upon a sample following the inclusion of each new subject.

As a consequence, sample measurements, such as means, medians, standard deviations, and proportions and percentages of categorical variables, tend to fluctuate in a very small range about a fixed value as more and more information is added to the sample. In addition, the degree of fluctuation decreases as sample size increases. This means, for example, that the error in a sample proportion for a sample size of 100 is smaller than the error in a sample proportion for a sample size of 50. This property of statistical measurements was used extensively in Chapter 6 on survey sampling techniques.

The example of Table 8–1 reveals that 19 patients had a mild form of the condition. This may seem to convey information, but it really does not. A reader needs to know the size of the sample on which this number is based. Knowing that 19 of 39 patients have been rated as having a mild form of the condition is very different from knowing that 19 of 246 patients have been rated as having a mild form of the condition. Sample size is *essential* to interpreting frequency data. Without sample size information, frequency data is less than meaningful. The far right column is the most essential and useful column in a frequency table. No frequency table should be constructed or printed without it.

Frequency tables also can be useful in the preliminary phases of data analysis to detect errors. They can be used to help a researcher check for punching and recording errors, for detecting possible biases in the study, and for detecting errors in data collection. The first time that the data were examined with respect to severity, frequencies other than those reported in Table 8–1 were obtained. The frequencies did not agree or match the frequencies reported. Instead, the frequencies were those reported in Table 8–2. The first impression that draws the viewer's attention is the appearance of "6" and "1" as possible values for severity. Because sever-

TABLE 8–1 ILLUSTRATION OF HAND TABULATION OF DATA WITH HOSPITAL ONE AS AN INDEPENDENT VARIABLE AND SEVERITY OF ILLNESS AS THE DEPENDENT VARIABLE

Variable	Tabulation	Frequency	Percent
1. Mild	⦀ ⦀ ⦀ ⦀	19	48.7
2. Moderate	⦀ ⦀ //	12	30.8
3. Severe	⦀ ///	8	20.5
Total		39	100.0

TABLE 8–2 HOSPITAL ONE AND SEVERITY OF ILLNESS: THE FIRST COMPUTER PRINTOUT ASSOCIATED WITH TABLE 8–1

Value	Frequency	Percent
1. Mild	17	44.7
2. Moderate	12	31.6
3. Severe	7	18.4
6	1	2.6
1	1	2.6
Total	38	99.9

ity was coded as 1, 2, or 3, clearly these are punching errors. Why they occurred is not known. The 6 could have appeared because it is above the 3 in the number block of the computer used for entering the data into the CRUNCH file used for storing the data. The 1 might be produced by mistaking the letter "l" for the number "1", but even this is speculation. Another error discovered at this point is that data for one of the patients in Hospital One were missing. Thirty-nine patients were in that hospital but data for only 38 were punched in. After some time and search, the error was corrected. Finally, one might think that the total of 99.9 for the percent column is in error. This is not an error. Rounding errors frequently produce totals that do not perfectly match theory.

As the example shows, frequency tables can be used to detect entering and data processing errors. It is recommended that early in the data analysis phase of a study, all data should be examined in terms of their frequency tables. It is best to find the errors before the data are analyzed, published, and distributed. It is embarrassing to have errors discovered by others. Many readers discredit what otherwise appears to be an excellent research report simply because errors have

been found in the data or in the analysis of the data. Researchers should not provide such opportunities to their readers or to their critics. A word to the wise is sufficient!

Frequency tables also can be used to check for experimental bias. In the postoperative teaching study, most of the surgery took place in a central city medical center where research on abdominal problems was conducted. A greater percentage of severe cases is likely to be found in Hospital Three. If this were not the case, one might suspect some bias. The overrepresentation of severe cases can be tested by examining the frequency tables for all three hospitals in one frequency table. The frequency table for this set of comparisons is provided in Table 8–3.

With respect to severity level 3, it is seen that the data agree with expectations. About 40% of the patients operated on in Hospital Three had been classified as having a serious condition. A rather unusual finding, however, is that the percent of severe cases in the rural hospital is higher than that of the suburban hospital. A careful nurse researcher would try to explain this finding. A possible explanation is that the persons doing the ratings in the three hospitals are using different standards in diagnosing severity. If true, using different criteria could be a source of bias, which should be taken into account. Perhaps the rural hospital may be the site of many emergency operations. If the hospital is located in a farming area, accidents on the farm or in the field may account for the larger percentage of severe cases. Certainly, this factor should be considered when the final evaluation of the data takes place.

Using frequency tables to provide checks on the representativeness of data is one of their important uses in nursing research. Under- or overrepresentation of specific subsets

TABLE 8–3 FREQUENCY TABLE OF SEVERITY OF PATIENT PREOPERATIVE STATUS ACCORDING TO THREE DIFFERENT HOSPITAL SITES

Severity	Hospitals					
	Rural		Suburban		Urban	
	No.	%	No.	%	No.	%
1. Mild	19	48.7	39	54.2	64	47.4
2. Moderate	12	30.8	29	36.1	31	23.0
3. Severe	8	20.5	7	9.7	40	39.6
Total	39	100.0	72	100.0	135	100.0

TABLE 8–4 DISTRIBUTION OF WEIGHTS OF THE 246 PATIENTS IN THE PREOPERATIVE TEACHING STUDY

Weight	True Upper Limit	Frequency	Cumulative Frequency	Percent
109	109.5	1	1	.41
110	110.5	1	2	.81
111	111.5	0	2	.81
112	112.5	1	3	1.22
113	113.5	1	4	1.63
114	114.5	0	4	1.63
115	115.5	0	4	1.63
116	116.5	0	4	1.63
117	117.5	1	5	2.03
118	118.5	0	5	2.03
119	119.5	3	8	3.25
120	120.5	5	13	5.28
121	121.5	2	15	6.10
122	122.5	3	18	7.32
123	123.5	0	18	7.32
124	124.5	1	19	7.72
125	125.5	2	21	8.54
126	126.5	2	23	9.35
127	127.5	5	28	11.38
128	128.5	2	30	12.20
129	129.5	2	32	13.01
130	130.5	1	33	13.41
131	131.5	1	34	13.82
132	132.5	4	38	15.45
133	133.5	3	41	16.67
134	134.5	3	44	17.89
135	135.5	5	49	19.92
136	136.5	4	53	21.54
137	137.9	9	62	25.20
138	138.5	5	67	27.24
139	139.5	5	72	29.27
140	140.5	2	74	30.08
141	141.5	2	76	30.89
142	142.5	4	80	32.52
143	143.5	3	83	33.74
144	144.5	5	88	35.77
145	145.5	9	97	39.43
146	146.5	7	104	42.28
147	147.5	5	109	44.31
148	148.5	1	110	44.72
149	149.5	6	116	47.15
150	150.5	9	125	50.81
151	151.8	1	126	51.22
152	152.5	4	130	52.85
153	153.5	7	137	55.69
154	154.5	8	145	58.94
155	155.5	10	155	63.01
156	156.5	7	162	65.85
157	157.5	4	166	67.48
158	158.5	6	172	69.92
159	159.5	1	173	70.33
160	160.5	3	176	71.54
161	161.5	2	178	72.36
162	162.5	4	182	73.98
163	163.5	5	187	76.02
164	164.5	5	192	78.08
165	165.5	3	195	79.27
166	166.5	5	200	81.30
167	167.5	1	201	81.71

TABLE 8–4 DISTRIBUTION OF WEIGHTS OF THE 246 PATIENTS IN THE PREOPERATIVE TEACHING STUDY *Continued*

Weight	True Upper Limit	Frequency	Cumulative Frequency	Cumulative Percent
168	168.5	3	204	82.93
169	169.5	3	207	84.15
170	170.5	4	211	85.77
171	171.5	0	211	85.77
172	172.5	2	213	86.59
173	173.5	2	215	87.40
174	174.5	1	216	87.80
175	175.5	0	216	87.80
176	176.5	2	218	88.62
177	177.5	1	219	89.02
178	178.5	0	219	89.02
179	179.5	0	219	89.02
180	180.5	2	221	89.04
181	181.5	1	222	90.24
182	182.5	0	222	90.24
183	183.5	1	223	90.65
184	184.5	0	223	90.65
185	185.5	1	224	91.06
186	186.5	0	224	91.06
187	187.5	1	225	91.46
188	188.5	3	228	92.68
189	189.5	0	228	92.68
190	190.5	1	229	93.09
191	191.5	2	231	93.90
192	192.5	0	231	93.90
193	193.5	0	231	93.90
194	194.5	0	231	93.90
195	195.5	0	231	93.90
196	196.5	0	231	93.90
197	197.5	0	231	93.90
198	198.5	0	231	93.90
199	199.5	0	231	93.90
200	200.5	1	232	94.31
201	201.5	2	234	95.12
202	202.5	0	234	95.12
203	203.5	0	234	95.12
204	204.5	2	236	95.93
205	205.5	1	237	96.34
206	206.5	1	238	96.75
207	207.5	0	238	96.75
208	208.5	0	238	96.75
209	209.5	0	238	96.75
210	210.5	0	238	96.75
211	211.5	0	238	96.75
212	212.5	1	239	97.15
213	213.5	0	239	97.15
214	214.5	2	241	97.97
215	215.5	0	241	97.97
216	216.5	0	241	97.97
217	217.5	2	243	98.78
218	218.5	1	244	99.19
219	219.5	0	244	99.19
220	220.5	0	244	99.19
221	221.5	0	244	99.19
222	222.5	0	244	99.19
223	223.5	0	244	99.19
224	224.5	1	245	99.59
225	225.5	1	246	100.00

can be readily discerned. It is recommended that each independent variable in a study be scrutinized early through examination of the frequency tables. Personal computer programs like CRUNCH (Bostrom 1986), used throughout this book, quickly and inexpensively generate frequency tables. It is a mistake not to perform these preliminary investigations before beginning the qualitative and quantitative analysis of data.

The main purpose of a table is to inform readers about the findings, and so a researcher should make the table as self-explanatory as possible. For journal publication and reporting purposes, all frequency tables should satisfy the following conditions:

1. They should have a complete title. The independent and dependent variables should be named in the title.

2. The target population of the study should be identified.

3. The total sample size should appear in the table, preferably at the bottom of the frequency column. If multiple groups are in a table, the sample sizes for each of the subgroups must be printed.

4. All frequency columns must be augmented by a percentage column. If these columns are omitted, the frequency table is worthless.

5. Every column must be carefully labeled. The reader of a table should understand clearly the source of all figures in the table.

6. A frequency table must be able to stand by itself. A reader should not have to refer to the text to find out what is in a table. Nor should a reader have to read the text to determine what a table has to say about the relationship between the independent and dependent variables of the study.

8–3. USING FREQUENCY TABLES TO ASSESS ACCURACY AND CONSISTENCY OF QUANTITATIVE DATA

Frequency tables can be used to check the accuracy and consistency of data. This use of a frequency table is illustrated with weight, one of the independent variables of the preoperative teaching study. In many research investigations, the reported reliability of this characteristic is doubtful for all subjects in a study. Weight data can be reported in many different ways. One way is for subjects to strip to the nude and then to be weighed on perfectly balanced scales at each site. As might be expected, this rarely happens. Even if it did, standardization of the weighing protocol and the scales across sites would be required.

Furthermore, duration of time between last food and fluid intake and between last bowel movement and time of weighing would need to be specified. Other factors that contribute to the hourly changes in body weight would also have to be considered if an accurate measurement of each person's weight is required.

In the hypothetical preoperative teaching study, it is certain that no standardization of weight measurement was even contemplated. Probably nurses and nurses' aides asked patients how much they weighed. Most likely, some patients reported their weight taken in the morning while in a nude or partially nude state, whereas others reported weights taken while fully clothed and wearing shoes. Others may have reported a weight which was corrected by subtracting five or ten pounds for the additional weight of clothes and shoes. Some might have guessed at their weights. In other cases, the weights may have been determined at hospital admission or at some later point before or even after an operation, either with or without clothes. Other sources of measurement errors most certainly exist.

If the weight data are free of bias, the last digit of each reported weight should appear with equal probabilities. This statement implies that the last digit of the reported weights should be randomly distributed across all patients. The final digits of reported weights should possess what statisticians call a *uniform distribution*. In a uniform distribution, all outcomes are equally possible. This means that the proportion of weights ending in 0, 1, 2, . . . ,9 are expected to be equal. In this case, the proportion of cases ending in k = 0, 1, 2, . . . ,9 all are equal to the common value of $p_k = .10$. Thus, there should be about

$$E(f_k) = NP_k = (246)(.10) = 24.6$$

patients whose weights end in 0, 1, 2, . . . ,9. The symbol $E(f_k)$ is called the *expected value* or *expected frequency* of the number of people whose weights end in the digit k. N is the total number of people in the study, and p_k is the expected proportion of people whose weights end in the digit k.

The distribution of weights is shown in Table 8–4. For the present discussion, ignore the columns headed *cumulative frequency* and *cumulative percent*. They are examined in Sections 8–5 and 8–6. As can be seen, the weights range from a low of 109 pounds to a high of 225 pounds. Consider the weights that end in the digit 9. The number of these is given as

$$f_9 = 1 + 3 + 2 + 5 + 6 + 1 + 3 = 21$$

a number not too deviant from the expected number of 24.6. The remaining frequencies are reported in Table 8–5. With these figures a researcher can test the hypothesis that the last digits are randomly distributed. The test statistic for testing this hypothesis is defined as

$$X^2 \sum_{k=1}^{K} \frac{[f_k - E(f_k)]^2}{E(f_k)}.$$

This statistic is called the Karl Pearson Chi Square Goodness of Fit Statistic (Hays, 1981). The sampling distribution of this statistic is chi-square, provided that the hypothesis of randomness is true. If this hypothesis is true, than X^2 tends to equal the expected value of $v = (K - 1)$, where K equals the number of categories. The number v is called the *degrees of freedom* of the

TABLE 8–5 FREQUENCY DISTRIBUTION FOR THE LAST DIGIT ON REPORTED WEIGHTS FOR ALL 246 SUBJECTS OF THE PREOPERATIVE TEACHING STUDY

Value of Last Digit	Frequency
0	29
1	13
2	23
3	22
4	28
5	32
6	28
7	29
8	21
9	21
Total	246

test, and is the parameter of the distribution of chi-square. Critical values for the chi-square distribution are reported in Table A–1. In this case $v = (10 - 1) = 9$. The determination of X^2 for the data of Table 8–5 is shown in Table 8–6. As reported in Table 8–6, $X^2 = 11.64$. This number does not deviate too much from the expected value of 9. If the observed X^2 had been statistically too large, for instance, greater than the upper 95th percentile of the chi-square distribution with $v = 9$, the hypothesis of randomness would be rejected. In this case, the 95th percentile of the chi-square distribution read from Table A–1 is given as 16.92. As indicated, the hypothesis of randomness is not rejected. The reported weights have passed this crude test of accuracy and consistency.

TABLE 8–6 WEIGHTS OF 246 PATIENTS IN THE PREOPERATIVE TEACHING STUDY: COMPUTATIONS FOR THE KARL PEARSON CHI-SQUARE STATISTICS OF GOODNESS OF FIT FOR THE DATA OF TABLE 8–5*

Value of Last Digit	Observed Frequency f_k	Expected Frequency $E(f_k)$	$f_k - E(f_k)$	$\dfrac{[f_k - E(f_k)]^2}{E(f_k)}$
0	29	24.6	4.4	0.7870
1	13	24.6	−11.6	5.4699
2	23	24.6	−1.6	0.1041
3	22	24.6	−2.6	0.2748
4	28	24.6	3.4	0.4699
5	32	24.6	7.4	2.2260
6	28	24.6	3.4	0.4699
7	29	24.6	4.4	0.7870
8	21	24.6	−3.6	0.5268
9	21	24.6	−3.6	0.5268
Total	246	246	0.0	11.6422

*$\chi^2_{9:0.95} = 16.92$

As an aside, the last column of Table 8–6 shows an interesting property about weight measurements based on self-reports. Weights ending in 0 and 5 occur more often than expected. There is weak evidence that this happened for weights ending in 5, but not for weights ending in 0. Also for some unknown reason, there is an underrepresentation of weights ending in 1. The expected number is 24.6; the observed number is 13. Note that this one outcome accounts for almost half of the total chi-square value. A reason for this underrepresentation is not clear. Finally, it should be noted that a tendency to report ages ending in 0 and 5 is common. An overrepresentation of ages ending in an even-numbered digit is not unusual.

8–4 USING FREQUENCY TABLES TO ASSESS ACCURACY AND CONSISTENCY OF QUALITATIVE DATA

Qualitative data that can be dichotomized can also be tested for randomness by using the Wald-Wolfowitz Runs Test (Hays, 1981). An an illustration, consider the following question asked of 20 nurses concerning their attitudes on going on strike.

If a strike is called, will you cross the picket line?

Yes___ No___

Suppose the responses are as shown in the chart at the bottom of this page.

By definition a run is a succession of identical letters. In this example, there are three runs of size 1, one run of size 2, two runs of size 3, one run of size 4, and one run of size 5 for a total of eight runs. At one extreme, if all the no responses were observed at the beginning of the series, the hypothesis of randomness would be suspect. This would also be true if all eight yes responses appeared at the beginning. At the other extreme, the hypothesis of randomness would be suspect if the no and yes responses alternated across all 20 nurses. Let the number of yes re-

sponses be n_1 and let the number of no responses be n_2. Tables have been constructed of the number of runs to be expected for various values of n_1 and n_2. The critical values for various sample sizes are reported in Table A–2. For 20 trials and $n_1 = 8$ and $n_2 = 12$, the critical values for $\alpha = .05$ are given by $R_{lower} = 6$ and $R_{upper} = 14$. The hypothesis of randomness is rejected when the number of runs is less than or equal to six or when the number of runs is greater than or equal to 14. In this case the number of runs is 8. The hypothesis of randomness is not rejected.

This example and that in the previous section were presented to show how statistical tests can be used in preliminary data analysis to check the accuracy and consistency of research data. Many such tests are available to a researcher. All that is needed is a little creativity and imagination to generate these types of tests. They do not provide answers to the original research questions, but they do aid in the defense of the integrity of a research investigation and the respective findings. They provide simple checks on the data with respect to potential biasing factors.

8–5 CUMULATIVE FREQUENCY TABLES FOR QUANTITATIVE DATA

Take another look at Table 8–4. This table contains two columns not included in the frequency tables examined in Section 8–2. The first of these two new columns is headed *Cumulative Frequency*. It is constructed from the *Frequency* column. It is found by adding the frequencies of the categories above and including the category being examined. If the investigator wants the cumulative frequency that is associated with category 4, the cumulative frequency is found by adding the frequencies of categories 1, 2, 3, and 4.

The interpretation of the numbers in the cumulative frequency column can be very tricky. For example, the number of patients

Nurse	1	2	3	4	5	6	7	8	9	10	11	12	13	14	15	16	17	18	19	20
Answer	Y	N	N	Y	Y	Y	N	Y	N	N	N	N	N	Y	Y	Y	N	N	N	N
Run	1	2		3		4	5		6					7			8			

whose weight is equal to 109 pounds is one. This is also the first number appearing in the cumulative frequency column, but here it has a different meaning. In this column, the cumulative frequency of one must be interpreted in the way weights are measured. Typically, weights are measured to the nearest pound with a scale divided into ounces. Under this measurement scheme, the patient with the reported weight of 109 could be as light as 108 pounds 8 ounces and as heavy as 109 pounds 8 ounces. Thus, when reading the cumulative frequency column, a mental addition of one half pound must be added to the weight column figures to provide a proper interpretation of the cumulative frequency and cumulative percentage columns. The use of these adjustments will become clearer in the discussion that follows.

The number of patients whose weight is less than 109.5 pounds is 1; the number of patients whose weight is less than 110.5 pounds is 2; the number of patients whose weight is less than 129.5 is 32, and so on. Although considerable information is contained in this column, it is not too useful to a reader or to a researcher for the same reason that frequency data are not useful when portrayed in a frequency table. Again a base figure is required to know what is meant by a cumulative frequency of 1, 2, . . . , 32, . . . , and so on. The solution, of course, is to convert the cumulative frequencies to percentages by dividing by the size of the sample—in this case, 246. These cumulative percentages are reported in the far right column of Table 8–4. Thus, the proportion of patients whose weights are less than 109.5, 110.5, and 129.5 are given by 0.41, 0.81, and 13.01, respectively.

8–6 PERCENTILES AND RELATED MEASUREMENTS OF A FREQUENCY TABLE

Frequency distributions can be used to estimate population characteristics about the center and spread of the relative frequencies in a population. The weight values and the cumulative percentages taken together give rise to a set of very useful statistical measurements called *percentiles*. The pth percentile of a frequency distribution is the value of the variable, P_p, which has the property that it divides the cumulative percentage distribution into two parts such that p% of the distribution is below P_p and $(1 - p)\%$ of the distribution is above P_p. Thus, the value closest to the 13th percentile of the distribution of weights of the 246 patients is read from Table 8–4 to be given as $P_{13} = 129.5$ pounds. Other percentile values can be determined in a similar fashion.

The *median* value of a distribution is identical with the 50th percentile. By definition the median is the value of the variable that divides a distribution so that 50% is below the median and 50% is above the median. The median is the preferred measurement of central tendency if the frequency distribution is skewed. A distribution is said to be skewed if it is not symmetrical about its median. If the tail extends to the left, the distribution is said to be negatively skewed. A positively skewed distribution has a tail extending to the right.

For the weight distribution of Table 8–4, the median is given by the value closest to $P_{50} = 150.5$ pounds. The 25th percentile is sometimes called the *first quartile*. For the weight distribution, the first quartile is given by the value closest to $P_{25} = 137.5$ pounds. The 75th percentile is sometimes referred to as the *third quartile*. For the weight distribution, the third quartile is closest to 163 pounds. Sometimes the median is called the *second quartile*. Notice that these three numbers convey meaningful summary information to a reader. Twenty-five percent of the patients weigh less than or equal to 137.5 pounds, 50% weigh less than or equal to 150.5 pounds, and 75% weigh less than or equal to 163 pounds.

With this type of information a reader and a researcher can compare this distribution with standard weight tables. The purpose of the comparison is to determine whether the sample is biased toward light or heavy patients or whether it is similar in form to the weights of the general population. This kind of information can provide credence to the accuracy and consistency of the weight measurements. Whenever sample data can be compared with an outside criterion such as standard weight tables, a researcher should do it. Both researchers and readers need to know how much trust can be placed in the conclusions drawn from a study, especially if the purpose of a study is to generalize to a larger population of subjects. External validity checks on the accuracy and consistency of the data should be made whenever possible.

The *tenth percentile* is sometimes called the *first decile*. In like manner, the 20th, 30th percentiles, and so on, are referred to as the second, third decile. The nine deciles of the weight distribution are given approximately by 126.5, 135.5, 139.5, 145.5, 150.5, 154.5, 158.5, 165.5, and 180.5, respectively.

8–7 GROUPED FREQUENCY TABLES FOR QUANTITATIVE DATA

Table 8–4 is a cumbersome table to use because of the large number of weight values. A smaller, more condensed table is generally preferred. A condensed table is certain to be preferred by most readers when done properly; it can convey more information than that provided by a complete listing of all values. This is demonstrated in Table 8–7. This table is set up by determining a set of equal width weight intervals.

Usually weights are reported to the nearest unit. Thus, a person with a reported weight of 109 pounds could actually have a true weight as low as 108.5 pounds or as high as 109.5 pounds. When using grouped frequency data, this *rounding* of data to the nearest unit must be considered. In this particular case, the smallest and largest weights are given by the reported weights of 109 and 225 pounds, respectively, so that the range of true weights is given as

$$R = 225.5 - 108.5 = 117$$

When setting up a grouped frequency table, it is recommended that the number of intervals be kept within a range of 8 to 12. Fewer than 8 is not advisable because a small number of intervals obscures the form of a distribution. More than 12 should be avoided because the distribution would appear to be very irregular and uneven, especially if the sample size is small. Also, when determining the widths of the interval, it is recommended that simple numbers be chosen. Thus, intervals of size 10 are preferred to intervals of size 13 or 17 or any other unusual number. In this case, intervals of size 10 are perfectly adequate; however, we chose to use intervals of size 12 to attain a range of 10 intervals.

The next problem that must be solved is placement of the bottom of the first interval. A good rule of thumb is to place the bottom of the first interval at a point where the smallest observed value is near the middle or slightly below the middle of the first interval. Such a choice keeps distortions of presentation to a minimum. The meaning of this suggestion will soon become clear.

With these caveats, the lower end points of the interval are given by the reported weight values of 106, 118, 130, 142, 154, 166, 178, 190, 202, and 214. The distribution is shown in Table 8–7. With this tabulation, weights are no longer being treated as having been measured to the nearest pound. Instead, weights are treated as though they were measured to the last pound. The reason for this shift in treatment is convenience. The arithmetic that follows is easier for measurement made to the last unit. As will be

TABLE 8–7 GROUPED FREQUENCY SHOWING THE DISTRIBUTION OF WEIGHTS OF 246 PATIENTS IN THE PREOPERATIVE TEACHING STUDY OF TABLE 8–4

Interval	Midpoint of Interval	Frequency	Percent per Interval	Cumulative Percentage
106–118	112	5	2.03	2.03
118–130	124	27	10.98	13.01
130–142	136	44	17.89	30.89
142–154	148	61	24.80	55.69
154–166	160	58	23.58	79.27
166–178	172	24	9.76	89.02
178–190	184	9	3.66	92.68
190–202	196	6	2.44	95.12
202–214	208	5	2.03	97.15
214–226	220	7	2.84	100.00

seen, corrections for this shift are easy to make. All that is necessary is to subtract 0.5 pound from the final measures.

As can be seen in Table 8–7, the distribution peaks in the interval given as

$$142 < Y < 154$$

This is not surprising because it has already been demonstrated that the median weight is 150.5 pounds. From this comment, it should *not* be concluded that the median is always in the interval with the largest frequency. That is true for the distributions that are fairly symmetrical but not for the distributions that are skewed.

Note the symbolism used to denote the interval with lower limit of 142 and upper limit of 154. The value of 142 is included in the interval but the value of 154 is not. The value of 154 is included in the interval directly above this one. This notation and interpretation are required because, as indicated, we are now treating the data as if the weights have been reported to the *last* pound.

In most cases, the distinctions between measurement to the *nearest* or *last* unit are not very important, because grouped frequency tables are used to convey quick visual impressions and are rarely used for analytical purposes. There is one important exception to this statement. In the United States, ages are always reported to the last birthday and never to the nearest, as, for instance, in England. Thus, when grouping ages for Americans the bottom of the intervals is always closed and the top is always open.

8–8 USING GROUPED FREQUENCY TABLES ANALYTICALLY

Sometimes grouped frequency tables can be used for analytical purposes. Suppose the frequency table reported as Table 8–4 were not available and that a researcher wished to determine the 25th or 50th percentile. A good estimate can be had by using the cumulative percentage column of Table 8–7 and the upper limits of the grouping intervals. This is done by *interpolation* in the cumulative percentage figures. In what follows, we will continue to assume that weight measurements were made to the last pound.

Under this assumption, the approximate 31st percentile is given as $Y_{31} = 142$ because 31% of the weights are below that value. In like manner, the approximate 13th percentile is at 130. Thus, the 25th percentile must be a weight between 130 and 142 pounds. An approximation to the 25th percentile can be obtained by setting up a working arithmetic table like the one shown in Table 8–8.

In this table, under the weight column are listed the end points of the interval containing the 25th percentile. The 25th percentile can be denoted by $P_{25} = 130 + X$. The cumulative percentages associated with the end points and the 25th percentile are reported in the cumulative percentage column. Under the assumption that the weights are uniformly distributed in the interval, the proportion of the interval is determined, which identifies the location of the 25th percentile. The weight interval is 12 pounds wide and the 25th percentile is X pounds into the interval. The interval contains 17.88% of the total frequency. The 25th percentile is associated with 13.01% of the distribution below 130 plus the lower 11.99% of the distribution of the interval containing the 25th percentile. To find the 25th percentile, solve the following proportional equation for X.

$$X/12 = 11.99/17.88$$

In this case,

$$X = 12(11.99/17.88) = 8.04$$

Thus, the 25th percentile is given as

$$P_{25} = 130 + 8.04 = 138.04$$

At this point, the correction for measurement to the nearest pound is made by subtracting 0.5 pound from 138.04 to give an

TABLE 8–8 WORKING ARITHMETIC TABLE FOR APPROXIMATING THE 25TH PERCENTILE OF THE DISTRIBUTION SUMMARIZED IN TABLE 8–7

	Weight	Cumulative Percentage	
12 $\begin{bmatrix}$ X $\begin{bmatrix} 130 \\ 130+X \\ 142 \end{bmatrix}$		$\begin{bmatrix} 13.01 \\ 25.00 \\ 30.89 \end{bmatrix}$ 11.99 $\end{bmatrix}$ 17.88	

adjusted 25th percentile value of 137.54 pounds. Examination of the figures reported in Table 8–4 shows that, under the assumption that weights are reported to the nearest half pound, 25.20% of the cases are below 137.5 pounds. The approximation is good.

To determine the median from the grouped data, it is seen that the median is in the interval bounded by 142 and 154. For this interval, the proportional equation is given by

$$X/12 = 19.11/24.80$$

with $X = 9.25$. With measurement to the last pound, the median is given as

$$P_{50} = 142 + 9.25 = 151.25$$

and with measurement to the nearest unit, the median is given as

$$P_{50} = 151.25 - .5 = 150.75$$

In Table 8–4 where weights are reported to the nearest pound, it is seen that 50.81% of the patients weigh less than 150.5. Again the approximation is quite good.

8–9 HIGHER ORDERED FREQUENCY TABLES

Often a researcher wants to show how two or more independent variables relate to a single dependent measure. An example is shown in Table 8–9. In this table, length of stay following operation is shown in terms of the hospital where the operation took place and the type of preoperative treatment given to the patients. As can be seen, it is a very extensive table rich with information. The frequencies and total sample sizes appear, and the table is carefully labeled. In the rural hospital, 13 patients were assigned to each of the three treatment conditions. In the suburban hospital, 24 patients were exposed to the three treatment conditions, and in the city research hospital 45 patients were placed in each of the three treatment conditions. Furthermore, it is seen that 39 patients were treated in the rural hospital, 72 in the suburban hospital, and 135 in the city research hospital.

Among the patients exposed to treatment one, none left the hospital on the day of the operation and three remained under treatment for nine days. Patients in the city hospital were released at an earlier date than patients at the other two hospitals. Fifty-eight percent of the patients in the city hospital were released on or before the fourth day following surgery. In the rural hospital only 39% were released on or before the fourth day following surgery. In the suburban hospital the corresponding percentage is 25%.

For treatment two, the corresponding percentages are given as 62% for the rural hospital, 63% for the suburban hospital and 56% for the city university hospital. Finally, for treatment three, the three percentage values are 46, 83, and 78%, respectively. Thus, it appears that treatment three is the most successful in speeding up the date of hospital

TABLE 8–9 LENGTH OF STAY FOLLOWING OPERATION ACCORDING TO TREATMENT AND TYPE OF HOSPITAL

	Treatment One						Treatment Two						Treatment Three					
	Rural		Suburban		City		Rural		Suburban		City		Rural		Suburban		City	
Days	Freq.	%	Freq.	%	Freq.	%	Freq.	%	Freq.	%	Freq.	%	Freq.	%	Freq.	%	Freq.	%
1	0	0.0	0	0.0	0	0.0	0	0.0	0	0.0	0	0.0	0	0.0	0	0.0	0	0.0
2	1	7.7	1	4.2	0	0.0	1	7.7	0	0.0	2	4.0	3	23.1	10	41.7	18	40.0
3	2	15.4	3	12.5	11	24.4	3	23.1	10	41.7	5	11.1	1	7.7	7	29.2	11	24.4
4	2	15.4	2	8.3	15	33.3	4	30.8	5	20.8	18	40.0	2	15.4	3	12.5	6	13.3
5	3	23.1	8	33.3	8	17.8	1	7.7	3	12.5	8	17.8	4	30.8	4	16.7	6	13.3
6	2	15.4	2	8.3	7	15.6	2	15.4	4	16.7	6	13.3	3	23.1	0	0.0	3	6.7
7	2	15.4	7	29.2	2	4.4	2	15.4	2	8.3	5	11.1	0	0.0	0	0.0	1	2.2
8	0	0.0	0	0.0	1	2.2	0	0.0	0	0.0	1	2.2	0	0.0	0	0.0	0	0.0
9	1	7.7	1	4.2	1	2.2	0	0.0	0	0.0	0	0.0	0	0.0	0	0.0	0	0.0
Total	13		24		45		13		24		45		13		24		45	

discharge. Rural and suburban hospitals tended to keep their patients in the hospital for a longer period of time than did the city teaching and research hospital.

Other information can be gleaned from this table. Very few patients stayed in the hospital for eight or nine days. Of the five that did, four had been exposed to treatment one. Among the treatment three patients only one remained for seven days; all of the others had been released on or before the sixth day.

This table has been set up to focus interest on hospital differences and not on treatment differences. Within each treatment, comparisons are emphasized across hospitals, even though comparisons between treatments within hospitals can be obtained. If the main interest had been on the treatment differences, the table should be redrawn so that the treatment columns are nested within the individual hospitals. This restructuring places fewer demands on a reader. In any case, a researcher must decide which is the best table for presenting the most interesting and pertinent information to the reader or user of a table.

Sometimes an investigator may wish to include a fourth variable in a higher order table that already has three variables. An example is given by the addition of the gender or sex of the patient. Other variables of interest in this study are age, drug use, and levels of uncertainty as measured by the uncertainty scale scores obtained on each patient. We advise against this practice. The information in Table 8–9 is already excessive. For most readers, it is at the point of information overload. The addition of another independent or dependent variable will make the ta-

ble too complex for most readers. Instead, it is recommended that extra tables be prepared in which those variables are separately examined. If treatment is of interest in other tabulations, it should certainly be included and reported.

Table 8–9 involves two independent variables, treatment and hospital, and one dependent variable, length of stay. Sometimes a researcher may want to cross-tabulate two dependent variables for the various levels of an independent variable. An example would be one in which length of stay is crossed with postoperative complications for each of the treatment conditions. In theory, this can be done. Unfortunately, it would not be very useful in this study, because the number of cells in the table would be so large that most cells would have zero frequencies. Little meaningful information would be conveyed to the reader or to the user of the table. When this happens, the researcher should collapse, in a meaningful manner, the categories used to define the variables. This is shown in Table 8–10 where length of stay is divided into two classes, four days or less and five days or more, and where number of postoperative complications is maintained as coded. The independent variable is treatment.

Among the patients given the training of treatment one, 68% had zero complication given for the reason why they remained in the hospital for four days or less. Among those who stayed five or more days, only 4% had no postoperative complications. Among those assigned to treatment two, 83% had no complications, provided that their stay in the hospital was four days or less. Whereas among their long-term cohort, about 27% had no complications. Finally, among those

TABLE 8–10 INTERACTION OF POSTOPERATIVE COMPLICATIONS AND LENGTH OF STAY FOLLOWING OPERATION FOR THE THREE TREATMENT CONDITIONS*

No. of Compli-cations	Treatment One				Treatment Two				Treatment Three			
	Length of Stay in Days				Length of Stay in Days				Length of Stay in Days			
	4 or Less	%	5 or more	%	4 or less	%	5 or more	%	4 or less	%	5 or more	%
0	25	67.6	2	4.4	40	83.3	9	26.5	47	93.4	9	42.9
1	8	21.6	16	35.6	6	12.5	7	20.6	3	4.9	5	23.8
2	2	5.4	14	31.1	2	4.2	13	38.2	0	0.0	5	23.8
3	2	5.4	13	28.9	0	0.0	5	14.7	1	1.6	2	9.5
Total	37		45		48		34		61		21	

*Each distribution is based on 82 patients.

patients assigned to treatment three, 93% of those who stayed for four days at the most had no complications following the operation. At the same time, the percentage of those with no complications who stayed in for five or more days increased to 43%. In essence, it appears that treatment three is the most successful in reducing postoperative complications for both long- and short-term patients. Short-term stay is defined as being confined to the hospital for four days or less following an operation. Success is measured as the absence of postoperative complication.

In this section, we have tried to demonstrate the construction of tables that can be useful to and can aid researchers and readers of journal articles and reports. Tables should be clearly labeled, sample sizes must be shown, and percentages should be reported. In addition, it is recommended that the number of variables in a table be limited to three. Table 8–9 was based on two independent variables and one dependent variable. Table 8–10 made use of two dependent variables and one independent variable. Finally, it is recommended that categories be collapsed to define a smaller set of categories when limitations in the sample sizes produce many zero frequency cells or when the number of categories is large. Remember that tables are made to convey information. They are printed not to overload a reader, and they are not made to obscure research findings. They should be a help and not a hindrance to potential readers and attendees at meetings and conferences.

Because the purpose of a graph is to provide a *quick and dirty* impression of the relationship between a set of independent and dependent variables, graphs should be simple, neat, and self-explanatory. There are extra bonuses if they are also eye-catching. Color is highly desirable. Sharp, clear printing is important. Because graphs can be used to deliberately distort research findings, a number of conventions have evolved to reduce the possibilities of inadvertently introducing *falsification* into scientific and professional graphing methods (Popper, 1959). Some suggestions are the following:

1. Each graph in a manuscript should be placed on a separate sheet of paper.
2. A title should appear at either the top or the bottom of the graph that bears the names of the independent and dependent variables.
3. The size or sizes of the samples used must be specified somewhere on the page.
4. The independent variable must be labeled clearly along the horizontal axis of the graph.
5. The dependent variable must be labeled clearly along the vertical axis of the graph.
6. A simple scale unit should be used on each scale.
7. The ratio of the vertical scale units to the horizontal scale units must be chosen carefully so as not to distort the research findings.

These guidelines are illustrated in the sections that follow.

8–10 GRAPHING DATA FOR EXPOSITION

Graphs also can be used to gain further understanding of collected data and are useful adjuncts to presenting data to readers. In the following sections, the presentation emphasizes the use of graphs. Results of a study are of no value unless they can be communicated to another interested person. Written communication is the best mode for describing research or evaluation findings. However, graphs are very useful adjuncts to providing pictorial presentations of research findings. Graphs are worth using for that reason alone!

8–11 THE BAR GRAPH FOR QUALITATIVE DATA

The most commonly encountered statistical graph is the *bar graph*. It is also the easiest to draw and interpret. The bar graph summarizing the data of Table 8–1 is shown in Figure 8–1. It provides a visual picture of the relationship between the distribution of severity for the patients operated upon in the rural hospital of the study. The levels of the independent variable (mild, moderate, and severe) are indicated along the horizontal axis, and the variable is named below the categories. The vertical axis is titled *percent of patients per level of severity*. Often, bar

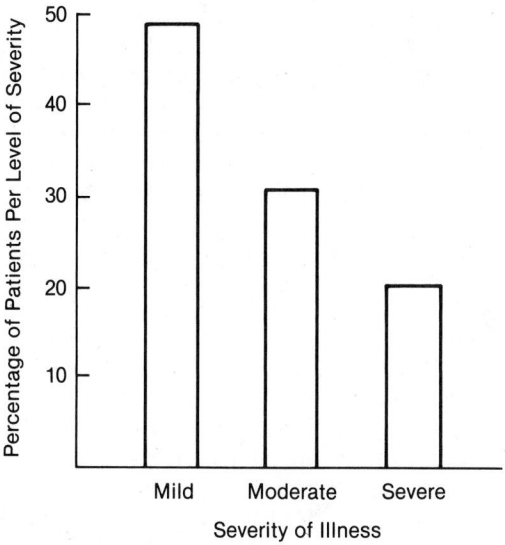

Figure 8−1. Bar graph of severity in the patients of Hospital One. N = 39.

graphs are seen with the vertical axis simply labeled *percent*. Because the purpose of a graph is to provide information to a reader, this latter simplification is not recommended. A gross error would be to report frequency or number of cases per category. Graphing frequencies is not recommended. The reader needs to know sample size and related frequencies because, for example, a frequency of 19 in 39 cases is different from

a frequency of 19 in 246 cases. A good place to report sample size is in the title.

Finally, there is the problem of distortion. Distortion can be introduced into a graph with ease by means of a poor choice of a scale for the vertical axis. The variation among the three levels of severity can be made to look small by changing the vertical scale. For example, in Figure 8−2, changing 10 percentage points to the inch to 20 percentage points to the inch would reduce the height of each bar by 50% and would provide a visual picture of similarity to the three severity levels. Furthermore, the differences could be exaggerated in the percentages by decreasing the vertical scale so that one inch represented 5% rather than 10%. This would double the height of each bar, making it look as if the differences between the three percentages are very large.

Note that a simple scale has been used for the vertical column. The scale marks for Figure 8−1 are at 10, 20, 30, 40, and 50. These are easy numbers to translate. It would not have been wrong to use scale marks at 8, 16, 24, 32, and 40, or at 7, 14, 21, 28, 35, and 42, except that they would make interpretation more complicated for most readers. Any scale division can be used, provided that the spaces between the marks are equal in length. Even so, the scale based on multiples of 10 is preferred because of its simplicity. In a bar diagram the bars are not joined but are separated from one another. This is not

Figure 8−2. Bar graph of severity in the patients of Hospital One. N = 39.

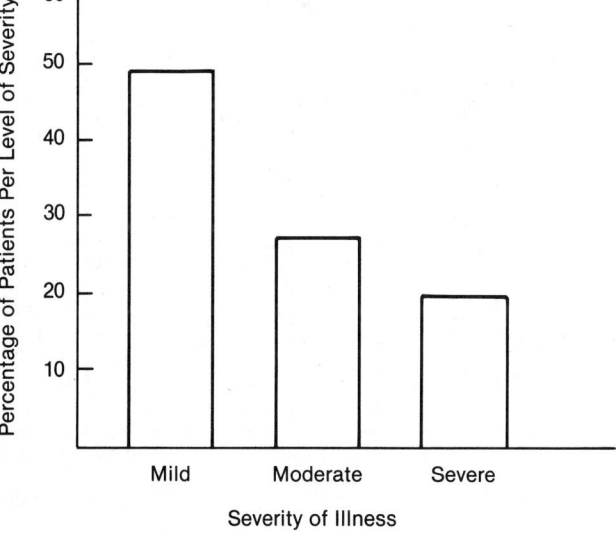

an absolute necessity, but again it is the preferred mode. The separation reminds the reader that the variable plotted along the horizontal axis is qualitative and not quantitative and is definitely not continuous.

Figure 8–3 is the graphic presentation of the data in Table 8–3 and provides a visual display of the relationship of the distribution of severity according to hospital. Actually, it is three bar graphs shown on one display. It provides a simple way to compare the hospitals. For example, it is clear that more than 50% of the patients in the suburban hospital had a mild abdominal problem, whereas the city hospital had almost 30% of its patients with severe abdominal problems.

Figures 8–1 and 8–3 provide an example of how important the scale units are in distorting the picture portrayed by a graph. Hospital one is shown in both graphs. There is a tendency to view the differences in bar heights in Figure 8–3 as being greater than those shown in Figure 8–1. This tendency is a result of the differences in the widths of the bars. The bars in Figure 8–3 appear to be tall and thin, whereas those in Figure 8–1 appear to be short and fat. In reality, they are the same height. From this it should be clear that bar graphs have no analytical value and should be used with caution.

Frequently bar graphs are represented as *pie charts*. An example is shown in Figure 8–4. This is a pie chart representation of the data shown in Figure 8–3. In this case, distances along the vertical axis are converted to angles. For example, a bar representing 25% of a distribution would be represented in a pie chart by a wedge covering 90 degrees of the full 360 degrees represented by the whole pie. One advantage to the pie chart is that it is difficult to distort. Regardless of the radius chosen for the pie, 90 degrees always represents 25% of the distribution. Thirty-three and one third percent is always represented by an arc along the circumference or angle at the center of 120 degrees.

Finally, it should be stated that bar graphs should be used only for nominal or qualitative data, whether the categories are ordered or unordered. Quantitative data are graphed using *histograms*. This type of graph is described in the next section.

8–12 THE HISTOGRAM FOR REPRESENTING GROUPED QUANTITATIVE DATA

Frequency distributions for quantitative variables that are discrete or continuous are best displayed as histograms. As a consequence, histograms are appropriate for variables measured on an interval or ratio scale

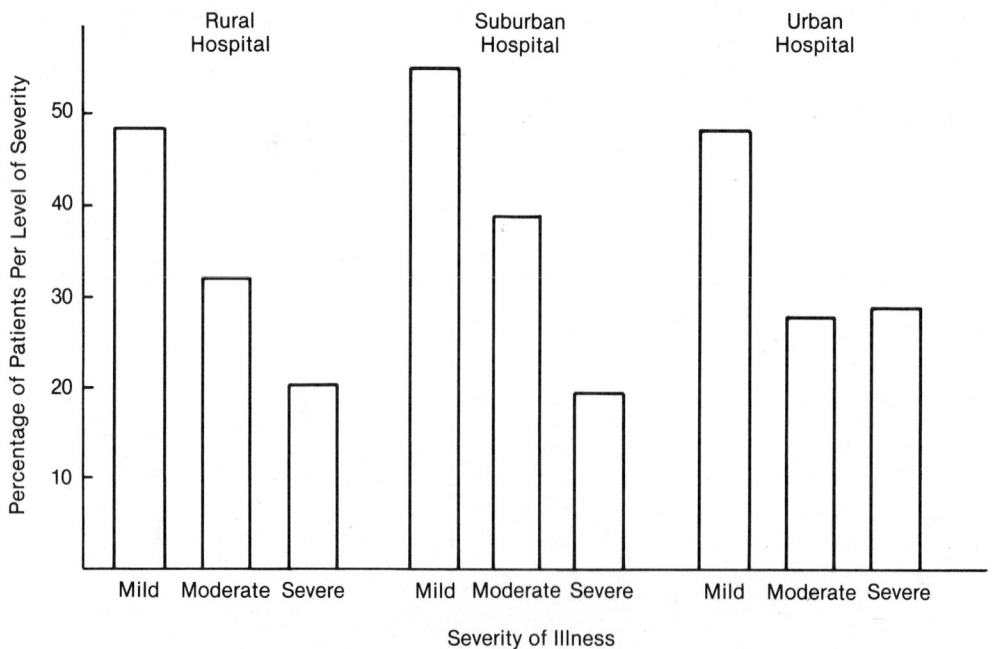

Figure 8–3. Bar graph of severity in 246 patients in three different hospitals.

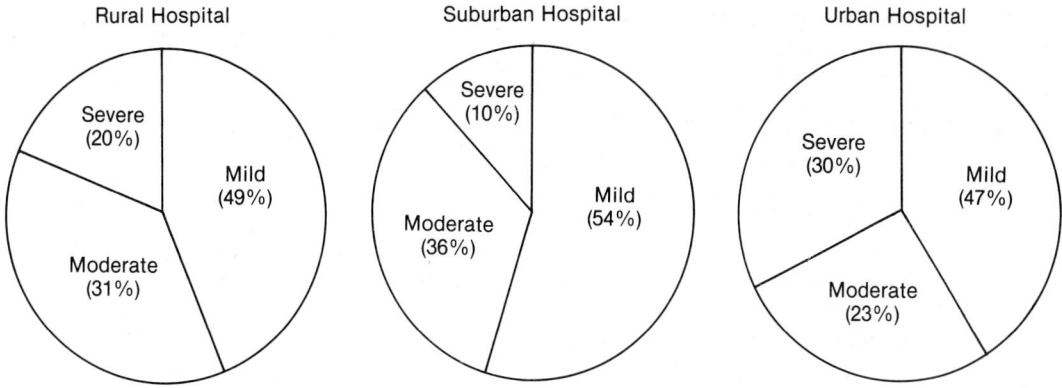

Figure 8–4. Distribution of severity in 246 patients in three different hospitals.

as well. A histogram is a pictorial display of a frequency table for grouped data. Thus, the starting point for a histogram is a frequency table for grouped data. The histogram for the frequencies of Table 8–7 is shown in Figure 8–5. Along the horizontal scale are listed values of the independent variable. Here, a researcher can label either the midpoints of the intervals or the end points. The choice is based on the way that the variable is measured and on making the graph easy to read by others.

In Table 8–7 weight has been measured to the last pound with the lower limit of the first interval being 106 pounds and the upper limit being 117.99999. . . . This means that the second interval begins at exactly 118 pounds and extends up to but does not include 130. If this is the case the midpoints of the first and second intervals are given as 112 and 124 pounds. With measurement to the last pound, either the midpoint values or the end point values may be listed along the horizontal axis. With end point plotting, the scale values would read 106, 118, 130, . . . , but with midpoint plotting the scale values would read 112, 124, 136, ...

Suppose weights had been measured to the nearest pound. Then these reported values would be in error. To see this, consider the first interval with lower limit 106. Anyone whose weight exceeds 105.5 pounds but is less than 106.5 pounds would have reported their weight at 106 pounds. Thus, the true lower limit is given as 105.5. With similar reasoning the true upper limit is given as 117.5 so that the midpoint would be given as 111.5. If one wanted to be exact, then the horizontal scales that are admissible are given as 105.5, 117.5, 129.5, . . . , for end point reporting or as 111.5, 123.5, 135.5, . . . , for midpoint reporting. Without doubt, the reporting of such numbers along the horizontal scale goes against the imperative of making the scale values simple. Histograms are used to generate a visual image of a distribution and are not used to perform analytical investigation. The rule of simplicity has a tendency to win over the rule of accuracy, and the incorrect whole number values are usually reported. This simplification is not mandatory. If desired, the exact values can be reported. More often than not, the simpler reporting convention is seen more frequently.

It has been found that one way to reduce possible distortions in a histogram presentation is to draw the histogram in a space that has a height-to-width ratio of about 2:3.

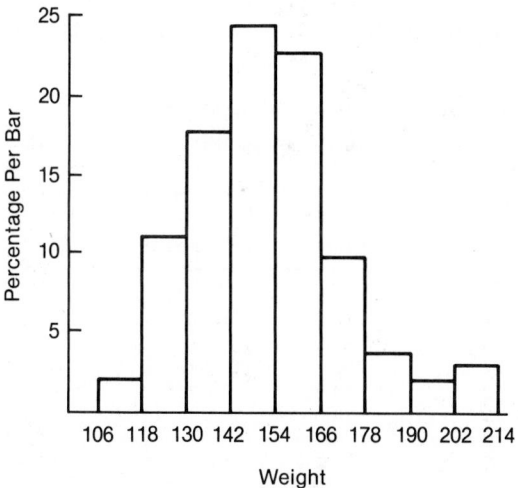

Figure 8–5. Distribution of weights of the 246 patients of the preoperative teaching study.

Technically speaking histograms are justifiable only for continuous variables, and for that reason the bars are joined. There is no space between the bars. It must be noted, however, that histograms are used for discrete variables as well. Consider the uncertainty scores of the preoperative teaching study. The scores are on a discrete scale that extends from a low of about 20 to a high of about 80. To treat a discrete variable as if it were a continuous variable, a correction for continuity is imposed on the measurement. For the uncertainty scale, the correction involves the convention that any discrete score, Y, actually represents measurement along a continuous interval that extends from a low value of $Y - .5$ to $Y + .5$. In drawing a histogram, this correction would be used in exactly the same manner as that used for weights measured to the closest unit. For graphing purposes, the exact midpoints or end point values could be used to represent position along the X scale. More frequently, the uncorrected values reported along the horizontal axis are more likely to be seen. Strictly speaking it is wrong, but everyone does it. The error is not grave, because as it is repeatedly pointed out, graphs are used to give visual images only.

8–13 RELATIVE FREQUENCY POLYGONS FOR QUANTITATIVE DATA

Histograms are used to describe the frequency distribution of a quantitative variable for a single sample. Often, a researcher

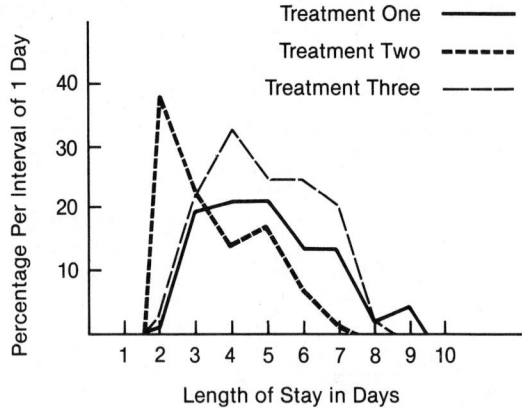

Figure 8–6. Distribution of days in the hospital for each of the preoperative treatments. Each distribution is based on 82 patients.

wishes to provide a visual comparison of two or more distributions. This is done by means of a graph called a *relative frequency polygon*. The numbers for the drawing of this graph are found in a frequency table. If the data are grouped, % frequencies are plotted against the midpoints of the intervals. The plotted points are joined by line segments to produce a polygon. The polygon is closed off at the bottom by extending the outer line segments to the horizontal axis at the lower and upper end points of the two extreme intervals. If the data are not grouped, a correction for continuity is assumed, and the graph is drawn under that assumption.

Figure 8–6 shows the relative frequency polygons corresponding to the data of Table 8–11. Here, the variable is discrete, the number of days remaining in hospital fol-

TABLE 8–11 FREQUENCY DISTRIBUTIONS OF DAYS IN HOSPITAL FOR EACH OF THE PREOPERATIVE TEACHING PROGRAMS*

Days in Hospital	Treatment One Frequency	Treatment One Percent	Treatment Two Frequency	Treatment Two Percent	Treatment Three Frequency	Treatment Three Percent
1	0	0.0	0	0.0	0	0.0
2	2	2.4	3	3.7	31	37.8
3	16	19.5	18	22.0	19	23.2
4	19	23.2	27	32.9	11	13.4
5	19	23.2	12	14.6	14	17.1
6	11	13.4	12	14.6	6	7.3
7	11	13.4	9	11.0	1	1.2
8	1	1.2	1	1.2	0	0.0
9	3	3.7	0	0.0	0	0.0
Total	82	100.0	82	100.0	82	100.0

*Each distribution is based on 82 patients.

lowing a surgical operation for each of the three treatments. This variable can take on the values 0, 1, 2, ... The interpretation of these numbers is more complicated than is apparent at first glance. The problem is easy to demonstrate.

Consider all patients whose length of stay is 2 days. Some of these patients will be released from the hospital 48.5 hours after termination of surgery. Others will be released at 50 hours, some at 55.25 hours, and some at 71.75 hours. Thus, we see that the discrete number 2 actually represents the continuous range of exactly 48 hours up to and not including 72 hours. The midpoint of this interval is 60 hours, which is equivalent to 2.5 days. Therefore, we see that 2 days represents the continuous interval of 2 up to and not including 3 days. The midpoint is 2.5 days. This is actually the mean length of stay for all patients who remain in the hospital following surgery for 2 days. This must be taken into account when drawing the relative frequency polygon. Operationally this means that the relative frequencies must be plotted against .5, 1.5, 2.5, and so on.

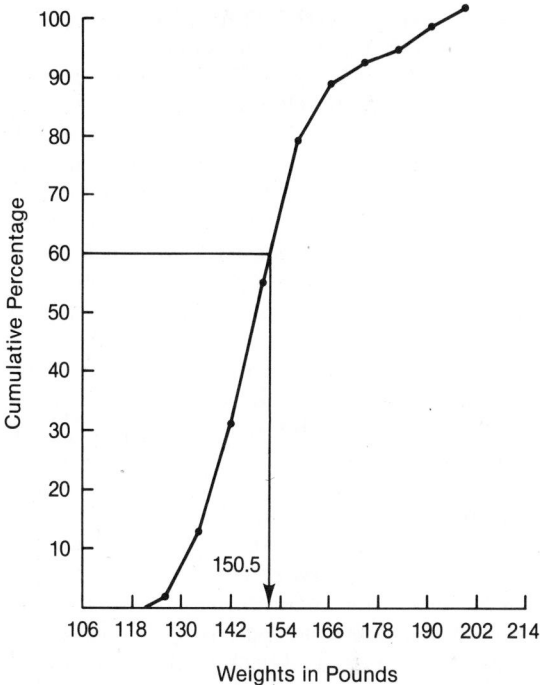

Figure 8–7. Cumulative distribution of weights of the 246 patients of the preoperative treatment study.

8–14 CUMULATIVE RELATIVE FREQUENCY POLYGON FOR QUANTITATIVE DATA

Cumulative relative frequency polygon graphs are not seen often in research articles or professional reports. In a sense, this is unfortunate because, of all the statistical graphs discussed in this chapter, the cumulative frequency polygon is the only one that can be used for analytical purposes. If it is drawn correctly, it can be used to determine the median, the first and second quartiles, and any percentile value of interest. An example is provided in Figure 8–7. This graph is based on the cumulative percentages shown in Table 8–4 and is the only graph described in this chapter that technically should be based on the correction for continuity in that the cumulative percentages are plotted against the upper end points corrected for continuity. The horizontal scale must be labeled to reflect the continuity correction provided that the graph is to be used to determine percentiles. If it is being used strictly for visual inspection purposes, then the correction is not required.

Figure 8–7 has been graphed without the correction. This is apparent in the determi-

nation of the median or 50th percentile value. Note that the vertical scale has a range of zero to 100%. The median is found by tracing a line from the 50% point to the curve and extending the line straight down to the horizontal axis to where it cuts the axis. This point is the median. In this case, the median is read to equal 150. In Section 8–6, it was reported that the median is equal to 150.5 when corrected for measurement to the nearest pound. If the points had been plotted with the half-pound correction for continuity, this value would have been obtained. Thus, if the correction is not used for making the graph, the corrected median and percentiles can be estimated by reading the values from the graph and adding the correction for continuity to the observed value. For these data, the estimated corrected median is

$$150.0 + .5 = 150.5.$$

We close this section by noting that other percentile values can be obtained in a similar fashion. For example, the 60th percentile not corrected for continuity is given as 154 and with the correction for continuity as 154.5. In like manner, the 40th percentile is given as 146 when uncorrected and 146.5 when corrected.

8–15 THE SCATTER DIAGRAM FOR REPRESENTING THE CORRELATION BETWEEN TWO QUANTITATIVE VARIABLES

A scatter diagram is a two-dimensional visual display of two interrelated variables. It is used to provide a pictorial impression of the correlation between two variables. It can also be used to make judgments concerning the valid use of the *Pearson Product Moment Correlation Coefficient*.

An example of a scatter diagram is provided in Figure 8–8. In this figure the relationship between the uncertainty scores and days in the hospital following operation is shown for the patients in the suburban hospital, who were given treatment three. As shown, there seems to be a positive relationship between the two variables; r = 0.53. Patients with low uncertainty scores leave the hospital sooner than patients with high uncertainty scores. The best fitting straight line for these data is given as

$$Y = -.90 + .085X.$$

From this equation it is seen that patients with uncertainty scores of 30 tend to leave the hospital in about

$$Y = -.90 + .085(30) = 1.65 \text{ days}$$

on the average, whereas patients with uncertainty scores of 55 tend to leave in about Y = 3.78 days.

Although the evidence is not overwhelming, there is reason to believe that patients with low uncertainty scores are expected to leave the hospital before patients with high

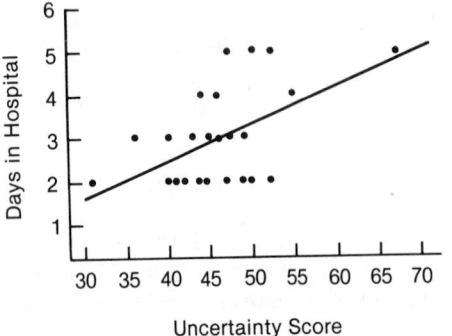

Figure 8–8. Scatter diagram of uncertainty and days in hospital and best-fitting straight line for the 24 patients of the suburban hospital who were given treatment three.

uncertainty scores. The mean length of stay for the 24 patients of Figure 8–8 is 3.04 days. Unless the scatter diagrams were investigated, it would not be known that people whose uncertainty score was 35 or less would be expected to leave in less than two days, and patients with uncertainty scores exceeding 46 would be expected to remain three or more days. Clearly, the scatter diagram provides information that can be useful to nurses and other care takers having to work with patients like those of Figure 8–8.

The nature of the scatter of the points in the two-dimensional space indicates that the correlation coefficient is a valid measure of association for these variables. The scatter of the points in the diagram shows the following properties:

1. The relationship between the two variables is linear.
2. There are no unusual or outlier values in the distributions of either variable.
3. Neither distribution appears to be truncated.
4. Variation about the regression line is *homoscedastic*.

Thus, there is no strong evidence against using the Pearson product moment correlation coefficient to assess the strength of the relationship between uncertainty and length of stay.

Whenever a researcher decides to use the Pearson product moment correlation coefficient as a measurement of association, the four conditions listed above should be satisfied.

Unless the relationship between the two variables is linear, the use of the Pearson product moment correlation coefficient cannot be justified. If the relationship is curved and not linear, the correlation coefficient as a measurement of association will be too small.

Also, the correlation coefficient is an invalid measurement of association if extreme values or outliers are in the sample. Outliers tend to inflate the correlation if both the X and Y values are jointly small or jointly large. Outliers tend to reduce the correlation coefficient if one measurement is unusually large and the other measurement is unusually small.

In addition, a researcher must assure that the scatter plot is not bounded at the top or bottom by floor or ceiling effects placed on the measurement of the two variables. This problem is compounded when a paper and pencil test is given in which the number of items is small. With a scale with only a small number of items, there is a tendency for people to bunch up at the top. With this bunching comes truncation and the correlation coefficient becomes an invalid measurement of association. Thus, it is a good idea to use a semantic differential scale, a Guttman scale, a Likert scale, and other psychometric devices that contain as many items as possible.

Homoscedasticity is the property in which the variability around the regression line is equal to a common value for all values of the independent variable. This assumption is almost always violated in growth or developmental studies. Subjects at the bottom end of a scale tend to be homogeneous, whereas subjects at the top end tend to be heterogeneous. In this case, the assumption of homoscedasticity is violated and the use of the Pearson product moment correlation coefficient is invalid.

8–16 TREATMENT OF OUTLIERS

Often the examination of a histogram, relative frequency polygon, or scatter diagram suggests to an observer that the data contain outliers. For example, the one value of Figure 8–8 at X = 67 has the appearance of an outlier. In this case, the nearest neighbor is X = 55. A number of statistical tests have been proposed to test a suspect observation as being one that should be excluded from the study. One such test has been designed by Grubbs (1969). For this test, the number of standard deviations between the mean of the sample and the suspected outlier is determined. If the distance is greater than chance would predict, the decision is made that the observation is an outlier. The Grubbs test is performed as follows.

1. Determine the mean and standard deviation of the full sample.
2. Determine the number of standard deviations between the suspected outlier and the mean of the sample.
3. Find the appropriate critical values in Table A–3 for the number of observations in the sample and the chosen risk of a type I error.
4. If the number of standard deviations between the outlier and the mean exceeds the

table value, conclude that the suspected observation is an outlier.

5. If the observation is named an outlier, remove it from the study and reduce the sample size accordingly, or replace it by its closest neighbor.
6. If the replaced observation is used for future statistical computations, subtract one degree of freedom from all associated error terms.

We apply Grubbs' test to X = 67. For these data, the mean value is 46.17 and the standard deviation is 6.98. The number of standard deviations between 67 and the mean is given as

$$Z = (67 - 46.17)/6.98 = 2.98.$$

For a risk of a type I error controlled at .05, the critical values read from Table A–3 are −2.80 and +2.80. Because Z = 2.98 is larger than the positive critical value, we conclude that the observation is an outlier. In this case, we would remove it from the study. If there was a need to maintain the sample size, the X = 67 could be replaced by X = 55, the nearest neighbor. This process is referred to as Winsorizing the mean (Dixon and Tukey, 1968).

8–17 TREATMENT AND ESTIMATION OF MISSING DATA

It is the rule rather than the exception for a researcher to encounter the problem of missing data in a study. For instance, consider the study in Chapter 7 in which nurses were asked to report their views about participation in a strike. Suppose 20 nurses were interviewed and upon examining the data, the researcher discovered that for some questions the data were not recorded or could not be coded. Suppose that upon examining the one question related to support or opposition to the strike, it was found that 12 of the 20 nurses moderately or strongly supported a strike and that 7 nurses were moderately or strongly opposed to the strike. The data for one nurse on this crucial item were missing. So as not to lose the remaining information from the interview of this one nurse, an investigator can estimate this sole piece of missing information so that the analysis of data can proceed on the full sample.

A number of methods have been proposed for estimating missing data. For data that possess a normal distribution, Bhoj (1978; 1984), Ekbohm (1976), and Wu (1989) have proposed methods for estimating missing data in the pretest-posttest design. Similar methods have been generated for dichotomous variables by Campbell (1984); Choi and Stablein (1982); Ekbohm (1982). Marascuilo, Omlich, and Gokhale (1987) describe procedures for estimating missing data and testing hypotheses for the pretest-posttest design with multiple groups and dichotomous dependent variables. Dempster, Laird, and Rubin (1977) and Little and Rubin (1987) describe procedures using a complex model called the EM Algorithm that is very effective for estimating missing data in survey research. Whereas their method is designed to produce unbiased estimates of missing data, the estimated data cannot be used for hypothesis testing because of inflated type I error rates and tendency to reject the null hypothesis too often (Wu, 1989). Marascuilo and Levin (1983) provide directions for estimating missing data using regression models. Cohen and Cohen (1982) describe estimation procedures for repeated measurement designs.

The simplest missing data estimation procedure is best exemplified in a study conducted as a survey sample. For example, consider the study of Chapter 6 on assessing nurses' attitudes toward working with AIDS patients. Each nurse in the study can be classified according to city, gender, age, marital status, religious orientation, number of years worked as a nurse, current employment with persons with AIDS (PWAs), attitude toward working with PWAs, willingness to work with PWAs, knowing or having gay or lesbian acquaintances, and current sexual orientation. The classification of each nurse into a precise, demarcated cell can be done through employment of cross-tabulation procedures available on many main frame and personal computer packages as SPSS (1986), BMDP (Dixon, 1983), and CRUNCH (Bostrom, 1986).

Suppose that, as a result of using one of these computer packages, it was found that five nurses in Los Angeles were classified as male, over the age of 35, single, Catholic, 10 years working as a nurse, currently working with PWAs, positive attitude toward PWAs, willing to work with PWAs, no gay or lesbian friends, and with a heterosexual orientation. Because the number of men in this particular cell is very small, a researcher would not want to discard any because of missing data. A proposed solution is to estimate the mean or the median value for any item of interest among the pieces of information available for these five subjects. If information is missing for any subject on a specific item, the mean or median of that cell is substituted for that particular missing value.

If the missing data are associated with a Likert or semantic differential scale, the median of the sample is suggested as the estimate in place of the mean, because the median will be a scale value like 1, 2, 3, 4, or 5. If a researcher plans to use the missing data in further studies involving hypothesis testing models, one degree of freedom must be subtracted from the total degrees of freedom before any test of hypothesis is performed.

Using a measure of central tendency as an estimator has one serious drawback. It tends to produce an overabundance of type I errors in hypothesis testing models. The reason for this is easy to show. Consider the following sample of Likert scale responses concerning support or opposition to the strike:

1 1 2 3 3 3 3 3 3 4 4 4 4 4 4 5 U U U U

The median of the 16 observations is equal to 3. If this value is substituted for the missing data, we have as a final sample for data analysis the following set of numbers:

1 1 2 3 3 3 3 3 3 3 3 3 3 4 4 4 4 4 4 5

The median of the sample is still equal to three, but the standard deviation of the completed sample has changed. The standard deviation of the completed sample is much reduced. In fact the standard deviation is reduced from 1.11 to .99. All the missing observations are assigned to the center of the distribution. This causes havoc in all statistical hypothesis testing procedures that can be applied to the data. The standard deviation is always placed in the denominator of t and F tests. With a spuriously low measurement of variation, many significant findings may well represent type I errors. In these cases, the investigator will draw false conclusions.

One solution to the problem of reduced variation is to estimate the standard deviation of the complete data and use this estimate to provide different estimates for each of the missing pieces of datum. The procedure is based on the use of a table of random normal numbers ($\mu = 0$ and $\sigma = 1$) in the following fashion. Each missing piece of information is replaced by the mean plus the product of a randomly selected random normal number and the standard deviation. With each missing piece of information, a different random normal number is used for the estimation process. With this model the mean and the standard deviation of the original sample are maintained and the chances of rejecting null hypotheses inappropriately are reduced.

For the example, the mean Likert score is 3.1875 and the standard deviation is 1.1087. We now enter Table A–4 of random normal numbers in the Appendix. In this case, the four numbers we selected at random are 0.151, 0.290, 0.873, and −1.289. These numbers are used as follows to estimate the four missing pieces of data.

$$U_1 = 3.1875 + 0.151(1.1087) = 3.35$$
$$U_2 = 3.1875 + 0.290(1.1087) = 3.51$$
$$U_3 = 3.1875 + 0.873(1.1087) = 4.16$$

and

$$U_4 = 3.1875 - 1.289(1.1087) = 1.79.$$

We now convert these to the nearest Likert values of 3, 4, 4, and 2, respectively. The completed sample is now given as

1 1 2 2 3 3 3 3 3 3 3 4 4 4 4 4 4 4 4 5

The standard deviation of this sample is equal to 1.06 and is larger than the sample that used only the measurement of central tendency to estimate the missing data.

In a correlational study, missing data can be estimated using the procedures described in this section. Some computer programs have an option known as *pairwise deletion.* If one observation is missing on a profile of data for one subject, it would be costly in terms of information loss to remove that one subject from the study. The problem is especially acute if one or two pieces of data on different variables are missing for a large number of subjects. The pairwise deletion solution for missing data is to compute the correlation coefficients on the pairs of complete data. In most cases, the estimation causes no problems. In some cases, a researcher may generate a *matrix* of correlation coefficients which cannot be analyzed. This happens when the resulting matrix of correlation coefficients is *singular,* and a message is usually provided on the computer printout. For the nurse researcher, this means that the data cannot be analyzed and that all numbers on the computer printout are suspect.

8–17 SUMMARY

In this chapter a presentation of rules, procedures, and conventions for the visual display of qualitative and quantitative data was offered. The advantages and disadvantages of using the various pictorial displays were provided. Suggestions were offered for independent verification or confirmation of the accuracy and consistency of collected data. In particular, bar graphs, pie charts, histograms, scatter diagrams, and cumulative relative frequency graphs were illustrated. It was shown how the scatter diagram can justify the measurement of the association between two variables in terms of the Pearson product moment correlation coefficient. Guidelines for handling of outliers or extreme numerical values were depicted. Lastly, illustrations were provided and alternatives were suggested for the treatment of missing data.

REFERENCES

Bhoj, D.S.: Testing equality of correlated variates with missing observations on both responses, Biometrika, *65:* 225–228, 1978.

Bhoj, D.S.: On difference of means of correlated variates with incomplete data on both responses, J. Stat. Comput. Sim., *19:* 275–289, 1984.

Bostrom, A.: CRUNCH Software. Oakland, CA, 1986.

Campbell, G.: Testing equality of proportions with incomplete correlated data, J. Stat. Planning Inf., *10:* 311–321, 1984.

Choi, S.C., and Stablein, D.M.: Practical tests for comparing two proportions with incomplete data, Appl. Stat., *31:* 256–262, 1982.

Cohen, J., and Cohen, P.: Applied Regression Analysis/Correlational Analysis for the Behavioral Sciences, ed. 2. New York, John Wiley & Sons, 1982.

Dempster, A.P., Laird, N.M., and Rubin, D.D.: Maximum likelihood from incomplete data via the EM algorithm, J. Royal Stat. Soc., Series B, *39:* 1–22, 1977.

Dixon, W.J., ed.: BMDP Statistical Software. Berkeley, CA, University of California Press, 1983.

Dixon, W.J., and Tukey, J.W.: Approximate behavior of the distribution of the Winsorized t. Technometrics, *10:* 83–98, 1968.

Ekbohm, G.: Comparing means in the paired case with incomplete data, Biometrika, *63*: 229–304, 1976.

Ekbohm, G.: On testing the equality of proportions in the paired case with incomplete data, Psychometrika, *47*: 115–118, 1982.

Grubbs, F.E.: Procedures for deleting outlying observations in samples, Technometrics, *11*: 1–21, 1969.

Hays, W.L.: Statistics, ed. 3. New York, Holt, Rinehart & Winston, 1981.

Little, R.J.A., and Rubin, D.A.: Statistical Analysis with Missing Data. New York, John Wiley & Sons, 1987.

Lin, P.E., and Stivers, L.E.: On difference of means with incomplete data, Biometrika, *61*: 299–304, 1974.

Marascuilo, L.A., and Levin, J.: Multivariate Methods for Social Science Research: A Researcher's Handbook. Monterey, CA, Brooks/Cole, 1983.

Marascuilo, L.A., Omelich, C.L., and Gokhale, D.V.: Planned and post hoc methods for multiple sample McNemar tests with missing data, Psych. Bull., 1987.

Popper, K.R.: The Logic of Scientific Discovery. New York, Basic Books, 1959.

SPSS, Inc.: SPSS* User's Guide, ed. 2. New York, McGraw-Hill, 1986.

Wu, P.: A Monte Carlo investigation of ten test statistics for testing the equality of two-group change parameters of quantitative variables with missing data, Unpublished doctoral dissertation, University of California at Berkeley, 1989.

Chapter 9

INFERENTIAL STATISTICS FOR UNIVARIATE DEPENDENT VARIABLES

9–1 ROLE OF THE NORMAL DISTRIBUTION IN STATISTICAL HYPOTHESIS TESTING ESTIMATION MODELS

The normal distribution plays the major role in statistical hypothesis testing and estimation theory. One way to understand this role is to perform a mental exercise or thought experiment, such as that used in the physical sciences to conduct a hypothetical investigation of an experiment, which, in fact, cannot be performed. The purpose of this thought experiment is to provide a justification for the hypothesis testing models described

throughout this text. This mental exercise provides a brief review of:

1. the normal distribution,
2. the central limit theorem,
3. the sampling distribution of a statistic,
4. standard statistical terminology,
5. type I and type II errors, and
6. statistical hypothesis testing and estimation theory.

For the mental exercise, consider the study in Chapter 1 on preoperative training given to 246 subjects about to undergo surgery. In particular, consider the 82 subjects that were assigned to treatment one. The length of stay in the hospital following surgery for these patients is given by the following set of numbers:

Patient Number 3067 2 days

Patient Number 2010 2 days

Patient Number 3070 6 days

$$\vdots \qquad \downarrow \qquad \downarrow$$

Patient Number 3082 4 days

These figures are taken directly from Table B–1. (See Appendix B.) If we let Y_1, Y_2, Y_3, . . . , Y_N represent the values 2, 2, 6, . . . , 4, then the mean number of days in the hospital following surgery is given as

$$\overline{Y} = \frac{1}{N} \sum_{i=1}^{N} Y_i = \frac{1}{N} (Y_1 + Y_2 + Y_3 + \ldots + Y_N)$$

$$= \frac{1}{82} (2 + 2 + 6 + \ldots + 4) = 4.89$$

The data of Table B–1 represent the first possible replication of a study in which 82 patients have been assigned to treatment one. From a theoretical point of view, it is possible to replicate the study with a new group of patients in a similar setting. This would generate a new set of data, which could be reported in a new table called Table B–2 and which would be similar to but not identical with Table B–1. For the 82 subjects assigned to treatment one of this second theoretical repetition, the mean value can be computed. Most likely, it would be a number other than 4.89.

There is no reason to limit the theoretical repetitions of the study to one extra replication. In one's mind, a third replication could be summarized in a table that could be denoted Table B–3. For this third theoretical repetition, the mean length of stay could be computed for the 82 patients assigned to treatment one. Most likely the mean value would be a number that differs from that of replications one and two. In theory the study could be replicated as often as desired. Each of these replications would produce a mean value for the number of days that the patient remained in the hospital following operation. If all these hypothetical mean values were tabulated, a histogram could be generated using the model described in Chapter 8.

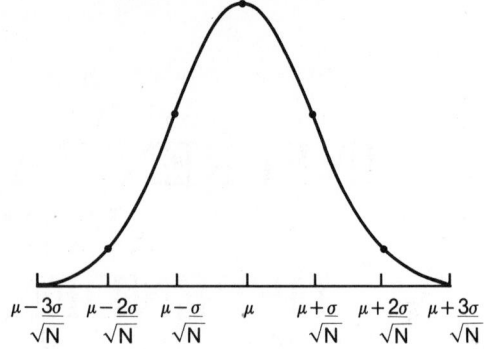

$$\mu - \frac{3\sigma}{\sqrt{N}} \quad \mu - \frac{2\sigma}{\sqrt{N}} \quad \mu - \frac{\sigma}{\sqrt{N}} \quad \mu \quad \mu + \frac{\sigma}{\sqrt{N}} \quad \mu + \frac{2\sigma}{\sqrt{N}} \quad \mu + \frac{3\sigma}{\sqrt{N}}$$

Figure 9–1. The sampling distribution of $\overline{Y}$.

If there were an exceedingly large number of replications of the study that were tallied in a large set of exceedingly narrow intervals, the histogram would look much like the idealized graph shown in Figure 9–1. This idealized curve is a graphic representation of the *normal distribution* and in this case is a theoretical graphic representation of the sampling distribution of the mean for samples of size N = 82.

Any normal distribution is defined by two numbers called *parameters*. One parameter defines the center of the distribution and the other parameter defines the degree of spread of the values from the center. The center is described as the *mean value* and is sometimes called the *expected value* of the distribution. It is identical with the *median* of the distribution because the normal distribution is symmetrical about its *mean value*. The parameter that defines the spread is called the *standard deviation*. Traditionally the mean value is represented by the Greek letter μ (mu) and the standard deviation is represented by the Greek letter σ (sigma). If the values of μ and σ are known, the percentiles of the distribution can be determined with ease. For example,

1. the .5th percentile is given as

$$P_{.005} = \mu - 2.58\sigma$$

2. the 1st percentile is given as

$$P_{.01} = \mu - 2.32\sigma$$

3. the 2.5th percentile is given as

$$P_{.025} = \mu - 1.96\sigma$$

4. the 5th percentile is given as

$$P_{.05} = \mu - 1.645\sigma$$

5. the 10th percentile is given as

$$P_{.10} = \mu - 1.28\sigma$$

6. the 16th percentile is given as

$$P_{.16} = \mu - \sigma$$

7. the 50th percentile is given as

$$P_{.50} = \mu$$

8. the 84th percentile is given as

$$P_{.84} = \mu + \sigma$$

9. the 90th percentile is given as

$$P_{.90} = \mu + 1.28\sigma$$

10. the 95th percentile is given as

$$P_{.95} = \mu + 1.645\sigma$$

11. the 97.5th percentile is given as

$$P_{.975} = \mu + 1.96\sigma$$

12. the 99th percentile is given as

$$P_{.99} = \mu + 2.32\sigma$$

13. the 99.5th percentile is given as

$$P_{.995} = \mu + 2.58\sigma$$

The remaining percentiles are reported in Table A–5. In theory, normally distributed variables are continuous. In practice, the normally distributed variables are associated with discrete variables like $\overline{Y}$.

9–2 LINEAR COMBINATIONS AND THE CENTRAL LIMIT THEOREM

A variable whose mathematical form consists of a weighted sum of other variables is called a *linear combination* (Hays, 1988). The sample mean is an example of a linear combination. It is a weighted sum of other variables. Each weight is equal to 1/N. If the number of algebraic terms in a linear combination is large, then the distribution of the linear combination over repeated sampling comes under the control of the *central limit theorem*. From an operational point of view, the central limit theorem can be stated as follows:

A linear combination based on the sum of a large number of algebraic terms has a sampling distribution that tends to have a normal distribution over multiple replications or sampling under identical experimental or observational conditions.

Thus, sample averages have over multiple replications of an experiment or sampling survey normal distributions for large samples. For all practical purposes, sample averages based on 30 or more observations are considered large enough for the operation of the central limit theorem and the justification for using the normal distribution for estimation of population parameters and statistical hypothesis testing.

9–3 STATISTICAL HYPOTHESIS TESTING THEORY

In practice, a study is performed only once. As a consequence, a researcher has only one mean value to examine. The problem facing a researcher is "Where in the theoretical normal distribution of means is the observed mean of a particular study? Is the observed mean near the 50th percentile value, the value most expected, or is it near the 1st or 99th percentile value, values that are not expected?" Strictly on the basis of lack of precise knowledge, it is hypothesized that the observed mean is near an assumed expected value. The hypothesis is tested and a conclusion is made to reject or to retain the hypothesis. The model used in statistical hypothesis testing is as follows.

1. Hypothesis Specification

There is a hypothesis to test. If the hypothesis is rejected, an alternative hypothesis is assumed to be correct. In the preoperative teaching study, the exact nature of the hypothesis to test is not obvious. There are few theoretical constructs, limited prior research, and ambiguous empirical evidence on which to base a hypothesis to test in this specific investigation. One solution is to examine research in related areas to learn what others have found in studies with different treatments but similar operational procedures.

Suppose that as a result of earlier research by others in different settings, it is learned that the mean time remaining in the hospital following operation amounted to $\mu = 5.5$ days and that the standard deviation for the number of days was $\sigma = 1.5$ days. On this basis, the following proposition could be tested.

H_0: The results of treatment one are no different from what earlier studies have shown about the average length of time remaining in the hospital following surgery.

In symbolic form, this hypothesis can be stated as follows:

$$H_0: \mu = 5.5.$$

From the researcher's perspective, it is hoped that treatment one produces a shorter hospital stay. Because there is no interest in adopting the treatment if the length of stay is too long, it is advisable to perform a *one-tailed* test of the hypothesis. This is made whenever the prediction or the desired outcome is known to be less than or greater than a prespecified numerical value. A *two-tailed* test is performed whenever the outcome can be either less than or greater than the prespecified numerical value. Another way to view a two-tailed test is simply to state that the alternative hypothesis is false.

The outcome predicted by theory or similar research is referred to as the *experimental hypothesis* or *alternative hypothesis*. The assumed hypothesis of no difference from theoretical considerations or previous studies is called the *null hypothesis* or the *hypothesis under test*. The hypothesis to be tested is denoted as H_0 and the alternative is denoted as H_1. In this example H_0 and H_1 are given as

$$H_0: \mu = 5.5$$

and

$$H_1: \mu < 5.5$$

2. Test Statistics

The observed mean value $\overline{Y} = 4.89$ is compared with the hypothesized value of $\mu = 5.5$. One way to make the comparison is to determine the number of standard deviations between the observed value and the hypothesized value. If it is larger than what would be predicted by chance, the hypothe-

sis is rejected. The number of standard deviations between the observed value and the hypothesized value is given as the numerical value of the following criterion variable:

$$Z = \frac{\overline{Y} - \mu}{\dfrac{\sigma}{\sqrt{N}}}$$

where N = the size of the sample used to determine $\overline{Y}$. Criterion measures such as Z are called *test statistics*. In this case, the numerical value of this test statistic is given as

$$Z = \frac{4.89 - 5.50}{\dfrac{1.50}{\sqrt{82}}} = -3.68$$

This number is used to make a decision as to whether H_0 should be retained or rejected.

3. The Sampling Distribution of Test Statistics

If the hypothesis that $\mu = 5.5$ is true, then with $\sigma = 1.5$ the *sampling distribution of the means* under all possible repetitions of the study with each replication based on $N = 82$ patients is as shown in Figure 9–2. This figure is based on the fact that mean values over replicated studies have a normal distribution because of the central limit theorem. Moreover, the mean value of this distribution, $\mu_{\overline{Y}}$, is equal to the mean number of days, μ_Y, that individual patients spend in the hospital following surgery. The standard deviation of

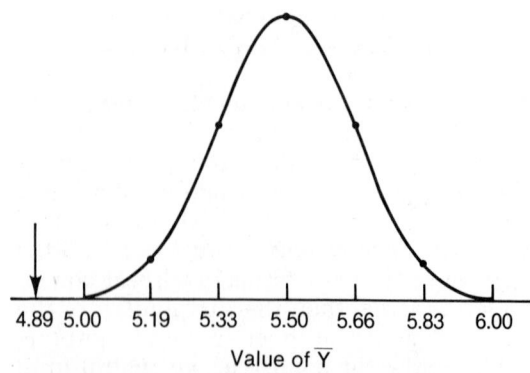

Value of $\overline{Y}$

Figure 9–2. Sampling distribution of $\overline{Y}$ with $\mu_{\overline{Y}} = 5.5$ and $\sigma_{\overline{Y}} = 0.1656$.

the distribution of the means is given as $\sigma_{\bar{Y}}$ = $\sigma_Y/\sqrt{N}$. For this example, it follows that

$$\mu_{\bar{Y}} = \mu_Y = 5.5$$

and

$$\sigma_{\bar{Y}} = \sigma_Y / \sqrt{N} = 1.5/\sqrt{82} = 0.1656$$

so that

1. the .5th percentile is given as

$$P_{.005} = 5.5 - 2.58(.1656) = 5.07$$

2. the 1st percentile is given as

$$P_{.01} = 5.5 - 2.32(.1656) = 5.12$$

3. the 2.5th percentile is given as

$$P_{.025} = 5.5 - 1.96(.1656) = 5.18$$

4. the 5th percentile is given as

$$P_{.05} = 5.5 - 1.645(.1656) = 5.23$$

As can be seen, the observed value of $\bar{Y} = 4.89$ is not very likely to have come from the normal distribution of replicated means. The smallest value to be expected is a mean greater than 5.00, provided that the true mean is 5.5. Because the value of 4.89 is so unlikely, it is reasonable to reject the hypothesis and conclude that the mean value is a number less than 5.5. Notice also that the 5th percentile is defined as $\bar{Y} = 5.23$. Values smaller than this could occur about 5% of the time under replications of the study even if the true mean is equal to 5.5. Thus, 4.89 could in theory appear but because it has such a low likelihood of coming from the normal distribution of Figure 9–1, it makes sense to say it does not belong to that distribution but to some other distribution.

4. Type I and Type II Errors

Unfortunately, no statistical decision can be made without running the risk of being wrong. If H_0 is rejected when it should be retained, an error is made. This error is called a *type I* error and is considered serious. Another type of error could be made if H_0 is retained when it should be rejected. This error is called a *type II* error and is less serious. Let us see why.

Suppose a type I error is made, and it is concluded that the average stay in the hospital following surgery is less than 5.5 days when in reality this decision is false. If one acts on the decision to reject H_0 and adopts the treatment to apply to future patients, the researcher would expect people to be out of the hospital in a shorter time period. Money would be spent to create a new program to train patients. Extra personnel to operate the program would have to be hired. After a period of time, the program would be seen to be operating with a mean length of time of 5.5 days or more. Money that could have been spent on more fruitful activities would have been wasted. A bad program would have been instituted that should have been scrapped.

Suppose that a type II error had occurred. In this case, it would be concluded that the new program is no better than previous programs, and so no money would be spent in its adoption. This decision would keep hospital administrative costs down, but patients undergoing abdominal surgery are likely to face unnecessary pain and suffering that could have been avoided if the denied program had been properly adopted. If the program had been adopted, days in the hospital would be reduced and savings in cost to the patients would also be expected. Which is more serious: wasting hospital money or increasing the length of potential pain and costs to patients? From the hospital's point of view and according to federal reimbursement priorities, wasting hospital funds is considered a more serious error.

Is there a way to eliminate the possibilities of these potential errors? Unfortunately, the answer is no. Strategies can be adopted to minimize the risks of making these errors. Possible strategies can be obtained by using properties of the normal distribution to define a *decision rule* that indicates when to reject H_0. This is achieved by specifying in advance of data collection the risk of a type I error that a researcher will tolerate or that is dictated by life and death situations. In the behavioral and nursing sciences, most researchers control the risk of a type I error at .05 or .01. Here, we will use .05. With this risk of a type I error, the decision rule is

Decision rule: reject H_0 if $\bar{Y} < 5.23$

The number that defines the limits of rejection is called the *critical value*. The set of numbers smaller than the critical value is called the *critical region*. The critical value for this study is 5.23 days. The critical region consists of all mean values of less than 5.23 days. With this rule the probability of making a type I error is given as $\alpha = .05$. It is sometimes called the α *(alpha)* error. It could be made smaller, but for a study like this it is usually left at 0.05. If the harm in making a type I error were serious, it would be reduced to a lower value. For example, in the testing of drugs, it would be reduced to a value like $\alpha = 0.00000001$. In many health sciences studies, it would be reduced to $\alpha = 0.001$.

As can be seen, the size of the risk of making a type I error is at the discretion of the researcher. It can be made as small as desired. When the consequences of a type I error are not serious, it is set at $\alpha = .05$. When the consequences are serious, it is made smaller. In theory, the size of the risk of a type II error can be controlled. To control it, one must know the alternative hypothesis *exactly*. In most studies, this cannot be done. In the case of nursing science, sufficient substantive research and knowledge about alternatives do not exist; consequently, an exact alternative hypothesis cannot be stated with a high degree of confidence. Thus, the risk of a type II error is not generally controllable.

One way to achieve partial control of a type II error is to take a *large* sample. The problem now is "What is the meaning of the word *large*?" No one has a definite answer, but a good rule of thumb is about 20 subjects per group. According to this rule, the preoperative teaching study should entail small risks of type II errors because treatment one is applied to 82 patients. Another way to reduce the risk of a type II error is to increase the risk of a type I error. Because type I errors are the more serious of the two errors, this modification should never be employed in studies using human subjects.

For completeness, it is noted that the risk of a type II error is called the β *(beta)* error. The probability of rejecting H_0 when it is false is called the *power of the test* and is given as $P = (1 - \beta)$. For an extensive discussion on power and its control, see Cohen (1977). For a less extensive discussion, see Marascuilo and Serlin (1988). Both sources provide directions for controlling power and determining sample sizes for many types of experimental designs and observational studies provided the risk of a type I error is controlled.

5. Decision Rules

In the previous paragraphs the decision rule was defined in terms of the mean values. In practice, this model is rarely followed because the tabled normal distribution values can be used directly to define the critical value. As indicated, the 5th percentile is given as $P_{.05} = \mu - 1.645\sigma$. This means that one can use the tabled value $Z = -1.645$ directly. Thus, the decision rule would be given as

Decision rule: reject H_0 if $Z < -1.654$

For the example, the numerical value of the test statistic is given as $Z = -3.68$. The hypothesis under test is rejected because the observed Z is in the critical region. The mean length of stay in hospital following surgery is less than 5.5 days, the value specified by the null hypothesis.

6. Summary of the Statistical Hypothesis Testing Model

In summary the hypothesis testing model is as follows:

a. A null hypothesis exists which can be tested against an alternative.

b. A test statistic is defined which connects the parameters of the null hypothesis to the sample statistics.

c. The size of the risk of a type I error is selected.

d. A decision rule is specified which connects the risk of a type I error to the distribution of the test statistic.

e. A decision is made to reject or retain the null hypothesis by comparing the value of the test statistic with the critical value defined by the decision rule.

9–4 CONFIDENCE INTERVAL THEORY

In addition to testing null hypotheses about parameters, statistical theory provides rules and guidelines for estimating the values of population parameters. Two different estimation models are employed for assessing research findings. These two models are referred to as *point* estimation and *interval* estimation. The theory on unbiasedness, efficiency, and consistency of point estimates is described in Chapter 6.

Here the use of *confidence intervals* as interval estimates of population parameters is examined. The null hypothesis provides a unique population value for comparison purposes. In the previous example, the null hypothesis value of $\mu = 5.5$ days served as the basis for comparing the observed mean value of $\overline{Y} = 4.89$ days. Most of the time such unique values cannot be specified in advance of data collection. To overcome this problem, all possible null hypotheses associated with a proposition can be defined on a post hoc basis. This can be achieved by providing a confidence interval that defines all possible null hypotheses that could give rise to the observed data. All two-tailed confidence intervals can be written in the following format:

(Estimate of the population parameter)
 − (The maximum error of the estimate)
  < The unknown population parameter <
(Estimate of the population parameter)
  + (The maximum error of the estimate)

Whenever a one-tailed test is contemplated, a one-tailed confidence interval should be used. In the preoperative teaching study, the one-tailed confidence interval would be given as

The unknown population parameter <
 (Estimate of the population parameter)
  + (The maximum error of the estimate)

For illustration, the confidence interval for the mean number of days remaining in hospital following surgery can be written as

(Observed mean) − (Maximum error)
 < Population mean <
 (Observed mean) + (Maximum error)

In this case,

$$(\text{Observed mean}) = \overline{Y} = 4.89 \text{ days}$$

In addition, it can be shown that with a risk of a type I error controlled at α, the maximum error is given as,

$$(\text{Maximum error}) = Z_{\alpha/2}\ \sigma/\sqrt{N}$$

With $\alpha = .05$, the maximum error is given as

$$\begin{aligned}(\text{Maximum error}) &= 1.96\ (1.50/\sqrt{82}) \\ &= 1.96\ (.1656) \\ &= .32 \text{ days}\end{aligned}$$

Thus, the 95% confidence interval for the mean number of days remaining in hospital following surgery is given as

$$4.89 - .32 < \mu < 4.89 + .32$$
$$\text{or } 4.57 < \mu < 5.21$$

Thus, the mean length of stay can be as low as 4.57 days or as high as 5.21 days. Finally, it should be noted that this interval defines all possible null hypotheses that are in agreement with the data collected on the $N = 82$ patients in the study. At no point in the determination of this interval was it necessary to know that previous research had a mean value of 5.5 days.

For the one-tailed confidence interval with $\alpha = .05$, the maximum error is given as

$$\begin{aligned}(\text{Maximum error}) &= 1.645\ (1.50 / \sqrt{82}) \\ &= 1.645\ (.1656) \\ &= .27 \text{ days}\end{aligned}$$

Thus, the one-tailed 95% confidence interval for the mean number of days remaining in hospital following surgery is given by

$$\mu < 4.89 + .27$$

or

$$\mu < 5.16$$

Thus, the mean length of stay can be as high as 5.16 days.

The information provided in a confidence interval should be of considerable interest to many researchers in nursing science. It provides a strategy for hypothesis testing that does not require advance knowledge of the null hypothesis. With this strategy the sample data are used to define all possible null hypotheses that could give rise to the observed data. In practice, a researcher need never test null hypotheses. Instead, null hypothesis testing can be bypassed and all research questions can be answered directly in terms of a confidence interval.

9-5 ANALYTICAL PROCEDURES FOR UNIVARIATE QUANTITATIVE VARIABLES

In the previous chapter, methods for tabular and graphic presentation of data were presented. We continue with analytical procedures for testing hypotheses about univariate quantitative variables. The t test is discussed and its extension to the F test of the one-way analysis of variance is illustrated. Interactions are introduced and the two-way analysis of variance is discussed. Linear contrasts are introduced and their relationship to questions in nursing research are illustrated. Interaction contrasts are described. The notion of a family type I error rate is examined and its role in the analysis of planned and post hoc comparisons is depicted. Distinctions between interaction contrasts and simple effect contrasts are made in the context of interaction and nested designs. Confidence intervals are introduced and their important role in nursing research is emphasized. Finally, an introduction to nonparametric tests using ranks is presented.

9-6 TWO SAMPLE TESTS FOR MEANS AND VARIANCES

The most commonly performed statistical test is the *two-sample t test*. It is used to test the hypothesis that two samples are selected from populations for which the mean values are equal. The alternative hypothesis is that the mean values are different. The test is based on four assumptions. They are:

1. The underlying variable is normally distributed.
2. The standard deviations in the two populations are equal to a common unknown numerical value.
3. The observations within each sample are independent or are uncorrelated with one another.
4. The observations between the two samples are independent.

As an example of this test, consider the data reported in Table 9-1. The numbers in this table have been generated from the CRUNCH (Bostrom, 1986) program. The dependent variable is the length of stay in the hospital following surgery. The 82 patients

TABLE 9-1 SAMPLE STATISTICS FOR THE TWO-SAMPLE t TEST APPLIED TO TREATMENTS ONE AND TWO OF THE PREOPERATIVE STUDY WITH THE LENGTH OF STAY AS THE DEPENDENT VARIABLE

Group	Mean	SD	Sample Size
One	4.890	1.618	82
Two	4.524	1.425	82

in treatment one had a mean stay of $\overline{Y}_1 = 4.890$, whereas the 82 patients in treatment two had a mean stay of $\overline{Y}_2 = 4.524$. The population standard deviations are unknown but they have been estimated from the data using the formula

$$S_Y^2 = \frac{1}{N-1} \sum_{i=1}^{N} (Y_i - \overline{Y})^2$$

S_Y^2 is called the *sample variance*. Its square root is called the *sample standard deviation*. It is an estimate of the population standard deviation. For the 82 patients of Table B-1 in treatment one,

$$S_{Y(1)}^2 = \frac{1}{82-1} [(4 - 4.890)^2 + (6 - 4.890)^2 + \ldots + (5 - 4.890)^2]$$
$$= 2.6179$$

so that

$$S_{Y(1)} = \sqrt{2.6179} = 1.618$$

For the patients in treatment two,

$$S_{Y(2)} = \sqrt{2.0306} = 1.425$$

One of the assumptions of the two-sample t test is that the population standard deviations are equal and unknown. The two-sample t test uses an estimate of the common value which is called the *pooled* estimate of the variance or the *mean square within* and denoted by MSW. It is defined as

$$MSW = \frac{(N_1 - 1) S_{Y(1)}^2 + (N_2 - 1) S_{Y(2)}^2}{(N_1 - 1) + (N_2 - 1)}$$

where

N_1 = number of observations in sample one

and

N_2 = number of observations in sample two

For the data of Table 9–1,

$$MSW = \frac{(82 - 1)(2.6179) + (82 - 1)(2.0306)}{(82 - 1) + (82 - 1)}$$
$$= 2.3242$$

The t statistic is defined in terms of the two mean values and the mean square within groups as

$$t = \frac{\overline{Y}_1 - \overline{Y}_2}{\sqrt{\dfrac{MS_W}{N_1} + \dfrac{MS_W}{N_2}}}$$

For our example,

$$t = \frac{4.890 - 4.524}{\sqrt{\dfrac{2.3242}{82} + \dfrac{2.3242}{82}}} = \frac{0.366}{0.2381} = 1.54$$

The numerator of this statistic is equal to the *mean difference* and the denominator is identical with the *standard error*. These numbers are used to determine the confidence interval for the mean difference in the population parameters. For large samples, the sampling distribution of t comes under the influence of the central limit theorem. Critical values taken from the normal distribution can be used to make a decision between H_0 and H_1. In small samples, the normal distribution cannot be used because the central limit theorem requires large samples for its application. Fortunately, the sampling distribution of t for small samples is known and its critical values have been tabled. A compact table of the critical values is reported in Table A–6.

The t distribution is symmetrical about zero. Whereas the normal distribution is defined by two parameters, its mean and standard deviation, the t distribution is defined by one parameter called the *degrees of freedom*. Whereas there exists one standard normal distribution with mean zero and standard deviation of one, there exists a family of t distributions each with its own parameter. For the family of t distributions, the parameters are defined in terms of the Greek letter ν (nu) and are given as

$$\nu = (N_1 - 1) + (N_2 - 1)$$

For the example,

$$\nu = (82 - 1) + (82 - 1) = 162$$

This number is used to define the rejection rule for testing the hypothesis of interest. Now let us examine the hypothesis.

Let the two population means be denoted by μ_1 and μ_2. Recall that population one serves as the control group for population two and that population two serves as the control group for population one. The null hypothesis states that the mean length of stay in the hospital for the two treatments is the same. In other words, neither of the two treatments is superior nor inferior to the other. If that is true, then the differences in the population means must be zero. Thus, the null hypothesis to be tested can be stated as

$$H_0: \mu_1 - \mu_2 = 0$$

Because there is no reason to predict a direction to the difference in mean values, the alternative hypothesis is

$$H_1: \mu_1 - \mu_2 \neq 0$$

Note that the alternative hypothesis could be written as

$$H_1: \mu_1 < \mu_2 \text{ or that } \mu_1 > \mu_2$$

Such hypotheses are called *two-tailed alternatives*. When an alternative hypothesis is two-tailed, the risk of a type I error is partitioned to cover the two tails of the corresponding criterion distribution. This means that if the risk of a type I error is controlled at $\alpha = .05$, then .025 of the risk is assigned to each tail of the null distribution.

The degrees of freedom for the t test for this example are given as $\nu = 162$. We enter Table A–6 with this value to determine the values of $P_{.025}$ and $P_{.975}$. As indicated, there are no entries for 162 but there are for 120 and for ∞ (infinity). The last column of Table A–6 corresponds to normal curve values. These are the values most researchers use whenever $\nu > 120$. When using 120 degrees of freedom for a test in which the degrees of freedom are larger, the test is said to be *conservative*. By this is meant that the risk of a type I error is smaller than the specified value of α. For example, if the tabled risk of a type I error is given as $\alpha = .05$, the actual risk may be a number like .0435.

For this example, the decision rule is given as

Decision rule: reject H_0 if $t < -1.98$
or if $t > +1.98$

With the less conservative position, the decision rule for rejecting H_0 is given as

Decision rule: reject H_0 if $t < -1.96$
or if $t > +1.96$

Because $t = 1.54$ is not in the critical region, the hypothesis is not rejected. It is concluded that μ_1 does not differ from μ_2. The effects of treatments one and two are not different in their impact on the average length of stay in the hospital following an operation.

In addition to reporting a test statistic value as being significant or not significant, a researcher can summarize the results of a statistical test in a confidence interval. For this example, the 95% confidence interval is given as

$\mu_1 - \mu_2$ = (Mean difference)
$\pm$ (Critical value)(Standard error)
= .366 ± 1.96(.2381) = .366 ± .467

As expected, zero is in the interval because the null hypothesis of no difference was not rejected. For a review of confidence intervals theory, see Section 9–4.

Consider the validity of the four assumptions in this example. The first assumption is that the underlying variable is normally distributed. In this case, the assumption is false. As shown in Figure 8–6, the distribution for length of stay for treatment one is positively skewed and the distribution for treatment two shows even greater skewness. In addition, recall that the length of stay is a discrete variable, whereas the normal distribution is defined for continuous variables. On these grounds alone, it is tempting to discard the decision as invalid. If the samples were small (less than 30), the decision would certainly be in doubt. When the samples are large, as they are in this example, the statistical decision is most likely correct because the t test is *robust* in its treatment of the violations of the assumptions of normality and the continuity of the variable. On the basis of empirical investigations, the robustness can be called on for justification of the t test if the total number of observations exceeds 30. In this case, the sample sizes are well

above this minimum standard. The decision not to reject the hypothesis of equal mean values is defensible.

The second assumption is that the population variances are equal. There is a statistical test which can be used to test this assumption. It is called the F test and is used to test the hypothesis,

$$H_0: \sigma_1^2 = \sigma_2^2$$

against the alternative

$$H_1: \sigma_1^2 \neq \sigma_2^2$$

The test statistic for this test is given as

$$F = \frac{S_{Y(1)}^2}{S_{Y(2)}^2}$$

The critical values for the F test are reported in Table A–7. The F distribution is defined by two parameters. They are

$$\nu_1 = N_1 - 1 \quad \text{and} \quad \nu_2 = N_2 - 1$$

For our example, $\nu_1 = 81$ and $\nu_2 = 81$. Because we have a two-tailed alternative, we divide the risk of a type I error equally between the two tails. Similar to that illustrated for the t test, no critical values for these particular degrees of freedom exist. If one adopts a conservative stance, one can use the values for $\nu_1 = 60$ and $\nu_2 = 60$. With these degrees of freedom, the decision rule read from Table A–7 is given as

Decision rule: reject H_0 if $F < .65$
or if $F > 1.53$

For the example,

$$F = 2.6179 / 2.0306 = 1.29$$

There is no reason to reject the hypothesis of equal variances because the sample F statistic is not in the critical region. The assumptions required to justify the F test of equal variance are identical with assumptions 1, 3, and 4 (normality, independence between and independence within samples) of the t test. With this form of the F test, assumption 2 of the t test (equal variance) is under examination.

The last two assumptions of both the t test and the F test, independence between and independence within samples, cannot be tested directly. These assumptions must be incorporated into the design of the study by the researchers. In this particular case, there should be no reason to doubt the existence of independent observations among patients. Pain and recovery are individual experiences. It is hard to see how one person's hospital recovery experience can influence another person's recovery experience. If this assumption can be questioned, then the decision not to reject the hypothesis of equal mean values can be challenged. Events unknown to the researcher could produce observations that violate the assumption of independence. For example, a specific nurse could have an exceedingly warm and supportive bedside manner and thereby influence patients collectively to a speedier recovery. In the preoperative teaching study, this is not possible because of the long periods of time required to conduct the study. On any one day, a nurse would be expected to care for only one or two preoperative patients. Interactions between many preoperative patients by a given nurse would be minimal.

Finally, it should be noted that competitors of the two-sample t test exist. Two such competitors are available on CRUNCH (Bostrom, 1986): the Welch-Aspin test (Welch, 1951) and the two-sample Wilcoxon test (1949). The Welch-Aspin test can be substituted for the t test when the population variances are not equal, and the Wilcoxon test can be used for nonnormal distributions, discrete variables, and small samples for which assumptions cannot be evaluated. The Welch-Aspin test is not described here but an in-depth discussion is found in Marascuilo and Serlin (1988). The Wilcoxon test is described in terms of the Kruskal-Wallis test (1952) in Section 9–17.

9–7 MULTIPLE TWO-SAMPLE t TESTS AND F TESTS

In the previous section a review of the two-sample t test for equal mean values and the two-sample F test for equal standard deviations were presented. These are the core tests of empirical research, and they are used repeatedly between and within studies. Within a study their repeated use is problematic because observations within subjects are correlated. As an example of a study in which multiple t tests or F tests might be of

interest, consider the data of Table 9–2. These data represent the summary statistics for the five dependent variables of the preoperative study. The five variables, (1) length of stay, (2) number of pain medications requested on the first day after surgery, (3) number of pain medications requested on the second day, (4) number of postoperative complications, and (5) number of days following release before a patient can proceed unassisted from residence are contrasted for treatments one and two. The five t values range from a low of 1.54 to a high of 6.46, whereas the five F values range from a low of .84 to a high of 1.17.

Consider the five t statistics. Because each subject is represented in each of the five test statistics, it follows that the statistics are correlated. As a consequence, if a type I error is made with any one of the dependent variables, there is an increased risk of encountering a type I error with another variable. Thus, a statistical model is required which takes into account the intercorrelations

TABLE 9–2 MULTIPLE TWO-SAMPLE t TESTS FOR THE DEPENDENT VARIABLES OF THE PREOPERATIVE STUDY FOR COMPARISON OF TREATMENTS ONE AND TWO*

Variable		Group One	Group Two	t Test	F Test
Length of Stay	$\overline{Y}$ S	4.890 1.618	4.524 1.425	1.54	1.17
Pain† Med. One	$\overline{Y}$ S	6.646 1.673	4.988 1.614	6.46	1.07
Pain‡ Med. Two	$\overline{Y}$ S	2.622 1.402	1.720 1.534	3.93	0.84
Postop.§ Comp.	$\overline{Y}$ S	1.232 1.103	0.707 0.975	3.23	1.13
Days‖ pdch	$\overline{Y}$ S	5.573 2.634	4.171 2.403	3.56	1.10

*Reported are sample means $\overline{Y}$, sample standard deviations S. Sample size: $N_1 = 82$ and $N_2 = 82$.

†Pain med. one = no. of pain medications requested on first day after surgery.

‡Pain med. two = no. of pain medications requested on second day after surgery.

§Postop. comp. = no. of postoperative complications.

‖Days pdch = no. of days spent at home before leaving unassisted.

Note: Mean differences are significant if $t < -2.58$ or if $t > 2.58$. Variances are significantly different if $F < .54$ or if $F > 1.84$.

among the five dependent measurements. Note that this discussion applies equally well to the five F tests.

As a first approach, a researcher might decide that each test should be performed with the decision rule used in Section 9–6. Many researchers do just that. A number of researchers do not recommend this practice (Dunn and Clark, 1974). Part of the disagreement among researchers can be traced to the meaning of a type I error when multiple intercorrelated tests are performed within a single study. When a single hypothesis is tested, the definition of a type I error is clear. A type I error occurs whenever a hypothesis under test is rejected when it should be retained. If the single decision rule of the previous section at $\alpha = 0.05$ is used to test all five hypotheses of equal mean values, a problem would arise because across all five hypotheses taken collectively, the type I error control is inflated. Let us see how this can happen.

The five hypotheses of equal mean values are said to represent a *family* of hypotheses (Ryan, 1962). They represent five similar interrelated hypotheses based on a single set of observations. Within a family of interrelated hypotheses, a type I error is said to occur when at least one of the individual tests leads to a rejection of a hypothesis that should have been retained. Thus, a type I error occurs in the family of five hypotheses if one, two, three, four, or five type I errors are made. It can be shown using theorems from probability theory that the maximum probability of making at least one type I error is given as

$$\alpha_T = \alpha_1 + \alpha_2 + \ldots + \alpha_Q = \sum_{q=1}^{Q} \alpha_q$$

where α_q equals the probability of making a type I error when testing hypothesis q. If Q = 5 and if each $\alpha_q = .05$, the maximum risk of at least one type I error in the five collective t tests is equal to $\alpha_T = Q\alpha_q = 5(0.05) = 0.25$. To many researchers this risk is too large. For these researchers, the family type I error rate needs to be controlled. Family error rate control is achieved by specifying the maximum error to be tolerated for the entire family and then partitioning that maximum risk equally among all the family hypothesis members. Tables have been provided for this partitioning by Dunn (1961). A shortened

version of critical values of Dunn's table is presented in Table A–8 for family controlled error rates of $\alpha = 0.05$ and $\alpha = 0.01$.

For the data of Table 9–2, with Q = 5 and $\alpha = .05$, Table A–8 is entered with a third parameter. The third parameter is v, the number of degrees of freedom associated with the mean square within for the corresponding t tests. For the data of Table 9–2 each $v = 162$. As noted for the t and the F tables, no critical values corresponding to $v = 162$ exist so one uses $v = \infty$. For Q = 5 and $\alpha = .05$, the critical value read from Table A–8 is given by t = 2.58. The critical values for the Dunn partitioning of the risk of a type I error are based on the t distribution, which is distributed symmetrically about zero. To save printing costs only the positive values are reported. Thus, in terms of the tabled value the decision rule for each of the t tests is given as

Decision rule: reject the hypothesis of
equal mean values
if t < −2.58 or if t > +2.58

Thus, it is concluded that mean values for treatments one and two are different for all variables except length of stay.

There are no published tables for family type I error control for two-sample F tests. Decision rules can be determined using the F table reported in Table A–7. In this case, five F tests are to be performed. If the family error rate is controlled at $\alpha_T = .05$, then each hypothesis should be tested at $\alpha_q = .01$. With $v_1 = 81$ and $v_2 = 81$ replaced by $v_1 = v_2 = 60$, the critical values found in Table A–7 are given as 0.54 and 1.84 so that the decision rule for each F test is given as

Decision rule: reject the hypothesis of
equal standard deviations
if F < 0.54 or if F > 1.84

None of the hypotheses of equal standard deviations is rejected.

When there are multiple t tests or F tests to be performed on a single set of subjects, it is recommended that type I error control be applied to the family of hypotheses and not to the individual hypotheses. This type of error control is closely connected to a model referred to as *planned analysis*. This topic is discussed in Section 9–12. When a researcher performs each test at an $\alpha = 0.05$ level, the set of hypotheses is said to be under *hypothesis error control*. This term is used to distinguish the testing from *family error control*. Hypothesis error rate control is the most frequently encountered error rate control model in the research literature. There are good reasons for its popularity. Journal editors publish only research findings that are statistically significant. Statistically significant findings can be seen more often using hypothesis error rate control. This is because critical values for hypothesis error rate control are smaller than those of family error rate control. In any case, for the nursing researcher there is a price to pay for the adoption of hypothesis error rate control. The chances of making type I errors are increased.

The assumptions for family error control are identical with those required for single hypothesis tests. They are normality for the underlying dependent variable or large samples, independence between samples, independence within samples, and, for the t test, equal population variances. Type I error rates can be partitioned for the Welch-Aspin and the two-sample Wilcoxon tests. These models are not described here, but an in-depth description can be found in Marascuilo and Serlin (1988).

9–8 STATISTICAL POWER FOR THE TWO-SAMPLE t-TEST

The biologist rates the strength of a microscope by specifying its magnification power. The statistician rates the strength of a statistical test by specifying its probability power. A 50-power microscope increases the dimensions of an object by a factor of 50. A 100-power microscope has twice the power of a 50-power microscope. A statistical test with a power of .40 has 40% chance of rejecting a null hypothesis that is false. A statistical test with a power of .80 has an 80% chance of rejecting a null hypothesis that is false. Like the biologist who would prefer to use the more powerful microscope, the statistician would prefer to use the more powerful test.

The power of the two-sample t test can be increased by increasing the risk of a type I error. As might be expected, this is not a viable solution. Another way to increase the power is to increase the sample size. If funds are available, this is the preferred procedure.

The determination of the sample sizes to use for the two groups in a t test is quite simple. In theory, a researcher begins by making an informed guess of the means and standard deviations of the two populations. As will be seen, this can rarely be achieved.

As an example, consider treatments one and two of the preoperative teaching study. Suppose we denote the mean for treatment one by μ_1 and the mean for treatment two by $\mu_2 = \mu_1 + Z\sigma$. With this formulation we can use the numbers of Table 9–3 to determine the sample sizes N_1 and N_2 for the study. The numbers in the body of the table are sample sizes for $N_1 = N_2$ for a risk of a type I error controlled at $\alpha = .05$ and for power levels of .70, .80, .90, and .95. The table is entered with an estimate of the treatment effect as defined in Chapter 15 for meta-analysis. In meta-analysis the treatment effect is defined as the standardized difference between the two population means where the standardization is based on the value of the standard deviation. Thus, the treatment effect measures the difference in mean population values in standard deviation units. In this case,

$$\delta = (\mu_1 - \mu_2)/\sigma = (\mu_1 - \mu_1 - Z\sigma)/\sigma = Z$$

Thus, the researcher need only specify the size of the treatment effect in standard deviation units.

If a treatment effect of $Z = 1$ standard deviation or a difference in means of $D = .5$ day in mean length of stay is expected between the two treatments, it is seen in Table 9–3 that the sample sizes for statistical powers of .70, .80, .90, and .95 are given as 50, 64, 85, and 105 per group. In the preoperative teach-

TABLE 9–3 SAMPLE SIZES FOR THE TWO-SAMPLE t TEST

Treatment Effect	Power Level for $N_1 = N_2$			
$\delta = (\mu_1 - \mu_2)/\sigma$	.70	.80	.90	.95
.10	1235	1571	2102	2600
.20	310	393	526	651
.30	138	175	234	290
.40	78	99	132	163
.50	50	64	85	105
.60	35	45	59	73
.70	26	33	44	54
.80	20	26	34	42
1.00	13	17	22	27

(Adapted with permission from Table 2.4.1, n to detect d-by-t test, in Cohen, J.: Statistical Power Analysis for the Behavioral Sciences. New York, Academic Press, 1977.)

ing studies, the sample sizes were set at 82. Thus, the power for detecting half of a standard deviation between the means of the two treatments is approximately equal to .90. Thus, if the mean length of stay for treatment one is given as 5.5 days, the researcher has a .90 chance of rejecting the null hypothesis of no difference if the mean length of time for treatment two is less than $5.5 - .5 = 5$ days.

Note that if the true difference is greater than one standard deviation, the statistical power is greater than .90. This suggests a strategy for determining sample size. The strategy is to specify the minimal mean difference that one would be interested in detecting and then to choose the sample sizes for the minimal effect size that is of interest. For example, suppose the minimal treatment effect of interest is given as Z = .30 of a standard deviation. The corresponding sample sizes for power levels of .70, .80, .90, and .95, respectively, are given as 138, 175, 234, and 290. Clearly, the sample sizes used for the preoperative teaching study are not large enough to detect such a small treatment effect.

Table 9–3 can be used to determine sample sizes for a minimal amount of explained variation deemed by a researcher to be of practical or theoretical value in the two-group study. Suppose that in the preoperative teaching study a researcher would like to know whether at least 10% of the variation in length of stay following operation can be attributed to the difference in effectiveness of treatments one and two. The sample sizes for answering this question are determined by entering Table 9–3 with

$$\delta = \sqrt{4E/(1-E)}$$

where E is the amount of explained variation of interest.

In this example,

$$\delta = \sqrt{4(.1)(1-.1)} = 2/3 = .67$$

Because δ = .67 is not in the table, one must interpolate. For δ = .60, the sample sizes for power levels of .70, .80, .90, and .95 are given as 35, 45, 59, and 73, and for δ = .70 the corresponding sample sizes are given as 26, 33, 44, and 54. By interpolation, the corresponding sample sizes are given as 29, 41, 55, and 68. Thus, for a power of 90% each treatment group should contain 44 subjects. In this case, more than sufficient power is available to detect 10% explained variation that can be attributed to the difference between the two treatments.

9–9 THE ONE-FACTOR ANALYSIS OF VARIANCE

The one-factor analysis of variance is the multiple sample analog to the two-sample t test. It is based on the same four assumptions as the two-sample t test. Valid conclusions require variables that are normally distributed, with equal population variances and independence of observations between and within samples. If the samples are large, the normality assumption can be relaxed and if the sample sizes are equal, the equal variance assumption can be relaxed. Whereas the t test is based on only two samples, the one-factor analysis of variance (ANOVA) is usually performed on three or more samples. If there are only two samples, the ANOVA model is still valid and can be used if desired. In the literature the two-sample tests are almost always presented under the t test model even though it is not wrong to perform an analysis of variance on two groups.

Because ANOVA hypothesis for K groups is an extension of the t test, it is reasonable to conclude that it is given as

$$H_0: \mu_1 = \mu_2 = \ldots = \mu_K$$

and that the alternative hypothesis is given as

$$H_1: \mu_1 \neq \mu_2 \neq \ldots \neq \mu_K$$

Unfortunately the hypothesis under test and the alternative are more complicated than indicated, but at this point it is difficult to state them in their correct statistical form. This is done later, in Section 9–11.

As an example of an ANOVA, consider the data reported in Table 9–4. These data provide mean values, standard deviations, and sample sizes for length of stay for the three experimental programs of the preoperative study. The data for treatments one and two were first reported in Table 9–1. The relative frequency polygons for these data were shown in Figure 8–6. As seen earlier, all distributions are skewed, with the most skewness shown by treatment three. Because the sample sizes are large, the lack of normality

TABLE 9–4 SAMPLE STATISTICS FOR THE THREE TREATMENTS OF THE PREOPERATIVE STUDY WITH LENGTH OF STAY AS THE DEPENDENT VARIABLE

Treatment	$\bar{Y}_k$	S_k	N_k
One	4.890	1.618	82
Two	4.524	1.425	82
Three	3.366	1.392	82
Total	4.260	1.613	246

can be ignored. The assumption of equal variance seems acceptable. None of the pairwise F tests of equal population standard deviations leads to rejection. The three F ratios for testing the equality of the variances are given as

$$F_{1-2} = (1.618/1.425)^2 = 1.29$$
$$F_{1-3} = (1.618/1.392)^2 = 1.35$$
$$F_{2-3} = (1.425/1.392)^2 = 1.05$$

No pairwise difference in variances is statistically significant. Finally, there is no reason to question the assumptions of independence among treatments nor among the patients within each treatment. The analysis of variance appears to be justified.

The test statistic of the analysis of variance has an F distribution if random sampling is employed and if the null hypothesis is true. The derivation of the test statistic is complex and is not shown. Instead, the test statistic is presented and its computation shown. In practice, very few researchers would perform the computations because they are readily carried out by programs such as CRUNCH (Bostrom, 1986), SPSS (1986), BMDP (Dixon, 1983), SAS (1985), and a host of other main frame and personal computer programs. The test statistic is given as

$$F = \frac{\text{Mean square between groups}}{\text{Mean square within groups}} = \frac{\text{MSB}}{\text{MSW}}$$

where

$$\text{MSB} = \frac{\text{SSB}}{K-1} = \frac{1}{K-1}\sum_{k=1}^{K} N_k(\bar{Y}_k - \bar{Y})^2$$

$$\text{MSW} = \frac{\text{SSW}}{N-K} = \frac{1}{N-K}\sum_{k=1}^{K} (N_k - 1)S_k^2$$

$$\bar{Y} = \frac{1}{N}\sum_{k=1}^{K} N_k\bar{Y}_k$$

and

$$N = N_1 + N_2 + \ldots + N_K$$

The numerator of the MSB is called the *sum of squares between groups* and is usually denoted by SSB. The numerator of the MSW is called the *sum of squares within groups* and is usually denoted by SSW. It can be shown that if the hypothesis under test is true, the sampling distribution of F is given as an F variable whose degrees of freedom are given as

$$\nu_1 = (K - 1) \quad \text{and} \quad \nu_2 = (N - K)$$

For the data of Table 9–4,

$$\nu_1 = (3 - 1) = 2 \text{ and } \nu_2 = (246 - 3) = 243$$

Because the alternative hypothesis is associated only with large values of F, the decision rule for ANOVA is always one-tailed. Thus, the $\alpha = 0.05$ decision rule is given as

Decision rule: reject the hypothesis if $F > F_{2,243;.95} = 3.00$

For the data of Table 9–4 equations 1 and 2 at the top of page 208 apply. In addition,

$$\text{MSB} = 103.8618/2 = 51.9309$$

and

$$\text{MSW} = 533.4878/243 = 2.1954$$

so that

$$F = 51.9309/2.1954 = 23.65$$

Because F = 23.65 is larger than the critical value of 3.00, the hypothesis is rejected. There are differences among the treatments concerning the mean length of stay remaining in the hospital following an operation.

The results of an analysis of variance are customarily reported in a table called *The Analysis of Variance Table*. The analysis of variance table for the data of Table 9–4 is shown in Table 9–5. This table has headings for the source of variance, the degrees of freedom associated with each source, the sum of squares and mean squares for each source, the F ratio, and a final column headed (eta square). This final column provides a statistic that offers an opportunity to assess the practical or scientific significance of the finding. This measurement specifies the

(1) $SSB = 82(4.890 - 4.260)^2 + 82(4.524 - 4.260)^2 + 82(3.366 - 4.260)^2 = 103.8618$

---

(2) $SSW = (82 - 1)(1.618)^2 + (82 - 1)(1.425)^2 + (82 - 1)(1.392)^2 = 533.4878$

---

amount of the variation that can be attributed to the effects of the treatment. In this case, $\hat{\eta}^2 = 0.16$. What does this figure mean?

First of all, note that the total variance reported in Table 9–5 is given as

$$S_Y^2 = SST/(N - 1) = 637.3496/245 = 2.6018$$

Part of this variance can be attributed to the variance among the patients within each of the treatment groups. This within group variance is measured by the MSW. Its numerical value is given as MSW = 2.1954. Suppose that the within group variance is subtracted from the total variance. When this is done, it follows that

$$2.6018 - 2.1954 = 0.4064$$

To what can this part of the total variance be attributed? It is attributed to the variation that exists among the groups; that is, it is the variance component produced by the three treatments of the study. As a percent of the total variance, this part of the variance is equal to

$$0.4064/2.6018 \times 100 = 15.62 \equiv 16$$

This suggests that $\hat{\eta}^2$ is a measurement of the amount of the variance in the total distribution of length of stay in the hospital that can be attributed to the effects of the differences among the three treatments. It is a measure-ment of *explained variance* and is usually computed as

$$\hat{\eta}^2 = SSB / SST$$

Of all of the numbers in the ANOVA table, $\hat{\eta}^2$ is the most important. It provides a way to evaluate the findings of the study. When the treatments have very minimal effects on the dependent variable, $\hat{\eta}^2$ is a number close to zero, but when the effect is strong, $\hat{\eta}^2$ is a number close to one. It equals zero when the treatment effect is completely null, and it equals one when the treatment effect explains all of the variance. In the social, behavioral, and health sciences, $\hat{\eta}^2$ tends to fluctuate around values ranging from 5% to 30%. The observed value of 16% is large for behavioral and health care variables and is of considerable practical significance. The large magnitude for $\hat{\eta}^2$ suggests that the treatments are having a relatively strong impact on the length of stay in the hospital following an operation. Unfortunately, not too many researchers examine the value of $\hat{\eta}^2$ and regrettably too many researchers are mesmerized by the value of the F ratio. This practice is to be avoided because F ratios are essentially devoid of meaning.

The research literature is rampant with phrases like "the result is highly significant" or "the result is significant beyond the p = .001 level of significance." Statements like

TABLE 9–5 THE ANALYSIS OF VARIANCE TABLE FOR THE DATA OF TABLE 9–3

Source	d/f	S of S	MS	F Ratio	$\hat{\eta}^2$
Between	2	103.8618	51.9309	23.65	0.16
Within	243	533.4878	2.1954		
Total	245	637.3496			

$F_{2,\infty:0.95} = 3.00$
Source = source of variance
d/f = degrees of freedom
S of S = sum of squares
MS = mean squares
$\hat{\eta}2$ = eta square

these should alert a reader to the fact that the author(s) of the study are less than precise in reporting the meaning of their statistical test. Statements like these show an incomplete comprehension of statistical hypothesis testing and the meaning of statistical power. In Section 9–8, the concept of statistical power is reviewed. There it is stated that the power of a test is equal to one minus the risk of a type II error, $P = (1 - \beta)$. As stated in Section 9–8 the risk of a type II error is hard to control, and the common solution for its control is to take a large sample. One objective of a research study is to obtain a test statistic that is contained in the critical region. Thus, a researcher wants the test statistic to be large. For the ANOVA Table 9–5, the value of the F statistic is 23.65 and this is considerably larger than the critical value of 3.00. In addition, according to the CRUNCH (Bostrom, 1986) printout, the probability of getting a value of F this large or larger is 0.0000—a very low probability indeed. From this probability level would a researcher conclude that a "highly significant difference" has been found or that "a result significant beyond the p = 0.00001 level of significance" has been found? Less than knowledgeable researchers would. We would not, nor would the discriminating researcher.

The numerical magnitude of all test statistics is influenced by at least two factors. The two most important factors are (1) the alternative hypothesis and (2) the size of the sample. These influences are apparent in the formula for the SSB. If the alternative hypothesis is true, the following deviations will be large:

$$(\overline{Y}_1 - \overline{Y}), (\overline{Y}_2 - \overline{Y}), \ldots, (\overline{Y}_K - \overline{Y})$$

When these numbers are squared, they become even larger. As a consequence, they can produce a large SSB. This is desirable. To compute the SSB, each of these squared numbers is multiplied by its corresponding sample size. Thus, if the sample sizes are large, the SSB is also large, but if the sample sizes are small, the SSB is also small. This is true when the treatment effects are small or when the treatment effects are large. Because the sample size has such a profound effect on the value of SSB and the resulting F statistic, the interpretation of F is devoid of meaning. A large F ratio might only reflect large sample sizes and nothing else.

This is probably the case in the preoperative teaching study. With 246 subjects, an F ratio of 23.65 was obtained. It can be shown that a study with half this number of subjects would produce an F ratio of about half the size of 23.65 or 11.82. On the basis of hindsight, it can be shown that with a sample one sixth the size of the present sample, the F ratio would be a number close to $(1/6)(23.65) \equiv 4.00$. This number would be larger than the $\alpha = 0.05$ critical value, and it would still lead to the decision to reject the hypothesis under test. What seems to be a highly significant finding for N = 246 subjects is reduced to a significant finding for N = 41 subjects. Certainly a procedure or view of statistical hypothesis testing that turns a "highly" significant finding into a significant finding is suspect. Fortunately, it is not the procedure that is suspect but the false logic used by many researchers who use p values for decision making. Remember that all test statistics are a function of sample size and therefore not indicative of the strength of the association. Measurements of association exist for all tests and consequently should be used to evaluate all research findings.

Because the mean values for each of the treatments are determined by the effectiveness of the independent variable, the mean values cannot be influenced by increasing or decreasing sample sizes. Treatment effects are unrelated to sample sizes. If they were a function of sample sizes, statistical hypothesis testing would have no usefulness in nursing research. Surely declaring findings to be highly significant on the basis of an F statistic alone is a fallacy. The hypothetical study with 246 subjects has a high statistical power and a low probability of making a type II error. The only measurement in a study that is not a function of sample size is the proportion of explained variation or eta square. This is the number that should be used to defend the statement that a highly significant difference has been found. Large samples and small samples have no effect on the numerical value of this statistical measurement of treatment effects.

The *correlation ratio* or eta square is a pure measurement of association influenced almost exclusively by the alternative hypothesis. For that reason it is truly the most important figure in an ANOVA table (Hays, 1988). This is the number that the nurse investigator should look for and use for interpreting the results of a rejected hypothesis.

The phrase *highly significant* can be applied to this number only. If an independent variable accounts for a large part of the variance in a dependent variable and leads to a rejection of the null hypothesis, then certainly a researcher has found a highly significant finding and the results should be considered important.

The analysis of variance has a major weakness. In the preoperative teaching study, the hypothesis under test has been rejected. It has been concluded that the independent variable accounts for a large part of the variance in the dependent variable. The sources of the differences or reasons for the rejection have not been identified. In Section 9–6, a t test was performed on the difference between the means of treatments one and two. This two group difference was not significant, and yet a significant difference was identified by the ANOVA test. Does the rejected ANOVA hypothesis then mean that

1. Treatment groups one and three are different or
2. Treatment groups two and three are different or
3. Treatments one and two taken collectively differ from treatment three?

The analysis of variance does not provide answers to these questions and other similar questions that are asked by a researcher. The F test is an *omnibus* test of a very complicated alternative hypothesis. This hypothesis needs to be examined in detail. What is stated about the ANOVA F test is valid for all omnibus hypotheses tested under other statistical models. The complex nature of the ANOVA hypothesis is illustrated in Section 9–11.

9–10 POWER AND SAMPLE SIZE FOR THE ANALYSIS OF VARIANCE

Sample sizes for the analysis of variance are reported in Table 9–6 for risks of a type I error controlled at $\alpha = .05$ and for power levels of .70, .80, .90, and .95. This table is entered with the numerator degrees of freedom of the F test and

$$f = \sqrt{E/(1-E)}$$

where E is the amount of explained variance associated with the independent variable of the study. As an example, consider the three treatments of the preoperative teaching

study. Suppose that a researcher wishes to find a significant difference only if the amount of explained variance exceeds a minimal value of 15%. For this situation, the numerator degrees of freedom are given by 2 and

$$f = \sqrt{(.15)/(1-.15)} = .42$$

For f = .40, the sample sizes for power levels of .70, .80, .90, and .95 are given as 17, 21, 27, and 33, and for f = .50, the sample sizes are 11, 14, 18, and 22. With interpolation the corresponding sample sizes are 16, 20, 25, and 31. Because each sample in the preoperative teaching study was set at 82, there is more than sufficient power to detect a minimal amount of explained variance set at 15%.

9–11 LINEAR COMBINATIONS AND CONTRASTS, AND SCHEFFÉ'S METHOD OF POST HOC COMPARISONS

In Section 9–2, it is stated that linear combinations tend to have a normal distribution if the number of terms in the combination is large. This statement needs to be expanded to better understand the exact form of the alternative hypothesis of the analysis of variance. A linear combination is a weighted sum of variables. For example, consider the variables $Y_1, Y_2, \ldots, Y_P$ and the weights $W_1, W_2, \ldots, W_P$. As defined in Section 9–2, a linear combination of the variables is given as

$$L = W_1Y_1 + W_2Y_2 + \ldots + W_PY_P$$

If P is a large number, a variable that possesses this structure has a normal probability distribution under repeated random sampling. The mean of a simple random sample has this structure. For the sample mean, all the weights are equal to 1/N.

Consider an ANOVA study involving K groups for which the unknown population means are given by $\mu_1, \mu_2, \ldots, \mu_K$. A linear combination of the population means is defined as

$$L = W_1\mu_1 + W_2\mu_2 + \ldots + W_K\mu_K$$

For example, a linear combination of the three treatment means of the preoperative study for which the weights are 3, 6, and 12 is given as

TABLE 9-6 SAMPLE SIZES FOR THE ANALYSIS OF VARIANCE AND REGRESSION ANALYSIS

Power Level	f	Degrees of Freedom for the Numerator							
		1	2	3	4	5	6	8	10
.70	.10	310	258	221	195	175	160	138	123
	.20	78	65	56	49	44	41	35	31
	.30	35	29	25	22	20	18	16	14
	.40	20	17	15	13	12	11	9	8
	.50	13	11	10	9	8	7	6	6
	.60	10	8	7	6	6	5	5	4
	.70	7	6	6	5	5	4	4	3
	.80	6	5	5	4	4	4	3	3
.80	.10	393	322	274	240	215	195	168	148
	.20	99	81	69	61	54	50	42	38
	.30	45	36	31	27	25	22	19	17
	.40	26	21	18	16	14	13	11	10
	.50	17	14	12	10	9	9	8	7
	.60	12	10	9	8	7	6	6	5
	.70	9	8	7	6	5	5	4	4
	.80	7	6	5	5	4	4	4	3
.90	.10	526	421	354	309	275	250	213	187
	.20	132	106	89	78	69	63	54	48
	.30	59	48	40	35	31	29	24	22
	.40	34	27	23	20	18	16	14	13
	.50	22	18	15	13	12	11	9	8
	.60	16	13	11	10	9	8	7	6
	.70	12	10	8	7	7	6	5	5
	.80	9	8	7	6	5	5	4	4
.95	.10	651	515	430	372	331	299	254	223
	.20	163	130	108	94	83	75	64	56
	.30	73	58	49	42	38	34	29	26
	.40	42	33	28	24	22	20	17	15
	.50	27	22	18	16	14	13	11	10
	.60	19	15	13	11	10	9	8	7
	.70	14	12	10	9	8	7	6	5
	.80	11	9	8	7	6	6	5	4

(Adapted with permission from Tables 8.4.4 to 8.4.5, n to detect f-by-F test at $\alpha = .05$, $\nu = 1, 2, 3, 4, 5, 6, 8$, and 10, in Cohen, J.: Statistical Power Analysis for the Behavioral Sciences, New York, Academic Press, 1977.)

$$L = 3\mu_1 + 6\mu_2 + 12\mu_3$$

As presented, this linear combination has no practical interpretation in the preoperative teaching study. Not all linear combinations are void of interpretive meaning. A special case, called a *linear contrast,* however, has practical significance for nursing research. In fact, linear contrasts are the operative components that make the analysis of variance a highly effective research model.

By definition a linear contrast is a linear combination whose weights sum to zero. Six linear contrasts that are interpretable in terms of the three treatments of the preoperative study are the following:

$$\psi_1 = \mu_1 - \mu_2$$
$$\psi_2 = \mu_1 - \mu_3$$
$$\psi_3 = \mu_2 - \mu_3$$

$$\psi_4 = \frac{82}{164}\mu_1 + \frac{82}{164}\mu_2 - \mu_3$$
$$= \frac{1}{2}(\mu_1 + \mu_2) - \mu_3$$

$$\psi_5 = \frac{82}{164}\mu_1 + \frac{82}{164}\mu_3 - \mu_2$$
$$= \frac{1}{2}(\mu_1 + \mu_3) - \mu_2$$

and

$$\psi_6 = \frac{82}{164}\mu_2 + \frac{82}{164}\mu_3 - \mu_1$$
$$= \frac{1}{2}(\mu_2 + \mu_3) - \mu_1$$

The first three *pairwise contrasts* when set equal to zero are the hypotheses for a three-family set of t tests. The remaining three contrasts are not so obvious. Contrast number four is a contrast based on pooling the 82 patients in treatment one and treatment two and treating the 164 patients as a single group to compare with the 82 patients in treatment three. It is said to be a *complex contrast*. Contrasts five and six have similar interpretations. Each of the six contrasts are interpretable, and they are the only ones that are in this study. Other contrasts exist that are not so meaningful. Here is one:

$$\psi_7 = 0.34\mu_1 + 7.49\mu_2 - 7.83\mu_3$$

There is no limit to the number of such meaningless linear contrasts. Their existence is the source of the problem in using the analysis of variance. The alternative hypothesis of ANOVA is actually a statement about the infinite set of contrasts including those that are meaningful and meaningless. The null hypothesis of the analysis of variance states that *all* linear contrasts are equal to zero, whereas the alternative states that at least *one* linear contrast exists that is different from zero. Symbolically we have

$$H_0: \text{All } \psi = W_1\mu_1 + W_2\mu_2 + \ldots + W_K\mu_K$$
$$= 0$$

and

$$H_1: \text{At least one } \psi \neq 0$$

This null hypothesis and this alternative hypothesis were first recognized by Scheffé (1959) and became the basis of the Scheffé Method of Post Hoc Comparisons.

Scheffé showed that the F test makes a search among the infinite set of possible contrasts and locates the one that is most different from zero. The most different from zero contrast is put to a statistical test of the null hypothesis. If the null hypothesis for the most extreme contrast does not lead to rejection, it is immediately known that no other contrasts are significantly different from zero. This includes all the pairwise contrasts and all the complex contrasts that have or do not have meaning. If the most deviant contrast is different from zero, Scheffé argued that others might be different from zero. Because of this, a post hoc search for other significant differences should be conducted.

In addition to these recommendations, Scheffé was able to determine the correct critical values used to control the risk of at least one type I error to the numerical level chosen by a researcher when performing the F test. The critical values are called Scheffé coefficients and are defined as

$$S = \pm \sqrt{\nu_1 F\nu_1, \nu_2 : 1 - \alpha}$$

Note that the Scheffé coefficient takes on two values: one with a positive sign and one with a negative sign.

The Scheffé coefficients are used for the decision rule for as many t tests that a researcher might wish to examine following the rejection of a tested ANOVA hypothesis. The individual t tests are performed using the following general formulas:

$$t = \frac{W_1\overline{Y}_1 + W_2\overline{Y}_2 + \ldots + W_K\overline{Y}_K}{\sqrt{MSW\left(\frac{W_1^2}{N_1} + \frac{W_2^2}{N_2} + \ldots + \frac{W_K^2}{N_K}\right)}}$$

The denominator of this statistic is called the standard error of the contrast. Sometimes t is written as

$$t = \frac{\hat{\psi}}{SE(\hat{\psi})}$$

This test statistic is used to test the following null hypothesis:

$$H_0: \psi = W_1\mu_1 + W_2\mu_2 + \ldots + W_K\mu_K = 0$$

against the alternative hypothesis:

$$H_1: \psi \neq 0$$

The decision rule is given as

Decision rule: reject H_0 if $t < -S$
or if $t > +S$

For our example the only contrasts that have meaning are the six already described. The post hoc analysis of these six contrasts is summarized in Table 9–7. For contrast number one, see equation 1 and for contrast number four, see equation 2, both at the top of page 213. In this case, $\nu_1 = 2$ and $\nu_2 = 243$ is replaced by ∞. Thus, the Scheffé coefficient is given as

$$S = \sqrt{2(3.00)} = 2.45$$

Thus all the contrasts except one and five are statistically different from zero.

① $$t = \frac{(+1)(\overline{Y}_1) + (-1)(\overline{Y}_2)}{\sqrt{MSW\left(\frac{(+1)^2}{N_1} + \frac{(-1)^2}{N_2}\right)}} = \frac{4.890 - 4.524}{\sqrt{2.1954\left(\frac{1}{82} + \frac{1}{82}\right)}} = 1.58$$

② $$t = \frac{\left(+\frac{1}{2}\right)\overline{Y}_1 + \left(+\frac{1}{2}\right)\overline{Y}_2 + (-1)\overline{Y}_3}{\sqrt{MSW\left(\frac{\left(+\frac{1}{2}\right)^2}{N_1} + \frac{\left(+\frac{1}{2}\right)^2}{N_2} + \frac{(-1)^2}{N_3}\right)}} = \frac{\frac{1}{2}(4.890) + \frac{1}{2}(4.524) - (3.366)}{\sqrt{2.1954\left(\frac{\frac{1}{4}}{82} + \frac{\frac{1}{4}}{82} + \frac{1}{82}\right)}} = 6.69$$

Many researchers prefer to use confidence intervals rather than test statistics when performing the Scheffé Method of Post Hoc Comparisons. As indicated in Section 9–4, statistical hypothesis testing is, from a theoretical point of view, equivalent to confidence interval estimation procedures. The two models can be used interchangeably because both provide answers to the same questions. In particular, a test of the null hypothesis in terms of a test statistic is identical with the examination of a confidence interval to determine whether the interval contains zero. If the confidence interval contains zero, the corresponding test statistic is not significantly different from zero. The converse of this statement is also true. If the test statistic is not significantly different from zero, the corresponding confidence interval contains zero. Thus, the Scheffé Method of Post Hoc Comparisons can be approached by the examination of post hoc confidence intervals.

The post hoc confidence intervals for the six contrasts across the three treatments for the preoperative teaching study have the following form:

(Population contrast) = (Sample contrast) ± (Scheffé coefficient) (standard error)

In this case, the six confidence intervals are shown at the top of page 214. As indicated, the first and fifth contrasts are not statistically different from zero because these intervals contain the null hypothesis value of zero.

There is reason to wonder why a researcher would prefer the confidence interval approach to the hypothesis testing approach when it is known that both can be used to answer the same questions. When one considers the extra information provided about the independent variable in the confidence interval approach, the preference is easy to understand. Consider, for example,

TABLE 9–7 POST HOC CONTRASTS FOR THE DATA OF TABLE 9–3

Contrast: ψ	$\hat{\psi}$	SE ($\hat{\psi}$)	t	Decision
$\mu_1 - \mu_2$	0.366	0.2314	1.58	N.S.
$\mu_1 - \mu_3$	1.524	0.2314	6.59	Sig
$\mu_2 - \mu_3$	1.158	0.2314	5.01	Sig
$(1/2)(\mu_1 + \mu_2) - \mu_3$	1.341	0.2004	6.69	Sig
$(1/2)(\mu_1 + \mu_3) - \mu_2$	-0.396	0.2004	-1.98	N.S.
$(1/2)(\mu_2 + \mu_3) - \mu_1$	-1.077	0.2004	-5.37	Sig

$$S = \sqrt{2F_{2F_{2,\infty:0.95}}} = \sqrt{2(3.00)} = 2.45$$

Contrast

$$\mu_1 - \mu_2 = 0.366 \pm (2.45)(0.2314) = 0.366 \pm .567$$
$$\mu_1 - \mu_3 = 1.524 \pm (2.45)(0.2314) = 1.524 \pm .567$$
$$\mu_2 - \mu_3 = 1.158 \pm (2.45)(0.2314) = 1.158 \pm .567$$
$$(1/2)(\mu_1 + \mu_2) - \mu_3 = 1.341 \pm (2.45)(0.2004) = 1.341 \pm .491$$
$$(1/2)(\mu_1 + \mu_3) - \mu_2 = -0.396 \pm (2.45)(0.2004) = -0.396 \pm .491$$
$$(1/2)(\mu_2 + \mu_3) - \mu_1 = -1.077 \pm (2.45)(0.2004) = -1.077 \pm .491$$

the significant contrast involving treatments one and three. The null hypothesis that states that treatment one and treatment three have equal mean values is false because the corresponding confidence interval does not contain zero. In addition, examination of the confidence interval shows that treatment one and treatment three differ, with the minimum mean difference being given as 1.524 − .567 = .957 days and with the maximum mean difference being given as 1.524 + .567 = 2.091 days. With this information, a researcher can make an informed assessment of the findings in terms of either practical or theoretical meaning.

In this case, treatment one, under the best scenario, requires as a minimum almost one additional day of hospital care. Under the least desired scenario, treatment one requires a little more than two extra days of hospital care. When this information is converted into a subjective evaluation of comfort and convenience to a patient, it is seen that treatment three is to be preferred. At the same time, if the extra days of hospital care are translated into a dollar and cents assessment, it is again seen that treatment three is highly desirable because of the cost savings that result from an earlier discharge from the hospital. Similar interpretations can be made for the remaining significant contrasts.

On the basis of this analysis it can be concluded that

1. Treatments one and two are not statistically different from one another in how they affect length of stay in the hospital following an operation.

2. Treatment three differs from both treatments one and two. Patients of treatment three tend to leave the hospital about 1.5 days sooner than those of treatment one and about 1.2 days sooner than those of treatment two.

3. When patients of treatments one and two are combined into a single group and compared with the patients in treatment three, it is seen that the patients in treatment three are released about 1.3 days sooner.

4. Treatment one is definitely the inferior treatment because when it is compared with the combined sample of treatment two and three patients, they are seen to remain in the hospital for about one extra day.

5. If a choice must be made between treatments two and three, treatment three should be selected.

9–12 POST HOC VERSUS PLANNED COMPARISONS

In the previous section directions were provided for a post hoc analysis following the rejection of a tested ANOVA hypothesis. The post hoc analysis was performed on six contrasts that were interpretable. One might wonder why the six hypotheses were not tested as a family of hypotheses using Dunn's critical values as described in Section 9–7. If this model were used, it would be said that a planned or a priori analysis had been performed. Sometimes a planned analysis is more powerful than a post hoc analysis. In this case, it would not be advisable. This is easy to show. For Q = 6, α = .05, and $\nu = \infty$, the critical value in the Dunn table is 2.64. This is larger than the Scheffé coefficient of 2.45. Are there times when a planned analysis is preferable to a post hoc analysis? The answer is yes, and it is almost always yes.

The analysis of variance test is an omnibus test that spreads the risk of at least one type I error across an infinite set of possible contrasts, most of which are uninterpretable in most research studies. It is clearly wasteful of type I error probability. This is not always true for a planned analysis that applies the probability of at least one type I error to the specific contrasts selected by the researcher. In the example, this was not true; the post hoc analysis was more powerful. The reason for this can be traced to the small value of K, the number of groups in the study. As soon as the number of groups increases beyond 3, planned analyses generally prove to be more powerful. For example consider a study with K = 6 and N = 126. The Scheffé coefficients for this post hoc analysis are given as S = ± 3.38. For the same amount of type I error protection a researcher can examine more than 50 planned comparisons. Thus, if a researcher only wanted to test 20 contrasts, the planned procedure would be more powerful.

Here is a useful strategy for choosing between a planned and a post hoc analysis. Compute the Scheffé coefficient that would be needed for a post hoc analysis of a rejected ANOVA hypothesis. Next, count the contrasts that focus *directly* on the research questions of interest. Determine the Dunn coefficient for this small number of contrasts. Use the method that provides the smallest critical value. A word of caution is in order if this strategy is adopted. The choice between a planned and a post hoc analysis must be made before any data are collected or before the analysis is performed. Many researchers frown on planned analyses because there are good reasons to believe that it has been abused by some investigators. It is very easy to perform the F test, applying Scheffé's method, and to discover that the research hypotheses have not been verified. At that point, it is even easier to substitute a planned analysis and thereby verify the hypotheses of interest by casting out all the results that were not significant by the Scheffé method. It is dishonest and it entails the risk of making a large number of type I errors. It is not to be done!

Tukey's Method of Paired Comparisons is another planned procedure that is frequently reported in the literature (1949). This method is preferred to the Dunn procedure provided that a researcher wishes to examine all the two-sample t tests. If this is what the researcher wishes to test, then the F test should not be performed nor should the Dunn procedure be adopted. For a complete discussion of the Tukey method, see Marascuilo and Serlin (1988).

Finally, there are alternative methods to the F test—the Scheffé method of post hoc comparisons, the Dunn method for a planned analysis, and Tukey's method.

These four models require normality for the dependent measurement or large samples, equal population variances, and independence between and within samples. If the underlying variables are not normally distributed or are skewed or if the samples are too small to permit an evaluation of the assumptions, a viable competitor is the Kruskal-Wallis test. This test is described in Section 9–17. For unequal variance distributions, extensions of the Welch-Aspin test are available. These models are described in detail by Marascuilo and Serlin (1988). For highly peaked distributions, competitors exist in terms of normal-score tests and multiple-sample median tests. These procedures are described by Marascuilo and McSweeney (1977).

9–13 MULTIPLE ANOVA F TESTS

In Section 9–7 procedures for multiple t tests were described. In this section multiple F tests are examined. For this examination consider the data reported in Table 9–8. These data summarize the five ANOVA F tests for the five dependent variables of the preoperative study. As can be seen, the amount of variance explained by the three treatments range from a low of 11% to a high of 30%. Whereas the treatment of multiple t tests is relatively straightforward, the treatment of multiple F tests is not so clear. We describe some of the strategies used in the literature by various researchers. Where we can, we point out the favorable and unfavorable features of each strategy.

Strategy One

The most commonly used strategy is *hypothesis control*. With this method, each F test is performed with an $\alpha = .05$, and each F test is evaluated in terms of the decision rule:

Decision rule:
$$\text{reject } H_0 \text{ if } F > F_{2,\infty:0.95} = 3.00$$

In this case, each hypothesis of no treatment effect is rejected for each variable. Each variable would now be analyzed using Scheffé's method of multiple comparisons.

The advantage in using this strategy is that

TABLE 9-8 MULTIPLE ANOVA F TESTS FOR THE DEPENDENT VARIABLES OF THE PREOPERATIVE STUDY

Variable	Group	Mean	N	$\dfrac{MSB}{MSW}$	F	$\hat{\eta}^2$
Length of Stay	1	4.890	82			
	2	4.524	82	$\dfrac{51.9309}{2.1954}$	23.65	0.16
	3	3.366	82			
Pain Med. One	1	6.646	82			
	2	4.988	82	$\dfrac{145.4309}{2.7190}$	53.49	0.30
	3	4.012	82			
Pain Med. Two	1	2.622	82			
	2	1.720	82	$\dfrac{30.8455}{2.0746}$	14.87	0.11
	3	1.451	82			
Postop. Comp.	1	1.232	82			
	2	0.707	82	$\dfrac{16.8415}{0.9123}$	18.46	0.13
	3	0.329	82			
Days pdch	1	5.573	82			
	2	4.171	82	$\dfrac{162.6870}{5.6987}$	28.55	0.19
	3	2.756	82			

each hypothesis is treated as a separate family so that the total risk of a type II error is kept low. The method has very good statistical power and of the strategies discussed here, it has maximum power. Many *significant* differences will be identified. The disadvantage with this strategy is that the risk of making at least one type I error in the entire set of hypotheses examined is increased. In this case the maximum risk of at least one type I error is $\alpha_T < 5(0.05) = 0.25$. To many researchers a risk of a type I error of this magnitude is too high. Because the five dependent variables are correlated with one another, type I errors are certain to be compounded. For example, if a type I error is made for length of stay on the contrast of treatment one with treatment two, it is likely that the same type I error would be made when this contrast is investigated for some of the other variables. The use of this strategy gives rise to some significant findings that may actually represent type I errors.

Strategy Two

Strategy two is based on treatment of the five hypotheses as one family of interrelated hypotheses. The total risk of a type I error is partitioned equally across the five families so that each hypothesis is tested with an $\alpha = (1/5)(0.05) = 0.01$. With this risk the decision rule for each F test is given as

Decision rule:

$$\text{reject } H_0 \text{ if } F > F_{2,\infty:0.99} = 4.61$$

In this case, the same decisions are reached about each of the omnibus F tests. Even so, note that if any of the F ratios had been in the range of 3.01 to 4.60, they would have led to rejection for strategy one but not for strategy two. In addition, if Scheffé's method is applied here, the numerical value of the Scheffé coefficient is given as S = 3.04, which is considerably larger than 2.45, the value used for individual variable hypothesis control.

The advantage with this method is that it provides a tighter statistical control on the making of type I errors. Its disadvantage is that the power is reduced and potentially significant findings are not identified.

Strategy Three

The third strategy is to perform a planned analysis. In this example, the six contrasts of Section 9-11 are tested for each of the five dependent measurements. For five dependent measurements, the total number of planned comparisons is given as Q = 6(5) = 30. With $\alpha = .05$ and $\nu = \infty$, the critical value read from Table A-8 is given as t = 3.15. In this case, this value is larger than the Scheffé critical value for strategy two, so that strategy two would be preferred to strategy three. This, however, is not always true. If the number of groups exceeds three, the Dunn method usually proves to be superior.

Strategy three usually provides the tightest statistical control on the risks of at least one type I error. In most situations it has more statistical power than strategy two but less than strategy one. It is the method that we recommend for most situations.

9–14 TWO-FACTOR INTERACTIONS IN ANOVA

Many research studies involve the joint examination of the effects of two independent variables acting in concert on a single dependent variable. As an example of such a study, consider the data shown graphically in Figure 9–3. This graph shows the joint relationship of the three treatments and the three hospitals have to the length of stay following operation. The first thing to note is that treatment three has the shortest postoperative hospital time period for all three hospitals. Treatment two has an intermediate position at Hospitals One and Two but not at Hospital Three. Finally treatment one is least favorable at Hospitals One and Two and, yet, in Hospital Three it is intermediate to treatments one and three. The effects of the treatments are not uniform in the various hospitals. It is said that treatments

interact with hospital. The analysis of variance is well suited to the study of interactions. The reason for this is easy to show.

Consider a study in which a group of patients are given two different drugs, drug A and drug B, which are known to be effective in producing sleep following surgery. Suppose that it is known that drug A produces an average of three hours of sleep and that drug B produces an average of four hours of sleep for patients on the first night following surgery. Because the two drugs are individually effective in producing sleep, a researcher could ask the question: "What are the effects on sleep when drug A and drug B are administered simultaneously to patients following surgery?" If the effects of the joint administration of the two drugs are equal to the simple effects of each drug (3 + 4 = 7), it is said that the two drugs do not interact. If, however, the total amount of sleep differs from the simple sum of seven hours, it is said that the two drugs interact. Let us now see how the testing for the existence of an interaction is related to the analysis of variance.

In order to test for the existence of an interaction, a minimum of four groups of comparison subjects are required for analysis. To help understand the basis of this requirement and the role played by the analysis of variance in assessing interactions, consider the design represented in Table 9–9 and represented graphically in Figure 9–4. In this figure the mean values are shown for four groups of patients given one of four experimental drug treatments following surgery. Let the four groups be denoted as (OO), (AO), (OB), and (AB). Let the mean values for the four groups be denoted as

1. $\mu(OO)$ for subjects in group 1 who are given a placebo,
2. $\mu(AO)$ for subjects in group 2 who are given drug A,
3. $\mu(OB)$ for subjects in group 3 who are given drug B, and
4. $\mu(AB)$ for subjects in group 4 who are given both drugs.

See Figure 9–4 for the relative location of these means with respect to hours of sleep.

The mean difference between the placebo group and the drug A group is given as

$$\delta(A) = \mu(AO) - \mu(OO)$$

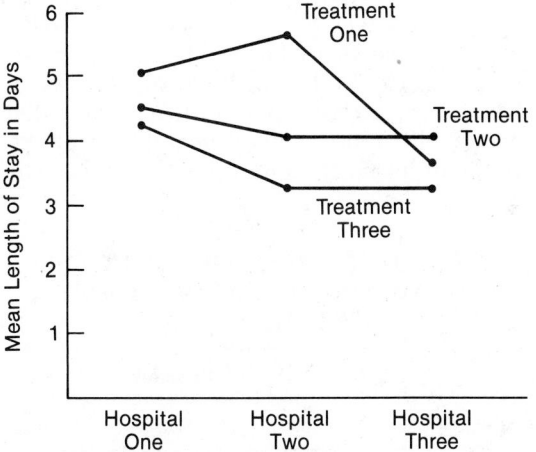

Figure 9–3. Mean length of stay according to treatment and hospital.

TABLE 9–9 TWO-FACTOR INTERACTION TABLE OF ASSESSING THE JOINT EFFECTS OF TWO DRUGS ON SLEEP FOLLOWING SURGERY

Drug A	Drug B Present	Drug B Not Present	δ
Present	μ(AB)	μ(AO)	
Not Present	μ(OB)	μ(OO)	μ(AO) − μ(OO)
δ	μ(OB) − μ(OO)		μ(AB) − μ(OO)

The mean difference between the placebo group and the drug B group is given as

$$\delta(B) = \mu(OB) - \mu(OO)$$

If the two drugs do not interact, then the outcome for the subjects given both drugs would be equal to the sum of the two effects. Mathematically, this means that

$$\mu(AB) = \mu(OO) + \delta(A) + \delta(B)$$
$$= \mu(OO) + (\mu(AO) - \mu(OO)) + (\mu(OB) - \mu(OO))$$

If all terms are transferred to the left-hand side of the equal sign, it follows that

$$\mu(AB) - \mu(AO) - \mu(OB) + \mu(OO) = 0$$

This is a contrast in the four cell averages of Table 9–9. As a consequence, we can test it for significant difference from zero. Contrasts based on matched row and column cells are called *tetrad* differences. For a more complete discussion on this topic, see Marascuilo and Levin (1970). Note that any tetrad difference can also be written as

$$\mu(AB) - \mu(AO) = \mu(OB) - \mu(OO)$$

In this form it is seen that a tetrad difference is used to determine whether the effects of drug B are the same for subjects given the placebo or given drug A. Also note that the contrast can be written as

$$\mu(AB) - \mu(OB) = \mu(AO) - \mu(OO)$$

In this form the contrast is used to test whether the effects of drug A are the same for the subjects given the placebo or given drug B. If in either case the paired differences are equal, there is no interaction.

Let us now examine possible interactions between treatments and hospitals in the preoperative teaching study and see how they jointly make an impact on length of hospital stay. The mean values used to construct Figure 9–3 are reported in Table 9–10. These numbers are based not on the full set of 246 subjects but on the 117 selected at random to provide 13 patients for the 9 cells of the study. This was done to equalize the number of subjects in each treatment-hospital combination. In this case, 13 was the size of the largest sample that could be generated across all nine treatment-hospital combinations to provide equal size samples. The

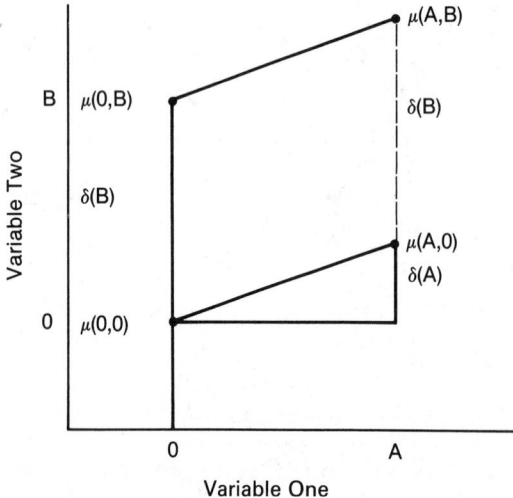

Figure 9–4. An illustration of no interaction for a 2 × 2 design.

TABLE 9–10 MEAN LENGTH OF STAY ACCORDING TO TREATMENT AND HOSPITAL

Treatment	Hospital One	Two	Three
One	5.077	5.769	3.769
Two	4.462	4.154	4.154
Three	4.231	3.308	3.308

$$t = \frac{(\overline{Y}_{11} - \overline{Y}_{12}) - (\overline{Y}_{21} - \overline{Y}_{22})}{\sqrt{MSW\left(\frac{(+1)^2}{N_{11}} + \frac{(-1)^2}{N_{12}} + \frac{(-1)^2}{N_{21}} + \frac{(+1)^2}{N_{22}}\right)}} = \frac{-1.000}{\sqrt{2.0370\left(\frac{4}{13}\right)}} = -1.26$$

method we are describing here is restricted to equal size samples. In Section 10–11 we describe procedures that are valid for unequal numbers of observations per cell.

Let us examine the tetrad difference that involves treatments one and two and Hospitals One and Two. This contrast is given as

$$\hat{\psi} = (\overline{Y}_{11} - \overline{Y}_{12}) - (\overline{Y}_{21} - \overline{Y}_{22})$$
$$= (5.077 - 5.769) - (4.462 - 4.154)$$
$$= -0.692 - 0.308$$
$$= -1.000$$

As shown in Table 9–11, the MSW for this study is given as

$$MSW = 2.0370 \text{ with } \nu = 108$$

In terms of this number, the equation at the top of this page applies. This contrast as well as the remaining eight tetrad differences involving all two levels of treatments and hospitals are summarized in Table 9–12. As a planned analysis with Q = 9, ν = 108, and α = .05, the critical value read from Table A–8 is given as t = ± 2.77. Thus, the decision rule for testing each contrast for statistical significance is given as

Decision rule: reject H_0: $\psi = 0$,
    if t < − 2.77 or if t > 2.77

None of the contrasts is statistically different from zero. It is concluded that treatment and hospital do not interact.

It should be noted that two of the contrasts generated t statistics that are slightly smaller than the planned critical value. The sample sizes are relatively small and so the tests may not have sufficient power to reject false hypotheses. It is probably for this reason that the analytical procedures do not support the visual picture portrayed in Figure 9–3. This example also shows how important statistical hypothesis testing is for the evaluation of empirical data. It is definitely more objective than a simple visual examination of a graph. Statistical procedures ensure that all re-

TABLE 9–11 ANALYSIS OF VARIANCE TABLE FOR THE DATA OF TABLE 9–10

Source	d/f	S of S	MS	F	$\hat{\eta}^2$
Treatment	2	30.7863	15.3932	7.56	0.11
Hospital	2	15.5043	7.7521	3.81	0.05
T × H	4	19.5214	4.8803	2.40	0.07
Within	108	220.0000	2.0370		
Total	116	285.8118			

TABLE 9–12 ALL POSSIBLE TETRAD INTERACTION TESTS

Treatments		Hospitals			t*
1	2	1	2	−1.00*	−1.26
1	2	1	3	1.000	1.26
1	2	2	3	2.000	2.53
1	3	1	2	−1.615	−2.04
1	3	1	3	0.385	0.49
1	3	2	3	2.000	2.53
2	3	1	2	−0.615	−0.77
2	3	1	3	−0.615	−0.77
2	3	2	3	0.000	0.00

$*t^{DUNN}_{9,108:0.95} = 2.77$

searchers come to the same conclusions for a given set of data. Visual impressions do not promise unity in the decision process.

9–15 THE TWO-FACTOR ANALYSIS OF VARIANCE

In the previous section, the procedure for a planned analysis of an interaction hypothesis was illustrated. Not many researchers use this model. Instead, they use a post hoc analysis, which is almost always less powerful. The two-factor ANOVA is based on partitioning the explained variance into preidentifiable components. For the data of Table 9–11, it is clear that treatment, hospital, and the interaction of treatment by hospital contribute to the amount of explained variance. For example, look at Figure 9–3 once again. Note that treatment three tends to have the lowest group means. In addition, treatment one seems to have the highest mean values. Certainly, treatment explains part of the variance. Also note that the mean values for Hospital One are generally higher than those of the other two hospitals. This suggests that hospital can be used to explain part of the variance. In the previous section it was suggested that with a larger sample, a significant treatment by hospital interaction could be identified.

The formulas used to achieve two-factor partitioning of the explained variance are not presented. The arithmetic required to do the analysis is not demonstrated. The reasons for not presenting these steps is that most researchers use computer programs to generate the test statistics and the corresponding analysis of variance table. This is exactly what was done using CRUNCH (Bostrom, 1986). The ANOVA table is reported in Table 9–11. As can be seen there are three sources of variance. They are treatment, hospital, and the interaction of treatment and hospital. There are three treatments with $\nu_T = 2$ degrees of freedom, there are three hospitals with $\nu_H = 2$ degrees of freedom. It can be shown that the degrees of freedom for the interaction is given as

$$\nu_{T \times H} = \nu_T \times \nu_H = 2 \times 2 = 4$$

The degrees of freedom for the MSW is given as $\nu_W = N - K$, where K is the number of unique groups in the study. In this case $K = 9$, so that $\nu_W = 117 - 9 = 108$.

Each source of variance can be tested by an omnibus F statistic which tests the null hypothesis that all contrasts about the parameters identified with a given source of variance are zero. This hypothesis is tested against an alternative which states that at least one contrast is different from zero. If any source of variance is found to be statistically different from zero, Scheffé's method of multiple comparisons would be applied. With each family of hypotheses tested at $\alpha = 0.05$, the decision rules for the three families are given as

Decision rule for treatment:
reject H_0 if $F_T > F_{2,108:0.95} = 3.08$

Decision rule for hospitals:
reject H_0 if $F_H > F_{2,108:0.95} = 3.08$

and

Decision rule for treatment by hospital interaction:
reject H_0 if $F_{T \times H} > F_{4,108:0.95} = 2.46$

The hypotheses for treatments and hospitals are rejected, but the hypothesis for the interaction is not. Scheffé's method would now be applied to the treatment means and to the hospital means. Note that the interaction just missed being significant. This could reflect the small sample sizes and might actually be a type II error. There is good reason to believe that an increase in sample sizes from 13 to 14 would have been enough to make the finding significant.

If the interaction had been significant, a post hoc analysis would need to be performed. The post hoc analysis would certainly entail an examination of the nine contrasts reported in Table 9–12. The critical value would be given as the Scheffé coefficient value of

$$S = \sqrt{\nu_{T \times H} F \nu_{T \times H} \nu_W : (1 - \alpha)} = \sqrt{4(2.46)}$$
$$= 3.14$$

This value is considerably larger than the planned contrast critical value of 2.77.

It should be noted that complex contrasts are covered by the omnibus F test of no interaction. Almost all these contrasts are uninterpretable. In this study, the only contrasts that seem to make much sense are the nine listed in Table 9–12. Because of this, it is unwise to carry out the omnibus analysis of variance F test for the interaction. It is recommended that interactions be examined in terms of a planned analysis.

9–16 NESTED OR SIMPLE COMPARISONS

Some researchers perform an analysis of variance without a true understanding of the research questions answered by the specific partitioning of the explained variation illustrated in Table 9–11. The analysis of variance shown in Table 9–11 has as its focus an examination of the interaction between hospital and treatment. Sometimes interaction hypotheses have little practical importance or are devoid of theoretical interpretation. An example of an interaction question

$$t = \frac{\overline{Y}_{11} - \overline{Y}_{12}}{\sqrt{MSW\left(\frac{(+1)^2}{N_{11}} + \frac{(-1)^2}{N_{12}}\right)}} = \frac{0.615}{\sqrt{2.0370\left(\frac{1}{13} + \frac{1}{13}\right)}} = 1.10$$

in the preoperative teaching study is as follows:

Is the mean length of stay between treatments one and three in Hospital One of .85 of a day statistically different from the corresponding difference in Hospital Three of .46 of a day?

If it were significant, what would it mean to patients, third party providers, and health care administrators? For patients the statistical significance of the finding has no practical use. From this type of finding the patient knows only that the mean length of stay for treatments one and three are more alike in Hospital Three than they are in Hospital One. With this information even an informed patient cannot choose between the best hospital nor between the better treatment. Even third party providers and health care administrators could not make much use of this information.

Two questions of greater interest to the patient who seeks a quick recovery are

Is the difference in mean length of stay between treatments one and three in Hospital One of .85 days statistically significant?

and as a second independent question,

Is the difference in mean length of stay between treatments one and three in Hospital Three of .46 days statistically significant?

With answers to these questions, a patient can make a decision as to which treatment to choose, given that the treatment is to take place in Hospital One or Hospital Three. Informed patients could avail themselves of the option to choose the treatment with the shorter length of stay. In addition, health care administrators at each hospital could argue for adoption of the method that produces the shorter length of stay in the hospital. Finally, administrators might more easily meet third party health insurance length of stay criteria for specific diagnostic related groups (DRGs) and thus support the preoperative teaching method most successful in meeting individual hospital length of stay reimbursement criteria. With the use of a nested analysis, each hospital is provided with the data on which to base important cost-effective programmatic decisions.

Contrasts within a hospital are called nested comparison or are referred to as simple effect comparisons (Winer, 1971). Simple effect comparisons do not cut across one of the independent variables. The comparisons remain completely nested in one of the variables. Perhaps of greater interest to most patients considering surgery is an analysis of a single treatment nested in a series of hospitals. Here informed patients could choose the hospital that has the shortest length of stay. As indicated, nested analyses can be performed in two directions. In this example, a researcher could nest treatments in hospitals or nest hospitals in treatments. The two designs answer different research questions.

For our example, there are three simple effect comparisons in Hospital One. They are given as

$$\hat{\psi}_1 = \overline{Y}_{11} - \overline{Y}_{12} = 5.077 - 4.462 = 0.615$$
$$\hat{\psi}_2 = \overline{Y}_{11} - \overline{Y}_{13} = 5.077 - 4.231 = 0.846$$
$$\hat{\psi}_3 = \overline{Y}_{12} - \overline{Y}_{23} = 4.462 - 4.231 = 0.231$$

The t statistic for the first of these comparisons is given in the equation at the top of this page. The remaining t values are reported in Table 9–13. Note that there are nine comparisons so that with a planned analysis comparisons less than −2.77 or larger than +2.77 are indicative of significant sources of variance.

Again it should be noted that confidence intervals can be used to assess the nine contrasts of Table 9–13. Because the sample sizes are all equal to a common value, the assessment is simple. In this case, any confidence interval is given as the following

(Population contrast) = (Sample contrast) ± (Critical value)(Standard error)

For a planned analysis with nine contrasts, the confidence intervals are given as

TABLE 9-13 ALL POSSIBLE SIMPLE COMPARISONS FOR TREATMENT NESTED IN HOSPITAL

Hospital	Comparisons	Contrast	t*
One	1 vs 2	0.615	1.10
	1 vs 3	0.846	1.51
	2 vs 3	0.231	0.41
Two	1 vs 2	1.615*	2.88*
	1 vs 3	2.461*	4.40*
	2 vs 3	0.846	1.51
Three	1 vs 2	−0.385	−0.46
	1 vs 3	0.461	0.82
	2 vs 3	0.846	1.51

*Significance for t
$t_{9,108:0.95}^{DUNN} = \pm 2.77$

Significance for the contrast
$2.77(.5598) = \pm 1.55$

(Population contrast) = (Sample contrast)
$\pm 2.77(.5598)$ = Sample contrast ± 1.55

For a post hoc analysis, the planned critical value of 2.77 is replaced by the Scheffé coefficient of 2.45. Again, two of the contrasts are significantly different from zero (treatment one versus treatment two in Hospital Two and treatment one versus treatment three in Hospital Two).

9-17 INTRODUCTION TO NONPARAMETRIC RANK TESTS

All the methods discussed in the previous sections have been based on the assumption that the underlying variables are normally distributed or that the sample sizes are large (greater than 30). If these conditions are not satisfied, the described methods should not be used. Instead, a researcher should consider the nonparametric statistical tests described in this section. The prototype of all nonparametric tests is the one-way analysis of variance on ranks or the Kruskal-Wallis test (1952). If the number of groups is equal to two, the Kruskal-Wallis test is equivalent to the two-sample Wilcoxon test (1949) and the two-sample Mann-Whitney U test (1947). The Kruskal-Wallis test is described in a form presented by Serlin, Carr, and Marascuilo (1982).

Consider the following hypothetical study. A group of patients suffering from migraine headaches was divided at random into two groups. The result of this division was to assign 10 subjects to one group and 10 to the other group. One group was given a standard drug that provided temporary relief from the pain. The second group was given a new experimental drug. Each patient was assigned a drug and told to take the drug as needed. In addition, each patient was told to keep a diary and record the number of hours that elapsed between the time that he or she took the drug until the appearance of the next migraine headache. They did not know whether the drug was the standard drug or a new experimental drug. They were given sufficient medication for a two-week period. At the end of the second week, each patient returned the completed diary to the research staff. Because the times at which the drugs needed to be taken varied by subjects, it was decided arbitrarily to use the second time that the drug was used as the test condition. Thus, the dependent variable of the study is the number of hours between the taking of the drug and the appearance of the next migraine headache. The results for the second administration of the drug are reported in Table 9-14. Through inspection of the data, visual evidence exists that the new drug offers more relief than the standard drug.

The hypothesis to be tested is that the mean difference in number of hours of pain relief between the two drugs is zero. Because of the small sample sizes, application of the two-sample t test would not be justified. Thus, we consider a transformation of the number of hours between administration of the drugs to ranks.

There are many ways to define the Kruskal-Wallis statistic. A very simple version has

TABLE 9-14 NUMBER OF HOURS OF PAIN RELIEF IN 20 PATIENTS GIVEN ONE OF TWO DRUGS FOR MIGRAINES*

Old Drug	New Drug	Rank for Old	Rank for New
5.5	10	1	5
7	17.5	2	8
7.5	20	3	9
9	21	4	10
12	24	6	13
17	24	7	13
21.5	29	11	15
24	30	13	16
35	48	17	19
36	60	18	20
Total		82	128

*Data refer to the second trial only.

been described by Serlin, Carr, and Marascuilo (1982). In this form, the Kruskal-Wallis statistic, H, is as follows:

$$H = (N - 1)\, \hat{\eta}^2,$$

where $\hat{\eta}^2$ is a measurement of the strength of association based on ranks that are equivalent to the correlation ratio of the analysis of variance. By definition,

$$\hat{\eta}^2 = \frac{\text{sum of squares explained}}{\text{sum of squares total}} = \frac{SS_E}{SS_T} = \frac{III - II}{I - II}$$

where

$$I = \Sigma r^2$$

$$II = \frac{(\Sigma r)^2}{N}$$

and

$$III = \frac{R_1^2}{N_1} + \frac{R_2^2}{N_2} + \ldots + \frac{R_K^2}{N_K}$$

and where R_1 is the sum of the ranks in sample one, R_2 is the sum of the ranks in sample two, and R_K is the sum of the ranks in sample K. In this case K = 2 and

$$III = \frac{82^2}{10} + \frac{128^2}{10} = 2310.8$$

In addition,

$$I = 1^2 + 2^2 + \ldots + 20^2 = 2858$$

and

$$II = (82 + 128)^2/20 = 2205, \text{ so that}$$

$$\hat{\eta}^2 = \frac{2310.8 - 2205}{2868 - 2205} = .1596$$

Finally the Kruskal-Wallis statistic is given as

$$H = (20 - 1)(.1596) = 3.03$$

This number is referred to the chi-square distribution with degrees of freedom given by $\nu = (K - 1)$. In this case, K = 2, so that $\nu = 1$. Thus, the 95% decision rule read from Table A−1 for rejecting the hypothesis of equal measures of central tendency is as follows:

Reject the hypothesis if H > 3.84.

The hypothesis is not rejected.

Existing computer programs for the analysis of variance can be used to obtain the sum of squares explained and the sum of squares total by computing the analysis of variance on the ranked data. With the output from the computer program, $\hat{\eta}^2$ can be computed by treating the sum of squares among the groups as the sum of squares explained. Planned and post hoc procedures for the Kruskal-Wallis test and other nonparametric tests exist for fully crossed ANOVA designs and can be found in Marascuilo and McSweeney (1977) and in Conover (1980). The illustration was based only on K = 2 groups. The test is not so restricting and can be used for K > 2 as well. When K = 2, the test is equivalent to the two-sample Wilcoxon test and the Mann-Whitney U test.

The two-sample Wilcoxon statistic is the sum of the ranks in the smaller sample. If the sample sizes are equal, either sample can be treated as the criterion sample. The test statistic is defined as

$$Z = \frac{\left(T_1 \pm \dfrac{1}{2}\right) - E(T_1)}{\sqrt{\text{Var}(T_1)}}$$

where

1. the smaller sample is denoted as N_1
2. T_1 is the sum of the ranks in the smaller sample

3. $E(T_1) = \dfrac{N_1(N_1 + N_2 + 1)}{2}$

4. $\text{Var}(T_1) = \dfrac{N_1 N_2}{N_1 + N_2 - 1} \dfrac{I - II}{N}$

and

5. 1/2 is added if $T_1 < E(T_1)$ and 1/2 is subtracted if $T_1 > E(T_1)$.

In this case,

$$N_1 = 10,\ T_1 = 82,\ E(T_1) = 10(21)/2 = 105,$$

and

$$\text{Var}(T_1) = \frac{10(10)}{19} \frac{2868 - 2205}{20} = 174.47$$

In addition, 1/2 is added so that

$$Z = \frac{\left(82 + \dfrac{1}{2}\right) - 105}{\sqrt{174.47}} = -1.70$$

If H_0 is true, the sampling distribution of Z is normal with a mean of zero and a standard deviation of 1. Thus, with $\alpha = .05$ the null hypothesis is not rejected because $Z = -1.70$ is not in the critical region defined by $Z < -1.96$ and $Z > 1.96$. For more on this test see Marascuilo and Serlin (1988).

9-18 SUMMARY

In this chapter, a number of parametric and nonparametric tests for comparative studies was described. The most commonly performed two-sample test is the t test based on the assumption of normality of distribution for the underlying variable and equality of variances in the populations. The test also assumes that the observations between and within samples are independent. Procedures for dependent measurements for randomized blocks and repeated measurement designs exist and can be found described in detail by Winer (1971) and Kirk (1982).

It was also shown that testing of the null hypothesis for significance is equivalent to examining a confidence interval for the inclusion of zero. For some researchers, confidence intervals have greater usefulness than tests of hypothesis. One advantage to the confidence interval approach is that the confidence interval identifies every possible null hypothesis that could have given rise to the data being analyzed. The limits of the interval provide information about the smallest and largest population values that might exist in the populations, given a specified risk of a type I error.

The extension of the two-sample t test to the multiple sample F test of the analysis of variance was described. Contrasts were described and planned and post hoc comparisons were illustrated. Interactions were introduced and it was shown how a tetrad difference could be used to assess the meaning of a two-factor interaction. Higher order interactions also can be examined and sometimes are useful for interpretative purposes. For alternative views on the treatment of interactions, consult Winer (1971) and Kirk (1982). In many studies, simple or nested comparisons are of greater usefulness than are interactions. For two contrasting views on this topic, see Winer (1971) and Marascuilo and Serlin (1988).

Nonparametric statistics has an extensive literature, and models exist for many situations in which small samples must be se-

lected. In this chapter, the Kruskal-Wallis test was described and illustrated. If the number of groups is equal to 2, the Kruskal-Wallis test reduces to the two-sample Wilcoxon or the Mann-Whitney U tests. For more on the applications of nonparametric procedures, consult Siegel and Castellan (1988) and Marascuilo and McSweeney (1977).

REFERENCES

Bostrom, A.: CRUNCH *Software*. Oakland, CA, 1986.

Cohen, J.: Statistical Power Analysis for the Behavioral Sciences. New York, Academic Press, 1977.

Conover, W.J.: Practical Nonparametric Statistics. New York, John Wiley & Sons, 1980.

Dixon, W.J., editor: BMDP Statistical Software. Berkeley, CA, University of California Press, 1983.

Dunn, O.J.: Multiple comparisons among means, J. Am. Stat. Assoc., 56: 52-64, 1961.

Dunn, O.J, and Clark, V.A.: Applied Statistics: Analysis of Variance and Regression. New York, John Wiley & Sons, 1974.

Hays, W.L.: Statistics, ed. 4. New York, Holt, Rinehart, & Winston, 1988.

Kirk, R.E.: Experimental Design, ed. 2. Belmont, CA, Brooks-Cole, 1982.

Kruskal, W.H., and Wallis, W.A.: Use of ranks in one-criterion variance analysis, J. Am. Stat. Assoc., 47: 583-621, 1952.

Mann, H.B., and Whitney, D.R.: On a test of whether one of two random variables is stochastically larger than the other. Ann. Math. Stat., 18: 50-60, 1947.

Marascuilo, L.A., and Levin, J.R.: Appropriate post hoc comparison for interactions and nested hypotheses in analysis of variance designs: the elimination of type IV errors, Am. Ed. Res. J., 7: 397-421, 1970.

Marascuilo, L.A., and McSweeney, M.: Nonparametric and Distribution Free Methods for the Social Sciences. Belmont, CA, Brooks-Cole, 1977.

Marascuilo, L.A., and Serlin, R.C.: Statistical Methods for the Social and Behavioral Sciences. New York, Freeman and Company, 1988.

Ryan, T.A.: The experiment as the unit for computing rates of error, Psych. Bull., 59: 301-305, 1962.

SAS, Inc.: SAS User's Guide: Statistics, version 5. Carry, NC, published by author, 1985.

Scheffé, H.: The Analysis of Variance. New York, John Wiley & Sons, 1959.

Serlin, R.C., Carr, J., and Marascuilo, L.A.: A measure of association for selected nonparametric procedures, Psych. Bull., 92: 786-790, 1982.

Siegel, S., and Castellan, N.J.: Nonparametric Statistics for the Behavioral Sciences, ed. 2. New York, McGraw-Hill, 1988.

SPSS, Inc.: SPSS* User's Guide, ed. 2. New York, McGraw-Hill, 1986.

Tukey, J.W.: Comparing individual means and the analysis of variance, Biometrics, 5: 99-114, 1949.

Welch, B.L.: On the comparison of several mean values: an alternative approach, Biometrika, 38: 330-336, 1951.

Wilcoxon, F.: Individual comparisons by ranking methods, Biometrics, 3: 119-122, 1949.

Winer, B.J.: Statistical Principles in Experimental Design, ed. 2. New York, McGraw-Hill, 1971.

Chapter 10

INFERENTIAL STATISTICS FOR CORRELATED VARIABLES

10–1 CORRELATED VARIABLES IN NURSING RESEARCH

In the previous chapter, methods for univariate dependent variables were described. In this chapter, comparable methods for correlated variables are presented. Bivariate data are graphically displayed in a *scatter diagram*. Next, rationales for interpreting correlation coefficients and regression equations are presented. This is followed by a discussion of one sample test for correlation coefficients and regression slopes. Next, procedures for testing multiple regression lines for parallelism are described. This test is often neglected by researchers who perform the analysis of covariance on experimental or nonrandomized studies. The theory of part and partial correlation is described and is used to introduce one of the most important measures of statistical theory, namely, the multiple correlation coefficient. This meas-

ure of association plays an important role in both nonrandomization and randomization studies. Its use is illustrated using the preoperative teaching study. Procedures are presented for testing independent variables for statistical significance, using simultaneous test procedures and stepwise regression. Dummy coding is introduced and its role in converting the analysis of variance into a regression model is illustrated for the one-way analysis of variance and the two-way analysis of variance involving unequal sample size. Finally, the analysis of covariance is introduced and illustrated using data from the preoperative teaching study.

10–2 THE BIVARIATE SCATTER DIAGRAM

For any sample of data, it is good practice to make a visual inspection of an appropriate graph. In addition to the graphs illustrated in Chapter 8, a researcher should know how to construct and interpret a graph that shows the relationship between two variables. For a quantitative dependent and independent variable, the appropriate graph is the *scatter diagram* or *scatter plot*. An example was provided in Figure 3–1, where split-half reliability was discussed. Another example is provided in Figure 10–1. This graph shows the relationship between weight at admission to hospital and length of stay for the subjects who were exposed to treatment one of the hypothetical study on preoperative teaching. The independent variable is weight and the dependent variable is length of stay. The independent variable is plotted along the horizontal axis and the dependent variable is plotted along the vertical axis. Each dot represents the joint observation of weight and length of stay for each patient. There are 82 dots on the graph, one dot for each patient. The sample statistics for this graph are reported in Table 10–1. As reported, the mean length of stay is 4.89 days. The mean value is valid for patients who weigh as little as 109 pounds and as much as 225 pounds. This constant value is represented by the broken line that runs across Figure 10–1 parallel with the horizontal axis of the graph. The correlation coefficient between weight and length of stay is given as $r_{XY} = .48$. This suggests that using 4.89 days for all patients may not be an efficient way to evaluate the effectiveness of the treatment, because length of stay is also influenced by the weight of the patients. A better model is to use the *regression equation* to evaluate length of stay.

The regression line for predicting Y from X is given as

$$Y = \alpha + \beta X$$

α (alpha) is called the *intercept* and β (beta) is called the *slope*. In all research studies these values are unknown and must be estimated from the data. The estimates are given as

$$B = r_{XY}\left(\frac{S_Y}{S_X}\right) \quad \text{and} \quad A = \overline{Y} - B\overline{X}$$

For the data of Table 10–1,

$$B = (0.4820)\left(\frac{1.618}{24.443}\right) = 0.0319$$

and

$$A = 4.890 - (0.0319)(156.768) = -0.1109$$

so that the regression equation is given as

$$Y = -0.1109 + 0.0319X$$

This equation has been plotted on the scatter diagram of Figure 10–1. As indicated, the regression line tends to increase as weight values increase. The increase in the line is measured by the slope. As the weights increase by one pound, the length of stay in the hospital increases by .0319 day. The in-

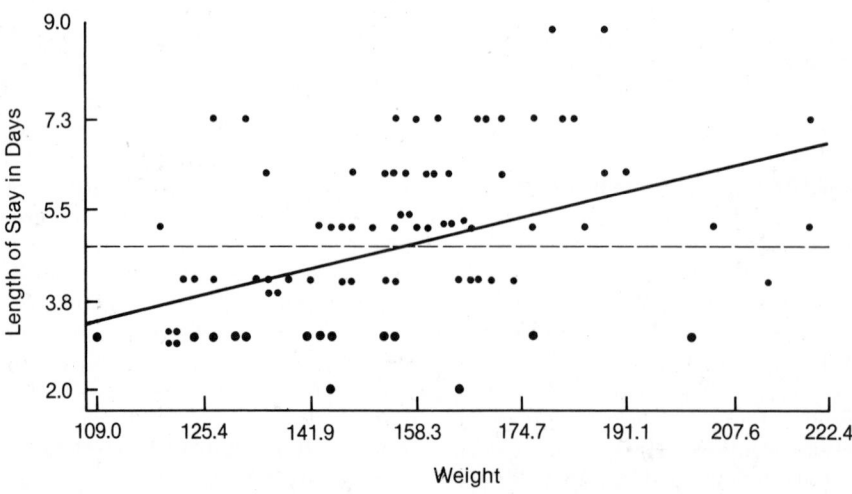

Figure 10–1. Scatter diagram showing relationship between weight at admission and length of stay of patients in treatment one.

TABLE 10−1 SAMPLE STATISTICS ASSOCIATED WITH THE SCATTER DIAGRAM OF FIGURE 10−1

Variable	Length of Stay	Weight
Mean	4.890 days	156.768 lbs.
Standard Deviation	1.618 days	24.443 lbs.
Correlation Coefficient		0.4820

tercept is not shown on the graph because the range in weight does not include anyone who weighs zero pounds. Rarely can the intercept be shown on a scatter diagram because in most cases no subject has an independent variable value equal to zero. If the regression equation is used to estimate mean length of stay in the hospital, it can be seen that the mean length of stay for patients who weigh 109 pounds is

$$Y_{110} = -0.1109 + 0.0319(109)$$
$$= 3.3662 = 3.37 \text{ days}$$

whereas for patients who weigh 225 pounds the mean length of stay is

$$Y_{225} = -0.1109 + 0.0319(225)$$
$$= 7.0666 = 7.07 \text{ days}$$

Certainly both values are different from the mean value of 4.89. This suggests that body weight is an important factor and predictor of length of stay in hospital for the patients assigned to treatment one. As such, the regression equation (solid increasing line of Fig. 10−1) should be preferred to the group mean (flat dotted line of Fig. 10−1).

10−3 INTERPRETING A CORRELATION COEFFICIENT

Throughout the earlier chapters, especially in Chapter 3, we have referred to and made extensive use of the Pearson Product Moment Correlation Coefficient, frequently referred to as a *zero order correlation coefficient*. We now wish to expand on the earlier presentations and describe what is meant by *explained variation*, a phrase used repeatedly in earlier sections. The idea of explained variation is simple, even though the

algebra can be taxing. Correlation coefficients can be generated under two statistical theories: (1) the bivariate correlation theory and (2) the univariate regression theory. We begin with the bivariate correlation theory and then examine univariate regression theory.

In *bivariate* correlation theory, two variables are correlated with one another. One of the variables, X, is the independent variable for the other variable, Y. At the same time Y is the independent variable for X. An example is provided in the joint relationship that exists between body length and weight at birth. As we all know, long babies tend to be heavy babies and short babies tend to be light babies; we also know that heavy babies tend to be long babies and that light babies tend to be short babies. Neither is body length the cause of body weight, nor body weight the cause of body length. The correlation that exists between these variables is caused by other variables associated with genetic and environmental factors. Because neither is the cause of the other, it is said that the variables, birth weight and length, are interrelated and share a *common* variance.

A basic assumption of bivariate correlation theory is that the two variables possess a joint bivariate normal distribution identified by five parameters. These parameters are the *mean values* of the two variables, the *variances* of the two variables, and the *correlation coefficient* that measures the strength of association between the two variables. For the scatter diagram of Figure 10−1 the *sample estimates* of these five parameters are reported in Table 10−1. The intercept and slope of the regression line were estimated using these five sample statistics.

A second assumption is that each variable is linearly related to the other in terms of equations called *regression equations*. A regression equation is used to predict length of stay from weight. A second regression equation is used to predict weight from length of stay. This equation can be found by reversing the roles of X and Y in the definitions of A and B. The procedure is not illustrated here.

A third assumption states that the variation about the regression lines that relate each variable to the other possesses the property of *homoscedasticity*. This property implies that the variation about a regression line is constant for any value of the independent variable. In the scatter plot of Figure 10–1, this assumption seems to be satisfied. If one chooses any two different weight values and determines the two corresponding standard deviations, it would be found that the two standard deviations do not deviate too much from each other. In other words, the variance about the regression line would be found to be constant for any weight value that is chosen. This property of *common variance* about the regression line for all values of the independent variable is the basis of the concept of *explained variation*. This property is now examined.

Denote the total variance in Y by Var(Y) and let the correlation between the two variables be denoted by ρ_{XY}. Under the assumption of homoscedasticity, it can be shown that the variance about the regression line is given by the following equation:

$$Var(Y|X) = Var(Y)(1 - \rho_{XY}^2)$$

The symbol Var(Y|X) defines the variance in Y for each specific value of X. Sometimes it is referred to as the variance in Y for fixed values of X or as the variance in Y where the effects of the variance in X are partialled out. As we know, ρ_{XY} is a number less than 1, and ρ_{XY}^2 is even smaller. The quantity $(1 - \rho_{XY}^2)$ serves as a multiplier to the Var(Y). As a consequence, it is known that Var(Y|X) is a number less than Var(Y) because it is multiplied by a number less than one. If the above equation is solved for ρ_{XY}^2 it is found that

$$\rho_{XY}^2 = \frac{Var(Y) - Var(Y|X)}{Var(Y)} = 1 - \frac{Var(Y|X)}{Var(Y)}$$

This equation states that the square of the correlation coefficient is the proportion of the total variance that remains when the variance about the regression line is subtracted. Variation about the regression line is natural variation that any variable possesses. Much of that variation is unexplainable. It results from a host of factors.

As an illustration, consider the birth length and weight example. In particular, consider all babies who are exactly 18 inches in length. Their birth weights vary. Some weigh less than 6 pounds and some weigh more than 10 pounds. A question that immediately arises about the variation in the weights at birth is, Why don't they all weigh the same amount? The question has no single answer; it has many. Some possible answers are that newborns differ in weight because:

1. in utero they were exposed to different nutritional prenatal environments because of different diet practices of their mothers,
2. they have parents with different genetic backgrounds,
3. the ages of their parents, especially that of their mothers, differed at time of conception,
4. their mothers differed in the use of coffee, tea, alcohol, cigarettes, marijuana, aspirin, and other drugs,
5. the health status of mothers varied over the length of the pregnancy,
6. there were differences in the type of work and exercise that mothers did while carrying the fetus.

The list is endless. The total list of possible sources of variation give rise to the variation that is termed *error variance*, *residual variance*, and more commonly, *unexplained variance*.

For the data of Table 10–1, the estimate of the total variance is given as

$$S_Y^2 = (1.618)^2 = 2.6179$$

This is the variance in Y if the relationship with X is completely ignored. It is known, however, the X and Y are correlated, and as a result, the variation about the regression line must be smaller. The *estimate* of this common variance is

$$S_{(Y|X)}^2 = S_Y^2(1 - r_{XY}^2)$$
$$= 2.6179(1 - 0.4820^2) = 2.0097$$

This estimate is valid for *all* values of X. As indicated, the variance about the regression line is smaller than the total variance. The total variance is equal to 2.6179, whereas the variance about the regression line is equal to 2.0097. This reduction in variance is due to the correlation that exists between the two variables. Finally, note that if the common variance is subtracted from the total variance and what is left over is divided by the total variance, it is seen that the proportion of explained variation is given as

$$r_{XY}^2 = (2.6179 - 2.0097)/2.6179 = 0.2323$$

Consider the square root of 0.2323. It is given as $r_{XY} = 0.4820$. This demonstrates that the square of the correlation coefficient is the proportion of the total variance that is explained variation.

Under this formulation, it is seen that

1. [Var(Y|X)/Var(Y)] is the proportion of variance that is unexplained and
2. [1 − Var(Y|X)/Var(Y)] is the proportion of variation that is explained variation.

Because this latter quantity is identical with $(1 − \rho^2_{XY})$, it is seen that ρ^2_{XY} is the proportion of the variance in Y that can be explained by the variance in X.

For example, suppose that the correlation coefficient between birth weight and birth length were equal to 0.7. It would be known immediately that $(0.7)^2$ or 49% of the variation in the birth weights can be attributed to the variation that exists in birth lengths. At the same time, it can be said that 49% of the birth lengths can be explained by the variation that exists in birth weights. When the relationship is reciprocal, the two variables *share* their variance. In this example, it is said that birth weight and length share 49% of their variance. The discussion on reliability presented in Chapter 3 was based on this property of correlation coefficients. All reliability and validity coefficients described earlier, as well as Cronbach's coefficient alpha, are special cases of the formulas for ρ^2_{XY} presented in this section.

The *univariate* model is now presented. In the univariate case, the same conclusions about explained variance can be reached by using a slightly different approach. In this model X is treated as the independent variable and Y is the dependent variable. The model is illustrated in Figure 10−2. Here each person's observed Y value can be subtracted from the mean value, $\overline{Y}$, of all of the observations. This difference is called the *total deviation* and can be denoted by T = $(Y − \overline{Y})$. It is represented by the difference of the plotted point from the dashed line, which represents the mean value of Y. If the two variables are correlated, the best guess of a person's *true score* is the value of the regression line determined at the value of X possessed by the person. Let this true score estimate be denoted by Y_T. This deviation is represented in Figure 10−2 by the deviation of the point to the regression line and is denoted by U = $(Y_T − \overline{Y})$. Note that it is only part of the total deviation. The other part of the deviation represents the distance of the regression line from the mean line and is denoted by E = $(Y − Y_T)$. If there were no cor-

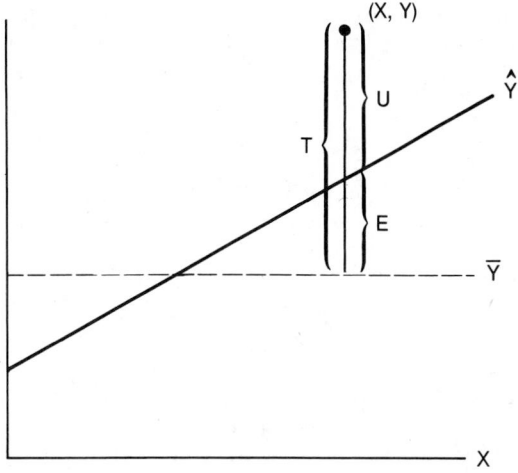

Figure 10−2. Decomposition of a total deviation into an explained and unexplained Y deviation for simple regression.

relation between the two variables, the latter deviation would be equal to zero because the regression line (solid line) and the mean line (dashed line) would be the same. Now consider the following equation:

$$T = (Y − \overline{Y}) = (Y − Y_T) + (Y_T − \overline{Y})$$

The first term on the right-hand side of the equal sign is the difference between the observed score, Y, and the estimated true score, Y_T. The question arises: Why is the difference not equal to zero? There is no simple or single answer to the question. As before, the collective answer is that the deviation of the observed value from the true value is *residual variation, error variation,* or *unexplained variation.* The second term on the right is the *explained deviation.* If we denote the total, explained, and unexplained deviations as T, E, and U, respectively, the latter equation can be written as:

$$T = U + E$$

If T, E, and U were computed for each person in a sample of size N, it could be shown that the square of the Pearson Product Moment Correlation Coefficient reduces to

$$r^2_{XY} = \frac{\Sigma E^2}{\Sigma T^2} = \frac{\Sigma (Y_T − \overline{Y})^2}{\Sigma (Y − \overline{Y})^2}$$

In this form, it is again seen that the square of the correlation coefficient identifies the proportion of the total variation that is explained variation. When there is no correlation between the two variables, each $E = 0$ so that $\Sigma E^2 = 0$, and $r_{XY}^2 = 0$; but if the correlation is equal to plus or minus one, each $E = T$ so that $\Sigma E^2 = \Sigma T^2$ and $r_{XY}^2 = 1$. The definition of reliability in Chapter 3 is a special case of this last formula.

This section ends with the comment that this discussion holds for any correlation coefficient. In the following sections part, partial, and multiple correlation coefficients are introduced. What is said here for *zero order correlation coefficients* holds equally well for all others. Thus, to determine the amount of variance that can be identified as explained variation, simply square the value of the correlation coefficient. The resulting number is the proportion of variation that is explained variation.

10–4 ONE-SAMPLE PROCEDURES FOR CORRELATION COEFFICIENTS AND REGRESSION SLOPES

In Section 10–2, it was stated that the regression line provides different estimates of the length of stay according to variations in patient's weights. The question can be asked: Are the estimates from the regression line more *efficient*, as described in Chapter 6, than the group mean of 4.89 days? The answer to the question is *yes*, provided that the correlation coefficient is statistically different from zero. Thus, a test of significance about the correlation coefficient is in order.

The test of the hypothesis,

$$H_0: \rho_{XY} = 0$$

against the alternative hypothesis,

$$H_1: \rho_{XY} \neq 0$$

is conducted with the following test statistic:

$$t = \frac{\sqrt{N - 2}\, r_{XY}}{\sqrt{1 - r_{XY}^2}}$$

If the hypothesis is true, this statistic has a t distribution with degrees of freedom given by $\nu = N - 2$. Thus, the $(1 - \alpha)$ percent decision rule for rejecting H_0 is given as

Decision rule: reject H_0 if $t < t_{\nu:\alpha/2}$

or if $t > t_{\nu:(1-\alpha/2)}$.

For the data of Table 10–1,

$$t = \frac{0.4820\sqrt{82 - 2}}{\sqrt{1 - (0.4820)^2}} = 4.92$$

With $N = 82$, $\nu = 80$ so that the 95% decision rule read from Table A–6 is given as

Decision rule: reject H_0 if $t < -2.00$
or if $t > +2.00$

The hypothesis is rejected. The correlation between length of stay and weight is significantly different from zero. Therefore the regression line provides a better description of the effects of treatment one than does the mean value of the number of days remaining in hospital after operation.

The test statistic for testing the hypothesis that a correlation coefficient is equal to zero was presented in terms of a t test. This is the way most researchers would test the hypothesis that ρ_{XY} is equal to zero. It is not the only way, however. One can also test the hypothesis in terms of an F statistic. In this case, the F statistic is simply related to the t statistic with $F = t^2$. In this case, $\nu_1 = 1$ and $\nu_2 = N - 2$. This latter form is used more frequently in multiple regression analysis than for the case of only one predictor. It is valid if and only if $\nu = 1$. This use will be seen in Section 10–9.

Another hypothesis that is of interest in a correlation and regression analysis is whether the slope of the regression line is different from zero. Because the slope of a regression line is determined directly from the correlation coefficient, the statistical test of the correlation coefficient is identical with the test of the slope being different from zero. In the example, it is known that the correlation coefficient is statistically different from zero. As a consequence, it is known immediately that the slope of the regression line is different from zero. For emphasis, testing a correlation coefficient for significance from zero is the same as testing the slope of a regression line for significance from zero.

Sometimes a nurse researcher may want to know how good is the estimate of the slope of the regression line. The answer to this question is provided in a confidence interval for the regression slope. The $(1 - \alpha)$ percent confidence interval for the slope of a regression line is given as

$$B + t_{\nu:\alpha/2}\, SE(B) < \beta < B + t_{\nu:1-\alpha/2}\, SE(B)$$

where the standard error of B in a single sample is given as

$$SE(B) = \frac{S_Y}{S_X} \sqrt{\frac{1 - r_{XY}^2}{N - 2}}$$

For the data of Table 10–1,

$$SE(B) = \frac{1.618}{24.443} \sqrt{\frac{1 - (0.4820)^2}{82 - 2}} = 0.0065$$

The 95% confidence interval for the slope is given as

$$0.0319 - 2.00(0.0065) < \beta < 0.0319 + 2.00(0.0065)$$
$$0.0189 < \beta < 0.0449$$

Note that the interval does not cover zero. This is not unexpected because a confidence interval defines all hypotheses compatible with the data. It has already been demonstrated that the slope of the regression line is statistically different from zero; therefore it is not surprising to learn that the confidence interval does not include zero.

Sometimes a nurse researcher may wish to place a confidence interval about a correlation coefficient. The process for this is more complex and requires the use of a transformation which was originally described by Sir R.A. Fisher (1948). A table of the transformation is provided in the Appendix as Table A–9. The variable in this table is traditionally denoted as z. The determination of the confidence interval is a two-step process. First, a confidence interval on the Fisher transformation scale is obtained and then on the scale of the original variable. The method is illustrated with the data of Table 10–1.

The $(1 - \alpha)$ percent confidence interval for the mean value of z is given as

$$z + Z_{\alpha/2} \frac{1}{\sqrt{N - 3}} < \mu_z < z + Z_{1-\alpha/2} \frac{1}{\sqrt{N - 3}}$$

where $Z_{\alpha/2}$ and $Z_{1-\alpha/2}$ are the $\alpha/2$ and $(1 - \alpha/2)$ percentiles of the standard normal distribution. For the example, the correlation coefficient between the two variables is equal to $r_{XY} = 0.48$. Table A–9 is entered with this value, and the value of the Fisher transformation is found to be equal to $z = .523$. With this value the confidence interval for the mean Fisher z value is given as

$$0.523 - 1.96 \frac{1}{\sqrt{82 - 3}} < \mu_z$$

$$< 0.523 + 1.96 \frac{1}{\sqrt{82 - 3}}$$

$$0.302 < \mu_z < 0.744$$

This confidence interval is on the Fisher z transformation scale and not on the scale of the correlation coefficient. To get to the scale of the correlation coefficient one must transform backward in the Fisher table. Thus, for $z = 0.302$ the lower limit is given as $\rho_{XY}^L = 0.29$ and for $z = 0.744$ the upper limit is given as $\rho_{XY}^U = 0.63$. Thus the 95% confidence interval for the correlation coefficient is given as

$$0.29 < \rho_{XY} < 0.63.$$

Special attention should be paid to the fact that the width of the confidence interval is very large. Correlation coefficients are very unstable statistics. They show a great deal of variation under random sampling. The only way to obtain a correlation coefficient that is a close estimate of a population correlation coefficient is to take an exceedingly large sample. Generally this cannot be done. As a consequence, an investigator must be prepared to contend with ambiguous results because correlation coefficients are very difficult to estimate accurately and precisely.

Finally note that the Fisher z transformation can be used to test the hypothesis that the correlation coefficient is equal to a specified value. Because this test rarely occurs, it is not described. The interested nurse can find it described in Marascuilo and Serlin (1988).

10–5 MULTIPLE SAMPLE PROCEDURES FOR CORRELATION COEFFICIENTS AND REGRESSION SLOPES

The preoperative treatment study involves three treatment groups. In the previous section we examined only the statistics for the patients assigned to treatment one. The same analysis can be performed for the remaining two treatment groups. Unfortunately, such an analysis does not result in a comparison of the three treatments. Guidelines are offered in this section for the nurse interested in making group comparisons.

A question that may arise in health care research is one that focuses on the equality of correlation coefficients across independent groups of subjects. There are a number of solutions to this problem. One solution is illustrated which should prove to be sufficient for most situations. Other methods can be found in Marascuilo and Serlin (1988). The solution described here is based on the Dunn (1961) method used extensively in Chapter 9. For the three treatment groups of the preoperative teaching study, the correlation coefficients between length of stay and weight are reported in Table 10–2. The hypothesis of interest is whether the three correlation coefficients for the three different treatments are equal to a common value. The null hypothesis is that the correlation coefficients are equal. The alternative that is examined with the Dunn procedure is that all pairwise comparisons between correlation coefficients are equal to zero. If the hypothesis should be rejected, it would be concluded that an interaction exists between treatment and weight.

The test procedure for comparing two correlation coefficients is based on the Fisher z transformation. The test statistic for a pairwise comparison involving groups one and two is given as

$$Z_{12} = \frac{z_1 - z_2}{\sqrt{\dfrac{1}{N_1 - 3} + \dfrac{1}{N_2 - 3}}}$$

The values of the test statistics for the three possible pairwise comparisons are given as

$$Z_{12} = \frac{0.523 - 0.510}{\sqrt{\dfrac{1}{82 - 3} + \dfrac{1}{82 - 3}}} = 0.08$$

$$Z_{13} = \frac{0.523 - 0.277}{\sqrt{\dfrac{1}{82 - 3} + \dfrac{1}{82 - 3}}} = 1.54$$

and

$$Z_{23} = \frac{0.510 - 0.277}{\sqrt{\dfrac{1}{82 - 3} + \dfrac{1}{82 - 3}}} = 1.46$$

TABLE 10–2 SAMPLE STATISTICS FOR TESTING EQUALITY OF CORRELATION COEFFICIENTS AND REGRESSION SLOPES*

Preoperative Teaching	Treatment		
	One	Two	Three
r_{XY}	0.4820	0.4722	0.2724
Z	0.523	0.510	0.277
B	0.0319	0.0310	0.0189
$SE(B_1)$	0.0065	0.0065	0.0075
$S^2_{(Y|X)}$	2.034	1.597	1.817
$SE(B_C)$	0.00614	0.00690	0.00749

*Sample size for each treatment is 82.

Because the total risk of a type I error is partitioned across three statistical tests, the critical values in the Dunn table are used. Because the normal distribution is a limiting distribution for the t distribution, Table A–8 is entered with an infinity degrees of freedom (see last column of Dunn's table). Thus, for C = 3 and $\alpha = .05$, the decision rule for evaluating each test statistic is given as

Decision rule: reject H_0 if $Z < -2.39$
or if $Z > +2.39$

In this case it is concluded that the correlation coefficients are not statistically different from one another.

In this example, the sample sizes are large. All three samples contain 82 subjects, and yet it is not possible to conclude that the difference between the two extreme correlation coefficients of size .27 and .48 are statistically different from one another. The point is that correlation coefficients are highly unstable and require large samples to be of theoretical or practical significance.

If desired, these estimates could now be combined to provide a more precise estimate of r_{XY} because there is evidence that all correlation coefficients are not statistically different from a common value. The procedure for pooling the correlation coefficients is as follows. First, find the weighted average, $\bar{z}$, of the Fisher z values. For K groups,

$$\bar{z} = \frac{(N_1 - 3)z_1 + (N_2 - 3)z_2 + \ldots + (N_K - 3)z_K}{(N_1 - 3) + (N_2 - 3) + \ldots + (N_K - 3)}$$

For the example,

$$\bar{z} = \frac{79(0.523) + 79(0.510) + 79(0.277)}{79 + 79 + 79} = 0.437$$

To find the average correlation, the second step involves looking into Table A–9 for the value of r_{XY}, which corresponds to $z = 0.437$. In this case, $\bar{r}_{XY} = .41$ is the best estimate of the common correlation between length of stay and weight which is valid for all three treatment groups.

Although the tests on one sample correlation coefficients and regression slopes are the same, this is not true for tests involving multiple samples. The reason for this is that the slope of a regression line is also a function of the ratio of the standard deviations of the two variables. Thus, regression lines can be parallel even if their correlation coefficients are unequal, and they can deviate from parallelism even if their correlation coefficients are equal. As in the situation for multiple correlation coefficients, there are many ways to address the question of significant differences among slopes. The approach based on pairwise comparisons is described. For other approaches, see Marascuilo and Serlin (1988).

An interesting question in health care and nursing research is that of testing regression lines for equal slopes. In Chapter 9 the notion of an interaction between two variables was introduced and procedures for testing interactions between two qualitative variables were presented. Unfortunately, the model is used in cases in which a regression model is more appropriate. For example, consider the three treatments of the preoperative training study and the variables, weight and length of stay. To determine whether treatment interacts with weight many researchers would divide the weight scale into three ordered classes labeled, *high*, *medium*, and *low*. They would then perform a two-way analysis of variance and test the hypothesis that weight and treatment did not interact. Such a design is not recommended because the high quality of measurement available in the weight measures has been replaced by a cruder measurement of weight, namely, high, medium, and low (Cronbach and Snow, 1977). The weight measures are on a scale with fine gradations based on pounds as a unit of measure. In comparison, the three-category classification scale is gross. The appropriate model is to use the weights as they are measured, to perform a regression analysis on each treatment group, and then to test the slopes of the regression lines for parallelism. If the lines are not parallel, it is concluded that weight and

treatment interact. Under this model, it is seen that testing regression lines for equal slopes is a test of interaction between a qualitative variable and a quantitative variable.

In the treatment and weight example, this translates into a question as to whether the preoperative training treatments interact with weight. If there is an interaction, the regression lines have different slopes and if the regression lines are graphed, they are seen to deviate from parallelism. If they deviate from parallelism and, moreover, if they cross, it would be concluded that a specific treatment should be used for patients of a certain weight range and that a different or other treatment be used for patients in a different weight range. This situation is illustrated in Figure 10–3. In this example, treatment three is preferred whenever $X < A$, treatment two is preferred for $A < X < B$, and treatment one is preferred if $X > B$.

In Figure 10–4 the three regression lines for the preoperative teaching study are graphed. As indicated, it appears that the lines do not differ significantly from parallelism. As a result, it would not be concluded that treatment interacts with the weight of the patients. As a first impression, it appears that treatment three is uniformly the most effective treatment.

The test statistic for testing the parallelism between the two regression lines of groups one and two is given as

$$t_{12} = \frac{B_1 - B_2}{\sqrt{SE^2(B_1) + SE^2(B_2)}}$$

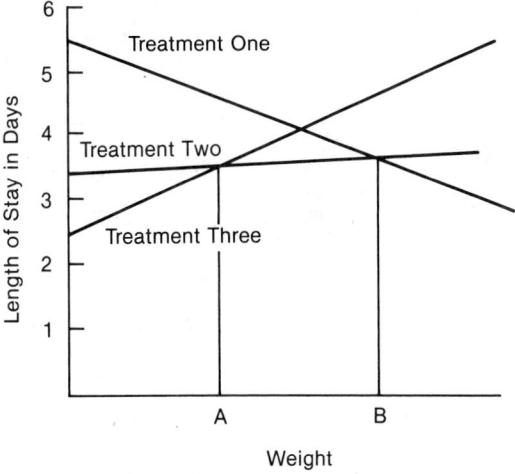

Figure 10–3. Treatment by covariate interaction for length of hospital stay and patient weight.

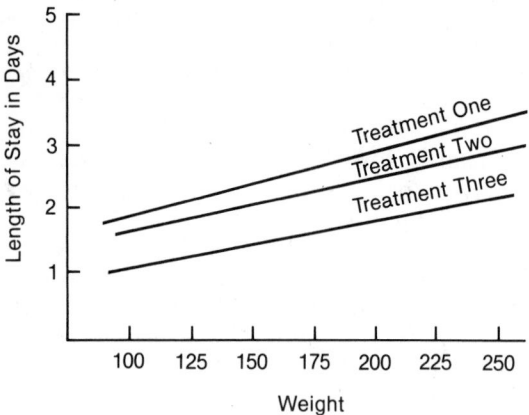

Figure 10–4. Regression lines for three preoperative teaching programs regressed on weights with length of stay as the dependent measurement.

where

$$SE^2(B_1) = \frac{\overline{S}^2_{(Y|X)}}{(N_1 - 1)S^2_{X1}}$$

$$\text{and} \quad SE^2(B_2) = \frac{\overline{S}^2_{(Y|X)}}{(N_2 - 1)S^2_{X2}}$$

and where S^2_{X1} is the variance in X for group one and S^2_{X2} is the variance in X for group two. These formulas for the squared standard errors for multiple samples differ from the formula for a single sample, as described in Section 10–3. The reason for the difference is that the methods of this section are based on the assumption that the variances about the regression lines are equal. Because the variances are assumed to be equal, a single estimate must be obtained to maintain the validity of the model being illustrated. In this case the $\overline{S}^2_{(Y|X)}$ is defined as the weighted average of the residual variances, $S^2_{(Y|Xk)}$, and where the weights are the sample sizes mi-

nus two. Thus, equation 1 below is true. The degrees of freedom associated with $\overline{S}^2_{(Y|X)}$ is given as

$$= (N_1 - 2) + (N_2 - 2) + \ldots (N_k - 2).$$

For the data of Table 10–2, equation 2 below applies.

Most computer programs do not provide estimates of the standard errors for the model being presented here. Instead, they provide the standard errors for the slopes of each regression line separately. To obtain the standard errors for this model simply perform the following arithmetic illustrated for treatment one. The standard error and residual standard deviation printed by CRUNCH (Bostrom, 1986) are given as

$$SE(B_1) = 0.0065 \text{ and } S_{(Y|X)} = \sqrt{2.034}$$
$$= 1.4262$$

These values are used with $\overline{S}_{(Y|X)} = \sqrt{1.816}$ = 1.3476 as follows to obtain the correct standard error:

$$SE(B_{1C}) = 0.0065 \left(\frac{1.3476}{1.4262} \right) = 0.00614$$

With the corrected standard errors reported in Table 10–2,

$$t_{12} = \frac{0.0319 - 0.0310}{\sqrt{(0.00614)^2 + (0.00690)^2}} = 0.21$$

$$t_{13} = \frac{0.0319 - 0.0189}{\sqrt{(0.00614)^2 + (0.00749)^2}} = 1.34$$

and

$$t_{23} = \frac{0.0310 - 0.0189}{\sqrt{(0.00690)^2 + (0.00749)^2}} = 1.19$$

①
$$\overline{S}^2_{(Y_iX)} = \frac{(N_1 - 2)S^2_{(Y_iX1)} + (N_2 - 2)S^2_{(Y_iX2)} + \ldots + (N_K - 2)S^2_{(Y_iXk)}}{(N_1 - 2) + (N_2 - 2) + \ldots + (N_k - 2)}.$$

②
$$\overline{S}^2_{(Y|X)} = \frac{(82 - 2)(2.034) + (82 - 2)(1.597) + (82 - 2)(1.817)}{(82 - 2) + (82 - 2) + (82 - 2)} = 1.816.$$

$$\overline{B} = \frac{\dfrac{0.0319}{(0.00614)^2} + \dfrac{0.0310}{(0.00690)^2} + \dfrac{0.0189}{(0.00749)^2}}{\dfrac{1}{(0.00614)^2} + \dfrac{1}{(0.00690)^2} + \dfrac{1}{(0.00749)^2}} = 0.0280$$

Because three tests are made with the familywise error rate of $\alpha = .05$, the decision rule for C = 3 and $v = 240$ is given as

Decision rule: reject H_0 if t < −2.39
and t > +2.39

Thus, it is concluded that the regression lines are parallel and that treatment and weight do not interact.

If desired, an average slope, $\overline{B}$ can now be computed because there is evidence that all three slopes are not statistically different from a common value. The average slope is found by weighting each slope by the reciprocal of its squared standard error. In this case, the equation above applies. The following are assumptions for the tests described in this section:

1. Observations within each sample are independent of one another.

2. Observations between samples are independent.

3. Regression lines are linear.

4. Variation about the lines is homoscedastistic.

5. Unexplained variances about each regression line are all equal to a common value.

These assumptions are common to the univariate and bivariate models. The tests for correlation coefficients require the residuals or error terms to have joint bivariate normal distribution or the sample sizes to be large (greater than 30). The tests for equal slopes can be justified if the latter assumption is satisfied. The test of equal slopes also can be satisfied for the univariate case if the errors for the dependent variable are normally distributed or if the sample sizes are large. In the example, the sample sizes are large, and so the tests are easy to justify.

In practice, it is very difficult to test these assumptions adequately. Assumptions 1 and 2 must be built into the design by the researcher. Assumptions 3, 4, and 5 can be evaluated by examining the scatter diagram. If the graph shows linear relationships with uniform variance about the lines for all values of X, the assumptions are most likely satisfied. In general, minor deviations are not serious and if the sample sizes are large, adherence to the assumptions is less important, because the tests are robust to violations of the assumptions.

10–6 PARTIAL AND PART CORRELATION THEORY

In the previous sections we have seen that the relationship of the treatments and the length of stay could be *confounded* by the relationship that exists between length of stay and weight of the patients. It frequently happens that one might like to study the relationship between two variables when the effects of a third, fourth, or more variables are controlled, removed, or *partialled* out. The measure of association that is used for this kind of an investigation is called a *partial* correlation coefficient, which is used when the effects of a confounding or set of confounding variables are removed from *both* of the variables to be correlated. If the unwanted variation is partialled out of only one of the variables to be correlated, the resulting measure of association is called a *part* correlation coefficient.

As an example, consider the relationship between Y: length of stay in hospital and X_1: uncertainty. This correlation can be measured directly. For the 246 subjects of the preoperative training study, this correlation coefficient is equal to $r_{YX_1} = 0.4067$. Unfortunately, the relationship between these two variables can be confounded by the correlations that exist between each of these variables with other variables. For example, the variable X_2: severity status of the patient at the time of operation is correlated with both length of stay and uncertainty. The values of the correlation coefficients are reported in Table 10–3.

Unfortunately, the high correlation between uncertainty and severity may account for some of the relationship that exists between length of stay and uncertainty. Fortunately, it is possible to remove statistically the effects of severity from both variables, and thereby have an unconfounded measurement of the relationship that exists between length of stay and uncertainty. The statistical measure used to estimate the unconfounded correlation is given by the equation,

$$r_{YX_1|X_2} = \frac{r_{YX_1} - r_{YX_2}r_{X_1X_2}}{\sqrt{1 - r_{YX_2}^2}\sqrt{1 - r_{X_1X_2}^2}}$$

where Y and X_1 are variables to be correlated and where X_2 is the variable to be controlled, held constant, or partialled out of both Y and X_1.

If we let Y represent length of stay, X_1 represent uncertainty, and X_2 represent severity, we have for the 246 patients of the preoperative training study that $r_{YX_1} = 0.4067$, $r_{YX_2} = 0.3189$, and $r_{X_1X_2} = 0.5602$, so that the partial correlation between length of stay and uncertainty with the effects of severity controlled is equal to

$$r_{YX_1|X_2} = \frac{(0.4067) - (0.3189)(0.5602)}{\sqrt{1 - (0.3189)^2}\sqrt{1 - (0.5602)^2}}$$
$$= .2905 = 0.29$$

In this case, it is seen that severity tends to increase the correlation between length of stay and uncertainty. It tends to raise the value of the correlation in the uncontrolled sample; but if the effect is statistically removed, it is seen that uncertainty and length of stay are less highly correlated.

The effects of any number of variables may be partialled out of the relationship that ex-

ists between two variables. Because the formulas are so complex, they are not provided. In practice, partial correlation coefficients are found using a computer. As a consequence, an investigator who wishes to examine partial correlation coefficients is advised to learn how to operate one or more of the prepared computer packages available for use on main frame computers or for desktop personal computers, such as the CRUNCH (Bostrom, 1986) program used in this book.

Another correlation coefficient that has the potential of greater use than the partial correlation coefficient is the *part* correlation coefficient. This measure is similar to a partial correlation coefficient except that it is based on removing the effects of a confounding variable from only one of the variables being correlated. For example, consider length of stay, uncertainty, and severity. Length of stay is positively associated with severity for patients who have a serious condition. Patients who have been classified as more severely ill prior to surgery are more apt to remain in the hospital for a longer period of time than patients whose severity level is mild. Unfortunately, the correlation between these two variables can affect the correlation between length of stay and uncertainty. To remove this confounding variable one can partial out severity from length of stay only and then correlate length of stay with uncertainty. It can be shown that the equation for this procedure can be achieved by using

$$r_{X_1(Y|X_2)} = \frac{r_{YX_1} - r_{YX_2}r_{X_1X_2}}{\sqrt{1 - r_{YX_2}^2}}$$

For the example,

$$r_{X_1(Y|X_2)} = \frac{(0.4067) - (0.3189)(0.5602)}{\sqrt{1 - (0.3189)^2}}$$
$$= 0.2406 = 0.24$$

Thus, it is seen that the correlation is lowered between length of stay and uncertainty after the effects of severity are removed on length of stay. This suggests that uncertainty has less of an impact on length of stay than indicated by the zero order correlation coefficient.

Part correlation coefficients are closely tied to partial correlations. In particular,

$$r_{X_1(Y|X_2)} = r_{YX_1|X_2}\sqrt{1 - r_{X_1X_2}^2}$$

TABLE 10–3 CORRELATIONS AMONG THE THREE VARIABLES*

	Y	X_1	X_2
Y	1.0000	0.4067	0.3189
X_1		1.0000	0.5602
X_2			1.0000

Y = length of stay in hospital; X_1 = uncertainty; X_2 = severity

This means that a part correlation can be different from zero only when its associated partial correlation coefficient is different from zero. Thus testing a partial correlation coefficient for significance from zero is the same as testing a part correlation coefficient for significance from zero. If the part correlation is equal to zero, so is the partial correlation coefficient, and vice versa.

Part correlations are useful in studying relationships where time or cause and effect relationships are thought to exist. For example, severity is expected to impact on length of stay directly. To determine the correlation between length of stay and uncertainty, it would be advisable to first partial out the effects of severity from length of stay. In this case, the part correlation is more meaningful than either the zero order correlation or the partial correlation coefficients, because the effects that severity have on length of stay have been removed.

Although the partialling out of only one variable has been illustrated, it should be noted that two, three, or any number of variables can be statistically controlled by partial and part correlation. For example, the correlation between Y and X_1 with X_2, X_3, and X_4 partialled out is generally denoted by $r_{YX_1|X_2X_3X_4}$, whereas the part correlation between Y and X_1 where X_2, X_3, and X_4 are partialled out of X_1 only, is generally denoted by $r_{Y(X_1|X_2X_3X_4)}$.

Partial correlations play a major role in understanding the relationships that exist among variables. Part correlations, however, provide a simple way to understand multiple regression and a host of designs in the analysis of variance. These are illustrated in the sections that follow.

Finally partial and part correlation coefficients can be tested for statistical significance. The equations presented in Sections 10–4 and 10–5 can be used directly as models. The only differences in the procedures are that the zero order correlation coefficients are replaced by the corresponding partial correlation measures. In addition the factors involving $(N - 2)$ or $(N - 3)$ in the formulas are replaced by other numbers. The replacement rule is easy to remember. Count the number of variables to be partialled out. Let the number be V. With this value, the factor $(N - 2)$ is replaced by $(N - V - 2)$ and the factor $(N - 3)$ is replaced by $(N - V - 3)$. The assumptions listed in Section 10–3

that are required for the bivariate case are required for the multivariate case but for P variables and not just two variables. As before, testing

$$\rho_{(YX_1|X_2)} = 0 \text{ is the same as}$$
$$\text{testing } \rho_{Y(X_1|X_2)} = 0.$$

10–7 THE MULTIPLE CORRELATION COEFFICIENT

In Table 10–3 it is seen that the correlation coefficient between length of stay and uncertainty is given as $r_{YX_1} = 0.4067$ and that the correlation between length of stay and severity is given as $r_{YX_2} = 0.3189$. A researcher might be interested in estimating the magnitude of the correlation between length of stay when uncertainty and severity are considered simultaneously as predictors of length of stay. The corresponding measure of association is called the *multiple correlation coefficient*. For Y predicted from X_1 and X_2, it is a measure of association between Y and X_1 and X_2 when taken together.

There are many ways to define this measure. One approach is described. Suppose that a decision was made to use uncertainty by itself as the only predictor for length of stay. The amount of explained variation for this single predictor is given as $r_{YX}^2 = (0.4067)^2 = 0.1654$. Now suppose that it is decided to add severity to the prediction model. Uncertainty is correlated with severity. Therefore, if severity is added directly, some of the explained variation possessed by uncertainty would be reproduced and counted a second time. To avoid this duplication of measurement, consider the part correlation of severity with length of stay where uncertainty, which is already in the model, has been removed from length of stay. This part correlation measures the variation between length of stay and severity that is free of uncertainty. The amount of this extra variation is given by the square of the part correlation between length of stay and severity where severity has been removed from uncertainty. This extra variation in length of stay explained by severity is given as $(0.1100)^2 = 0.0121$. Finally, the total amount of explained variation is given as

$$R^2 = (0.1654) + (0.0121) = 0.1775$$

The square root of this number is called the *multiple correlation coefficient* and is denoted by $R_{Y|X_1X_2}$. In this case,

$$R_{Y|X_1X_2} = 0.4213 = 0.42$$

With this example as a model, the multiple correlation coefficient for P predictors is now presented.

Consider a dependent variable Y and the set of independent variables $X_1, X_2, \ldots, X_P$. The square of the multiple correlation coefficient between the variable being predicted and the set of predictors is given as

$$R^2_{Y|X_1X_2\ldots X_P} = r^2_{YX_1} + r^2_{Y(X_2|X_1)} + r^2_{Y(X_3|X_1X_2)}$$
$$+ \ldots + r^2_{Y(X_P|X_1X_2\ldots X_{P-1})}$$

Note that the multiple correlation coefficient for our example could have been determined by using the correlation coefficient of length of stay and severity and the part correlation coefficient of length of stay with uncertainty but where severity was partialled out of uncertainty. Under this model

$$r^2_{YX_2} = (0.3189)^2 = 0.1017$$
$$\text{and } r^2_{Y(X_1|X_2)} = 0.0758$$

so that

$$r^2_{Y|X_1X_2} = 0.1017 + 0.0758 = 0.1775$$

The interrelationships that exist among zero order correlation coefficients, partial, part, and multiple correlation coefficients can be illustrated in terms of a Venn diagram. A Venn diagram consists of a series of intersecting circles that can be used to identify components of variances among correlated variables. For the data of Table 10–3, the corresponding Venn diagram is presented in Figure 10–5. In this figure, the area of each of the circles is set equal to one. Because the area of the circles are set equal to one, area is equivalent to percent variance. As shown in Figure 10–5,

1. The square of the zero order correlation between Y and X_1 is given as

$$r^2_{YX_1} = B + C = .0758 + .0896 = .1654$$

2. The square of the zero order correlation between Y and X_2 is given as

$$r^2_{YX_1} = C + D = .0896 + .0121 = .1017$$

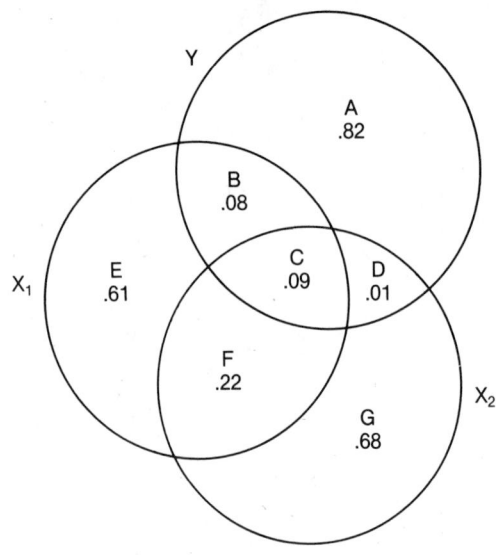

Figure 10–5. Venn diagram representation of unexplained and explained variance for simple, partial, part, and multiple correlation. E + F = 1 − .17 = .83 F + G = 1 − .10 = .90

3. The partial correlation between Y and X_1 with X_2 removed from both variables is given as

$$r^2_{YX_1|X_2} = B/(A + B) = .0758/(.8225 + .0758)$$
$$= .0844$$

4. The partial correlation between Y and X_2 with X_1 removed from both variables is given as

$$r^2_{YX_2|X_1} = D/(A + D) = .0121/(.8225 + .0121)$$
$$= .0145$$

5. The part correlation between Y and X_1 with X_2 removed from X_1 is given as

$$r^2_{Y(X_1|X_2)} = B = .0758$$

6. The part correlation between Y and X_2 with X_1 removed from both variables is given as

$$r^2_{Y(X_2|X_1)} = D = .0121$$

and

7. The multiple correlation between Y and X_1 and X_2 is given as

$$R^2_{Y|X_1X_2} = B + C + D$$
$$= (B + C) + D$$
$$= .1654 + .0121 = .1775$$
$$= (C + D) + B = .1017 + .0758$$
$$= .1775$$

Item number 7 illustrates the manner in which the multiple correlation coefficient is determined as the sum of the square of a zero order correlation and squared part correlations. For the first illustration (B + C) is the squared zero order correlation of uncertainty with length of stay and D is the squared part correlation of severity with length of stay after the correlation of severity with uncertainty removed.

Examination of the Venn diagram of Figure 10–5 also helps to show how a part correlation is a component of a total correlation. For example, the squared correlation between length of stay and uncertainty is given as (B + C). The part correlation of uncertainty with length of stay after the correlation with severity has been removed from uncertainty is B.

After the multiple correlation coefficient has been estimated from the sample data, what is its usefulness as an estimate of the unknown population value? In other words, is the sample value reliable as an indicator of the strength of the association of Y with its predictors in the population? This question is answered by testing the hypothesis that the population multiple correlation coefficient is statistically different from zero. The test of the hypothesis,

$$H_0: R_{Y|X_1X_2...X_P} = 0$$

against the alternative,

$$H_1: R_{Y|X_1X_2...X_P} \neq 0$$

is made in terms of the test statistic:

$$F = \frac{N - P - 1}{P}\left(\frac{R^2_{Y|X_1X_2...X_P}}{1 - R^2_{Y|X_1X_2...X_P}}\right)$$

If H_0 is true, then the sampling distribution of F has an F distribution with $v_1 = P$ and $v_2 = (N - P - 1)$. For length of stay predicted from uncertainty and severity, the test of significance of the multiple correlation coefficient is given as

$$F = \frac{82 - 2 - 1}{2}\left(\frac{0.1775}{1 - 0.1775}\right) = 26.22$$

The decision rule for $\alpha = 0.05$ and $v_1 = P = 2$ and $v_2 = N - P - 1 = 246 - 2 - 1 = 243$ is given as

Decision rule: reject the hypothesis if
$$F_{2,\infty:0.95} > 3.00$$

The hypothesis of no association is rejected. Length of stay is correlated with uncertainty and severity when they are taken in union.

Regression analyses are often summarized in an analysis of variance table. For this presentation the sum of squares total is given as

$$SS\ (Total) = (N - 1)S^2_Y$$

with

$$SS\ (Regression) = SS(Total)R^2_{Y|X_1X_2...X_P}$$

and

$$SS\ (Residual) = SS(Total)(1 - R^2_{Y|X_1X_2...X_P})$$

For our example,

$$
\begin{aligned}
SS\ (Total) \quad &= (246 - 1)(1.6129)^2 \\
&= 637.3500 \\
SS\ (Regression) &= (637.350)(0.1775) \\
&= 133.1296
\end{aligned}
$$

and

$$
\begin{aligned}
SS\ (Residual) &= (637.350)(0.8225) \\
&= 524.2203
\end{aligned}
$$

The ANOVA table is reported in Table 10–4. Note that in multiple regression theory,

$$\hat{\eta}^2 = R^2_{Y|X_1X_2...X_P} = \frac{SS(Regression)}{SS(Total)}$$

This is demonstrated in Table 10–4.

The statistical test that the multiple correlation coefficient is equal to zero can be justified under the correlation model and regression model described in Section 10–3. The only difference is that the models must hold for P variables instead of two variables. Unfortunately, it is almost impossible to verify the assumptions when P is large. A safe rule is to choose a large sample, where large means a sample size that exceeds 20P. Thus, a study with P = 2 predictors should be based on at least 40 subjects. For a more complete discussion on sample size and statistical power, consult Cohen (1977).

Often a researcher wants to test the hypothesis that two multiple correlation coefficients from independent groups of subjects are equal to a common value. There is no statistical test of this hypothesis. A little thought shows why. Two multiple correla-

TABLE 10–4 ANOVA TABLE FOR LENGTH OF STAY IN HOSPITAL PREDICTED FROM UNCERTAINTY AND SEVERITY

Source of Variation	d/f	SS	MS	F	$\hat{\eta}^2$
Regression	2	113.1296	56.565	26.72*	0.1775
Residual	243	524.2203	2.157		
Total	245	637.3500			

*Significant at $\alpha = 0.05$

tion coefficients could be equal to a common value for different reasons. The multiple correlations for the two sets of zero order correlations reported in Table 10–5 are equal even though the relationships reported are different. As this example demonstrates, testing for equality of multiple correlation coefficients does not produce information that is meaningful. One solution to the problem of determining whether two multiple correlation coefficients are based on the same *correlation structure* is to test the zero order correlation coefficients one by one for significance in a set of pairwise comparisons, as illustrated in Section 10–5. If any pair leads to rejection, then it is known that the correlation structures are different from one another. There is, however, a problem with this approach. If P is large, the risk of at least one type I error approaches 1 in numerical value. One way to avoid this problem is to count the number of pairwise comparisons and then to use the Dunn tables to achieve the proper statistical control. For P variables, the number of pairwise comparisons is given as $C = P(P - 1)/2$.

There are other ways to introduce multiple correlations. Examples are provided in Marascuilo and Levin (1983). The approach presented in this chapter is used directly in the following sections. It should be emphasized that any attempt to perform a multiple regression analysis without a computer is not recommended.

10–8 THE MULTIPLE REGRESSION EQUATION

When there is one predictor, the regression equation is defined as $Y = \alpha + \beta X$ and is estimated in a sample as $Y = A + BX$. For P predictors the *multiple regression equation* is defined as

$$Y = \alpha + \beta_1 X_1 + \beta_2 X_2 + \ldots + \beta_P X_P$$

and is estimated as

$$Y = A + B_1 X_1 + B_2 X_2 + \ldots + B_P X_P$$

The formulas required to estimate the *beta weights* are very complicated and are not reported here. For the example, the multiple regression equation for predicting length of stay from uncertainty and severity taken for the computer printout of the CRUNCH (Bostrom, 1986) program is given as

$$Y_T = 0.3452 + 0.0691 X_1 + 0.2659 X_2$$

These values are reported in Table 10–6.

The intercept is given by $A = 0.3452$. It represents the mean length of stay for patients who have a severity level of zero and whose uncertainty score is zero. No such patients exist in the study, and so the measure lacks interpretation. This is true in most studies. In most studies, a researcher is advised to ignore the value of this coefficient. The slope for uncertainty is given as $B_1 = 0.0691$. It shows that as the uncertainty

TABLE 10–5 DIFFERENT CORRELATION STRUCTURES WITH EQUAL MULTIPLE CORRELATION COEFFICIENTS

	Group One				Group Two		
	Y	X_1	X_2		Y	X_1	X_2
Y	1.00	0.70	0.30	Y	1.00	0.30	0.70
X_1		1.00	0.20	X_1		1.00	0.20
X_2			1.00	X_2			1.00

TABLE 10–6 SAMPLE STATISTICS FOR TESTING BETA WEIGHTS

Variable	Slope	Standard Error	t Statistic
Uncertainty	0.0691	0.0146	4.73*
Severity	0.2659	0.1407	1.88
Intercept	0.3452		

*Significant at $\alpha = 0.05$

scores increases by 1 point, the mean length of stay increases by .0691 days. Thus, two people whose uncertainty scores differ by 10 points are expected to differ in mean length of stay with the person with the higher score staying an extra 0.691 or 0.7 of a day.

The interpretation of the slope for the severity variable is more complicated because of the way the variables were reported and scaled. Remember that severity was defined by the ordered classes: mild, moderate, and severe and was scored by the numbers 1, 2, and 3. The slope of $B_2 = 0.2659$ represents the change in the length of stay as one moves one class up the scale. The mean difference in length of stay for patients who differ by mild and moderate levels of severity is 0.2659 days or about one fourth of a day. This is also true for patients who differ in moderate and severe classifications. The mean difference between mild and severe patients is 0.5318 or a little more than an extra half-day stay in the hospital. Care is required when trying to interpret beta weights. If the original variable is quantitative, the interpretation is simple; but if the measured variable actually represents a numerical code for an ordered qualitative variable, care is required.

This example demonstrates a very flexible property of regression analysis. Variables with a small number of outcome values can be used for predictive and explanatory purposes. Normality is not required and continuity of variables can be ignored, provided that the sample size is large.

10–9 TESTING BETA WEIGHTS FOR STATISTICAL SIGNIFICANCE

After a multiple regression equation has been determined, a researcher might want to know whether

1. all of the variables in the equation are necessary,
2. all of the variables are true predictors of the dependent measure and,
3. any of the variables can be removed to provide a simpler explanation of the findings?

There are many ways to answer these kinds of questions. Some are provided by Marascuilo and Levin (1983), Marascuilo and Serlin (1988), and Draper and Smith (1981). One

model is presented here, which is perhaps the most commonly used model in the behavioral sciences. This model reduces to the performance of a series of t or F tests on the slopes of the regression line. It is based on the test described in Section 10–4, with the exception being that the degrees of freedom of the test are not given as

$$\nu = N - 2$$

but by

$$\nu = N - P - 1$$

As an example, consider predicting length of stay from uncertainty and severity. The basic statistics are provided in Table 10–6. The figures are copied from a computer printout generated by CRUNCH (Bostrom, 1986). There are two slopes to test. The values of the test statistics for the two slopes are given as

$$t_1 = \frac{B_1}{SE(B_1)} = \frac{0.0691}{0.0146} = 4.73$$

and

$$t_2 = \frac{B_2}{SE(B_2)} = \frac{0.2659}{0.1407} = 1.88$$

If each test is performed with $\alpha = 0.05$ the decision rule for rejection based on

$$\nu = N - P - 1 = 246 - 2 - 1 = \\ 243 \text{ degrees of freedom}$$

is given as

Decision rule: reject the hypothesis if
$$t < -1.96 \text{ or if } t > +1.96$$

In this case the hypothesis that the slope is equal to zero is rejected for uncertainty but not for severity. Thus, severity is not necessary in the prediction equation. This agrees with the data. Recall that the $r^2_{Y|X_1X_2} = 0.1775$ and that

$$r^2_{YX} = r^2_{YX_1} = (0.4067)^2 = 0.1654$$

By itself, uncertainty accounts for 16.54% of the variation. When severity is added, the increase to 17.75% is a miniscule 1.21%. This is not enough to be considered important.

Each of the t tests could be performed as F tests. In this case,

$$F_1 = (4.73)^2 = 22.87 \text{ and}$$
$$F_2 = (1.88)^2 = 3.53$$

Under this model, rejection of the hypothesis of zero slope would be made if $F > F_{1,243:0.95} = 3.84$. As before, the null hypothesis that uncertainty is not a significant predictor of length of stay is rejected.

Frequently a researcher has a number of multiple regression equations to be compared. For example, a regression equation could be generated for each of the three treatments and the question could be asked as to whether the slopes for each of the variables across the regression equations were equal to a common value. The procedures for testing equal slopes described in Section 10–5 could be used to make these comparisons. This analysis provides a test of the hypothesis that the three treatment groups interact with the predictors. The assumptions that were required for the single sample case would have to be assumed to justify the analysis for the multiple sample case.

10–10 STEPWISE REGRESSION

Whereas the model of Section 10–9 is used most frequently, other models have been developed for determining which dependent variables are important in a regression equation. Even though it was not illustrated, one advantage of using the model of Section 10–9 is that Dunn's method can be applied to control the risk of making at least one type I error. The model to be described in this section does not have this feature. It is based on a logical approach to decision making that may have intuitive appeal. The method is called *stepwise regression*. Even though it uses decision rules based on the F distribution, the risks of making type I errors are unknown; yet, it is a very popular and useable model. It must be used with care because only the risk of a type I error associated with

the first step is valid. Type I error rates for all subsequent tests are unknown because all remaining tests are conditionally correlated (Cohen and Cohen, 1983). Even so, Cohen and Cohen recommend stepwise regression under the following stringent conditions:

1. The research goal is primarily predictive and not explanatory.
2. The ratio of sample size N to number of variables P is at least 40 to 1.
3. The results are cross-validated or replicated on a second sample.

Other reasons for using care in the performance of a stepwise regression are that in studies with a large number of independent variables, some could be statistically significant only on the basis of chance and might inadvertently be included in the regression equation. There is very little assurance that a second sample will include the same variables if they are entered into the equation in the same order. If two independent variables are highly correlated, only one is likely to get into the equation because of the high redundancy in information between the two variables. For further discussion on these topics, see Wampold and Freund (1987).

There are many forms of stepwise regression. An excellent presentation can be found in Draper and Smith (1981). In this section a model that is commonly referred to as *forward selection* or simply *forward stepwise regression* is described. It is illustrated with data from the hypothetical preoperative teaching study.

Consider the variables that are thought to be antecedent to prognosis following operation. In this case, the complete set is defined by sex, age, severity, education, income, weight, smoking history, alcohol usage, drug abuse status, exercise, and score on the uncertainty scale. Consider correlating length of stay with these variables. The analysis of variance table for this is presented in Table 10–7. As indicated, these variables collectively explain about 39% of the total varia-

TABLE 10–7 ANOVA TABLE FOR PREDICTING LENGTH OF STAY FROM 12 INTERRELATED ANTECEDENT VARIABLES

Source	d/f	SS	MS	F Ratio	$\hat{\eta}^2$
Regression	12	249.013	20.751	12.451*	0.3907
Residual	233	388.337	1.667		
Total	245	637.350			

*Significant at $\alpha = 0.05$

tion. The t tests for these 12 predictors are given, respectively, as 2.97, 1.94, −1.02, 0.76, 0.83, −0.48, 3.75, 4.90, 0.79, 0.00, 2.87, and 4.06 and reported in Table 10−8. As indicated, only five variables have test statistics that are in the rejection region defined by the decision rule.

Decision rule: reject if $t < -1.96$
or if $t > +1.96$

The remaining seven variables apparently contribute little to the magnitude of the correlation with length of stay. We should note that the maximum risk of at least one type I error with this hypothesis testing model is given as $\alpha_T < P\alpha$. In this example, P = 12, so that the maximum risk of at least one type I error is given as $\alpha_T = 12(.05) = .60$. Many researchers would find this an exceptionally high risk of error.

The predictor with the largest t value is *smoking*. It is identified as the main predictor of length of stay. The next largest t value is associated with *uncertainty*. If uncertainty is added to smoking as a predictor, a researcher might like to know whether the addition is large enough to improve the prediction. Improved prediction is always guaranteed if the part correlation of uncertainty with length of stay with the effects of smoking removed from uncertainty is statistically different from zero. Although improvement is ensured, the additional improvement may prove to be miniscule. In any case, the test of a partial correlation by a stepwise regression approach is illustrated here.

At *step one*, an examination is made of the correlation coefficients between each of the predictors and the dependent variables. These correlations are reported in Table 10−9 for the example. As indicated, the largest correlation with length of stay is smoking. Length of stay is now regressed on smoking. This analysis is summarized in Table 10−10. As indicated, smoking explains about 24% of the variance. The amount explained is significantly different from zero because F = 76.64 is in the critical region defined by

$$F > F_{1,244:0.95} = 3.84$$

The remaining 15% of the explained variation must be associated with the remaining 11 dependent variables. At this point in the stepwise process, the goal is to identify the variable that explains the most of this variation.

At *step two*, smoking is partialled out of each of the prospective second predictors, and the part correlation of each of the variables with the dependent variable is determined. The variable with the largest part correlation is identified and placed in the regression equation. In practice, this is not done because it is easier to compute and ex-

TABLE 10−8 TESTS OF THE SLOPES OF THE 12 PREDICTORS USED IN THE ANALYSIS OF VARIABLE TABLE 10−7

Variable	Slope	t Test	F Test
1. Sex	0.5661	2.97*	8.80*
2. Age	0.0240	1.94	3.73
3. Severity	−0.1370	−1.02	1.03
4. Education	0.0188	0.76	0.58
5. Provider	0.1568	0.83	0.69
6. Income	−0.0337	−0.48	0.23
7. Weight	0.0178	3.75*	14.04*
8. Smoking	0.4622	4.90*	23.99*
9. Alcohol	0.0818	0.79	0.63
10. Drug abuse	−0.0170	0.00	0.00
11. Exercise	0.7423	2.87*	8.21*
12. Uncertainty	0.0546	4.06*	16.52*

*Significant at $\alpha = 0.05$

TABLE 10−9 THE CORRELATION COEFFICIENTS OF EACH OF THE 12 PREDICTORS OF TABLE 10−7 WITH LENGTH OF STAY

Variable	Correlation Coefficient
1. Sex	0.02
2. Age	0.42
3. Severity	0.32
4. Education	−0.11
5. Provider	−0.08
6. Income	−0.05
7. Weight	0.40
8. Smoking	0.49
9. Alcohol	0.07
10. Drug abuse	−0.06
11. Exercise	−0.04
12. Uncertainty	0.41

TABLE 10−10 STEP ONE IN THE STEPWISE REGRESSION ON LENGTH OF STAY

Source	d/f	SS	MS	F Ratio	$\hat{\eta}^2$
Regression	1	152.348	152.348	76.64*	0.2390
Residual	244	485.002	1.988		
Total	245	637.350			

*Significant at $\alpha = 0.05$

amine the partial correlation coefficients directly. As stated in Section 10–6, part correlations are related to partial correlation coefficients. Part correlation coefficients differ from zero only if their associated partial correlation coefficient differs from zero. The partial correlation coefficients of each of the potential second predictors are shown in Table 10–11. Also reported are the corresponding t and F statistics. As indicated, the variable with the highest partial correlation coefficient is uncertainty. This variable is joined with smoking on the second step and the stepwise process continues. The results of this are summarized in Table 10–12.

As indicated, the proportion of variation explained by X_8 (smoking) and X_{12} (uncertainty) is given as

$$R^2_{Y|X_8X_{12}} = 0.3049$$

The additional amount of explained variation is given as

$$r^2_A = 0.3049 - 0.2390 = 0.0659$$

Now it is necessary to determine whether this additional amount of explained variation is significantly different from zero. This is done in terms of the following test statistic, which is frequently called the *F added test*:

$$F = \frac{(N - p - 1)r^2_A}{1 - r^2_{Y|X_1X_2...X_p}}$$

TABLE 10–11 THE PARTIAL CORRELATION COEFFICIENTS OF EACH PREDICTOR WITH LENGTH OF STAY WHERE SMOKING HAS BEEN PARTIALLED OUT OF EACH VARIABLE

Variable	Partial Correlation	t Statistic	F Statistic
1. Sex	0.0805	1.26	1.59
2. Age	0.2106	3.36*	11.28*
3. Severity	0.1201	1.89	3.56
4. Education	−0.0326	−0.51	0.26
5. Provider	0.0114	0.17	0.03
6. Income	−0.0067	−0.10	0.01
7. Weight	0.2768	4.49*	20.16*
9. Alcohol	0.0509	0.79	0.63
10. Drug abuse	−0.0364	0.57	0.32
11. Exercise	0.0339	0.53	0.28
12. Uncertainty	0.2943	4.80*	23.04*

*Significant at $\alpha = 0.05$

TABLE 10–12 ANOVA TABLE WITH SMOKING AND UNCERTAINTY AS PREDICTORS

Source	d/f	SS	MS	F Ratio	$\hat{\eta}^2$
Regression	2	194.356	97.178	53.306*	0.3049
Residual	243	442.993	1.823		
Total	245	637.349			

*Significant at $\alpha = 0.05$

where p is the number of variables in the equation including the one being evaluated for addition to the regression equation. Under random sampling this statistic has an F distribution with $v_1 = 1$ and $v_2 = N - p - 1$. In this case with smoking and uncertainty in the equation, p = 2, so that

$$F = \frac{(246 - 2 - 1)(0.0659)}{(1 - 0.3049)} = 23.04$$

Because

$$F > F_{1,243:0.95} = 3.84$$

the hypothesis that the additional amount of explained variance is equal to zero is rejected. Note that the value of this test statistic is identical with that reported in Table 10–11 for the test of the partial correlation associated with uncertainty. With most computer programs the test of additional variance need not be performed because it is identical with the test of the partial correlation coefficient performed on the previous step.

At *step three*, the remaining partial correlation coefficients are tested for significance to determine which variable should be included next. The partial correlations are reported in Table 10–13. The largest F statistic is associated with X_7 (weight). This is the variable added to the regression equation at step three. The ANOVA table for this step is shown in Table 10–14. As indicated, the total amount of explained variance has increased from 0.3049 to 0.3458.

On *step four*, sex is added to the regression equation. Because the increase in the squared multiple correlation coefficient is so small, the stepwise regression process is terminated at this point. The regression equation for predicting Y (length of stay) from X_8 (smoking), X_{12} (uncertainty), and X_7 (weight) is given as

TABLE 10–13 THE PARTIAL CORRELATION COEFFICIENTS OF EACH PREDICTOR WITH LENGTH OF STAY WHERE SMOKING AND UNCERTAINTY HAVE BEEN PARTIALLED OUT OF EACH VARIABLE

Variable	Partial Correlation	F Statistic
1. Sex	0.0520	0.66
2. Age	0.1652	6.79*
3. Severity	−0.0268	0.17
4. Education	0.0452	0.50
5. Provider	0.0288	0.20
6. Income	0.0232	0.13
7. Weight	0.2424	15.11*
9. Alcohol	0.0737	1.32
10. Drug abuse	−0.0499	0.60
11. Exercise	0.0833	1.69

*Significant at $\alpha = 0.05$

TABLE 10–14 REGRESSION ANALYSIS BASED ON SMOKING, UNCERTAINTY, AND WEIGHT USED AS PREDICTORS OF LENGTH OF STAY

Source	d/f	SS	MS	F Ratio	$\hat{\eta}^2$
Regression	3	220.397	73.466	42.64*	0.3458
Residual	242	416.952	1.723		
Total	245	637.349			

*Significant at $\alpha = 0.05$

$$Y = -1.6258 + 0.4753X_8 + 0.0493X_{12} + 0.0160X_7$$

The F added test has been described in terms of measurements of explained variance. This practice is not followed by all computer program authors. Some use sum of squares added in the F tests. This is not important because both models lead to the same conclusions. In practice, measurements of explained variance are used more frequently in multiple regression studies, whereas in the analysis of variance models sums of squares are preferred.

Occasionally an independent variable that enters at an early step in the process fails to maintain explanatory properties, because other variables appearing at a later step mask its correlation with the dependent variable. This can be detected by the F statistic associated with the corresponding partial correlation coefficient. If the F statistic is in the nonrejection region, the variable is removed on the next step. Many computer programs provide an option for making these kinds of deletions. It did not happen in the example because the number of variables finally retained was small. If many independent variables are used in a stepwise regression analysis, deletions may occur.

This example illustrates a common occurrence in social, behavioral, and health care science research. The process of stepwise regression halts after the first few steps. The reason for early termination in the process is that independent variables tend to be highly intercorrelated and, thus, share redundant information about the dependent measure. Independent variables should be selected based on prior research, theoretical rationales, and empirical knowledge. In the absence of these conditions, a recommended strategy is to choose variables that are highly correlated with the dependent variable but poorly correlated with the other independent variables included in the study.

10–11 DUMMY CODING OF VARIABLES AND THE ANALYSIS OF VARIANCE FOR UNEQUAL SAMPLE SIZES

Stepwise regression is one of the most efficient and flexible statistical models available to a nurse investigator. In Chapter 9, the analysis of variance was described for the case in which the number of subjects in each cell of the design was equal to a common value. This rarely occurs in practice, and so the models described in Chapter 9 are somewhat limiting. Stepwise regression can be used effectively to perform an ANOVA when sample sizes vary across the groups. The way to achieve this goal is to introduce new variables into the design called *dummy variables*.

Dummy variables are actually *coding variables* that permit a quantitative scoring of the categories of qualitative variables. There are many ways to code variables. For discussions of this topic, see Cohen and Cohen (1983), Pedhazur (1982), Marascuilo and Levin (1983), and Marascuilo and Serlin (1988). A coding scheme that is easy to use is described for a one-way analysis of variance for length of stay and the three treatment groups of the hypothetical preoperative teaching study.

Binary codes are assigned to each of the three treatments. In particular, this coding is achieved with two dummy variables. If there had been six treatment groups, five dummy variables would be needed. In general, if there are K groups to be coded, K − 1 dummy variables are required. For the first dummy variable the following code is assigned. Let $D_1 = 1$ if the subject is a member of treatment one and 0 otherwise. For the second dummy variable, let $D_2 = 1$ if the subject is in treatment two and 0 otherwise. This generates the following code scheme:

Treatment	D_1	D_2
One	1	0
Two	0	1
Three	0	0

As indicated, subjects in treatment one are dummy coded as (1,0), subjects in treatment two are dummy coded as (0,1), and subjects in treatment three are dummy coded as (0,0).

The dummy variables are now used as predictor variables for a multiple regression analysis described in Section 10−7. The results of this analysis are reported in Table 10−15. As indicated, the F ratio is given as F = 23.65. If the figures of this table are compared with those of Table 9−4, it is seen that the tables are identical. The multiple regression equation that connects length of stay to the two dummy variables is given as

$$Y = 3.3658 + 1.5244D_1 + 1.1585D_2$$

The mean values for the three treatments can be determined from this equation by substitution for the dummy coded values. Thus,

$$\overline{Y}_1 = 3.3658 + 1.5244(1) + 1.1585(0) = 4.89$$

$$\overline{Y}_2 = 3.3658 + 1.5244(0) + 1.1585(1) = 4.52$$

$$\overline{Y}_3 = 3.3658 + 1.5244(0) + 1.1585(0) = 3.37$$

These means may now be submitted to a post hoc analysis as shown in Chapter 9.

As this example shows, the analysis of variance is a special case of multiple regression theory in which the categories of a qualitative variable have been transformed to a quantitative form. This transformation is achieved by dummy coding.

The real advantage in using dummy coding is found in factorial designs with unequal sample sizes. As an example, consider the design illustrated in Table 10−16. Represented is a two-factor fully crossed design in which the independent variables are treatment and sex. As indicated, the cell sample sizes range from a low of 30 to a high of 52. To perform the analysis we have to generate dummy codes for each main effect and for the interaction. The number of dummy variables for

1. the main effect for sex is given as $v_S = S − 1$ where S = number of levels of sex,
2. the main effect for treatment is given as $v_T = T − 1$ where T = number of treatment groups, and
3. the two-factor interaction is given as $v_{SxT} = (S − 1)(T − 1)$.

For this example, S = 2 and T = 3 so that the number of dummy variables needed for each source of variance is 1, 2, and 3, respectively.

Because dummy variables have already been defined for treatment, only codes for sex and the interaction need to be defined. For sex, define the dummy variable as D_3. It equals 0 if the subject is male and 1 if the subject is female. The codes for treatment and sex are listed according to cell membership. To obtain the dummy variables for the interaction, simply multiply the dummy variables across the two sets of main effects. Thus, $D_4 = D_1 \times D_3$ and $D_5 = D_2 \times D_3$. The coding scheme is as follows:

TABLE 10−15 ANOVA ON TREATMENT USING DUMMY CODES TO PREDICT LENGTH OF STAY

Source	d/f	SS	MS	F Ratio	$\hat{\eta}^2$
Regression	2	103.862	51.931	23.65*	0.1630
Residual	243	533.488	2.195		
Total	245	637.350			

*Significant at $\alpha = 0.05$

TABLE 10−16 DISTRIBUTION OF PATIENTS ACCORDING TO SEX AND TREATMENT

	Treatment Group			
Sex	*One*	*Two*	*Three*	**Total**
Male	30	35	35	100
Female	52	47	47	146
Total	82	82	82	246

Cell in the Design	Treatment		Sex	Interaction	
	D_1	D_2	D_3	D_4	D_5
Male × treatment one	1	0	0	0	0
Male × treatment two	0	1	0	0	0
Male × treatment three	0	0	0	0	0
Female × treatment one	1	0	1	1	0
Female × treatment two	0	1	1	0	1
Female × treatment three	0	0	1	0	0

Because the sample sizes are unequal, care must be taken to run the stepwise regression correctly. The solution that has gained the most acceptance operates as follows and is based on recommendations of Carlson and Timm (1974), which is based on sums of squares rather than measures of explained variation. To determine the sum of squares associated with each source of variance a *forced stepwise regression* model is used. In this model, every dummy variable except the variables of interest are forced into the regression equation at step one. At step two the variables of interest are inserted simultaneously. The sum of squares associated with the source of interest is found by subtraction.

To find the sum of squares associated with sex, dummy variables D_1, D_2, D_4, and D_5 are entered at step one. The sum of squares at this step is given as 115.544. At step two, D_3 is entered. The sum of squares at this step is given as 121.364. Thus, the sum of squares associated with sex is read from the printout and is given as

$$\text{SS (Sex)} = 121.364 - 115.544 = 5.82$$

To find the sum of squares associated with treatment, dummy variables D_3, D_4, and D_5 are entered at step one. The sum of squares at this step is given as 33.456. Thus, the sum of squares associated with treatment is taken from the printout and is given as

$$\text{SS (Treatment)} = 121.364 - 33.456$$
$$= 87.908$$

To find the sum of squares associated with the interaction of sex with treatment, dummy variables D_1, D_2, and D_3 are entered at step one. The sum of squares at this step is read from the printout and is given as 103.875. Thus the sum of squares associated with the interaction is given as

$$\text{SS (Sex × treatment)} = 121.364 - 103.875$$
$$= 17.489$$

The mean square residual can be found at any of the final steps for the three separate computer runs. In this case, the sum of squares residual is given as SS (Residual) = 515.986.

The complete ANOVA table is reported in Table 10–17. Both the treatment and the sex by treatment interaction are statistically significant because both F statistics are larger than $F_{2,\infty:0.95} = 3.00$. Sex is not significant because the F ratio is smaller than the 95th percentile value of 3.84. The regression equation relating the dummy variables to length of stay is given as

$$Y = 3.0571 + 2.3094D_1 + 1.3429D_2$$
$$+ 0.5386D_3 - 1.2899D_4 - 0.3216D_5$$

This equation can be used to determine the cell means. To determine the mean value for the males in treatment one, the dummy code values of $D_1 = 1$, $D_2 = 0$, $D_3 = 0$, $D_4 = 0$, and $D_5 = 0$ are used. With these values

$$\overline{Y}_{\text{males × treatment one}} = 3.0571 + 2.3094(1)$$
$$+ 1.3429(0)$$
$$+ 0.5386(0)$$
$$- 1.2899(0)$$
$$- 0.3216(0)$$
$$= 5.3665 = 5.37 \text{ days}$$

TABLE 10–17 ANOVA TABLE FOR TREATMENT BY SEX WITH LENGTH OF STAY AS THE DEPENDENT VARIABLE

Source	d/f	SS	MS	F
Sex	1	5.820	5.820	2.71
Treatment	2	87.908	43.954	20.44*
S × T	2	17.489	8.745	4.06*
Residual	240	515.986	2.150	
Total	245	627.203†		

*Significant at $\alpha = 0.05$

†Total is not 637.350 because of the unequal sample sizes.

TABLE 10–18 MEAN VALUES FOR THE DESIGN OF TABLE 10–6

Sex	Treatment Group			Total
	One	Two	Three	
Male	5.3665	4.4000	3.0571	4.22
Female	4.6152	4.6170	3.5957	4.28
Total	4.89	4.52	3.37	4.26

The remaining mean values are reported in Table 10–18. Because the hypotheses for treatment and the sex by treatment interaction are significant, post hoc contrasts, as illustrated in Chapter 9 would now be performed.

10–12 THE ANALYSIS OF COVARIANCE

The analysis of covariance (ANCOVA) was developed by R.A. Fisher originally to reduce error variance in experimental studies and has been described in detail by Cochran (1957). Recently the model has been adopted by social scientists to provide statistical control in quasi-experiments. Among some researchers there is doubt that the latter use of ANCOVA is justified (Porter and Raudenbush, 1987). According to Porter and Raudenbush, social scientists have overused ANCOVA to reduce bias in nonrandomized studies and underused it to increase the statistical power of a test. Because the model is based on exceptionally strong assumptions, it is easy to misuse. Some researchers pay insufficient attention to these restrictive assumptions. At times, information is extracted indiscriminately from computer program printouts contributing to the continued misuse of ANCOVA.

The main purpose of the preoperative teaching study is to determine which of the three treatments is superior to the remaining two. Under certain conditions, the null hypothesis of no difference in mean values can be tested using the analysis of variance as described in Chapter 9. The ANOVA could be justified if it were known (1) that the three groups of subjects were comparable or (2) that no other independent variables could affect the dependent variable.

In this case, however, it was demonstrated that the second condition was not satisfied because smoking, uncertainty, and weight explain 39% of the variation in length of stay. Thus, to evaluate the differences in the three treatments, the effects of smoking, uncertainty, and weight *must* be considered. The model most frequently used to achieve statistical control is the *analysis of covariance*.

In any study making use of the analysis of covariance, there are three sets of variables. They are

1. the independent variables;
2. the dependent variables;
3. the covariates.

In the preoperative teaching study there is only one independent variable. It consists of the three treatments. There are five dependent measures: (1) number of pain medications given during the first 24 hours, (2) number of pain medications given during the second 24 hours, (3) number of postoperative complications, (4) length of stay in the hospital following surgery, and (5) number of days at home until being able to leave unassisted. The covariates are sex, age, severity, education, provider, income, weight, smoking, alcohol, drug abuse, exercise, and uncertainty. The covariates are potential confounding or nuisance variables that can vary across subjects and produce group differences that exist before the treatments are instituted and the effects of the independent variable(s) are assessed.

For expository reasons only, the ANCOVA adjustment procedure is illustrated for only one variable. In practice, multiple covariates would normally be employed. In the preoperative teaching study, the most likely candidates to use as covariates to achieve a higher level of statistical control are smoking, uncertainty, and weight. These variables were shown to explain 39% of the variance in the length of stay. If the effects of these variables are partialled out of length of stay, the ANCOVA would be employed in the sense that it was originally conceived by Fisher. Here the goal would not be to correct for differences in mean levels on the covariates but to use the covariates to increase the statistical power of the corresponding test statistics.

For example, in the preoperative teaching study none of the variables should introduce bias because a systematic sampling scheme was used to assign subjects to treatments. Consider the variable uncertainty as an individual difference variable whose numerical value is determined by individual psychological experiences and attitudes toward illness and the anticipated outcome. It should cause no problem in the preoperative teaching study because the variable should be equally distributed across the three treatment groups. But, if the distributions were unequal, uncertainty could be a source of a bias that disrupts the findings of the study.

One use of the analysis of covariance to correct for a potential bias is to create *adjusted* values for the dependent variable that are used for testing for statistical significance. The adjustment is achieved by determining the uncertainty score for an *average* patient and using this average person as a standard. With this as a standard, all other uncertainty scores are adjusted by determining what each uncertainty score should be if each person were like the average person.

As shown in Section 8–15, the regression equation that relates uncertainty to length of stay is given as

$$\hat{Y} = -.90 + .085X$$

and as shown in Section 8–16 the average uncertainty score is given as $\overline{X} = 46.17$. This mean value is now treated as representing the *average* person in the study. For this average person, the predicted length of stay is given as

$$\hat{Y} = -.90 + .085\overline{X}$$
$$= -.90 + .085(46.17)$$
$$= 3.02 \text{ days}$$

Consider patient number 3121 of Table B–1. The uncertainty score for this patient is $X = 60$ and the length of stay is $Y = 6$ days. Note that this patient has a high uncertainty score that is one standard deviation above the scale average of 50 and has a corresponding high length of stay. The predicted length of stay for this patient is given as

$$\hat{Y} = -.90 + .085X$$
$$= -.90 + .085(60)$$
$$= 4.20 \text{ days}$$

For some reason, this patient stayed $6 - 4.2 = 1.8$ days beyond the predicted value. If this patient were similar to the *average* patient, the uncertainty score would be given as $X = 46.17$ and the adjusted length of stay would be given as

$$\overline{Y}_A = 3.02 + 1.80 = 4.82 \text{ days}$$

This adjustment process would be applied to the remaining 245 subjects and the adjusted values would now be put to a statistical test that states that the adjusted means across the three treatments are equal to a common value.

The adjustment procedure for removing bias has been illustrated for one covariate only. It is also valid when the groups are similar and the covariate is highly correlated with the dependent variables. In this case, its use is to increase the statistical power of the F test. In the preoperative teaching study, it was shown in Section 10–10 that smoking, uncertainty, and weight are correlated with length of stay. Together they accounted for 39% of the variance in the distribution of length of stay. This is a large component of variance that could be removed statistically from the error variance and thereby improve the power of the test that the treatment effects are null. For this application of ANCOVA the multiple regression equation for predicting Y (length of stay) from X_8 (smoking), X_{12} (uncertainty), and X_7 (weight) is given as

$$Y = -1.6258 + 0.4753X_8$$
$$+ 0.0493X_{12} + 0.0160X_7$$

This equation is used to make the adjustments.

There are many ways to perform the necessary computations for this model. Each computer program reflects the preference of its author so that a researcher must read carefully the manuals provided for the operation of an ANCOVA analysis. One of the easiest algorithms to use is stepwise regression as described by Cohen and Cohen (1983). At *step one* a multiple regression analysis based on the potentially confounding or correlated variables is performed. After it is completed, the variables of interest are entered as dummy variables. The resulting F test of the additional amount of explained variance is the analysis of covariance test statistic. It is used to test that the treatment effects are zero after the effects of the possible confounding or correlated variables have been partialled out.

For the example, the first step in the stepwise regression is summarized in Table 10–14. As indicated, the sum of squares associated with smoking, uncertainty, and weight is given as 220.397. If the dummy variables for treatment, D_1 and D_2, are entered on the second step, the sum of squares (SS) explained increases to 297.029, so that the amount attributable to treatment is given as

$$SS \text{ (Treatment)} = 297.029 - 220.397$$
$$= 76.632$$

The analysis of variance table for this design is shown in Table 10–19. As can be seen, the hypothesis that treatment has no effect is rejected because F = 27.02 is larger than the critical value of $F_{2,240:0.95} = 3.00$. Treatment accounts for an extra 12% of the variation in length of stay. For health science variables, that is a large amount of explained variance.

The mean values of the three treatments can be determined from the regression equation:

$$Y = -2.2050 + 0.4322X_8 + 0.0473X_{12}$$
$$+ 0.0159X_7 + 1.2527D_1 + 1.1154D_2$$

The mean values determined from this equation are used to determine the *adjusted means*. The adjusted means can be submitted to a post hoc analysis. The procedure is complicated and described by Marascuilo and Serlin (1988). It requires a computer program and knowledge of matrix multiplication.

The analysis of covariance is a very delicate statistical model and is difficult to justify. It is based on the following assumptions:

1. The observations between samples are independent.
2. The observations within samples are independent.
3. The regression lines are linear.
4. The regression lines are parallel.
5. The variation about each regression line is homoscedastistic.
6. The residual variances about each regression line are equal to a common value.

7. The deviations from the regression lines have a normal distribution or the sample sizes are large.

These assumptions should be examined whenever this model is adopted. If it can be justified, it is an excellent model, but if it cannot be justified, it should be avoided.

Glass, Peckham, and Sanders (1972) have shown that the analysis of covariance is robust to violations of normality and common variance, provided that the sample sizes are large and equal. The independence assumptions cannot be violated for if they are, the resulting statistical test does not have an F distribution. Violation of the assumption of equal slopes invalidates the test of equal adjusted means because an interaction exists between the covariate and the treatment. This potential interaction can be detected using the methods of Section 10–5 to test regression lines for parallelism. These tests should always be performed before the performance of an analysis of covariance. If the test of parallelism is rejected, it is known that the treatment has an effect that varies with values of the covariate. The researcher should report the effects for each group separately using the regression lines. The adjusted mean values are less than meaningful when the lines are not parallel, and so the analysis of covariance should not be performed.

In a study using multiple covariates, a researcher should not choose variables that are highly correlated with one another because they serve as surrogates of one another. Instead, variables should be selected that are uncorrelated with one another and maximally correlated with the dependent variable. Note that in the example of the preoperative teaching studies 12 covariates were identified but only three were collectively related to the dependent measure in a statistically significant way. Together, they accounted for 39% of the variance which was

TABLE 10–19 ANCOVA TABLE FOR TREATMENT AND LENGTH OF STAY WITH SMOKING, UNCERTAINTY, AND WEIGHT PARTIALLED OUT

Source	d/f	SS	MS	F	$\hat{\eta}^2$
Smoking, Uncertainty, and Weight	3	220.397	73.466		
Treatment	2	76.632	38.316	27.02*	0.1202
Residual	240	340.321	1.418		
Total	245	637.350			

*Significant at $\alpha = 0.05$

partialled out for the ANCOVA test. A researcher rarely needs more than three variables as covariates. Typically one or two are satisfactory because covariates are usually strongly related to the treatment outcome. After the *best* covariates have been identified, the additional covariates contribute little fresh information about the treatment outcome (Porter and Raudenbush, 1987).

It is important that a researcher give serious consideration to the possible use of an outcome variable as a covariate. If an outcome variable is considered a potential covariate, it should not be used if it is correlated with the treatment. If it were used under these conditions, it would tend to dilute the treatment effects. With the dilution of the treatment effect, the potential for a type II error increases.

In the analysis of variance, total variability is partitioned into explained and unexplained variance. For the preoperative teaching study, the proportion of explained

variance is equal to 12% with the unexplained proportion being equal to 88%. Thirty-nine percent of the unexplained variation can be attributed collectively to smoking, uncertainty, and weight. When the variance is partialled out from the unexplained variation, the residual variance for the ANCOVA hypothesis test is reduced to 49%. This reduction in error variance generates an ANCOVA test that has greater power than the corresponding ANOVA test. A comparison of the partitioning of the total variance for the ANOVA and ANCOVA is shown in Figure 10–6.

Pretest-posttest studies on multiple groups are common in nursing research. For example, a researcher may obtain specific information on patients before treatment is instituted and then gather similar information following the administration of the treatment. Often such studies are analyzed in terms of gain scores. If the groups are initially different on the pretest, there is a ten-

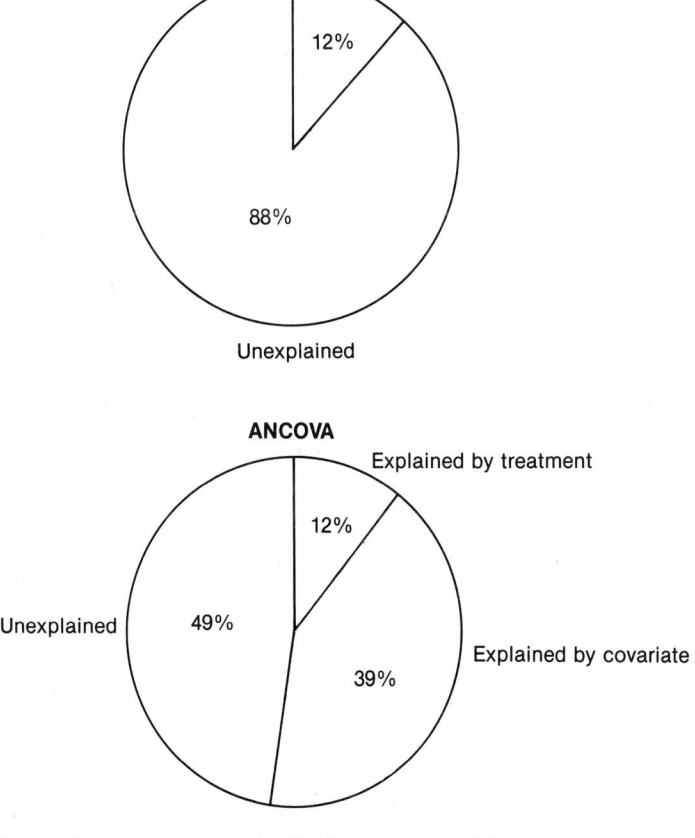

Figure 10–6. The distribution of variance in ANOVA and ANCOVA for the preoperative teaching study.

dency to adopt the ANCOVA model to handle the differences that exist on the pretest. An insightful discussion on this issue is provided by Elashoff (1969). As shown by Rogosa, Brand, and Zimowski (1982), there is no solution to the problem if measurement is made only at two times. These authors provide a solution based on measurements taken at multiple times.

Researchers would like to use the analysis of covariance to correct for the bias that results when two or more groups are statistically different from one another on the covariate. This use of covariance adjustment is not recommended when the groups are initially far apart. The reason for this is that the adjustment frequently produces an error term that is not very different from that found in the corresponding analysis of variance. According to Porter and Raudenbush (1987, p. 392) when random assignment cannot be employed, "a solution is to take multiple measures over time so that change or growth is separated from the effects of treatment."

10–13 SAMPLE SIZES AND POWER FOR THE PEARSON PRODUCT MOMENT CORRELATION COEFFICIENT

Sample sizes for detecting statistically significant correlation coefficients are reported in Table 10–20 for risks of a type I error controlled at $\alpha = .05$ and with power levels of

TABLE 10–20 SAMPLE SIZES FOR TESTING THE PEARSON PRODUCT MOMENT CORRELATION COEFFICIENT FOR STATISTICAL SIGNIFICANCE

Value of the Correlation Coefficient	Power Level			
	.70	*.80*	*.90*	*.95*
.10	616	783	1046	1308
.20	152	193	258	322
.30	66	84	112	139
.40	37	46	61	75
.50	23	28	37	46
.60	15	18	24	30
.70	10	12	16	19
.80	7	9	11	13
.90	5	6	7	8

(Adapted with permission from Table 3.4.1, n to detect r-by-t test, in Cohen, J.: Statistical Power Analysis for the Behavioral Sciences. New York, Academic Press, 1977.)

.70, .80, .90, and .95. Suppose that a researcher were interested in the correlation between uncertainty score and length of stay following surgery only if the correlation were greater than .30. The sample sizes needed for power levels of .70, .80, .90, and .95 are 66, 84, 112, 139, respectively. In this case, the samples of size 82 used in the study provide a power level of .80 of detecting a correlation coefficient of .30 or larger.

10–14 POWER AND SAMPLE SIZE FOR MULTIPLE REGRESSION

Table 9–6 can be used to determine sample size for multiple regression provided that a slight modification is made. Suppose that a researcher wishes to regress length of stay on uncertainty, weight, age, smoking, alcohol usage, and sex. The numerator for the F test is equal to the number of independent variables in the regression equation. In this case P = 6. Because R^2 is a direct statement of explained variance f reduces to

$$f = \sqrt{R^2/(1 - R^2)}$$

Suppose that a researcher is interested only in multiple regressions for which R^2 is greater than .30. For this case,

$$f = \sqrt{(.30)/(1 - .30)} = .65$$

The sample sizes for power levels of .70, .80, .90, and .95 are 4.5, 5.5, 7.0, and 8.0. In this case, these are not the sample sizes for the regression analysis. These are given as

$$N = n(P + 1)$$

Thus, the sample size for a power level of .70 is

$$N = 4.5(6 + 1) = 31.5 \text{ or } 32$$

For the remaining three power levels, the corresponding sample sizes are 30, 49, and 56. For the preoperative teaching study there is more than sufficient power for detecting R^2 values of .30 or greater.

10–15 SUMMARY

This chapter has presented methods for analyzing correlated variables in nursing research. Various approaches to the analysis and interpretation of zero order, part, partial, and multiple correlation coefficients were presented. All these measures can be used in experimental, quasi-experimental, survey, and observational studies. Examples of the use of multiple regression were provided using data from the preoperative teaching studies. The important question of deciding how to choose variables to enter into a prediction equation using multiple independent variables was illustrated for both simultaneous test procedures and for stepwise models. In addition, power and sample sizes for simple and multiple regression were illustrated.

The analysis of covariance was presented and illustrated. This is one of the most misused statistical procedures in the social, behavioral, and health care sciences. The ANCOVA test is based on stringent assumptions quite difficult to meet. One of the more common oversights made in using this model is that researchers often fail to test the hypothesis of identical slopes for the regression lines generated for each group in the study. If the lines are not parallel, the ANCOVA hypothesis should not be tested because it is known that the treatment and the covariate interact. Under such situations a researcher is advised to discuss each treatment independently in terms of the covariates used.

Guidelines were given for selecting covariates to use in an analysis of covariance. Too often researchers use the analysis of covariance to adjust groups that differ on the covariate. Sometimes the adjustment process is successful in correcting the bias and in increasing the statistical power of the test. If the groups are far apart on the covariate, adjustment might not be adequate and lead to increased risks of type II errors. Thus, a researcher is advised to select groups for an analysis of covariance that do not deviate significantly from one another on the covariate. If multiple covariates are to be used, a researcher should select variables that are highly correlated with the dependent variable but weakly correlated with each other.

REFERENCES

Bostrom, A.: CRUNCH Software. Oakland, CA, 1986.

Carlson, J.E., and Timm, N.H.: Analysis of nonorthogonal fixed-effects designs, Psychol. Bull., 81: 563–570, 1974.

Cochran, W.G.: Analysis of covariance: its nature and uses, Biometrics, 13: 261–281, 1957.

Cohen, J.: Statistical Power Analysis for the Behavioral Sciences. New York, Academic Press, 1977.

Cohen, J., and Cohen, P.: Applied Multiple Regression/Correlation Analysis for the Behavioral Sciences, ed. 2. Hillsdale, NJ, Erlbaum, 1983.

Cronbach, L.J., and Snow, R.E.: Aptitudes and Instructional Methods: A Handbook for Research on Interactions. New York, Irvington, 1977.

Draper, N.R., and Smith, H.: Applied Regression Analysis, ed. 2. New York, John Wiley & Sons, 1981.

Dunn, O.J.: Multiple comparisons among means, J. Am. Stat. Assoc., 56: 52–64, 1961.

Elashoff, J.D.: Analysis of covariance: a delicate instrument, Am. Ed. Res. J., 6: 383–401, 1969.

Fisher, R.A.: Statistical Methods for Research Workers, ed. 10. New York, Hafner, 1948.

Glass, G.V., Peckham, P.D., and Sanders, J.R.: Consequences of failure to meet assumptions underlying the analysis of variance and covariance, Rev. Ed. Res., 42: 237–288, 1972.

Marascuilo, L.A., and Levin, J.: Multivariate Statistics in the Social Sciences. Belmont, CA, Wadsworth, 1983.

Marascuilo, L.A.., and Serlin, R.C.: Statistical Methods for the Social and Behavioral Sciences. New York, Freeman, 1988.

Pedhazur, E.J.: Multiple Regression in Behavioral Research, ed. 2. New York, Holt, Rinehart, & Winston, 1982.

Porter, A.C., and Raudenbush, S.W.: Analysis of covariance: its model and use in psychological research, J. Counseling Psychol., 34: 383–392, 1987.

Rogosa, D.R., Brand, D.N., and Zimowski, M.: A growth curve approach to the measurement of change, Psychol. Bull., 90: 728–748, 1982.

Wampold, B.E., and Freund, R.D.: Use of multiple regression in counseling psychology research: a flexible data-analytic strategy. J. Counseling Psychol., 34: 372–382, 1987.

Chapter 11

MULTIVARIATE METHODS

11–1   AN OVERVIEW OF MULTIVARIATE METHODS FOR NURSING RESEARCH

In this chapter, an introduction to multivariate methods is presented. The presentation is not exhaustive because the number of multivariate methods is exceedingly large. Instead, the most commonly encountered models which are found to have the most usefulness to researchers in the social and biomedical sciences are described. It is important to note that the models are not interchangeable because each model is used to provide answers to specific questions or issues. Thus, a nurse researcher must know what questions are asked and answered by each model. With this understanding, a selection of the correct model is facilitated.

The first model to be described is *principal component analysis*. Its main application is found in reducing a large set of variables to a smaller, more manageable and meaningful set of variables. It is used most effectively when a researcher has collected information from each subject on a set of correlated data that is believed to measure a single unifying concept such as pain, anxiety, fear, anger, or any other psychological or psychophysiological construct. The model was originally proposed to obtain unifying measures of intelligence from a battery of items designed to tap components of intelligence. Its success has prompted researchers to apply it to many other contexts inside and outside of psychology for theory construction, test construction, data reduction, and data analysis. The model was first proposed by Hotelling (1933). It was not widely used until computer programs were written enabling the model to be put into practice. The arithmetic involved with the model is exceedingly tedious and lengthy, but with computer software availability the model is easy to execute. The model can be used to evaluate the measurement of many constructs at one time and has been so used, mainly by American psychologists, to study the *dimensions* of intelligence. It has also been used to study the dimensions of anxiety, homophobia, attitudes toward minority groups, and so on. It is a model that should be considerably useful to a research nurse investigator.

Closely allied to principal component analysis, and actually its precursor, is *factor analysis*. A general discussion of this model is presented but not illustrated. The *many* variants of this model are not described in this chapter because some are based on assumptions that may not hold for many of the constructs considered in nursing research. For a discussion of these models, see Harmon (1976) and Rummel (1970). Another reason why they are not described is that a principal component analysis produces results very similar to those of factor analysis. Because principal component analysis is based on simpler assumptions and because it so often parallels the results of a factor analysis, it is recommended.

One problem associated with principal components and factor analysis is *dimensionality*. For example, some psychologists view intelligence as a single unifying characteristic, whereas others see intelligence as being composed of unique components that collectively define it. This difference in viewpoint gives rise to a second problem referred to as *rotation* of factors to a meaningful structure. These two problems have generated many solutions, one of which is described in this chapter. The solution most commonly used to handle the two identified problems is that created by Kaiser's (1958) *varimax rotation* procedure. Kaiser's solution is described and illustrated in this chapter.

In principal component analysis and factor analysis, no clearly specified independent and dependent variables or sets of variables exist; however, such sets exist in some investigations and the goal of the research is to relate the independent and dependent variables to one another in a manner like that of simple or multiple regression. The model used for this situation is *canonical correlation theory*. Simple and multiple regression are special cases of this all-inclusive model. In canonical correlation a set of dependent measures are correlated collectively with a set of independent measures. When a canonical correlation analysis is performed, components similar to those of principal component analysis are developed and used for theory building, data reduction, and data analysis. It is a powerful method. When ca-

nonical correlation analysis can be justified, it proves to be effective for analyzing two sets of correlated multivariate data.

Another special case of canonical correlation theory is *discriminant analysis*. In its simplest form, a researcher has a control and experimental sample on which multivariate or profile data have been collected. The object is to weight the variables in order to produce a single index that can be used to score and rank order each subject in a way that produces maximum separation between the two groups. As a by-product, this index, which is called a *linear discriminant function*, can be used to determine whether a new subject is a person like those in the control or experimental group. This use of the model is described in detail by Marascuilo and Levin (1983). In most situations, discriminant analysis is used when the number of groups being compared is two or more. In the special two-group case, the model is often referred to as Hotelling's T^2 (1931). It is used to identify the variables that best differentiate two samples of subjects. Hotelling's T^2 is not described because it is identical with the more general multivariate analysis of variance involving exactly two groups.

Closely allied to linear discriminant function theory is the *multivariate analysis of variance*. This is the extension of the univariate analysis of variance model to the case, in which multiple dependent variables have been measured on each subject. As will be seen, it is a special case of canonical correlation theory and discriminant analysis.

As stated, other models exist but these models are primarily used today by researchers in the social and biomedical sciences. The next section begins with the presentation of principal component analysis.

11–2 PRINCIPAL COMPONENT ANALYSIS

The main use of principal component analysis is to reduce a large set of intercorrelated variables into a smaller, more manageable, and hopefully more meaningful set of variables for further investigation. The variables generated from the reduction process are called *principal components* and are popularly referred to as *factors*. Principal component analysis is also used to study the structure that exists among many different variables to provide a way for understanding how hypothetical variables relate to one another in a specific population.

As an example of how the principal components model might be useful to a nurse researcher, consider the preoperative teaching study used in the previous chapters. Five variables are used to measure postoperative recovery following surgery. These are

Y_1—length of stay in hospital following surgery,

Y_2—number of pain medications requested on the first day following surgery,

Y_3—number of pain medications requested on the second day following surgery,

Y_4—number of postoperative complications,

Y_5—number of days patients spent at recovery before being able to leave the recovery environment unassisted.

The correlations among these variables are reported in Table 11–1. As can be seen, the correlations are high and fairly uniform in value, ranging from a low of 0.51 to a high of 0.66. The purposes of using principal component analysis on these data are

1. to reduce the five variables to a smaller set of linear combinations that can be used to score and rank order each patient with respect to postoperative recovery and

2. to use the resulting scores as the dependent variable in an analysis of variance to assess the effects of the three treatments on patient recovery following surgery.

In particular, a reduction of the five variables to one measure of postoperative recovery is expected or anticipated.

Whenever a principal component analysis is being considered, the first set of data to examine is the matrix of correlation coeffi-

cients. If most of the correlations are high (0.30 to 0.80 in absolute value), principal component analysis will be effective because the model clusters together subsets of the variables that are highly correlated with one another. If most of the correlations are low (0.00 to 0.20 in absolute value), abandon the adoption of the model because principal component analysis will prove to be a waste of time and the clustered variables will not hold together in a meaningful fashion.

In the example, there are only five measures of postoperative recovery, but in other studies the number of measures can be exceedingly large. This is true in the AIDS survey of Chapter 6, in which each questionnaire contained about 25 separate items. In that study, high correlations among subsets of the variables would be expected, and principal component analysis could be used to reduce each set of 25 variables to a smaller set. It is worth noting that principal component analysis was used to generate the three-dimensional model of homophobia, which provided the theoretical basis for the construction of the three questionnaires used to measure nurses' attitudes toward the treatment of AIDS patients (Herek, 1984).

For an effective principal component analysis, the variables should partition into unique sets of highly correlated variables (0.30 to 0.80 in absolute value), but the correlations between the sets must be low (0.00 to 0.20 in absolute value). For example, in the AIDS survey, suppose 15 items are selected for a principal component analysis. Consider that items 1 through 10 have a median correlation of 0.70 and items 11 through 15 have a median correlation of 0.55. For the principal component analysis to be fruitful, the correlations between the 10 item set and the 5 item set should be close to zero. If they

TABLE 11–1 CORRELATION MATRIX, MEAN VALUES, AND STANDARD DEVIATIONS FOR THE FIVE POSTOPERATIVE RECOVERY VARIABLES

Variable	Y_1	Y_2	Y_3	Y_4	Y_5
Y_1: Length of stay	1.00	0.63	0.64	0.64	0.66
Y_2: Pain med. one*		1.00	0.63	0.51	0.58
Y_3: Pain med. two†			1.00	0.53	0.57
Y_4: Postop. comp.‡				1.00	0.56
Y_5: Days at home					1.00
Mean value	4.26	5.22	1.93	0.76	4.17
Standard deviation	1.61	1.97	1.52	1.02	2.64

*Y_2: Pain med. one = number of pain medications requested on the first postoperative day

†Y_3: Pain med. two = number of pain medications requested on the second postoperative day

‡Y_4: Postop. comp. = number of postoperative complications

are not, the data reduction to two clearly defined components may not be satisfactory. As indicated, correlation coefficients within clusters of variables should be high and at the same time, the correlation coefficients between clusters of variables should be low. Such a situation is ideal. Unfortunately, it is rarely achieved.

The primary objective of principal component analysis is to reduce a large set of P variables to a smaller set that capture the essence of the original P variables. When all the correlations are equal to a common value, only one principal component is generated. In the postoperative recovery example, all P = 5 variables are used to measure the single concept, *postoperative recovery*. It would be anticipated that the five variables would reduce to one composite variable. In this case, there is good reason to believe that this will happen because all of the correlations tend to be nearly equal in numerical value.

11–3 DETERMINATION OF PRINCIPAL COMPONENTS WEIGHTS

From a mathematical point of view, a principal component is a linear combination of the *standard scores* of the P original variables. Thus,

$$P = W_1 Z_1 + W_2 Z_2 + W_3 Z_3 + W_4 Z_4 + W_5 Z_5$$

See Section 9–2 for a discussion of standard scores and linear combinations. In terms of the means and standard deviations of the five variables reported in Table 11–1 the first principal component, P_1, is defined as the weighted sum of standard score variables.

$$P_1 = W_1 \left(\frac{Y_1 - 4.26}{1.61} \right) + W_2 \left(\frac{Y_2 - 5.22}{1.97} \right)$$
$$+ \cdots + W_5 \left(\frac{Y_5 - 4.17}{2.64} \right)$$

The principal component weights are unknown and must now be determined. The calculation of the weights is extremely complex because of the associated matrix algebra. The solution can be read from a principal component computer printout. For the data of Table 11–1 the weights are given as

$$W_1 = 1.1428$$
$$W_2 = 1.2258$$

$$W_3 = 1.2198$$
$$W_4 = 1.2750$$
$$W_5 = 1.2202$$

Thus, the first principal component is defined as

$$P_1 = 1.1428\ Z_1 + 1.2258\ Z_2$$
$$+ 1.2198\ Z_3 + 1.2750\ Z_4 + 1.2202\ Z_5$$

Consider a patient who

1. has a long length of stay,
2. receives many pain drug administrations in the first 48 hours,
3. has postoperative complications,
4. requires a long stay at home.

This patient has a large value for P_1 because all five standard scores are large and positive. Thus, the positive end of this scale is associated with patients who have a difficult postoperative recovery. The negative end of the scale is associated with patients who have a speedy and efficient postoperative recovery. For these patients all five standard scores should be large and negative, producing a large and negative value for P_1.

Note that all the weights are nearly equal to one another. This characteristic of weights being nearly identical always occurs when the correlation coefficients among the variables are nearly equal to one another. When this happens, the equation can be simplified by setting all of the coefficients equal to unity (Wainer, 1976). With this transformation, a simple linear combination that can be used to measure postoperative recovery is given as

$$P_1 = Z_1 + Z_2 + Z_3 + Z_4 + Z_5$$

In practice, this composite or linear combination of the five original variables can be taken as an operational definition of postoperative recovery.

11–4 DETERMINATION OF THE NUMBER OF MEANINGFUL PRINCIPAL COMPONENTS

From a mathematical perspective, P variables produce P principal components. At this point only one of the five principal components that could be generated by the data has been examined. We now explain why. The reason for this is that the remaining four variables are meaningless. Notice the unities in the diagonal of the correlation matrix, and recall that principal component analysis is based on standard scores and not on the original variables. The unities are the variances of the standard scores because standard scores have a mean of zero and a standard deviation and variance of 1. Thus, the total variance is equal to P = 5, the number of variables. In general, the total variance in any principal component analysis is equal to P.

In this study, five units of variance can be distributed to the five principal components. After the component scores of each subject are determined, the variance of the P components can be computed using the familiar formula for the sample variance. If this were to be done using the principal component weights, it would be found that the variance across all 246 subjects of P_1 is given as $Var(P_1) = 3.3851$. Of the five units of variance available to the five components, P_1 uses $[3.3851 / 5] \times 100\% = 67.7\%$ of the total. This means that only 32.3%, or $(5 - 3.3851) = 1.6149$ is left to distribute to the remaining four components for an average variance of $1/4(1.6149) = 0.4039$. As we see, the remaining components have, on the average, smaller variances than any of the original five variables used to measure recovery.

One of the objectives of principal component analysis is to create a variable that maximizes the separation between closely related subjects. Because variables with large variances provide a larger separation between subjects than do variables with small variances, it does not make sense to replace a single variable discriminator with a composite discriminator whose variance is smaller. For that reason, none of the other components is treated as meaningful. This decision is based on a commonly employed rule that is used to evaluate the importance of a principal component. According to this rule, only components with a variance greater than 1 are retained as having important measurement properties. This rule is referred to as *Kaiser's Rule* (Kaiser and Hunka, 1973).

In practice, variances associated with a principal component do not need to be computed directly; they are reported on the printouts associated with almost all computer programs. On most computer printouts, variances are rarely referred to as variances. Instead they are called *eigen values*. In principal components analysis, eigen values are synonymous to principal component variances.

TABLE 11–2 STRUCTURE MATRIX FOR THE DATA OF TABLE 11–1

Variable	Structure Correlation
Y_1	0.88
Y_2	0.81
Y_3	0.82
Y_4	0.78
Y_5	0.82

When a principal component analysis generates more than one principal component with eigen values greater than one, a researcher has the added problem of trying to deduce what the components are measuring. One solution, which has been proposed and is easy to execute, is to compute the correlation coefficient between each of the original variables and the scores generated by the principal components. Such correlations are called *structure correlations* or *loadings* and are always given on the computer printout. If the loading associated with a specific variable is large, the variable is said to be loaded on the component and is maintained as a variable that defines the component. The structure correlations for the five postoperative recovery variables are reported in Table 11–2. As can be seen, each of the five variables is highly correlated with the first principal component indicating that all variables load on P_1. Because each variable has a large loading, each is used to define P_1 as an *operational definition* of postoperative recovery. Note that the loadings are essentially equal to one another. When this happens, a researcher can replace a complicated form of the linear combination with a simple unweighted sum of the standard scores.

Principal components should always be referred to as components, but popular usage has seen the term *components* replaced by *factors*. Factor analysis generates factors and factor scores. Principal components analysis generates components and component scores.

11–5 SIMPLE STRUCTURE AND ROTATION FOR PRINCIPAL COMPONENTS

A decision a researcher is sure to have to make is to identify and to name the resulting components generated by a principal component analysis. Because a researcher would like to have factors that are interpretable, measurement experts have established different criteria which components should satisfy to achieve interpretability. A criterion that is most commonly used is that of *simple structure*, first defined by Thurstone (1947). According to Rummel (1970), there are five components to simple structure. We provide a description of them here.

1. Each variable should show small correlations with at least one component.
2. If Q components are retained on the basis of Kaiser's Rule, each component should show small correlations with Q variables.
3. For each pair of retained components, small correlations with the variables should be found for one of the components.
4. Each pair of components should be uncorrelated with most of the variables.
5. For each pair of variables, a small number of variables should correlate with each component.

As might be expected, these idealized conditions are rarely satisfied exactly for most investigations, but approximate satisfaction is frequently encountered. If *orthogonality* of the factors also is required, close approximations to simple structure can be attained. The property of orthogonality is that the correlation coefficient between two components be equal to zero. If this condition is satisfied and if the assumptions for simple structure are satisfied, the components are statistically independent. This means that information contained in a component is completely unrelated to the information contained in another component. As can be surmised, orthogonality is a desirable property and should be considerably useful in nursing investigations. One way to achieve orthogonal factors with simple structure is to *rotate* the components. The problem is a mathematical one and is not described. There are many solutions to the problem, but the most frequently used solution is *Kaiser's Varimax Rotation* (1958). This rotation model is illustrated in Section 11−7.

11−6 USING PRINCIPAL COMPONENTS AS DEPENDENT VARIABLES IN NURSING RESEARCH

Treating the first principal component as a dependent variable, a researcher could use the analysis of variance to determine whether the average values of the postoperative recovery components across the three treatment groups were significantly different from one another. Rejection of the null hypothesis of no difference in mean values P_1 warrants the conclusion that one method produced more effective recovery than the others. Planned and post hoc contrasts can be investigated, confidence intervals can be established, and measurements of explained variance can be assessed for P_1, as illustrated in Chapter 9. If it were of theoretical interest or of empirical importance, the principal component would be regressed on drug usage, smoking, age, or any other independent variable of interest using the methods of Chapter 10. By using this composite variable, the researcher would not have to make separate analyses on the five individual recovery measures as illustrated in Section 9−13.

The major research question associated with the preoperative teaching study is whether treatment three will be superior to the remaining two treatments. This can be tested by using P_1 as the dependent variable in a one-way analysis of variance. For this analysis, each of the 246 subjects are scored using the derived recovery measure based on equal weights. In particular,

$$P_1 = Z_1 + Z_2 + Z_3 + Z_4 + Z_5$$

is used. The resulting F ratio for testing the hypothesis

$$H_0: \mu_1 = \mu_2 = \mu_3$$

against

$$H_1: H_0 \text{ is false}$$

is given as F = 40.12. For comparison purposes, the individual F ratios for the five original recovery measures are reported in Table 11−3. As can be seen, the F ratio for the principal component scoring is larger than the average of the F ratios for the individual recovery variables. The average of the five F ratios is equal to 27.81. In addition to the increase in statistical power arising from using the composite of the five recovery measures as a single criterion, the potential problem of making multiple type I errors is eliminated because five separate F tests are reduced to one F test. If desired, a post hoc analysis on the mean scores can be conducted using the method of Section 9−11.

TABLE 11-3 F RATIOS FOR THE ORIGINAL FIVE RECOVERY MEASURES AND THE FIVE VARIABLE COMPOSITE MEASURES

Variable	F Ratio	Explained Variance
Y_1	23.65	0.16
Y_2	53.49	0.31
Y_3	14.89	0.11
Y_4	18.46	0.13
Y_5	28.55	0.19
P_1	40.12	0.24

For the unweighted linear combination, the three treatment mean values read from a computer printout are

$$\overline{P}_1 = 2.565$$
$$\overline{P}_2 = -0.143$$

and

$$\overline{P}_3 = -2.441$$

with the mean square within groups given as MSW = 12.8331 and the mean value of all component scores given as $\overline{P} = 0$.

It is worth noting that the average amount of explained variation of the five recovery variables is 0.18, whereas the explained variation associated with the composite variable is 0.24. The composite variable explains more variance between the treatments than the average explained variance across the five original variables.

Because the scale of the composite variable is not easily interpretable, many computer programs report results in standard deviation units. In terms of this type of rescaling, the mean for the patients of treatment one is

$$\overline{Z} = (\overline{P}_1 - 0)/\sqrt{\text{MSW}} =$$
$$2.565/\sqrt{12.8331} = 0.716$$

Thus, the patients of treatment one are on the average 0.716 standard deviations above the mean of all 246 patients. The corresponding values for patients in treatments two and three are, respectively, -0.040 and -0.682 standard deviations below the mean. In terms of the composite variable, the three groups are well separated from one another. For completeness, we provide a post hoc analysis of the pairwise differences on the standardized means.

For the standardized means, the MSW = 1.000, and the Scheffé coefficient is given as

$$S = \sqrt{\nu_1 \, F\nu_1, \nu_{2:(1-\alpha)}}$$
$$= \sqrt{2(3.00)} = 2.45$$

With these values,

$$\hat{\psi}_{12} = [0.7816 - (-0.040)]$$
$$\pm 2.45\sqrt{1.000[1/82 + 1/82]} = 0.756 \pm 0.383$$

$$\hat{\psi}_{13} = [0.716 - (-0.682)]$$
$$\pm 2.45\sqrt{1.000[1/82 + 1/82]} = 1.398 \pm 0.383$$

and

$$\hat{\psi}_{23} = [-0.040 - (-0.682)]$$
$$\pm 2.45\sqrt{1.000[1/82 + 1/82]} = 0.642 \pm 0.383$$

Because none of the confidence intervals contains zero, each treatment mean is statistically different from the other two. Also, a clear ordering of the treatments is indicated. Patients in treatment one have the least satisfactory postoperative recovery, and patients in treatment three have the most satisfactory recovery. The number of standard deviations between these two means on the scale of the standardized principal components is 1.40. For behavioral and health care variables this is a very large difference.

11-7 A PRINCIPAL COMPONENT ANALYSIS USING MANY INTERRELATED VARIABLES

The previous example of a principal component analysis was based on an ideal set of research data which reduced to a single unifying dimension, namely, postoperative recovery following major surgical intervention. Rarely does the reduction of a multivariate set of data reduce so efficiently. One reason for the clean and clear results is that the analysis is based on a small number of variables. In reality, most research studies involve numerous interrelated variables. As an example, let us reexamine the postoperative study data and include in the analysis some of the remaining variables such as sex, age, drug usage, and so on. With many interrelated variables, a researcher is tempted to place all of them—conceptually related or not—through a principal component analysis. Frequently the final results are not meaningful, and for good reason. Unless variables are conceptually or theoretically related to one another they do not cluster as a meaningful component.

Unlike many research studies, it should be noted that in the preoperative teaching study, the variables selected were conceptually or empirically linked to one another prior to data collection. Because of preplanning, a principal component analysis based on these variables has a high probability of producing meaningful results.

The variables used for this second principal component analysis include the five postoperative recovery variables augmented by Y_6: sex, Y_7: age, Y_8: severity, Y_9: weight, Y_{10}: smoking, Y_{11}: alcohol usage, Y_{12}: drug usage, Y_{13}: exercise, and Y_{14}: uncertainty. The correlation matrix for these 14 variables is reported in Table 11-4.

As before, the five recovery variables are highly correlated with one another and as a consequence should cluster together as a factor. These variables also show moderate correlations with Y_7: age, Y_8: severity, Y_9: weight, Y_{10}: smoking, and Y_{14}: uncertainty. Thus, we might expect these risk variables to show some clustering with the recovery variables. Patients at low risk should show efficient recovery, whereas patients at high risk should show difficult recovery. Also, we might expect that the risk variables could generate a factor unto themselves because they show moderate correlations with one another. For example, the correlation coefficient between Y_7: age and Y_9: weight is equal to 0.52. The others are similar in numerical value. Except for these associations, the re-

maining correlation coefficients are relatively close to zero. Note that the correlations with Y_6: sex, Y_{11}: alcohol usage, Y_{12}: drug usage, and Y_{13}: exercise are all close to zero. We would be surprised to find them clustering with any of the other variables. From these points of view, we would expect to find one factor clustering the recovery and risk variables together, or else we might expect to find two factors, one clustering the recovery variables and one clustering the risk variables.

The results of the principal component analysis are reported in the left-hand columns of Table 11-5. As indicated, five components were identified by the application of Kaiser's Rule. This is three more than were identified from a visual inspection of the correlation matrix. The numbers in the left-hand columns of Table 11-5 are the structure correlations or loadings. No universally accepted rule exists as to how large a factor loading must be in order to be considered theoretically meaningful. In this case, it was arbitrarily decided to set the minimal level to .40 to provide definers of each factor. As shown, all but four of the variables load on the first principal component. The variables that do not are Y_6: sex, Y_{11}: alcohol usage, Y_{12}: drug usage, and Y_{13}: exercise.

The general loading of most variables on the first factor is a typical finding in principal component analysis. The first principal component usually absorbs most of the P units of variance by loading on most of the variables. Often the first principal component is referred to as a general factor. In this example, the second component is charac-

TABLE 11-4 CORRELATION MATRIX FOR A PRINCIPAL COMPONENT ANALYSIS BASED ON FIVE RECOVERY VARIABLES AND NINE RISK VARIABLES

	Y_1	Y_2	Y_3	Y_4	Y_5	Y_6	Y_7	Y_8	Y_9	Y_{10}	Y_{11}	Y_{12}	Y_{13}	Y_{14}
Y_1	1.00	.63	.64	.64	.66	.02	.42	.32	.40	.49	.07	−.05	−.04	.41
Y_2		1.00	.62	.51	.58	.24	.23	.37	.25	.28	.03	−.03	−.05	.37
Y_3			1.00	.53	.57	.15	.26	.28	.30	.33	.11	.07	−.08	.25
Y_4				1.00	.56	.00	.39	.29	.49	.33	.06	.08	−.03	.29
Y_5					1.00	.03	.50	.50	.39	.47	.05	.02	−.13	.39
Y_6						1.00	−.10	.02	−.31	−.10	−.12	−.12	−.24	.06
Y_7							1.00	.36	.52	.54	.03	−.07	−.28	.33
Y_8								1.00	.31	.46	.01	.04	−.13	.56
Y_9									1.00	.37	.16	−.03	−.15	.27
Y_{10}										1.00	.06	−.05	−.14	.34
Y_{11}											1.00	.07	−.03	−.04
Y_{12}												1.00	−.01	.02
Y_{13}													1.00	−.19
Y_{14}														1.00

TABLE 11−5 STRUCTURE MATRIX FOR THE UNROTATED AND ROTATED PRINCIPAL COMPONENTS FOR THE DATA OF TABLE 11−4

Variable	Unrotated Factors					Rotated Factors				
	P_1	P_2	P_3	P_4	P_5	P_1^r	P_2^r	P_3^r	P_4^r	P_5^r
Y_1	0.82*	0.12	0.23	−0.15	−0.06	0.81*	0.29	0.16	−0.04	−0.09
T_2	0.71*	0.44*	0.21	−0.04	0.02	0.83*	−0.05	0.21	0.06	−0.03
Y_3	0.71*	0.30	0.34	0.08	−0.12	0.84*	0.06	0.02	0.09	0.08
Y_4	0.73*	0.02	0.31	−0.02	−0.05	0.73*	0.31	0.07	−0.05	0.06
Y_5	0.82*	0.07	0.06	−0.01	0.05	0.69*	0.31	0.31	0.07	0.02
Y_6	0.02	0.82*	−0.27	0.11	−0.22	0.26	−0.61*	0.08	0.55*	−0.22
Y_7	0.65*	−0.36	−0.32	−0.08	−0.17	0.24	0.68*	0.28	0.25	−0.15
Y_8	0.62*	−0.05	−0.33	0.10	0.40*	0.27	0.27	0.70*	0.11	0.14
Y_9	0.61*	−0.51*	0.02	−0.04	−0.19	0.29	0.76*	0.03	0.03	0.00
Y_{10}	0.65*	−0.26	−0.22	−0.11	0.03	0.30	0.56*	0.38	0.09	−0.10
Y_{11}	0.10	−0.29	0.33	0.43*	−0.48*	0.14	0.33	−0.55*	0.22	0.36
Y_{12}	−0.01	−0.10	0.28	0.77*	0.42*	0.01	−0.09	0.09	−0.03	0.92*
Y_{13}	−0.21	−0.08	0.62*	−0.45*	0.44*	0.05	−0.16	−0.10	−0.89*	−0.02
Y_{14}	0.59*	0.06	−0.36	0.10	0.30	0.27	0.18	0.70*	0.17	0.10
Eigen value	4.90	1.54	1.35	1.07	1.04	3.46	2.85	1.37	1.16	1.07

*Structure correlations greater than 0.40 used as definers of the factors

terized mainly as Y_6: sex and to a lesser degree as Y_2: pain med. one (number of pain medications requested on the first postoperative day) and Y_9: weight. Note that weight has a negative correlation with the factor. It is not clear what the factor represents, but it could reflect a bipolar factor associated with overweight women on one end of the scale who request a large number of pain relievers during the first day following surgery and with lighter weight men on the other end of the scale who request none. To identify and name a factor, it is a good rule to describe the type of subjects who are found at each end of the scale generated by the factor.

Component three is amorphous, with many correlation coefficients hovering about plus or minus 0.30. The largest correlation is with Y_{13}: exercise. This factor is hard to characterize. Component four is defined mainly as Y_{11}: drug usage and to a lesser extent as Y_{12}: alcohol usage and Y_{13}: exercise, variables which show little correlation with anything. Because Y_{13}: exercise appears with a negative correlation, these three variables may be focusing at one end of the scale on male drug users who smoke but do not exercise and at the other end of the scale on male nondrug users who do exercise. Finally, component five is not easy to define because the four largest correlations involve Y_8: severity, Y_{11}: alcohol usage, Y_{12}: drug usage, and Y_{13}: exercise. The negative correlation with drug usage makes the interpretation of this factor very difficult. For completeness,

notice in Table 11−5 the numerical values of the eigen values. Except for the first one, the others are small and close to unity, suggesting that the factors associated with these eigen values may not be meaningful. The latter comment is especially true for principal components four and five with eigen values of 1.07 and 1.04, respectively.

As indicated earlier in Sections 11−4 and 11−5, the naming of principal components is not easy. One solution is to rotate the components to simple structure, using a varimax rotation as described in Section 11−5. The results of a varimax rotation are reported in the right-hand columns of Table 11−5. Here, a very close approach to simple structure with orthogonal components is demonstrated. In terms of the five criteria of simple structure,

1. Each of the 14 original variables has at least one small correlation with the 5 components.
2. Each of the 5 components is uncorrelated with more than 5 of the original 14 variables.
3. For each of the 14 original variables, 1 large and 1 small correlation are found for each pair of components.
4. Most of the correlation coefficients across pairs of components are very small.
5. Only one variable, Y_6, shows a correlation with 2 or more components.

The first orthogonal rotated component is identical with the first component in the five-variable principal component analysis. This second larger study using 14 variables serves as a validation of the smaller study using five variables. Thus component one is clearly a *postoperative recovery* measure. The principal component defined by the summed unweighted Z values across the five recovery variables defined earlier is certainly valid here.

The second rotated component is defined as Y_6: sex, Y_7: age, Y_9: weight, and Y_{10}: smoking. Because sex is negatively correlated with the factor, it suggests that this bipolar component of risk is defined at one end by females who are overweight and are heavy smokers and at the other end by men who are not overweight and do not smoke. This component is identified as *risk factor one*, based on Y_6: gender, Y_9: weight, and Y_{10}: smoking.

Component three is defined as Y_8: severity, Y_{11}: alcohol usage, and Y_{14}: uncertainty. It seems to be defined at one end by those who use alcohol, have a severe abdominal condition, and show uncertainty and fear in undergoing surgery. At the opposite end of the scale, are nonalcohol users with less severe problems and low levels of uncertainty. This component is labeled as *risk factor two*, based on Y_8: severity, Y_{11}: alcohol usage, and Y_{14}: uncertainty.

Component four is defined mainly as Y_6: sex and Y_{13}: exercise. It probably separates males and females according to exercise activity. At one end of the scale are found males who exercise and at the opposite pole are found females who do not exercise. This component is called *risk factor three*, based on Y_6: gender and Y_{13}: exercise activity.

Finally, component five is defined as Y_{12}: drug usage. This component is named *risk factor four*, based on drug usage alone.

As a whole, these five constructs make conceptual sense within the boundaries of the preoperative teaching study. These five new hypothetical variables can now be used in place of the original 14 variables. Note that in the structure matrix some of the correlation coefficients are negative. This means that these variables are negatively correlated with the remaining variables and would generate negative standard scores when the standard scores for the other variables on the component were positive. This problem was discussed earlier in Section 5–12 for treating Likert scales with different positive and negative poles. There, it was pointed out that

the scale could be corrected by simple reversal of the scale. Here, the reversal can be achieved by multiplying by −1 all variables that show negative correlations in the structure matrix. In particular, if the signs of the structure correlations are used as multipliers to each of the standard scores, the five hypothetical variables are defined mathematically by the following unweighted linear combinations:

$$P_1 = Z_1 + Z_2 + Z_3 + Z_4 + Z_5$$
$$P_2 = -Z_6 + Z_7 + Z_9 + Z_{10}$$
$$P_3 = Z_8 - Z_{11} + Z_{14}$$
$$P_4 = Z_6 - Z_{13}$$
$$P_5 = Z_{12}$$

Many researchers prefer to use *component scores* rather than summed unweighted standard scores or Z values. Component scores are, of course, more precise and directly associated with the principal component analysis. Unfortunately, few principal component programs generate component scores for other statistical uses. Because summed unweighted Z scores give very similar results, the summed scores are recommended. For directions on how to obtain component scores see Marascuilo and Levin (1983) and Wainer (1976) for a discussion on the use of summed unweighted Z scores.

The CRUNCH (Bostrom, 1986) program provides component scores upon request. This was done for the five rotated principal components. The component scores were then used to test group differences across the three treatments. The F ratios for the five component scores are reported in Table 11–6. The only component that shows a significant difference across the three treatment

TABLE 11–6 ANALYSIS OF VARIANCE TABLE FOR THE FIVE ROTATED FACTORS BASED ON THE PRINCIPAL COMPONENT ANALYSIS OF THE DATA OF TABLE 11–4

Factor	F Ratio	Amount of Explained Variance
One	42.50*	0.26
Two	0.24	0.00
Three	0.15	0.00
Four	0.76	0.01
Five	1.72	0.01

*Significant at $\alpha = .05$

conditions is factor one which is essentially identical with the summed unweighted Z score component for the principal component analysis based on the five recovery measures in Section 11-5. This agreement in statistical findings identified through two different statistical procedures provides empirical support to using the simple summed unweighted Z scores as a meaningful measure of postoperative recovery.

A post hoc analysis is now performed on the component means for the three treatment groups. The mean values, as reported by CRUNCH (Bostrom, 1986) are

$$\overline{P}_1 = 0.634,$$
$$\overline{P}_2 = -0.023$$

and

$$\overline{P}_3 = -0.610$$

These means are on a scale with a variance of 0.7470. Treatment group one is 0.6336 standard deviation above the mean for all 246 subjects. Group two is slightly below the mean of zero, and treatment group three is 0.6101 standard deviation below the mean. For the post hoc analysis $v_1 = 2$, $v_2 = 243$. Because the 95% critical value is given as

$$F_{2,243:0.95} = 3.00$$

the Scheffé coefficient is given as

$$S = \sqrt{2(3.00)} = 2.45$$

The within group variance on the standard score scale is given as MSW = 0.7470. Thus, any pairwise difference exceeding

(Critical value) (Standard error) =
$$2.45\sqrt{0.7470[1/82 + 1/82]} = 0.331$$

represents a statistically significant difference. In this case, the post hoc confidence intervals are given as

$$\hat{\psi}_{12} = [0.634 - (-0.023)]$$
$$\pm 2.45\sqrt{0.747[1/82 + 1/82]} = 0.657 \pm 0.331$$

$$\hat{\psi}_{13} = [0.634 - (-0.610)]$$
$$\pm 2.45 \quad 0.747[1/82 \pm 1/82] = 1.244 \pm 0.331$$

and

$$\hat{\psi}_{23} = [-0.023 - (-0.610)]$$
$$\pm 2.45 \quad 0.747[1/82 + 1/82] = 0.587 \pm 0.331$$

Thus, treatment one differs from treatments two and three, and treatment two differs from treatment three as is shown here. Notice how similar these results are to those obtained by the simple summed unweighted Z scores of the analysis based on the five recovery variables in Section 11-6. The agreement in the two F ratios and the two sets of standardized means arises because the rotated first principal component for the analysis based on 14 variables is defined, for the most part, by the five recovery variables and by nothing else. Thus, this example supports the position of using simple summed unweighted Z scores instead of exact component scores. In most cases, the two summary measures produce very similar results. Of course, the final choice is up to the individual researcher.

11-8 PSYCHOMETRIC FACTOR ANALYSIS

In the previous sections a detailed discussion of principal component analysis was presented. Some researchers confuse principal component analysis with factor analysis. The confusion is easy to understand because of the joint use of common terms for the two models. Principal component analysis has its theoretical base in multidimensional geometry and has no true or theoretical relationship to behavioral or health care data. In principal component analysis, the goal is to define a reference system for a multidimensional scatter diagram or swarm of data points. Factor analysis is a psychometric model that postulates the existence of behavioral constructs or concepts that are measured indirectly through a series of interrelated variables measuring different facets of the concepts. It is hypothesized that the constructs are measured partially by each of the interrelated behavioral variables. The variance of the collection of the variables is factored into explained or *common variance* and unexplained or *residual components*. The common variance is then aggregated across variables to provide an estimate or operational definition of the factor or hypothetical variable.

In principal component analysis the data matrix contains unities in the main diagonal. The unities represent the variances of the various variables. As such, they contain both explained and unexplained variances. In factor analysis, only the explained portions are used. This presents a psychometric issue for the researcher who wishes to perform a factor analysis because to date no satisfactory solution exists as to how to estimate the explained variance. Guttmann (1956) suggested that a lower bound on the variance be used. He showed that the lower bound for each variable is given by the squared multiple correlation coefficient of each variable regressed on the remaining variables in the analysis. Thus, in a factor analysis it is recommended that the diagonal unities in the correlation matrix be replaced by the squared multiple correlation coefficients of each variable regressed on the remaining variables. This option is used most by researchers and is available on most computer programs for factor analysis.

Tinsley and Tinsley (1987) state that one goal of factor analysis is to satisfy the scientific canon of parsimony, that is, use of the smallest number of explanatory concepts to explain the maximum amount of common variance in a correlation matrix of many variables. Factors are hypothetical constructs or theories that can be used by an investigator to interpret or discern consistent meaning in any particular set of data generated on a large sample of persons. Factors provide a meaningful organizational structure which can be used to assess and derive understanding from a variety of behaviors in terms of providing the most parsimonious explanations.

In the latter sense, factor analysis is an inappropriate model to be applied to the preoperative teaching study. One reason why factor analysis would be inappropriate for these data is that the unities in the correlation matrix would have to be replaced by an estimate of the common variance. Consider the common variance for smoking. If Guttman's lower bound were used, it would have to be estimated by regressing the smoking data on the remaining eight covariate risk variables and the five dependent variables of postoperative recovery. Certainly, it is not theoretically sound or empirically meaningful to predict or measure the variation in an antecedent variable, such as smoking behavior, from postoperative recovery variables that may be caused by variations in smoking habits. This is true also for the remaining risk variables in the preoperative teaching study.

Consider an example in which factor analysis is a valid multivariate procedure. Questionnaire 2 of Chapter 6 was designed to measure nurses' attitudes toward working with dying patients. The items of the questionnaire were purposely constructed to elicit unique pieces of information about the general concept, *working with dying patients*. It is hypothesized that each item extracts a portion of the information about the concepts, working with dying patients. The goal of factor analysis is to factor out the common variance from each of the items to produce a small set of constructs that best define this hypothetical variable. If a multiple set of constructs is generated, the factors can be used to explain or describe how the items, when pooled together, form underlying meaning about working with dying persons.

On Questionnaire 2, fifteen of the twenty questions were identified as measuring different aspects of the concept of working with dying patients. In an examination of the scaling properties of the questions, six questions are on Likert scales, two are on quantitative scales, one is qualitative, and six are dichotomous in nature. All but the one qualitative variable can be used directly in a factor analysis. When the qualitative variable is dummy coded, it can be added to the data set for study.

The AIDS data set is unlike the data set used in the preoperative teaching study. In the latter study, the variables were selected because they were thought to be possible confounding variables that might produce biased results with respect to the three treatment programs. Here, all the variance of the 14 variables was used in the principal component analysis to achieve data reduction. From a different perspective, the nine covariates included in the principal components analysis could be viewed as measures of preoperative risk. As such, they could be submitted to a factor analysis with the purpose of identifying the minimal number of risk factors that influence a person's ability to recover quickly following an operation. The five dependent measures could be submitted to a second factor analysis because collectively they are thought to measure preoperative recovery.

As indicated, factor analysis is a psychometric model that is actually limited in applications. It is valid for factor analyzing the semantic differential scales described in Section 5–14 because the paired adjectives are hypothesized to measure three underlying behavioral constructs called evaluation, activity, and potency. It is also valid for factor analyzing instruments based on Likert scales (Section 5–12), Thurstone scales (Section 5–11), and related scales.

11–9 CRITERIA FOR PERFORMING AND EVALUATING A FACTOR ANALYTIC STUDY

A number of criteria should be examined before performing a factor analytic investigation. The following are some of the major criteria:

1. The data have been generated from a single sample.
2. There are no missing data on any one subject.
3. An adequate sample size is available.
4. The distribution of each variable has a large dispersion.
5. The distribution of each variable is not highly skewed.
6. The variables are not mathematically related or functions of one another.
7. A number of correlation coefficients in the data matrix are significantly different from zero.
8. A small number of dichotomous variables are used.
9. The quantitative variables include a large range of possible values.
10. The biserial or tetrachoric correlation coefficients are few in number in the correlation matrix.

In order to carry out the computational algorithms for a factor analysis, the data must come from one sample and complete information must be available for each subject in the study. Some computer programs have an option for estimating correlation coefficients using pairwise deletion methods (described in Section 8–17). Such methods must be used with care because they can introduce a singularity in the correlation matrix and produce computations that result in nonmeaningful factors.

There are no universally accepted rules concerning sample size. Comrey (1973) suggested that a sample size of 100 is poor, 200 is fair, 300 is good, 500 is very good, and 1000 is excellent. According to Tinsley and

Tinsley (1987) a factor analytic study should employ a minimum of 300 respondents. They also indicate that a factor analytic study based on 5 to 10 subjects per variable or item up to a sample size of 300 is acceptable. For instance if a scale contains 14 items, a minimal sample size between 70 and 140 is required. Guertin and Bailey (1970) suggest a minimum of 100 for Pearson Product Moment Correlation Coefficients and 400 for tetrachoric correlation coefficients. The bigger the sample, the better the sample is a simple rule to follow in most situations.

Normality of the underlying distributions is not a condition for a valid factor analysis. Psychometric factor analysis is not a statistical model that results in t or F tests. Thus, multivariate normally is not an assumption. Variables with restricted ranges should not be included. If the subjects are highly homogeneous on a variable, the variable should be removed from the data matrix. The goal is to use variables with large standard deviations. Variables with small standard deviations can result in correlation coefficients that are close to zero. Variables that are highly skewed with most subjects appearing at the bottom or top of the scale also should be removed because such variables can generate correlations with values close to zero.

Variables that are related to one another in direct mathematical form should not be included in the analysis. For example, in the analysis of the five preoperative teaching dependent variables, their sum, the sum of any two, the sum of their squares, or any transformation of the original data should not be included. Thus, it would be an error to include pain med. one and pain med. two and their sum in a single factor analysis. Variables of this type introduce what is called a *collinearity* in the correlation matrix and complications in the computational procedures that can lead to meaningless factors. Collinearities can be introduced inadvertently into a factor analysis by using *ipsative variables*. Ipsative variables are frequently encountered in studies in which subjects are asked to rank a set of stimuli. For example, a subject could be asked to rank four wines according to quality. After the ranks of 1, 2, and 3 are assigned, the rank of 4 must go to the last remaining wine. Thus, the ranks are correlated and the total sum of the ranks for each subject is equal to $1 + 2 + 3 + 4 = 10$. Such ipsative measures automatically introduce collinearities into the correlation matrix.

A potential problem exists for the researcher who employs 5-point Likert scales or two valued dichotomous variables. Empirical practice fortunately suggests that factor analytic techniques can be used successfully on Likert scaled items or dichotomous items provided that the sample size is large. Horst (1965) provides methods for the dichotomous case.

If the correlation coefficients fluctuate around zero, it is possible that a meaningless factor analysis could result. Armstrong and Soelberg (1968) have demonstrated that interpretable factors from a data matrix obtained by correlating random numbers can be generated. In order to reduce the risk of making such errors a researcher should test correlation coefficients for statistical significance using the Dunn method (described in Section 10–5). Because biserial correlation coefficients and tetrachoric correlation coefficients are biased upward from zero, they should not be used in large numbers in a factor analysis. If dichotomous variables are kept to a minimum, the problem is not severe. Note that dichotomous variables could be a problem in the factor analysis of the AIDS questionnaire.

Other decisions associated with factor analysis include selection of the best commonality estimate, identification of the appropriate extraction method, selection of factors to rotate, identification of the appropriate factor rotation to employ, and the estimation of factor scores. For a concise summary of the various types of factor extraction procedures, see Tinsley and Tinsley (1987). Most researchers use Kaiser Varimax Rotation model to achieve simple structure and Kaiser's Rule to determine the number of factors to retain (1958). (These models were described in Section 11–5. For other criteria see Tinsley and Tinsley, 1987).

Factor scores are extremely difficult to determine and one must be careful in choosing a computer program that does the computations correctly. A factor score is a composite score based on each variable's contribution to the factor. Individual scores on each variable are multiplied by the associated factor score coefficient. The products are summed across the variable to yield a factor score. The model is described by Marascuilo and Levin (1983).

In summary, factor analysis is a very useful multivariate method for nursing research. It should be used in studies in which it is known that a large number of interrelated variables are serving as surrogate measures for a theoretical construct that cannot be measured directly. It provides indirect measures for variables like fear and anger or attitude toward working with dying patients. Factor analysis is not a substitute for principal component analysis even though the results of a principal component analysis are often very similar to that of a factor analysis. Because the solutions are so often alike, researchers can be easily seduced into using a principal component analysis when a factor analysis is the more appropriate procedure for parsimoniously identifying meaningful underlying theoretical constructs. Many of the facets of principal component analysis such as varimax rotation, simple structure, Kaiser's Rule, structure correlations, and others can be employed in factor analysis.

11–10 CANONICAL CORRELATION THEORY

Principal components and associated forms of factor analysis are perhaps the most frequently used mathematical models for reducing a larger set of interrelated variables to a smaller, more manageable and meaningful set of hypothetical variables that can be employed for further model building and data analysis. Other models exist, with canonical correlation theory probably being the most prominent. We say that it is the most prominent because the two sample t test models, the K sample F test of the analysis of variance, simple regression, multiple regression, the multivariate analysis of variance, and the Karl Pearson tests of homogeneity and independence all constitute special cases of the general canonical correlation model. The connections among these more familiar statistical models and canonical analysis theory are described by Knapp (1978) and illustrated in Marascuilo and Levin (1983).

One of the main features of principal component analysis and factor analysis is the lack of a clearly defined set of independent and dependent variables. In principal component analysis and factor analysis they do not exist. This is unlike the situation in canonical correlation analysis. Here, P independent variables, $X_1, X_2, \ldots, X_P$ and P dependent variables, $Y_1, Y_2, \ldots, Y_Q$ where Q < P. If P is less than or equal to Q, simply interchange the role of the independent and dependent set of variables, because the mathematics of the model are unrelated to the distinction between independent and dependent variables. Canonical correlation theory reduces to simple regression theory if P = Q = 1 and it reduces to multiple regression theory if P > 1 and Q = 1.

As pointed out by Cooley and Lohnes (1971), the canonical correlation model reduces the dimensionality of the two sets of variables to a few linear functions of the measurements studied. In contrast, the factor analytic models identify linear functions of variables that have maximum variances or maximum discriminations between subjects, which are limited to the restrictions of orthogonality. The canonical model identifies pairs of linear functions—one from each set—which have maximum covariances between the independent and dependent variables, again restricted to the specifications of orthogonality. The canonical model describes the extent to which individual subjects occupy the same relative positions in the set of independent variables as they do in the set of dependent variables.

An example of the applicability of canonical theory is the preoperative recovery study. Here, the covariates are treated as independent variables; they are hospital, treatment, sex, age, severity, education, provider of health insurance, family income, weight, smoking habits, alcohol usage, drug usage, exercise practices, and uncertainty about surgical treatment. The outcome or dependent variables for this study are length of stay in hospital following surgery, the number of pain relief medicines administered one day and two days after surgery, the number of postoperative complications, and the number of days patients spend recuperating before being able to leave their place of recovery without assistance. Of course, separate principal component analyses or factor analyses could be performed on the two sets. A decision to perform separate data reduction analyses is always justified, because the two sets of variables are believed to be measuring different concepts; however, in this case there is a disadvantage to this approach to data analysis. The disadvantage arises because the variables are not only correlated

within each set but they are also correlated across the sets. A principal component analysis or factor analysis based on the joint collection of the independent and dependent variables does not maintain the separation between the two sets of correlation coefficients. In fact, the between set correlations are completely ignored. Canonical analysis, however, does maintain the separation between the two sets of correlations and for this reason can be justified. In a study with clearly defined independent and dependent variables such as the preoperative teaching study, a single canonical analysis is preferred and recommended in place of two principal component analyses or factor analyses applied to the independent and dependent variables separately.

As a justification for the use of the canonical correlation model, it is presumed that certain risk factors serve as predictors of the rate of speed and success with which the patient responds to one of the three treatment conditions. Although treatment is an independent variable, it is not included in the canonical analysis because the treatment is assigned to each patient for reasons of study and hypothesis testing. The researcher wants to know which of the three treatments is to be preferred and recommended for future use. Thus, a researcher should not include in the canonical analysis any variable that serves as a *domain of study* for hypothesis testing.

If a researcher wants to make comparisons across drug users and drug abstainers, the variable that measures drug use must also be excluded from the analysis. In this context, drug usage serves as an independent variable to predict and explain recovery. In other words, drug usage becomes a domain of study for statistical hypothesis testing. This would also be true for alcohol use, exercise patterns, smoking habits, and even weight, provided, of course, that one wished to test hypotheses on these independent variables. Thus, it becomes important to define independent variables, which can serve as domains of study for further research, and covariates, which are believed to have an impact in some way on the dependent variables. In some cases, this identification may produce problems in selection. However, every researcher must make these decisions before contemplating a canonical correlation analysis.

Let us return to the example. We begin by

defining the dependent variables. In this instance, the five variables of Table 11−1 serve as the dependent variables. They clearly measure the effects of the three treatment procedures. For the independent set, hospital, education, provider of insurance, and family income are excluded because they cannot serve as risk factors that influence speed and degree of recovery. The independent variables that may have an impact on the five recovery or dependent variables are X_1: sex, X_2: age, X_3: severity, X_4: weight, X_5: smoking, X_6: alcohol use, X_7: drug use, X_8: exercise, and X_9: uncertainty. It is important to note that none of these variables can now be used as a domain of study for any other research questions. To make comparisons across the various subgroups of smoking, using the derived canonical variables, it is necessary to repeat the entire analysis deleting smoking from the set of independent variables.

There is a misconception that canonical analysis can be justified only when the underlying variables have a multivariate normal distribution. This is not the case. As pointed out by Kerlinger and Pedhazur (1973, p. 8), variables that are dichotomous or qualitative can be incorporated into the

analysis using dummy coding. This model has been used in multiple regression in Section 10−8 and in the use of dummy codes in the analysis of variance and covariance in Sections 10−11 and 10−12. It was also employed in the principal component and factor analysis models described in Sections 11−7 and 11−8. Cooley and Lohnes (1971) provide an example in which dichotomous response variables to a personal activities inventory are used in a canonical analysis.

Before embarking on a canonical analysis, the nurse researcher is advised to examine the correlation matrix to determine whether the analysis will prove to be fruitful. This is done most easily by examining three submatrices of the total correlation matrix. The three matrices for the postoperative recovery study are reported in Table 11−7.

The first submatrix to examine consists of correlation coefficients among the dependent set of variables. This matrix is identical with the correlation matrix of Table 11−1, which also appears in Table 11−4. As indicated, the correlations in this submatrix are large. This is important. If the correlations were all close to zero, the analysis would not be fruitful. For a canonical analysis to be successful, a fairly large number

TABLE 11−7 CORRELATION MATRICES FOR A CANONICAL ANALYSIS BASED ON FIVE RECOVERY VARIABLES AND NINE RISK VARIABLES

	Y_1	Y_2	Y_3	Y_4	Y_5
Y_1	1.00	.63	.64	.64	.66
Y_2		1.00	.62	.51	.58
Y_3			1.00	.53	.57
Y_4				1.00	.56
Y_5					1.00

	X_1	X_2	X_3	X_4	X_5	X_6	X_7	X_8	X_9
X_1	1.00	−.10	.02	−.31	−.10	−.12	−.12	−.24	.06
X_2		1.00	.36	.52	.54	.03	−.07	−.28	.33
X_3			1.00	.31	.46	.01	.04	−.13	.56
X_4				1.00	.37	.16	−.03	−.15	.27
X_5					1.00	.06	−.05	−.14	.34
X_6						1.00	.07	−.03	−.04
X_7							1.00	−.01	.02
X_8								1.00	−.19
X_9									1.00

	X_1	X_2	X_3	X_4	X_5	X_6	X_7	X_8	X_9
Y_1	.02	.42	.32	.40	.49	.07	−.05	−.04	.41
Y_2	.24	.23	.37	.25	.28	.03	−.03	−.05	.37
Y_3	.15	.26	.28	.30	.33	.11	.07	−.08	.25
Y_4	.00	.39	.29	.49	.33	.06	.08	−.03	.29
Y_5	.03	.50	.50	.39	.47	.05	.02	−.13	.39

of high valued correlations should be present among the dependent variables. The second submatrix to examine is the one that consists of correlation coefficients among the independent set of variables. The same statements hold for the correlations among the independent variables. These correlations are reported in Table 11-7. Here, it is seen that X_2: age shows moderate positive correlations with X_3: severity, X_4: weight, X_5: smoking, and X_9: uncertainty. At the same time, X_3: severity is correlated with X_4: weight, X_5: smoking, and X_9: uncertainty. In addition, X_4: weight and X_5: smoking are correlated, as are X_5: smoking and X_9: uncertainty. These large correlations are favorable signs that the analysis has the potential for producing meaningful results.

Finally, the last correlation matrix to examine involves the correlation of each X variable with each Y variable. This correlation matrix also appears in Table 11-7 and Table 11-4. The correlation table must have as a minimum a number of moderately large correlations; otherwise the whole process will fail. If there are not many large correlation coefficients in this submatrix, the optimum approach would be to perform two separate principal component analyses or factor analyses on the independent set of variables and the dependent set of variables. Here, fortunately, eight correlation coefficients are larger than .40. Both length of stay and days following surgery before patient can ambulate freely show moderate positive correlations with X_1: sex, X_2: age, X_3: severity, X_4: weight, X_5: smoking, and X_9: uncertainty. Pain med. one shows some correlation with X_3: severity and X_9: uncertainty, and postoperative complications show some correlation with X_2: age and X_4: weight. These are excellent signs that the analysis has the potential of being successful.

These between set correlations are the most important because canonical analysis uses the correlations between the independent and dependent sets of variables (X,Y) to define pairs of hypothetical variables that are linear combinations of the X set and the Y set. In canonical analysis, the weights that define the two paired linear combinations are determined in order to maximize the correlation coefficient that exists between the two derived X and Y variables. The two weighted linear combinations that maximize the correlation between the hypothetical variables are called the *first pair of canonical variates*. The correlation that exists between the two variables is called the *first canonical correlation coefficient*. The reason that the adjective first appears in the named variables is that other pairs also are generated from the analysis. In fact, Q pairs are generated as are Q canonical correlation coefficients. The first pair generates the largest correlation coefficient, with subsequent pairs being sequentially smaller in numerical value. In addition, the pairs are so constructed that the correlation coefficient between pairs is zero. Thus, the pairs are uncorrelated or orthogonal with one another.

The results for the preoperative teaching study are reported in Tables 11-8 and 11-9. Table 11-8 provides the statistical tests that are used to determine how many pairs of canonical variates are statistically significant. The decisions are based on critical values selected from the F distribution. The required information needed by the nurse researcher appears on computer printouts. The figures of Table 11-8 have been read directly from such a printout. As indicated, four pairs of canonical variates are statistically significant because the first four F ratios are larger than the critical values defined by $\alpha = 0.05$. Because a canonical cor-

TABLE 11-8 TESTS OF HYPOTHESES TO DETERMINE THE NUMBER OF STATISTICALLY SIGNIFICANT PAIRS OF CANONICAL VARIATES

Canonical Pair	Value of R	Numerator, Degrees of Freedom	Denominator, Degrees of Freedom	F Ratio	Critical Value
1	0.69	45	1041	6.55*	1.34
2	0.40	32	861	3.72*	1.44
3	0.36	21	672	3.60*	1.56
4	0.34	12	470	3.42*	1.75
5	0.20	5	236	1.97	2.21

*Significant at $\alpha = 0.05$

TABLE 11-9 PATTERN AND STRUCTURE MATRICES FOR THE DATA OF TABLE 11-7

	Standardized Pattern Coefficients				Structure Correlation Coefficients			
	Y^1	Y^2	Y^3	Y^4	Y^1	Y^2	Y^3	Y^4
Y_1	0.31	−1.32	0.07	−0.90	0.87*	−0.31	0.18	−0.33
Y_2	0.04	0.95	0.33	−0.77	0.67*	0.48*	0.29	−0.45*
Y_3	−0.01	0.26	0.51	0.29	0.67*	0.22	0.37	−0.04
Y_4	0.30	−0.03	0.62	0.98	0.80*	−0.03	0.41*	0.35
Y_5	0.52	0.37	−1.22	0.30	0.91*	0.18	−0.38	0.02
	X^1	X^2	X^3	X^4	X^1	X^2	X^3	X^4
X_1	0.29	0.58	0.68	−0.21	0.04	0.63*	0.34	−0.41*
X_2	0.30	−0.09	−0.56	0.31	0.74*	−0.21	−0.37	0.22
X_3	0.16	0.88	−0.66	0.18	0.66*	0.47*	−0.41*	−0.08
X_4	0.43	0.00	0.89	0.49	0.70*	−0.22	0.24	0.44*
X_5	0.31	−0.52	0.10	−0.40	0.73*	−0.32	−0.21	−0.19
X_6	0.04	0.01	0.09	−0.08	0.10	−0.06	0.13	0.08
X_7	0.10	0.20	0.20	0.52	0.02	0.20	0.11	0.51*
X_8	0.20	0.06	0.33	−0.13	−0.13	0.16	0.20	−0.08
X_9	0.22	−0.28	0.25	−0.67	0.62*	0.05	−0.05	−0.45*

*Structure correlations greater than 0.40 used as definers of the factors

relation analysis requires large samples for justification, it is possible to obtain statistically significant results by just the use of a large sample and not because of scientific or practical significance. Cooley and Lohnes (1971, p. 176) do not recommend the use of statistical hypothesis testing to determine the number of significant pairs of canonical variables. Instead, they state that as a rule of thumb only canonical correlations of .30 or higher should be judged as having potential theoretical or practical significance.

Although statistically significant pairs of canonical variates have been identified, a researcher must now face the problem of defining these new constructs. As will be seen, this is not easy. Similar to the procedure used in principal component analysis, use is made of the structure matrix to solve one of the most difficult problems of multivariate analysis. The *pattern and structure matrix* for the canonical analysis is reported in Table 11-9. The numbers used as multipliers to the Z scores are referred to as the *pattern coefficients* and are used to compute the canonical variate scores. The *structure correlation coefficients* are used to define the variates. There is a tendency to focus on the pattern matrix when trying to name canonical variates. This practice is not recommended. The procedure recommended by psychometricians is use of the structure matrix. The reason for this will be seen in the discussion that follows.

For the first set of canonical variates, the first canonical correlation coefficient is equal to 0.69. Note that the amount of variation in the first Y variate explained by the first X variate is given as $(0.69)^2 = 0.48$. For behavioral and health care variables, that is a large amount of explained variability. In this example, $Y^{(1)}$ is similar to the principal component based on the five dependent variables. It defines a general recovery dimension. Note that the agreement between principal components and canonical analysis is not always expected. The equation for this canonical variate, defined in terms of standard scores for the five dependent variables, is

$$Y^{(1)} = 0.31Z_1 + 0.04Z_2 - 0.01Z_3 + 0.30Z_4 + 0.52Z_5$$

From this equation, it could be concluded that Z_2 and Z_3 do not weight or load on $Y^{(1)}$. If one were to conclude this, the decisions would be in serious error because the structure matrix indicates the opposite. Notice that the five correlations of each of the dependent variables with the newly constructed $Y^{(1)}$ are 0.87, 0.67, 0.67, 0.80, and 0.91, indicating that all five variables are definers of $Y^{(1)}$.

From the structure matrix, it is seen that $X^{(1)}$ is correlated with X_2: age, X_3: severity, X_4: weight, X_5: smoking, and X_9: uncertainty. At one end of the scale are patients who are advanced in age, who possess high levels of severity, who have excess weight, with high risk smoking habits, and who reveal high levels of uncertainty. They tend to show poor recovery experiences. At the opposite end of the scale are their counterparts who are younger, who possess lower levels of severity, who have acceptable weights, who are nonsmokers, and who reveal lower levels of uncertainty. They tend to recover with speed and efficiency. This analysis suggests that the $X^{(1)}$ factor is a bipolar general risk factor associated with age, severity, poor health factors, and fear of surgery. From a practical and theoretical point of view, the two variables, $X^{(1)}$ and $Y^{(1)}$, go together and their connection to one another is interpretable.

Consider the second set of canonical variates for which the correlation coefficient is 0.40 and for which the amount of explained variability is $(0.40)^2 = 0.16$. The amount of explained variation in $Y^{(2)}$ afforded by its correlation with $X^{(2)}$ is not very large. The high level of interpretability encountered for the first set of canonical variates may not materialize for these two new hypothetical correlated variates. $Y^{(2)}$ is defined primarily by pain med. one and $X^{(2)}$ is defined by X_1: sex and X_3: severity. On one end of the $X^{(2)}$ scale are women with severe abdominal conditions, whereas at the other end of the $X^{(2)}$ scale are men with minor abdominal problems. This scale is less easy to interpret and is probably best defined as a gender severity scale.

The connection between the third and fourth sets of variates is not clear. As a consequence, we would not use these variables for further study.

Now that the analysis and evaluation of the canonical variates is completed, canonical variate scores would be determined for the 246 subjects in the study for the first two sets of canonical variates. These derived scores would be used to make comparisons across the three treatment groups and across relevant variables of interest that were not used in the canonical analysis.

11–11 MULTIVARIATE ANALYSIS OF VARIANCE

Research in the behavioral and health care sciences is rarely univariate in its assessment of treatment and other independent variable effects. Typically, a researcher selects multiple dependent variables to study, which are almost always correlated with one

another. One historical option, which seems to be the rule, is to study each variable separately and never collectively. Many studies in the nursing research literature treat multiple dependent variables in exactly this manner. This is unfortunate because such analyses are almost certain to involve elevated type I and type II error rates. In addition, the correlational structure that exists among the variables is not used effectively to extract salient information from the data. The resulting redundancy in information contained in multivariate measures is thoroughly ignored. These design issues and reasons for using multivariate analysis of variance (MANOVA) are examined and discussed by Haase and Ellis (1987).

Multivariate analysis of variance is a special case of canonical analysis, based on the use of independent variables that are dummy coded to express or define group membership. When the model was first introduced, it was assumed that the dependent variables had to be discrete or continuous quantitative variables. Later, it was shown that categorical and dichotomous measures can be incorporated into the model with appropriate dummy codes. Examination of Knapp's (1978) discussion of dummy coding for canonical analysis shows that dummy codes can be used for both the independent and dependent set of variables. Cohen and Cohen (1983) provide an extensive discussion of this substitution for the univariate case. What is true for the univariate case also is true for the multivariate case. As will be seen, MANOVA provides an extension of the univariate analysis of variance to a model in which mean values across many interrelated dependent variables can be examined collectively. As shown by Knapp (1978), when K = 2 and Q = 1, multivariate analysis of variance reduces to the two-sample t test and when K > 2 and Q = 1, it reduces to the one-way analysis of variance. If K = 2 and if Q > 1, the multivariate analysis of variance is equivalent to Hotelling's T^2. Because Hotelling's T^2 is a special case, it is not described. (See Marascuilo and Levin (1983) for a discussion of this special case.)

The hypothesis tested by the multivariate analysis of variance F test is that the mean profile of Q dependent variables across K groups of subjects are equal. In particular, let the dependent variables be denoted as Y_1, $Y_2, \ldots, Y_Q$, and let their means be denoted as μ_{qk} where q = 1, 2, . . . ,Q and k = 1, 2,

. . . ,K. The hypothesis tested by the multivariate F test is

$$H_0: \begin{matrix} \mu_{11} = \mu_{12} = \cdots = \mu_{1K} \\ \mu_{21} = \mu_{22} = \cdots = \mu_{2K} \\ \downarrow \quad\quad \downarrow \quad\quad\quad \downarrow \\ \mu_{Q1} = \mu_{Q2} = \cdots = \mu_{QK} \end{matrix}$$

According to this representation of the null hypothesis, the K means of variable Y_1 are equal to a common value, the K means for Y_2 are also equal to a common value, the K means of variable Y_3 are equal to a common value, and so on, for the remaining variables. This is a very complex hypothesis and can be rejected for any number of reasons. If the hypothesis is not rejected, it can be concluded immediately that the mean values or profiles across the K groups are equal, variable by variable. But if the hypothesis is rejected, very complicated post hoc comparisons may need to be investigated.

As an example of where the multivariate analysis of variance could be used, consider the three treatment conditions of the preoperative teaching study and the five dependent variables of Table 11-1. The mean profiles on the five dependent variables for the three treatment groups are summarized in Table 11-10. The hypothesis tested by the multivariate F test is H_0: the three profiles are identical. The alternative hypothesis is H_1: the profiles are not identical. Inspection of the three empirical profiles suggests that the means are not equal, variable by variable. In fact, it appears that treatment one is the least effective. All five mean values of treatment one are larger than the corresponding means of treatments two and three. In addition, it appears that treatment three is most effective. Its five mean values are the lowest. For completeness and for post hoc compari-

sons, the mean square errors also are reported in Table 11-10.

Unlike the univariate analysis of variance F test, the testing of the hypothesis of identity of profiles can be approached from a number of different solutions. With exceedingly large samples, the methods are equivalent and interchangeable. With small samples, they are not. For this reason, it is recommended that multivariate analysis of variance be performed on large samples only. This leads to the question, "What constitutes a large sample?" No one seems to know. For a conservative rule, it is recommended that a large sample be defined as one in which $N > 10(K + Q)$, where K is the number of treatments and Q is the number of dependent measures. Thus, for the example, a large sample exists if N is larger than $10(3 + 5) = 80$. In this case, N is given as N $= 246$.

Four different solutions to MANOVA have been proposed by Pillai (1960), Hotelling (1931), Wilks (1932), and Roy (1957). Explicit mathematical formulations of these criteria are not presented because of their complexity. The numerical values can be read directly from computer printouts, as were the numbers appearing in Table 11-11. The Roy solution is not presented because it requires extensive tables and charts. It is described by Marascuilo and Levin (1983). The Pillai, Hotelling, and Wilks solutions can be approximated by use of the F distribution and corresponding critical values. The F distribution approximations are reported in Table 11-11. As indicated, all three criteria lead to rejection of the hypothesis that the mean profiles across the three treatment groups are identical. The F ratios for testing the identity of the three profiles are given by the three criteria values of F = 12.78. 14.29, and 13.54. All lead to rejection of the hypothesis of identity of mean profiles. Rarely do the three criteria disagree.

TABLE 11-10 MEAN PROFILES FOR THE THREE TREATMENT GROUPS OF THE POST-OPERATIVE RECOVERY STUDY WITH DEPENDENT VARIABLES OF TABLE 11-1

Variable	Treatment One	Treatment Two	Treatment Three	Mean Square Error
Y_1	4.89	4.52	3.37	2.20
Y_2	6.65	4.99	4.01	2.72
Y_3	2.62	1.71	1.45	2.07
Y_4	1.23	0.71	0.33	0.91
Y_5	5.57	4.17	2.76	5.70

TABLE 11–11 TEST STATISTICS FOR EVALUATING THE MEAN PROFILES OF TABLE 11–10

Criterion	Numerator, Degrees of Freedom	Denominator, Degrees of Freedom	F Ratio	Critical Value for $\alpha = 0.05$
Pillai	10	480	12.78	1.83
Hotelling	10	476	14.29	1.83
Wilks	10	478	13.54	1.83

Now that the hypothesis of identity of mean profiles has been rejected, the next step would be to perform a post hoc analysis on the mean values. The simplest post hoc procedure is to perform a variable by variable analysis on the means using as critical value the Scheffé coefficient defined as

$$S = \sqrt{\nu_1 \, F\nu_1, \nu_{2:(1-\alpha)}}$$

which, in this case, is given as

$$S = \sqrt{10(1.83)} = 4.28$$

For length of stay, the three pairwise contrasts are given as

$$\hat{\psi}_{12} = (4.89 - 4.52)$$
$$\pm 4.28\sqrt{2.20[1/82 + 1/82]} = 0.37 \pm 0.99$$

$$\hat{\psi}_{13} = (4.89 - 3.37)$$
$$\pm 4.28\sqrt{2.20[1/82 + 1/82]} = 1.52 \pm 0.99$$

and

$$\hat{\psi}_{23} = (4.52 - 3.37)$$
$$\pm 4.28\sqrt{2.20[1/82 + 1/82]} = 1.15 \pm 0.99$$

Because the confidence interval does cover zero, it is concluded that treatments one and two are not statistically different from one another. Both, however, are statistically different from treatment three. Thus, it makes sense to examine on a post hoc basis the contrast that combines treatments one and two and compares the combined sample mean to the mean of treatment three. This contrast is given as

$$\hat{\psi}_{(12)3} = [1/2(4.89 + 4.52) - 3.37]$$
$$\pm 4.28\sqrt{2.20[(1/2)^2/82 + (1/2)^2/82 + (-1)^2/82]}$$
$$= 1.335 \pm 0.909.$$

The post hoc hypothesis is supported. Similar contrasts can be examined on the other four dependent measures.

Whereas pairwise contrasts and a complex contrast within *single* variables have been examined, the intercorrelations among the variables have been completely ignored by the previous variable by variable post hoc analysis. The multivariate F test incorporates multivariate tests of variables that make use of the correlations across variables and the redundancy in information contained in correlated measures. Thus, it also examines weighted means across variables. In this case, differential weighting of two or three variables may not be meaningful, but summing standardized variables across all five variables makes sense. The rationale for summing the five standardized variables was provided in Section 11–7, in which it was seen that the first principal component for the five variables was interpretable as a postoperative recovery measure and could be estimated by Wainer's (1976) unweighted sum of standardized variables. This was done and reported in Table 11–3 for the mean values defined by the principal components. The F statistic for that test was F = 40.12.

Contrasts defined by the principal components, the canonical variates, and other linear combinations of the variables also are covered by the multivariate F test and can be examined on a post hoc basis, if desired. In the next section, linear discriminant functions can be seen to define contrasts that are also covered by the multivariate F test.

An important issue in evaluating any rejected null hypothesis centers on assessing the amount of variance explained in the dependent set of variables by the independent variables in a study. Cramer and Nicewander (1979) favor the arithmetic average of the squared canonical correlation as a measurement of explained variation. Serlin (1982) has shown that this criterion is a natural generalization of Pillai's trace criterion. (For more on MANOVA see Haase and Ellis (1987).)

11-12 LINEAR DISCRIMINANT ANALYSIS

Closely allied to multivariate analysis of variance is linear discriminant function analysis. Linear discriminant analysis is the flip side of multivariate analysis of variance. Each provides a different way to solve the same problem. Multivariate analysis of variances emphasizes group differences, and linear discriminant analysis emphasizes the estimation of the linear combination that maximizes group differences. This procedure was proposed by R.A. Fisher (1948) and later shown to be a part of multivariate analysis of variance. According to Betz (1987), linear discriminant analysis can be used

1. to describe, summarize, and understand the differences between or among groups on mean profiles and contrasts,
2. to determine which set of variables best captures or characterizes group differences with respect to mean profiles,
3. to describe the dimensionality of group differences, not in terms of structure, as in principal component analysis or factor analysis, but in terms of group profiles on means and contrasts,
4. to test theories that use stage concepts or taxonomies as independent variables,
5. to examine the nature of group differences following a null hypothesis rejected by a MANOVA F test.

The problem that Fisher set out to solve can be described easily in terms of the preoperative teaching study. Here, five variables characterize the effects of the three treatments on speed and efficiency of recovery. Each variable by itself can be used to test for differences in the populations. As indicated in Section 11-11, such variable by variable analysis is not recommended because of its possible elevation of type I and II errors and because of the complete lack of attention to the correlations that exist among variables. Thus, it is appropriate to ask the question, "Can the variables in concert provide a better evaluation of group differences than any one variable individually?"

Fisher approached the question by assuming that a linear combination of the variables would provide a more efficient discriminator than each variable individually. Thus, he proposed that a variable of the form,

$$L = W_1 Z_1 + W_2 Z_2 + W_3 Z_3 + W_4 Z_4 + W_5 Z_5$$

would provide a better measure than any of the variables singly. With this formulation, the linear discriminant analysis problem reduces to one of choosing the weights that provide the maximum discrimination between the three treatment groups. The weights that do the job most efficiently are the weights of the first canonical variate provided that the group memberships are *dummy coded* as described in Section 10-11. Fisher called the resulting linear combination the *linear discriminant function*.

Today, the Fisher linear discriminant function is often referred to as the *first canonical variate* and is most useful when the resulting linear combination is described in standard score form. Later, it was discovered that the multivariate approach gives rise to multiple discriminant functions in the same way that canonical analysis gives rise to multiple sets of canonical variables. Thus, a linear discriminant analysis gives rise to multiple discriminant functions and corresponding problems in dimensionality.

When Fisher first approached the problem, he considered the data in their original state. Later, it was found that the analysis could be simplified if standard scores were used in place of the originally scaled values. The model, based on standard scores, is used in all of the major computer programs. Also, note that the purpose of discriminant function analysis is to provide maximum discrimination between group centers or profiles. This purpose in focus is different from principal component analysis. There the goal is to provide maximum discrimination between the subjects in a single group. Thus, principal components analysis provides maximum within group discrimination, whereas linear discriminant analysis provides maximum between group discrimination.

Based on the discussion of canonical analysis, multiple canonical variates can exist. If Q variables are used to define the linear discriminant function and if there are K groups of subjects, then the number of discriminant functions is given as s, the smaller of (Q − 1) or (K − 1). Thus, for the preoperative teaching study with K = three treatment groups and Q = five variables, the number of discriminant functions is (K − 1) = 2. The two discriminant functions, the corresponding structure correlations, and the associated F tests are reported in Table 11-12.

As indicated, the first linear discriminant

TABLE 11–12   PATTERN AND STRUCTURE MATRICES FOR THE LINEAR DISCRIMINANT ANALYSIS FOR THE MEAN PROFILES OF TABLE 11–10

Variable	Pattern Coefficients		Structure Correlations	
	L_1	L_2	L_1	L_2
Y_1	0.159	1.400	0.56*	0.60*
Y_2	−0.888	−0.296	0.98*	−0.04
Y_3	0.218	−0.757	0.48*	−0.20
Y_4	−0.209	−0.335	0.54*	0.05
Y_5	−0.381	0.049	0.67*	0.21

*Structure correlations greater than 0.40 used as definers of the factors

function is defined as all five variables, with pain med. one showing the largest correlation with the first linear discriminant function. Thus, it is very similar to the first principal component except that pain med. one plays a more important role in its definition. The second linear discriminant function is defined primarily by length of stay. For all practical purposes, the single variable, length of stay, is equivalent to the more complicated second linear discriminant function which includes the addition of all five variables. This means that little analytical power is gained by using the second linear discriminant function in place of length of stay alone.

Now that the two linear discriminant functions have been defined, each patient can be scored in terms of the weights and standardized scores. The mean scores for the three treatments are reported in Table 11–13. The analysis of variance table for the first linear discriminant function across the three treatment groups is summarized in Table 11–14. As shown, the null hypothesis of identity of mean linear discriminant function scores is rejected because F = 61.94 is significant at $\alpha = 0.05$ with numerator degrees of freedom given as $\nu_1 = 2$ and numerator degrees of freedom given as $\nu_2 = 243$. Notice that this F ratio is larger than any of the others

reported in Table 11–3 and 11–6. This maximization of the F statistic is expected because the weights were determined to provide maximum group discrimination.

It is not unusual to find a multivariate F test to be exceptionally large, as illustrated in this example. Because the F ratio is related to the number of dependent measures and the sample sizes, large F ratios may have little substantive meaning. Here, as in the univariate case, a measure of explained variance is of interest. As shown by Serlin (1982), the appropriate measure of association for the multivariate test of the null hypothesis of no group differences is given by $\hat{\eta}^2 = V/s$, where V is the Pillai criterion and s is the minimum of (K − 1) and Q. In this example, the value of the Pillai criterion read from computer printouts is .4205 and s = 2. Thus, the amount of variance explained by the two discriminant functions is given as $\hat{\eta}^2 = .21$. This number can be compared with the average amount of variance explained separately by each variable. These measures of association are reported in Tables 9–6 and 11–3. The average values of these five measures is .18. As indicated, the discriminant functions explain .03 more of the variance.

The multivariate null hypothesis of identity of group means was tested in the previous section by the Pillai, Hotelling, and Wilks test statistics. When the hypothesis of identity of profiles was rejected, the hypothesis that the mean discriminant scores across the three groups is equal to zero was also rejected. The two hypotheses are interchangeable. Rejection of one null hypothesis implies rejection of the other. If desired, post hoc comparisons could be made across the mean values on the discriminant function reported in Table 11–13. The appropriate critical value is given as S = 4.28, the value reported in the previous section. For the three pairwise contrasts,

TABLE 11–13   MEAN VALUES ON THE FIRST DISCRIMINANT FUNCTION FOR THE THREE TREATMENT GROUPS ON THE POSTOPERATIVE STUDY AND THE FIVE DEPENDENT MEASURES OF TABLE 11–1

Treatment Group	Mean Value
One	−0.78
Two	0.11
Three	0.68

TABLE 11-14 ANALYSIS OF VARIANCE TABLE FOR THE FIRST LINEAR DISCRIMINANT FUNCTION ACROSS THE THREE TREATMENT GROUPS

Source of Variation	Degrees of Freedom	Sum of Squares	Mean Square	F Ratio
Treatment	2	88.87	44.44	61.94*
Residual	243	174.33	0.72	
Total	245	263.20		

*Significant at $\alpha = .05$

$\hat{\psi}_{12} = (-0.78 - 0.11)$
$\pm 4.28\sqrt{0.72[1/82 + 1/82]} = -0.89 \pm 0.57$

$\hat{\psi}_{13} = (-0.78 - 0.68)$
$\pm 4.28\sqrt{0.72[1/82 + 1/82]} = -1.46 \pm 0.57$

and

$\hat{\psi}_{23} = (+0.11 - 0.68)$
$\pm 4.28\sqrt{0.72[1/82 + 1/82]} = -0.57 \pm 0.57$

Except for the comparison involving treatments two and three, it can be concluded that treatment one differs from two and three. The most probable reason for the difference in the post hoc analysis based on the first linear discriminant function is the large weight (-0.888) given to pain med. one. It is an important definer of the weighted linear combination as indicated by the large structure correlation coefficient of .98. Another reason may be the large value of the Scheffé coefficient.

Finally, the results of a linear discriminant analysis can be portrayed vividly in graphic form. Figure 11-1 provides the distributions of the first linear discriminant function scores for the three treatment groups. As is apparent, of the three treatments, treatment three provides the quickest and speediest recovery. The least favorable treatment is treatment one. Similar graphs can be obtained for the second canonical variate or second linear discriminant function, if desired. However, for this second derived variable the graph should be very similar to the graph obtained for length of stay.

11-13 ASSUMPTIONS AND SAMPLE SIZE REQUIREMENTS FOR MULTIVARIATE METHODS

When the multivariate models described in this chapter were developed by mathemati-

cal statisticians, they began with very strong assumptions which are rarely satisfied by behavioral and health care data. The strongest assumption is that the variables possess multivariate normal distributions. This classic assumption suggests that only quantitative variables can be used as dependent measures, and that dichotomous variables, qualitative variables, and discrete number scales cannot be used. It might be concluded from this discussion that behavioral data would rarely meet the stringent conditions established by this assumption.

Multivariate normality also implies the following:

1. The variables are linearly related to one another in pairs.
2. Each two variable regression line possess homoscedasticity.
3. The multivariate distribution contains no outliers.
4. None of the variables is truncated.

Further conditions must be satisfied when multiple groups are employed. These assumptions are the following:

5. The variances across groups must be equal to one another for each variable and each pair of variables.
6. The correlations across groups must be equal to one another.
7. The observations between and within samples must be statistically independent.

If these assumptions are satisfied, all of the *statistical* tests described in this chapter are valid, and if orthogonal components are generated, they also are statistically independent.

If a researcher is not interested in hypothesis testing and only in data description, these assumptions are not required except for the assumption of independent observations. Even if the assumptions are not satisfied, all is not lost. Upon reflection, it is apparent that some of the assumptions were

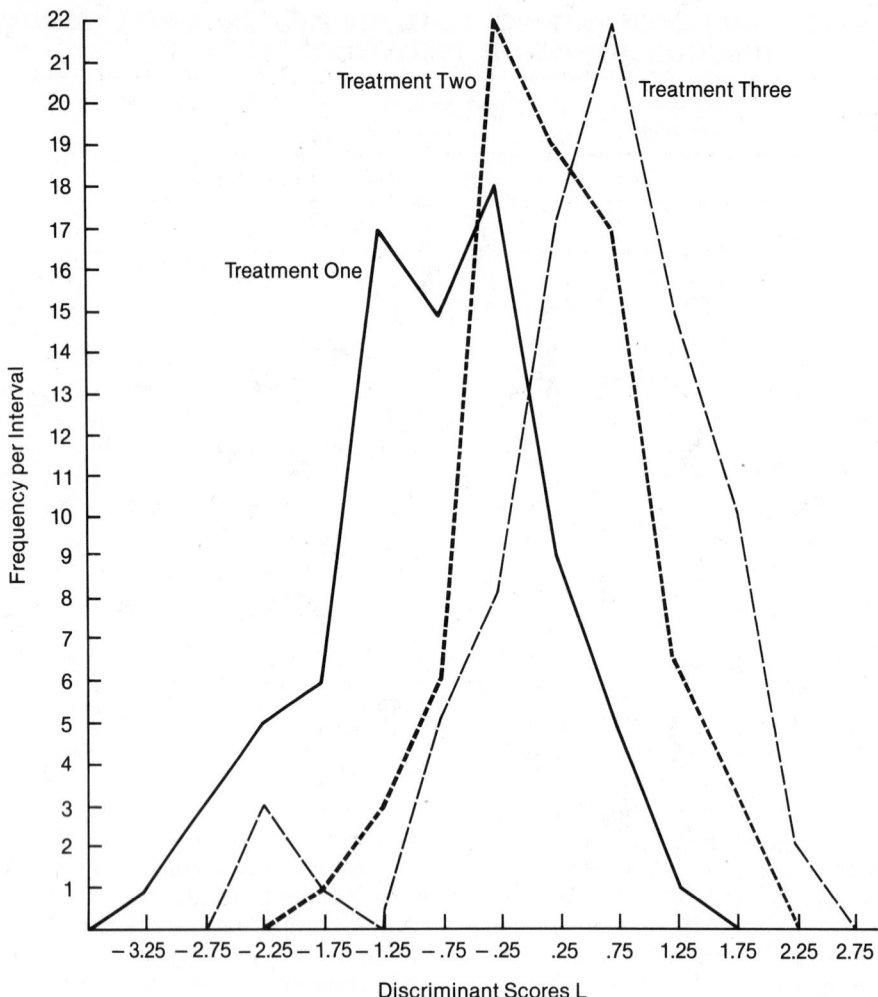

Figure 11-1. Linear discriminant scores for the three treatments.

violated from the presented examples. Dichotomous variables were employed as were qualitative and discrete measures. No investigation was made of the assumptions of linearity, homoscedasticity, truncation, and outliers. No tests were made of equality of variances and correlation coefficients across groups. It is natural to wonder how important these assumptions are to justify the use of these models.

The assumptions are vital if the sample sizes are small. If the sample sizes are large, the assumptions for statistical hypothesis testing can be relaxed because the multivariate analog to the *Central Limit Theorem* operates. If the number of variables in the linear combinations used to define principal components, canonical variates, and linear discriminant function is large, the resulting scores tend to have a normal distribution

even when the original variables are not necessarily normally distributed. This is especially true when P is large. Under this condition the distribution of scores comes under the purview of the Central Limit Theorem. Thus, if P is large, component scores, canonical variate scores, and linear discriminant function scores can be used directly for studies based on the analysis of variance, the analysis of covariance, and multiple regression analysis.

Guidelines can be proposed to assist researchers in selecting adequate sample sizes for multivariate analytical techniques. Not all methodologists agree with these recommendations:

1. For principal component analysis based on P variables, it is recommended that N = 10P subjects be employed. For the pre-

operative teaching study, a principal component based on P = 14 variables was illustrated. The recommended number of subjects for this study is 140. The number used is 246.

2. For canonical correlation analysis based on P + Q variables, it is recommended that N = 10 (P + Q) subjects be used. For the preoperative teaching study, P = 9 and Q = 5. The recommended number of subjects is 140. The number used is 246.

3. For linear discriminant analysis with K groups and P variables, the recommended number of subjects is given as N = 10(Q + K) subjects. For the example with K = 3 and Q = 5, N = 80 are recommended. The study used 246. Because multivariate analysis of variance is another way to approach the linear discriminant analysis, the same recommendations apply to MANOVA and to Hotelling's T^2.

11−14 SUMMARY

In this chapter the most commonly encountered multivariate models have been described. These models are

1. principal component analysis
2. psychometric factor analysis
3. canonical correlation analysis
4. multivariate analysis of variance
5. linear discriminant analysis

Each of these models provides answers to different research questions.

Principal component analysis is used when a researcher's main goal is to reduce a large set of correlated variables to a smaller more manageable and interpretable set of variates, which are linear combinations of the original variables. After the reduction is achieved, the component scores can be used as variates in an analysis of variance or regression. In hypothesis testing, the component scores can assume the role of a dependent or independent variable, depending on the goals and purposes of the investigation. If the weights on the principal component are nearly equal to one another, a simplification can be achieved by replacing each weight by unity. The loss in information, from adopting this simplification, is usually small.

Factor analysis is a measurement model very similar to principal components analysis except that it is based on the assumption that the multivariate variables all are measures of a single set of hypothetical constructs, which are best defined by linear combinations of the originally collected variables. In principal components, there is no assumption that the variables are necessarily conceptually related to one another. Because this is a basic assumption of the many forms of factor analysis, factor analysis is used to derive factors, factor weights, and factor scores. The model was described in this chapter but not illustrated.

In both principal component analysis and factor analysis, there is the added problem of assigning names to the constructed variables. One procedure used to provide empirical meaning to the components and factors is to rotate the variables to simple structure and orthogonal or uncorrelated factors and components. One way to achieve this is to use Kaiser's Varimax Rotation. The model was described and illustrated in this chapter.

Unlike principal component analysis and factor analysis, canonical analysis is used when variables can be divided into sets of independent and dependent variables. Its purpose is to define sets of paired correlated variables. Canonical analysis is useful when the correlations within the sets are large and when the correlations between the sets also are large. If the between set correlations are low, the interest and desire in performing a canonical analysis should be resisted. In such cases, it is a model that can produce spurious results.

Of the multivariate statistical models available, the multivariate analysis of variance is probably the most useful. It provides an extension of univariate analysis of variance to the simultaneous investigation of many correlated variables. It has a sound post hoc model for investigating contrasts within variables and across variables. The model was illustrated in this chapter.

Hotelling's T^2 is a special case of the multivariate analysis of variance. In fact, it is the multivariate analysis of variance for two groups, and for that reason it was not illustrated.

Linear discriminant function analysis is also a special case of the multivariate analysis of variance. It is a special case of the MANOVA model in which linear combinations of the variables produce maximum group discriminations. In this chapter, post

TABLE 11–15 COMPARISON OF THE STATISTICAL POWER IN TERMS OF t STATISTICS ASSOCIATED WITH THREE DIFFERENT LINEAR COMBINATIONS OF THE FIVE VARIABLES USED TO MEASURE RECOVERY ACROSS THREE TREATMENT GROUPS

Contrast	Summed Z Scores	Varimax Rotated Factor Scores	Linear Discriminant Scores
1 vs 2	4.85*	4.87*	6.85*
1 vs 3	8.96*	9.22*	11.23*
2 vs 3	4.12	4.35*	4.38*

*Significant at $\alpha = .05$; $t < -4.28$ or $t > 4.28$

hoc pairwise comparisons across the three treatment groups using summed Z scores, varimax rotated factor scores, and linear discriminant function scores were illustrated. The three sets of pairwise contrasts are summarized in Table 11–15 in terms of test statistics defined as $t = \hat{\psi}/ \text{SE}(\hat{\psi})$ for comparative purposes. As can be seen, the summed Z scores and varimax rotated factor scores give similar results. At the same time, the largest t values are found with the linear discriminant function scores.

REFERENCES

Armstrong, J.S., and Soelberg, P.: On the interpretation of factor analysis, Psychol. Bull., 70: 361–364, 1968.

Betz, N.E.: Use of discriminant analysis in counseling psychology research, J. Counseling Psychol., 34: 393–403, 1987.

Bostrom, A.: CRUNCH Software. Oakland, CA, 1986.

Cohen, J., and Cohen, P.: Applied Multiple Regression/Correlation Analysis for the Behavioral Sciences, ed. 2. Hillsdale, NJ, Erlbaum, 1983.

Comrey, A.L.: A First Course in Factor Analysis. New York, Academic Press, 1973.

Cooley, W.W., and Lohnes, P.R.: Multivariate Data Analysis. New York, John Wiley & Sons, 1971.

Cramer, E.M., and Nicewander, A.: Some symmetric invariant measures of multivariate association, Psychometrika, 44: 43–54, 1979.

Fisher, R.A.: Statistical Methods for Research Workers, ed. 10. New York, Hafner, 1948.

Guertin, W.H., and Bailey, J.P., Jr.: Introduction to Modern Factor Analysis. Ann Arbor, MI, Edwards Brothers, Inc., 1970.

Guttman, L.: Best possible systematic estimates of communalities, Psychometrika, 21: 273–285, 1956.

Haase, R.F., and Ellis, M.V.: Multivariate analysis of variance, J. Counseling Psychol., 34: 404–413, 1987.

Harmon, H.H.: Modern Factor Analysis, ed. 3. Chicago, University of Chicago Press, 1976.

Herek, G.M.: Beyond "homophobia": a social psychological perspective on attitudes toward lesbians and gay men, J. Homosexuality, 10: 1–21, 1984.

Hotelling, H.: Generalization of student's ratio, Ann. Math. Stat., 2: 360–378, 1931.

Hotelling, H.: Analysis of a complex of statistical variables into principal components, J. Ed. Psychol., 24: 417–441, 498–520, 1933.

Horst, P.: Factor Analysis of Data Matrices. New York, Holt, Rinehart, & Winston, 1965.

Kaiser, H.J.: The varimax criterion for analytic rotation in factor analysis, Psychometrika, 23: 187–200, 1958.

Kaiser, H.J., and Hunka, S.: Some empirical results with Guttman's stronger lower bound for the number of common factors, Ed. Psych. Measurement, 33: 99–102, 1973.

Kerlinger, F.N., and Pedhazur, E.J.: Multivariate Regression in Behavioral Research. New York, Holt, Rinehart, & Winston, 1973.

Knapp, T.: Canonical correlation analysis: a general parametric significance-testing system, Psychol. Bull., 85: 410–416, 1978.

Marascuilo, L.A., and Levin, J.: Multivariate Statistics in the Social Sciences. Belmont, CA, Wadsworth, 1983.

Pillai, K.C.S.: Statistical Tables for Tests of Multivariate Hypotheses. Manila, Statistical Center University of the Philippines, 1960.

Roy, S.N.: Some Aspects of Multivariate Analysis. New York, John Wiley & Sons, 1957.

Rummel, R.J.: Applied Factor Analysis. Evanston, IL, Northwestern University Press, 1970.

Serlin, R.C.: A multivariate measure of association based on the Pillai-Bartlett procedure, Psychol. Bull., 91: 413–417, 1982.

Thurstone, L.L.: Multiple-factor Analysis. Chicago, University of Chicago Press, 1947.

Tinsley, H.E.A., and Tinsley, D.J.: Uses of factor analysis in counseling psychology research, J. Counseling Psychol., 34: 414–424, 1987.

Wainer, H.: Estimating coefficients in linear models: It don't make no nevermind, Psych. Bull., 41: 213–217, 1976.

Wilks, S.S.: Certain generalizations in the analysis of variance, Biometrika, 24: 471–474, 1932.

Chapter 12

ALTERNATIVE MULTIVARIATE METHODS

12-1 AD HOC NONSTATISTICAL AND NONMEASUREMENT BASED MULTIVARIATE METHODS

A number of specialized multivariate methodological models have appeared in the general and the nursing research literature. These models have been spurred on because of the significant advances in computer science and the possibilities that the computer offers in the analysis of large complex data sets. In particular, these new multivariate analytical models have been developed and adopted by researchers in such diverse fields of inquiry as economics, genetics, biology, medicine, psychology, and related social sciences. The following four multivariate methods that are gaining popular use in the behavioral and nursing science research are described and illustrated in this chapter:

1. Path analysis
2. Linear structural equation models
3. Multidimensional scaling
4. Cluster analysis

These four methods have received considerable attention over the past few years and show some promise in the study of certain research questions in nursing science. None of the methods fits into the mainstream multivariate models of Chapter 11, in which models based on a priori theoretical statistical and measurement principles are described. The models presented here are based on ad hoc procedures designed to treat very specialized situations arising in many types of research. To some investigators, the models discussed here are designed primarily to serve and assist in the building of models for studying human behavior and related phenomena.

Although some of the developers and users of these alternative multivariate methods claim that the methods can be used in hypothesis testing modes, most applications that appear in the literature show that the procedures have been used almost exclusively to create models that are in theory testable with new data collected in new settings with new subjects. The alternative methods are most useful in observational and nonexperimental nursing investigations in which large masses of data are collected on large samples. The methods are used for outlining the structure of large data bases and for creating groups of subjects, objects, items, concepts, and so on, which can be studied by means of the more familiar statistical models described in the earlier chapters.

None of these models is examined in terms of null hypothesis testing procedure, mainly because the statistical theory behind the procedures is not well defined. Instead, researchers assess the findings using their knowledge of the specific questions being examined in terms of measures of statistical *stress*. Stress is measured by examining the difference between observed data and fitted data. The fitted data are estimated from the *model* that best describes the data. The Karl Pearson statistic is often used as a measure of stress. When observed and theoretical frequencies are close to one another, the chi-square goodness of fit statistic is close to zero and the fit is said to be *good*. If the chi-square statistic is large, the goodness of fit is said to be poor. It should be noted that many different measures of stress have been defined and are used for specialized functions. Some are discussed in this chapter.

12-2 INTRODUCTION TO PATH ANALYSIS

The main purpose of path analysis is to generate theoretical models that describe antecedent events, intervening factors, and subsequent outcomes or consequences based on the interaction of both independent and intervening variables on a single dependent measure. For this model, a *causal ordering* or *path* is presumed to exist leading to a description and eventual prediction of phenomena on only one outcome measure. In its most restrictive form, path analysis can be viewed as an ordered system of presumed causal connections among variables. From a pictorial perspective, the causal connections can be seen as a temporal ordering of one-way arrows representing the presumed causal connections among variables. In its least restrictive form, the connections among prior independent, intervening, dependent, and outcome variables can be representative of correlational connections and not causal relationships among the variables. In pictorial form, the correlation model is represented by connections with double-headed arrows among sets of variables.

From a pictorial perspective, the causal ordering model can be seen as a graph with directed arrows pointing the way and ordering the presumed causal relations, and the correlational model can be seen as a graph with double-headed arrows indicating correlation only. Three path analytic models for two antecedent variables and one outcome variable are presented in Figure 12-1. Figure 12-1A represents a causal model where X_1 causes Y and X_1 causes X_2, which in turn causes Y; thus, both X_1 and X_2 cause Y. Figure 12-1B is a model in which both X_1 and X_2 are correlated with Y and with each other. Figure 12-1C is a path model where X_1 and X_2

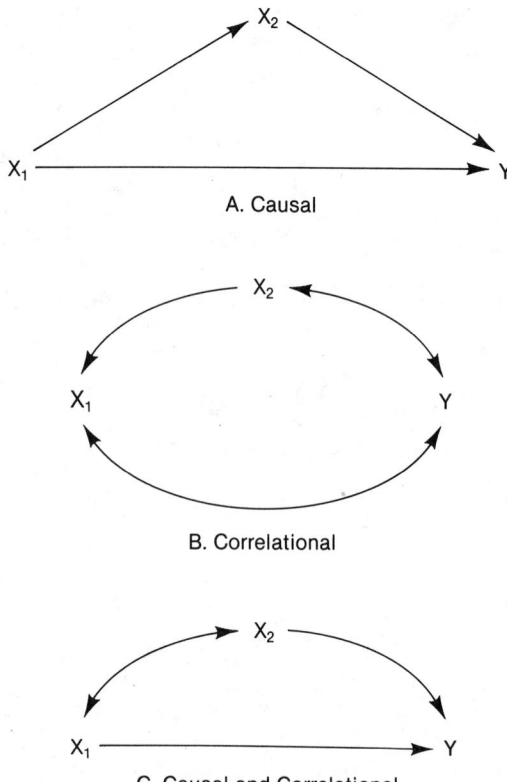

Figure 12-1. Three examples of path analysis with causal and correlational connections.

are correlated and where both X_1 and X_2 cause Y.

In order to perform a path analysis, a researcher must have substantive knowledge and insight into the research issues under investigation. The path analyst must accurately and precisely describe the salient variables thought to be precursors or antecedents to the phenomena under investigation. Detailed explication of independent variables thought to affect the outcome of health or behavioral indices must be provided.

After a researcher has specified the presumed causal direction and worked out the structure of the system under study, a preliminary model is diagrammed, reflecting a causal ordering of the connections among the variables. This means that the arrows are arranged on the path diagram representation from left to right, indicating the particular effects of antecedent and independent variables and their effects on subsequent variables in the path diagram.

As the data analysis proceeds, the path analyst must be prepared to review and reformulate the interrelationships among the selected variables to be studied when presumed relationships are not supported or are at variance with the data. Frequent modifications and realignment of variables should be expected in order to fashion a more theoretically defensible and empirically meaningful model of human behavior. There is little place for the amateur or dilettante in this complex data analytic approach to model building. After a model has been agreed on, information is collected on the variables selected for study. The principal statistical technique used at this juncture involves a set of multiple and simple regression analyses on the collected data as those described in Chapter 10.

Before a researcher can begin a path analysis some issues need to be resolved. Because variables with large variances can overpower an analysis, it is recommended that path analytic studies use only standardized variables. In some studies, this could be a disadvantage because all variables are given equal weights by this standardization. If some variables are assessed based on theoretical grounds or are assessed from prior research as being more important than others, the use of standardized variables reduces their importance and impact on the final analysis.

A path analysis should be performed only on large samples because the estimation procedures are based on correlation coefficients known to be very unstable in small samples. Also, large samples are required because of the large number of parameters that need to be estimated in the final analysis. A conservative rule often suggested is that 20 subjects should be used for each variable in the study.

It is recommended that all statistical tests be ignored because the risks of type I errors for path analysis are unknown. If a researcher needs a decision rule for assessing significance, a conservative rule would be to treat any path coefficient that is more than two standard errors from zero as being important in the analysis and in the path structure. Admittedly, even this rule is weak because with large samples, small differences from zero can be encountered quite frequently. It is also recommended that measures of association be examined carefully and that judgments based on their magnitude should receive priority over statistical tests of significance.

Marascuilo and Levin (1983) offer the following steps for conducting a path analysis:

1. Draw the path diagram with presumed causality or time extending from the left to the right.
2. Use directed arrows to represent causal relationships.
3. Use double-headed arrows to represent correlational relationships among variables.
4. Regress the dependent measure on all of its predictors.
5. Regress each independent variable on all of the variables that precede it in time.
6. Graph the results and write the final analysis and report.

The following path analysis is based on treatment one of the preoperative teaching study and illustrates the basic ideas and methods in performing a path analysis. The path structure to be examined is shown in Figure 12–2. Here, the input variables are X_1: weight, X_2: smoking, X_3: uncertainty, X_4: postoperative complications, X_5: pain med. one, and X_6: pain med. two. The outcome variable is Y: length of stay.

In this analysis, variables X_1, X_2, and X_3 are hypothesized to impact directly on X_4 and Y and indirectly on X_5 and X_6 through X_4. Because double-headed arrows are drawn among X_1, X_2, and X_3, it is hypothesized that these variables are correlated with one another and do not necessarily relate to one another in causative relationships.

Because the computations are so involved, only the results are reported in Table 12–1. These results were obtained by using the LISREL (Joreskog and Sorbom, 1986) program. Because the analysis is based on standardized variables, the path coefficients have simple interpretations.

The path coefficients are reported also in Figure 12–2. For example, the largest path coefficient between the input variables and X_4: postoperative complications is found for X_1: weight. In particular, $\beta_{4.1} = .44$. Thus, for each standard deviation change in weight, the number of postoperative complications changes by .44. In this case, the standard deviation for weight is given as 24.44 pounds, and the standard deviation for postoperative complications is 1.23. Thus, as weight increases by 24.44 pounds, the number of postoperative complications increases by .44(1.23) = .54, or as weight increases by 45 pounds the number of postoperative complications increases by

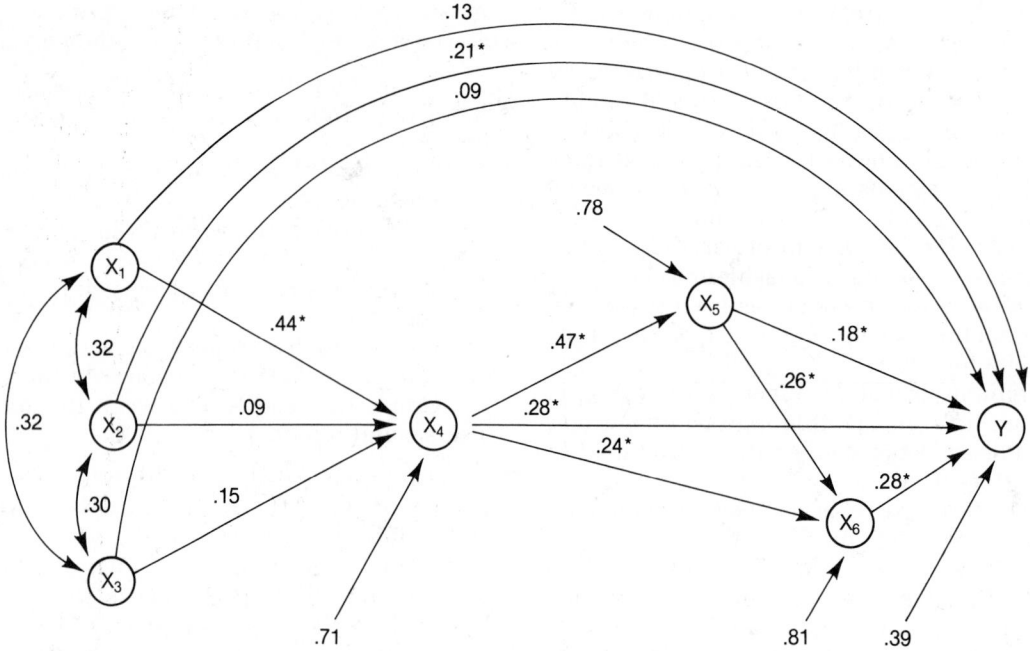

Figure 12–2. Path diagram connecting length of stay for treatment one of the preoperative teaching study with six predictors.

*Estimates differ from zero by at least two standard errors.

1(24.44/.54 = 45)

The remaining path coefficients can be interpreted similarly.

As indicated,

1. X_1: weight has the largest impact on X_4: postoperative complications, with $\beta_{4.1} = .44$.

2. X_3: uncertainty has the next largest impact, with $\beta_{4.3} = .15$.

3. X_2: smoking has the least effect on X_4: postoperative complications, with path coefficient of $\beta_{4.2} = .09$.

4. The largest path coefficient is between X_4: postoperative complications and X_5: pain med. one with $\beta_{5.4} = .47$. For each one

TABLE 12–1 PATH COEFFICIENTS AND t TESTS FOR THE THREE TREATMENT GROUPS OF THE PREOPERATIVE TEACHING STUDY

Path	Treatment One		Treament Two		Treatment Three	
	Coefficient	t Value	Coefficient	t Value	Coefficient	t Value
X_1 to X_4	.44	4.22*	.43	4.34*	.33	2.99*
X_2 to X_4	.09	.89	.25	2.49*	.08	.65
X_3 to X_4	.15	1.44	.03	.27	.21	1.99
X_4 to X_5	.47	4.74*	.47	4.68*	.21	1.93
X_4 to X_6	.24	2.11*	.39	4.97*	.30	3.45*
X_5 to X_6	.26	2.28*	.54	6.88*	.54	6.23*
X_4 to Y	.28	2.95*	.29	2.42*	.24	2.65*
X_5 to Y	.18	2.15*	.22	3.04*	.13	1.38
X_6 to Y	.28	3.61*	.24	2.01*	.28	2.83*
X_1 to Y	.13	1.53	.06	0.74	−.03	−0.33
X_2 to Y	.21	2.76*	.21	2.82*	.21	2.40*
X_3 to Y	.09	1.10	.07	0.96	.23	2.81*

*Values higher than 2.00.

standard deviation change in the number of postoperative complications, the number of pain medications requested on the first day changes by .47 requests.

5. The remaining path coefficients of $\beta_{6.4}$ = .24, $\beta_{6.5}$ = .26, $\beta_{Y.4}$ = .28, $\beta_{Y.5}$ = .18, and $\beta_{Y.6}$ = .28 are also large when it is noted that they are defined in standard deviation units.

6. Finally, variables X_1, X_2, and X_3 all impact directly on Y: length of stay with path coefficients of $\beta_{Y.1}$ = .13, $\beta_{Y.2}$ = .21, and $\beta_{Y.3}$ = .09, respectively.

7. The path coefficients among X_1, X_2, and X_3 are equal to $\beta_{1.2}$ = .32, $\beta_{1.3}$ = .32, and $\beta_{2.3}$ = .30.

8. The remaining four reported values are not path coefficients. They are measurements of unexplained variation. For example, the .71 associated with X_4: postoperative complications is simply the residual standard deviation for X_4.

The t statistics for each path coefficient are reported in Table 12–1. Of the 12 reported coefficients, 8 have t values higher than 2.00. These are starred on the path diagram and are the ones of most interest. Results for treatments two and three are also summarized in Table 12–1. Examination of the three sets of t values suggests that the interrelationships that exist among the variables are valid for all three treatments. In particular, note the following:

1. Weight is a strong causative factor of postoperative complications for all three treatments. As weight increases, postoperative complications increase.

2. As postoperative complications increase, pain relief requests increase for both day one and day two, with the largest increases associated with day one.

3. Increases in postoperative complications and requests for pain relief on day one and day two cause the length of hospital stay to increase.

4. Smoking has a direct impact on how long a patient remains in the hospital following surgery.

As indicated in Figure 12–2, smoking has a *direct* impact on length of stay, with a path coefficient of $\beta_{Y.2}$ = .21. At the same time, smoking has an *indirect* impact on length of stay through the following indirect paths:

1. X_2 to X_4 to X_5 to Y
2. X_2 to X_4 to X_5 to X_6 to Y
3. X_2 to X_4 to Y
4. X_2 to X_4 to X_6 to Y

The effects of X_1 through these indirect paths is found by multiplying the corresponding path coefficients and then summing the final results. Thus, the total effects of X_2 on Y is given in the equation below.

Thus, we see that the direct path accounts for the greatest part of the variable effect with a value of .21, whereas the four indirect paths pick up another .04 of the total effect. This means that as smoking increases by one standard deviation the number of days in hospital increases by .25 of a standard deviation. The treatment effects for the remaining input variables can be found in a similar fashion and are given as follows:

1. .33 for weight
2. .25 for smoking
3. .15 for uncertainty
4. .25 for pain med. one
5. .28 for pain med. two
6. .47 for postoperative complications

These values appear on the LISREL (Joreskog and Sorbom, 1986) printout.

Although inferential statistical tests are used to evaluate null hypotheses and statistical models, no such tests exist for path analysis. Instead, the researcher must rely on the evaluation of statistical measures of *stress*. A number of statistical stress measures can be used to evaluate the goodness of fit between the data and the model. If the stress measurements are small, the data are said to provide a good description of the model but if the stress measurements are large, the analysis should be discarded and a new model should be hypothesized and investigated.

The most commonly used measure of stress is a chi-square goodness of fit statistic with degrees of freedom given by ν = $T(T + 1)/2 - P$, where T is the number of variables in the model and P is the number

---

$$E = .21 + .09(.47)(.18) + .09(.47)(.26)(.28) + .09(.28) + .09(.24)(.28)$$
$$= .21 + .00 + .00 + .03 + .01 = .25$$

of parameters estimated from the data. In this example, T = 6 + 1 = 7, P = 22. There are 15 path coefficients and 7 residual standard deviations to estimate making P = 22. Thus, $\nu = 7(8)/2 - 22 = 6$. For treatment one, the value of the chi-square goodness of fit measure is given as $X^2 = 10.91$, which is smaller than the 95th percentile of the chi-square distribution of 12.59. This suggests that the fit is good. For treatments two and three, the goodness of fit statistics are given as 10.79 and 22.18, respectively. The fit is not acceptable for treatment three.

Another measure of stress that is used is the *goodness of fit index*. The closer this index is to one, the better is the fit. In this case, the goodness of fit index is equal to .97, again suggesting that the fit between data and model is good. For treatments two and three, the goodness of fit indices are .97 and .94, respectively. With this index, the fit is acceptable for treatment three.

According to Joreskog and Sorbom (1986), the most obvious way of assessing the goodness of the model is to examine the results. If the parameter estimates, standard errors, squared multiple correlation coefficients, coefficients of determination, and correlation coefficients of parameter estimates are reasonable, one should behave as if the fit is good. Warning signs include negative variances, correlation coefficients greater than one, correlation and covariance matrices that are not positive definite. Whenever such things happen the program prints a warning message which should be heeded. Other warning signs are negative squared multiple correlation coefficients or coefficients of determination that are negative. Also dangerous are very large standard errors and t statistics close to zero.

In general, path analysis solutions are very easy to explain, and this may account for their popularity among researchers in the social sciences. Unfortunately, the model is based on very powerful assumptions and if these assumptions do not hold, the entire model is invalid and worthless. The strongest assumption involves the causation among the variables. If they are not causally related, the entire analysis provides a futile attempt at explanation. In addition, the goodness of fit statistics are based on the following assumptions:

1. The observations are selected at random from a multivariate normal distribution.

2. The analysis is based on the sample variance-covariance matrix and not on the correlation matrix.

3. The sample size is large.

None of these assumptions is satisfied for treatment one. Smoking is not a quantitative variable with a large number of possible outcomes. Thus, the appearance of smoking places the normality assumptions in question. In addition, the analysis was based on standardized variables so that a correlation matrix is employed. With 22 parameters to estimate a sample size of $22 \times 10 = 220$ is recommended by Bentler (1985). The model must be used with care.

In a study such as the preoperative teaching study in which three treatments are under investigation, it is useful to make a visual inspection of the parameters for the various treatments. If the results appear to be similar between treatments, then a pooled correlation matrix should be determined and the entire analysis should be repeated on the larger sample. In this example, this would increase the sample size to 246 and thereby become closer to the 220 recommended by Bentler. In addition, variables with small t values should be removed from the analysis. In this case, none of the variables would be eliminated from further analysis.

12-3 LINEAR STRUCTURAL RELATIONSHIPS

Path analytic models have been extended in recent years to take into account clusters of independent and dependent variables that are believed to measure common *latent* variables or constructs such as those generated by principal component analysis, factor analysis, and canonical analysis. In this model, the same principles used to generate a path analysis are used to generate a model that relates clusters of variables together simultaneously. In addition to the appearance of latent variables, another major difference between path analysis and linear structural relationship models is that all paths are assumed to be causal in nature. None of the paths represents simple correlational associations. Because the algorithms for linear structural modeling are so complex, most researchers use the LISREL program of Joreskog and Sorbom (1986).

The LISREL program consists of a measurement component and a structural equation component. The measurement component provides a description of how the latent variables or hypothetical constructs are measured in terms of the observed variables. Furthermore, this component is used to describe psychometric properties, such as validity and reliability, contained in the observed variables. The structural equation component is used to specify the presumed causal relationships among the latent variables. It is also used to describe the causal effects and the amount of unexplained variance in the structural equation system. For a discussion of the properties of the measurement and structural equation models, see Fassinger (1987).

Because each structural equation in the model represents a causal link rather than an empirical association, the structural parameters do not coincide with coefficients of regression among observed variables as do the path coefficients of path analysis. This is another difference between structural equation modeling and path analysis. The structural parameters represent relatively unmixed, invariant, and autonomous features of the mechanisms that generate the observable variables. As a consequence, structural equation models go well beyond conventional regression analysis and analysis of variance.

In a structural equation model, the latent variables are represented by circles and the observable variables by rectangles. The circles are used to remind the reader that these variables are hypothetical and unobservable constructs or concepts. Some variables are called *exogenous* and do not provide hypothesized causes in the path analysis. *Endogenous variables* have at least one hypothesized cause in the path analysis. Most structural equation modeling contains both types of input variables. If there are no latent variables, structural equation modeling reduces to path analysis as described in the previous section. If all independent variables have a simultaneous impact on the dependent variable, path analysis reduces to multiple regression as described in Chapter 10.

Like path analysis the risks of type I errors for structural equation modeling are unknown. The most commonly used computer program for this model, LISREL (Joreskog and Sorbom, 1986), provides *goodness of fit* tests that must be used with care. With large samples these tests can lead to a decision to reject the hypothesis of goodness of fit of the

data to the theory, not because the fit is poor but because the sample is large. Because of this, it might be advisable to ignore the statistical tests and use judgments based on theory and empirical facts known about the variables used in the analysis.

According to Bentler (1985), no structural equation modeling should be attempted unless the number of subjects is 10 times the number of parameters to be estimated from the data. When it is realized that even a modest path requires 20 to 30 estimators, it is readily seen that large samples are required. As stated by Fassinger (1987), sample size requirements of structural equation modeling are so prohibitive in cost that few studies ever continue with adequate follow-up investigations when modifications are proposed by the analysis. The testing of modified models based on new sets of data are rarely encountered. Few researchers follow the scientific dictate that requires that new data be used to test theories generated from a prior set of data. Verification of an adjusted model on the original data is always suspect because the original data provide the evidence for the adjustment and so are certain to provide an excellent fit to the new model.

Actually the use of goodness of fit statistics in model building is a problem for researchers that seems to have an inadequate solution. According to the Popper (1959) point of view of science, theories can be disproved and never proven. This is the model under which null hypothesis testing operates. A null hypothesis can be rejected and thereby be considered as disproved. The null hypothesis is never accepted. The most that can be said about a null hypothesis with a small statistical value is that the hypothesis is not rejected. For this reason, goodness of fit statistics must be used with care in model building. It should not be concluded that just because a certain set of data fits a predetermined theoretical model, the data fit only that one model. Many other models most likely can be used to describe the structure in a given set of data. Nonrejection of a model is no proof of its scientific truth. This problem in model building has been examined by Freedman (1987) and Cliff (1983).

The LISREL program is flexible and also can be used to analyze multiple samples of data taken from several populations simultaneously. For example, the preoperative teaching study could be submitted to a LISREL analysis. Differences in treatments can be analyzed in terms of latent outcome and latent input variables. In addition, hypotheses can be tested for equality of covariance matrices, equality of correlational matrices, equality of slopes of regression lines, and equality of factor patterns and structures. Simplified models for doing these types of analyses were presented in Chapters 10 and 11.

Structural equation modeling should be of interest to the researcher who conducts a quasi-experimental or correlational study. According to Hughes, Price, and Marrs (1986), structural modeling can be used

1. to explicate theory from other sources more clearly and succinctly for testing,
2. to provide a means for testing a theory directly, and
3. to gain a more thorough explanatory understanding of the data.

The model is illustrated with the example taken from the preoperative teaching study. The model to be examined is shown in Figure 12–3. In this model, data for treatment one are examined. In particular, it is seen that

1. Variables X_1: age, X_2: severity, X_3: weight, X_4: smoking, and X_5: uncertainty are hypothesized to collectively measure a latent construct, X: preoperative risk.
2. Preoperative risk is hypothesized to have an impact on a second hypothetical construct, Y: postoperative recovery.
3. This latter construct is measured collectively by Y_1: length of stay, Y_2: pain med. one, Y_3: pain med. two, Y_4: postoperative complications, and Y_5: length of stay at home before being able to leave residence unassisted.

The three conditions just mentioned describe the canonical analysis model of Chapter 11. In this case, the methods of that chapter can be used directly instead of the LISREL program. On the basis of this example, it should not be concluded that all structural equation models are equivalent to canonical analysis. We begin with an analysis based on standardized variables with means of zero and standard deviations of one. This is similar to the canonical correlation model of Chapter 11. For this reason, comparisons and contrasts are provided to help understand the differences in the two models for the used data set.

In LISREL, the number of estimates to be specified is up to the researcher. This decision is based on the researcher's theoretical model about the nature of the relationships among the latent traits and observed variables. Here, a general or nonspecific model is fitted to the data. For this model, 22 parameters need to be estimated.

The estimates include

1. ten structural correlation coefficients,
2. one correlation coefficient between the two latent variables,
3. ten residual variances for the original variables, and
4. one residual variance for the latent endogenous variable.

This estimation of so many parameters immediately places the analysis under suspicion because the total sample size is given as N = 82 giving a ratio of sample size to parameters of less than 4. According to Bentler (1985), the ratio should exceed 10.

One goal of LISREL is to evaluate how well the researcher's choice of models fits the original data. Specifically, LISREL attempts to reproduce the initial set of T(T + 1)/2 correlation coefficients or the covariances

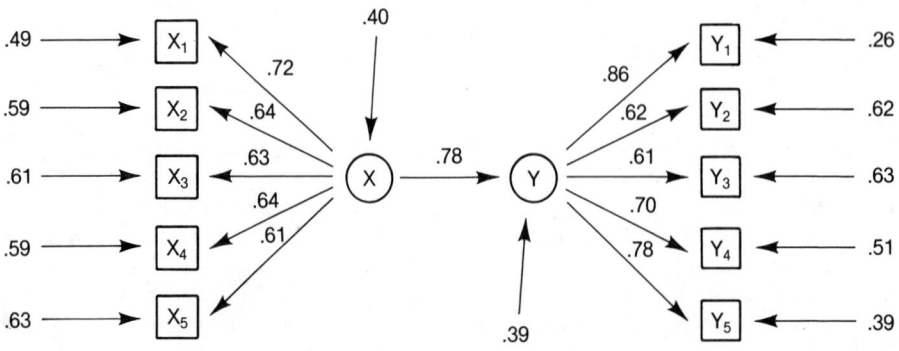

Figure 12–3. Structural equation model for treatment one.

① $Y = .40Y_1 + .12Y_2 + .11Y_3 + .16Y_4 + .24Y_5 + .06X_1 + .04X_2 + .04X_3 + .04X_4 + .04X_5$

② $X = .13Y_1 + .04Y_2 + .04Y_3 + .05Y_4 + + .08Y_5 + .25X_1 + .19X_2 + .18X_3 + .19X_4 + .17X_5$

among the T = 10 variables under study based on the LISREL estimators and then to test in order to see how well these "reproduced" correlations match the original correlations. If they do not fit well, then the researcher's original model or theory may not be correct.

The estimates of the parameters of the model are reported in Table 12–2 for the canonical analysis of Chapter 11 and for a solution based on maximum likelihood estimation theory. This theory is not described here.

As indicated, the two solutions are very similar but not identical. All input variables load on the preoperative risk factor and all output variables load on the postoperative recovery factor. The LISREL correlation coefficient of $R_{XY} = .78$ is large, suggesting that the hypothesized cause and effect relationship is strong. The residual variance for the endogenous latent variables is given as

$$(1 - R_{XY}^2) = (1 - .78^2) = .39$$

The residual variances for each of the standardized values is found in a similar fashion. For example, the residual variances for Y_1 is given as $(1 - .86^2) = .26$. Results are summarized on the diagram of Figure 12–3.

The LISREL program also determines the regression equations that can be used to score each subject on the latent variables. For this example, equations 1 and 2 at the top of this page apply.

Note that the Y factor is weighted primarily by the exogenous variables, whereas X is defined by the endogenous variables. Although these variables are not path coefficients, they are similar and can be viewed as analogs to the beta weights of path analysis. In any case, these coefficients can be applied to the standard scores of the 10 X and Y variables and used to score the 82 subjects on the latent variables. The correlation between these two latent variables is given as .78. The resulting scores can be used for any other analysis deemed important by the researcher. For example, a researcher can now score each subject on the X and Y latent variables and perform t tests to see whether males and females differ on the two latent variables.

As mentioned, LISREL provides statistical measures of stress (sometimes referred to as fit) that can be used for evaluation. For example, the chi-square goodness of fit statistic for treatment one is $X^2 = 84.36$. This is referred to a chi-square distribution with $\nu = T(T + 1)/2 - P$, where T is the number of

TABLE 12–2 COEFFICIENTS FOR THE STRUCTURAL MODEL FOR MAXIMUM LIKELIHOOD ESTIMATES (MLE) AND CANONICAL ANALYSIS ESTIMATES (CAE)*

Parameter	Treatment One	
	MLE	CAE
Y_1: stay	.86	.87
Y_2: pain med. one	.62	.55
Y_3: pain med. two	.61	.38
Y_4: postop. comp.	.70	.75
Y_5: days at home	.78	.85
X_1: age	.72	.85
X_2: severity	.64	.64
X_3: weight	.63	.74
X_4: smoking	.64	.71
X_5: uncertainty	.61	.67
Canonical correlation	.78	.70
Residual Variance		
Y:	.39	
Y_1: stay	.26	
Y_2: pain med. one	.62	
Y_3: pain med. two	.63	
Y_4: postop. comp.	.51	
Y_5: days at home	.39	
X:	.40	
X_1: age	.49	
X_2: severity	.59	
X_3: weight	.61	
X_4: smoking	.59	
X_5: uncertainty	.63	
Goodness of fit	84.36	

*Represented by the diagram of Figure 12–3 with Var(X) = 1.00 Var(Y) = 1.00.

variables in the model and P is the number of parameters estimated from the data. In this example, T = 5 + 5 = 10 and P = 22, so that ν = 10(11)/2 − 22 = 33. The 95th percentile of the chi-square distribution with 33 degrees of freedom is 47.30. Because the goodness of fit statistic exceeds the critical value, it must be concluded that the fit between the model and the data is not acceptable.

The LISREL program provides a number of other measures that can be used for evaluation purposes. One set of measures consists of the reliabilities of the variables. These are simply the multiple correlation coefficient between each variable in the model and the remaining variables in the set. It can be shown that this measure of reliability provides a lower bound on the true reliability. In this case, the reliabilities range from a low of .38 to a high of .74. These relatively low reliabilities may account for the poor fit. At the same time, other indicators are positive. For example, the LISREL program reports the values of normalized residuals between the observed correlations and the fitted correlation. In this case, all are smaller than 1.58 so that none exceeds 2 standard deviations from zero. In terms of this criterion, the fit is acceptable. A plot of the normalized residuals is also acceptable and indicative of a favorable fit. Thus, the researcher is forced to make subjective decisions concerning the acceptability of the fit. This is not unusual; the researcher has to bring to the situation his or her knowledge of the variables to assess the adequacy of the fit.

For completeness, the analysis for treatments two and three were also performed. The goodness of fit statistics for treatments two and three are given as 76.22 and 93.19, respectively. The fits are not acceptable for these two treatments either. Because the three analyses were so similar, the data could be pooled, and a single analysis can be performed using a different model with different parameter specifications. This also would ameliorate the sample size problem because with pooling across the three treatments the total sample size would be increased to 246. In any case, because of the differences that exist among the treatments on the various input and output variables, the analysis should be performed on the pooled within correlation matrix and covariance matrix. In addition, it is highly recom-

mended that the services of a consultant be obtained.

Another option that seems to be popular is that of fixing the variance of some of the original variables to unity (Joreskog and Sorbom, 1986). Specifically, some researchers set one observed variable for each latent variable equal to unity. This practice, sometimes called *congeneric measurement*, is fraught with difficulty. The primary reason for its use is that without some restrictions placed on the parameters, solutions may not be possible. In the previous example, restrictions were placed on the parameters of the variances of the latent measures. In particular, the variances of X and Y were set equal to one.

For a second method for fixing parameters, suppose that it is decided to fix the variance of length of stay and age at unity. The results of this analysis are summarized in Table 12−3. Note that the two resulting latent variables seem to be very highly correlated with an apparent correlation coefficient of R_{XY} = .94, which is very close to one. Unfortunately, such is not the case. This measure is not a correlation coefficient. It is a covariance! It is easy to see how a researcher could become excited about this analysis in preference to the one in which the variance of X and Y are set equal to unity. All the *structure* coefficients are larger. Unlike the analog to the canonical correlation coefficient, not one of these measures is a correlation coefficient. All these measures are confounded by the variability associated with all of the variables in the model. When the estimates are in terms of covariances and not correlations, social science interpretations for these measures are not clear. It is much easier to interpret LISREL results when the data are reported in standardized (correlational) form.

The remaining parameters are reported in Table 12−3 for the three treatments. Also shown are t statistics, which are valid for the results of Table 12−2. Any t statistic that exceeds 2 standard errors is generally treated as representing a statistically significant finding. Note that the parameter estimates for smoking in treatment two and treatment three are greater than unity. This shows that these parameters are not correlation coefficients as they are when the variances of X and Y are set equal to unities. These coefficients also involve the variability associated

TABLE 12–3 STRUCTURE COEFFICIENTS FOR THE LINEAR STRUCTURAL MODEL WHERE THE VARIANCE OF LENGTH OF STAY AND AGE ARE SET EQUAL TO UNITY*

Parameter	Treatment One		Treatment Two		Treatment Three	
	Coefficient	t Value	Coefficient	t Value	Coefficient	t Value
Y_1: stay	1.00	.00	1.00	.00	1.00	.00
Y_2: pain med. one	.72	5.81[+]	.88	8.15[+]	.74	5.32[+]
Y_3: pain med. two	.70	5.70[+]	.94	8.92[+]	.89	6.52[+]
Y_4: postop. comp.	.81	6.83[+]	.84	7.55[+]	.69	4.97[+]
Y_5: days at home	.90	7.86[+]	.84	7.54[+]	.82	6.01[+]
X_1: age	1.00	.00	1.00	.00	1.00	.00
X_2: severity	.89	5.05[+]	.87	4.34[+]	1.14	4.86[+]
X_3: weight	.87	4.96[+]	.86	4.28[+]	.88	4.01[+]
X_4: smoking	.90	5.10[+]	1.14	5.27[+]	1.15	4.88[+]
X_5: uncertainty	.85	4.85[+]	.75	3.81[+]	1.01	4.47[+]
Canonical covariance	.94		.96		1.05	

Residual Variance

Y:	.29		.35		.25	
Y_1: stay	.26	3.84[+]	.25	4.24[+]	.33	4.16[+]
Y_2: pain med. one	.62	5.84[+]	.41	5.37[+]	.64	5.75[+]
Y_3: pain med. two	.63	5.86[+]	.34	4.99[+]	.48	5.15[+]
Y_4: postop. comp.	.51	5.52[+]	.47	5.59[+]	.68	5.85[+]
Y_5: days at home	.39	4.98[+]	.47	5.59[+]	.55	5.46[+]
X_1: age	.49	4.93[+]	.56	5.18[+]	.62	5.52[+]
X_2: severity	.59	5.44[+]	.67	5.61[+]	.51	5.03[+]
X_3: weight	.61	5.50[+]	.68	5.65[+]	.70	5.80[+]
X_4: smoking	.59	5.41[+]	.43	4.38[+]	.49	4.98[+]
X_5: uncertainty	.63	5.57[+]	.75	5.88[+]	.61	5.50[+]

*Represented by the diagram of Figure 12–3.
[+]Statistically significant finding, as t exceeds 2 standard deviations.

with the other variables in the model and confound behavioral interpretation. Coefficients greater than 1 are also noted for severity in treatment three and for the canonical covariance of treatment three. Although the analysis is valid, its interpretation is difficult and, for that reason, we do not recommend its use.

The assumptions required for path analysis are also required here. Because severity and smoking represent classification variables and are not measured variables like age, weight, and uncertainty, the assumption of multivariate normality is not satisfied. In addition, the correlation matrix was used instead of the variance-covariance matrix. Because of this, the measures of stress are invalid and not interpretable. Finally, sample sizes are much smaller than that recommended by Bentler (1985). For additional discussions concerning structural equation modeling employing LISREL, see Boyd, Frey, and Aaronson (1988), Hayduk (1987), and Bentler (1988).

12–4 MULTIDIMENSIONAL SCALING

Multidimensional scaling is a general term for a set of procedures that can be used to represent spatially the interrelations that exist among a set of objects, items, concepts, and so on. The typical data for this class of techniques are a collection of numbers that reflect object similarity or *proximity*. Object proximity is measured by any numerical index that describes a relationship among objects. Examples of such numerical indices include correlation coefficients, similarity judgments, co-occurrence frequencies from free sorts, amount of communication and interaction among persons in a group, measures of stimulus confusability, euclidian distance, profile similarity, and like indices. The proximity measures provide an indication of how alike or dissimilar every measured object is to every other measured object. A multidimensional scaling analysis results in an indication of spatial configuration or cognitive map which pictorially displays the relationships among the measured sets of objects.

Two purposes mentioned by Rounds and Zevon (1983) for multidimensional scaling are *configural verification* and *dimensional representation* of a hypothesized set of dimensions that can be used to explain some theoretical phenomena. Configural verification is a strategy used to confirm stated a priori theoretical expectations. Here, the researcher assumes a set of relationships based on prior research and a theoretical model or models. The attributes representing the objects are examined in light of their configuration or representation in a multidimensional space as they relate to the theoretical model. Dimensional representation provides a much more exploratory investigative strategy. Here, the attributes of the objects are examined in relationship to how they fall in a two- or more dimensional space. The task of the investigator is then to derive meaning from the display and to establish a tentative theoretical explanation about the relationship of these objects to one another. (For more on this model, see Fitzgerald and Hubert, 1987.)

An instance in which a researcher might be interested in a multidimensional scaling investigation is offered in the analysis of the semantic differential scales described in Section 5–14. The goal would be to see how the bipolar adjectives arranged themselves in a three-dimensional space consisting of evaluation, potency, and activity. With such a display, a researcher would have a clearer understanding of how these paired adjectives relate to the characteristics under study.

Some forms of multidimensional scaling are referred to as *nonmetric*. By this is meant that the algorithm used to perform the scaling focuses on ordered relationships only among the proximity measures. In addition, most computer programs provide goodness of fit tests applied to external criteria that are termed measures of stress or discrepancy. (For a more complete discussion on various measures of discrepancy, see Linhart and Zucchini, 1986.) When the stress is low, the data are said to provide an adequate fit to the model. What was said about goodness of fit tests in the discussion of linear structural equation modeling applies equally well to this model. The model is illustrated with an example taken from Chapter 3. This example is based on the data of Table 3–1, which consists of the Likert scoring of 10 descriptors used to measure pain by 25 subjects. The proximity measure used in this example consists of the euclidian distance between the descriptors. For example, the euclidian distance between *sharp* and *excruciating* is given as

$$D = (4 - 4)^2 + (4 - 4)^2 + (1 - 1)^2 +$$
$$(4 - 1)^2 + \ldots + (1 - 1)^2$$
$$= 7.48$$

The remaining proximity values are reported in Table 12–4. The results of the multidimensional scaling are reported in Table 12–5 and shown graphically in Figure 12–4.

In this example, the interpretation of the two-dimensional array is not easy because the terms selected for evaluation are essentially synonyms of one another and are not broad descriptors of pain. As we see, hurt, harsh, and spasm cluster together as do sharp, pulsate, scream, and blinding. Inflamed and severe cluster together and excruciating seems to cluster with none of the other descriptors. It appears that dimension

TABLE 12–4 PROXIMITY VALUES FOR THE 10 DESCRIPTORS OF TABLE 3–1 USED TO MEASURE PAIN ACROSS 25 SUBJECTS

Descriptor	(2)	(3)	(4)	(5)	(6)	(7)	(8)	(9)	(10)
1. Sharp	7.48	6.71	7.28	8.31	8.31	5.57	6.48	6.24	6.63
2. Excruciating		5.39	6.08	6.71	8.18	6.40	4.47	5.92	4.47
3. Hurt			3.16	4.90	6.78	5.83	5.92	6.00	5.92
4. Harsh				4.69	6.16	6.32	6.24	6.78	6.56
5. Spasm					7.21	6.00	6.86	7.21	7.55
6. Inflamed						7.07	6.86	5.83	7.55
7. Pulsate							5.00	4.90	5.74
8. Scream								3.61	2.82
9. Blinding									4.12
10. Severe									

TABLE 12–5 SCALE VALUES FOR THE 10 DESCRIPTORS USED TO MEASURE PAIN

Dimension One			Dimension Two		
Descriptor Scale	SPSS*	Transformed	Descriptor Scale	SPSS	Transformed
Spasm	−1.84	0.0	Inflamed	−1.89	0.0
Inflamed	−1.30	1.5	Severe	−0.78	3.3
Harsh	−1.05	2.0	Sharp	−0.29	4.7
Hurt	−0.66	3.1	Pulsate	−0.18	5.0
Excruciating	0.22	5.3	Scream	0.03	5.7
Pulsate	0.44	5.9	Harsh	0.22	6.2
Severe	0.51	6.1	Blinding	0.41	6.8
Scream	0.65	6.5	Spasm	0.43	6.8
Blinding	1.02	7.4	Hurt	0.55	7.2
Sharp	2.02	10.0	Excruciating	1.50	10.0

*SPSS-Statistical Package for the Social Sciences.

one measures pain quality and that dimension two measures pain intensity.

The first thing that a researcher should investigate is the measure of stress, which ranges from a low of zero to a high of one. At the first iteration of the algorithm, the measure of stress is equal to .27 and at the end of the seventh iteration, the measure of stress is equal to .19. The closer the stress is to zero, the better is the scaling process. In this case, the measure of stress is defined by Kruskal's Stress Formula 1 (Kruskal, 1964) and is small, indicating that the scaling proc-

ess is adequate (SPSS[x], 1986). Another measure of stress is the goodness of fit between the observed discrepancies and the fitted discrepancies as defined by the Pearson Product Moment Correlation Coefficient. In this case, r = .94. This suggests that the quality of the multidimensional scaling is excellent.

The results of the scaling are reported in Table 12–5. As indicated for dimension one, the ordered words and their scaled values are given as spasm (−1.84), inflamed (−1.30), harsh (−1.05), hurt (−0.66), excruciating

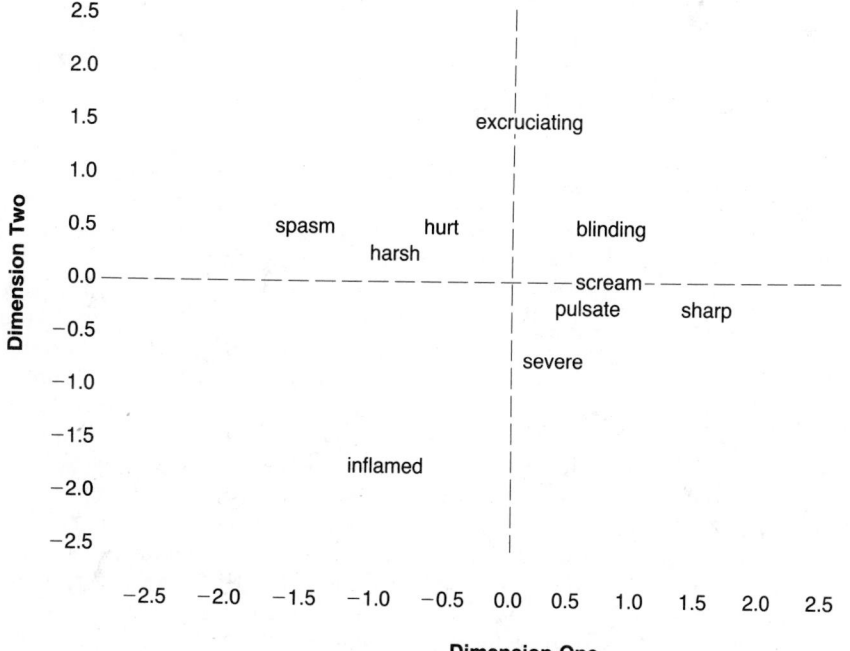

Figure 12–4. Two-dimensional display of the scales of the 10 descriptors used to measure pain by 25 subjects.

$$\text{Scale value} = \frac{\text{Observed value} - \text{Lower limit}}{\text{Upper limit} - \text{Lower limit}} \times 10$$

(0.22), pulsate (0.44), severe (0.51), scream (0.65), blinding (1.02), and sharp (2.02). For this dimension, the poles are defined as spasm and sharp. It is also clear that the descriptors are not equally spaced along the scale of the measurement probably reflecting the near identity of meaning of the 10 terms.

The scaled values can be used as reported, or they can be transformed to a more familiar scale such as zero to 10. This transformation is achieved with the linear transformation at the top of this page.

Thus, for spasm the transformed value is given in equation 1 at the top of page 295. For inflamed, the scaled value is given in equation 2 at the top of page 295.

The remaining values are reported in Table 12–5. Note that on dimension one, pulsate, severe, and scream are very similar in scaled values. This suggests that these adjectives are not effective discriminators of pain. Any one of the three can be used to measure the same degree of pain. The scaled values demonstrate how to define the pain scale using discriminating terms. For example, a six-point pain scale with a rough approximation to equal intervals could be defined as

0.0 Spasm
2.0 Harsh
5.3 Excruciating
6.5 Scream
7.4 Blinding
10.0 Sharp

with interval distances of 2.0, 3.3, 2.2, 0.9, and 2.6. A four-point scale with nearly equal intervals, 3.1, 3.4, and 3.5, is given as

0.0 Spasm
3.1 Hurt
6.5 Scream
10.0 Sharp

A similar analysis can be made for the second scale. In this case, the transformed scale and its ordered values are given as inflamed (0.0), severe (3.3), sharp (4.8), pulsate (5.0), scream (5.6), harsh (6.2), blinding (6.8), spasm (6.8), hurt (7.20), and excruciating (10.0). Here, scream, harsh, blinding, and spasm possess poor discriminating proper-

ties. The descriptors that can be used to provide a four-point scale with near equal intervals is given as

0.0 Inflamed
3.3 Severe
6.8 Blinding
10.0 Excruciating

Here, the distances between the terms are given as 3.3, 3.5, and 3.2. Thus, a patient could be given the two sets of descriptors:

Spasm
Hurt
Scream
Sharp

and

Inflamed
Severe
Blinding
Excruciating

and asked to choose the two descriptors that best describe his or her pain. For example, if a patient selected hurt and excruciating, he or she would be scored on quality of pain with a scored value of 3.1 and on intensity would be scored a 10. These would be used as dependent variables for further analysis.

12–5 CLUSTER ANALYSIS

Cluster analysis is a classification technique for forming homogeneous groups within complex data sets. The major difference between cluster analysis and multidimensional scaling is that cluster analysis is used primarily to group persons or objects, whereas multidimensional scaling techniques are used to spatially relate concepts or items on a scale in a pictorial form. The typical purpose of cluster analysis is to identify homogeneous subtypes of individuals or objects within a multivariate set of data. Often a researcher does not know in advance the natural or typical grouping of subtypes. One goal of cluster analysis is to identify specific subgroups or subtypes of persons in a data

① Spasm value = $[\{-1.84 - (-1.84)\}/\{2.02 - (-1.84)\}]10 = 0.0$

② Inflamed value = $[\{-1.30 - (-1.84)\}/\{2.02 - (-1.84)\}]10 = 1.5$

set. Consequently, a primary function of cluster analysis is to develop classification schemas, taxonomies, or typologies of persons, which represent different patterns in the data set.

Cluster analysis also is useful in exploratory studies, confirmatory studies, and very complex studies requiring simplification before primary statistical analyses can be performed. If a researcher is not certain about the structure and interrelationships that exist among people or objects, cluster analysis can help a researcher to understand multivariate data by producing a summary picture of the underlying structure. It can be used to confirm an a priori structure generated from other theoretical or empirical studies. Finally, if the grouping of subjects or objects is humanly difficult or impossible, a computer application of a cluster analysis program can be used to provide a first step in simplification of data for further analysis.

Cluster algorithms are written to search among the data for persons or objects that can be partitioned into relatively distinct groupings. In multidimensional scaling, a map of the items is of primary concern and serves as the end product of the scaling. In cluster analysis, the division of the objects or subjects into a set of mutually exclusive subsets is the final goal. In some perspectives, clustering can be viewed as an ad hoc data analytical procedure for combining persons or objects for other statistical analyses. If a researcher had prior knowledge about the specific types of persons and their groupings, more conventional techniques such as linear discriminant function analysis and MANOVA would be used immediately without clustering. These methods were described in Chapter 11. (For a further description of clustering techniques and alternative clustering methods, see Borgen and Barnett, 1987 and for an example involving the clustering of health locus of control types of subjects, see Rock, Meyerowitz, Maisto, and Wallston, 1987.)

An example is provided in Table 12−6 of the clustering of the treatment effect measures of Table 15−1 using a method developed by Hubert and explicated in detail by Hubert and Baker (1976). This method does not require a computer and can be done by an experienced person in 10 to 20 minutes.

TABLE 12−6 ILLUSTRATION OF THE COMPLETE LINK METHOD OF CLUSTER ANALYSIS USING THE TREATMENT EFFECTS OF TABLE 15−1

Study Number	3	12	11	8	7	13	14	10	2	15	9	4	6	1	5
	.03	.14	.21	.26	.26	.31	.40	.50	.50	.70	.71	.81	1.43	1.45	2.39
3	—	.11	.18	.23	.23	.28	.37	.47	.47	.67	.68	.78	1.40	1.42	2.36
12		—	.07	.12	.12	.17	.26	.36	.36	.56	.57	.67	1.29	1.31	2.22
11			—	.05	.05	.10	.19	.29	.29	.49	.50	.60	1.22	1.24	2.15
8				—	.00	.05	.14	.24	.24	.44	.45	.55	1.17	1.19	2.10
7					—	.05	.14	.24	.24	.44	.45	.55	1.17	1.19	2.10
13						—	.09	.19	.19	.39	.40	.50	1.12	1.14	2.05
14							—	.10	.10	.30	.31	.41	1.03	1.05	1.96
10								—	.00	.20	.21	.31	.93	.95	1.86
2									—	.20	.21	.31	.93	.95	1.86
15										—	.01	.11	.73	.75	1.66
9											—	.10	.72	.74	1.65
4												—	.62	.72	1.55
6													—	.02	.96
1														—	.94

The data in Table 12–6 represent the differences between the treatment effects for the 15 studies on pain used in the meta-analysis of Chapter 15. The numbers in the table are *proximity* measures of the simplest type. The numbers are simply the differences in the treatment effect measures for each pair of studies. A statistical post hoc grouping of the studies is illustrated in Chapter 15 using the methods of Hedges and Olkin (1985). The method described here also can be used to group the studies on a post hoc basis.

The clustering method is based on the *complete link method*. For the complete link clustering method, any new object considered as an addition to an already existing cluster is added to the cluster only when it is completely linked with all objects in the cluster. This differs from the *single link method*. As stated by Aldenderfer and Blashfield (1984), the single link method adds a new object to an already existing cluster if the object can be linked to at least one member of the existing cluster. The single link method tends to produce clusters that are linear in form, whereas the complete link method tends to produce clusters that are circular in shape.

For the Hubert method, the data are first transferred to three-by-five-inch cards with the study numbers, the values of the proximity measures, and the rank position of each ordered pair according to the proximity measures. The ranked data for this example are shown in Table 12–7.

There are as many steps in clustering as there are three-by-five-inch cards. At the beginning of the clustering process, each study is treated as a complete cluster. Thus, in this example, one begins with the following 15 clusters:

{1} {2} {3} {4} {5} {6} {7} {8} {9} {10} {11} {12} {13} {14} {15}

In the next step, the two clusters that are closest together are combined into one cluster. Here, two clusters consisting of studies 7 and 8, and 2 and 10 are both identified at rank 1.5, the average of ranks 1 and 2. For these clusters, the treatment effects are .26 and .50, respectively, and their corresponding proximity measures both are equal to zero. After these clusters are formed, the total set of clusters is reduced to:

{7,8} {2,10} {1} {3} {4} {5} {6} {9} {11} {12} {13} {14} {15}

TABLE 12–7 PAIRED STUDIES, PROXIMITY VALUES, AND RANK VALUES OF THE PROXIMITY VALUES FOR THE DATA OF TABLE 15–1

Paired Studies	Proximity Value	Rank
2,10	.00	1.5
7,8	.00	1.5
9,15	.01	3
1,6	.02	4
7,11	.05	6.5
7,13	.05	6.5
8,11	.05	6.5
8,13	.05	6.5
11,12	.07	9
13,14	.09	10
2,14	.10	12.5
4,9	.10	12.5
10,14	.10	12.5
11,13	.10	12.5
3,12	.11	15.5
4,15	.11	15.5
7,12	.12	17.5
8,12	.12	17.5
7,14	.14	19.5
8,14	.14	19.5
12,13	.17	21
3,11	.18	22
. . .	. . .	. . . .

At the next step, each study is now compared with the new clusters by examining the proximity measures to determine whether any complete linkages are formed. For example, for cluster {1} to be joined with {7,8}, object 1 must be linked with both 7 and 8. In this case, this does not happen. In fact, no one object links with either of the two existing object clusters. Objects (9 and 15) at rank 3, (1 and 6) at rank 4, (11 and 12) at rank 9, and (13 and 14) at rank 10 cluster before any one single object is clustered with any cluster containing two elements. With the clustering of (9 and 15), (1 and 6), (11 and 12), and (13 and 14), the set of clusters is reduced to:

{7,8} {2,10} {9,15} {1,6} {11,12} {13,14} {3} {4} {5}

At rank 15.5, {4} becomes linked to cluster {9,15}, completing the linkage begun at rank 12.5. Thus at rank 15.5, study 4 becomes completely linked with cluster {9,15} to make cluster {4,9,15}. At this point, the clusters are:

{7,8} {2,10} {4,9,15} {1,6} {11,12} {13,14} {3} {5}

At rank 15.5, clusters {7,8} and {11,12} become completely linked with one another to give the following set of clusters:

{7,8,11,12} {2,10} {4,9,15} {1,6} {13,14} {3} {5}

As the process continues, the following sets of clusters are formed:

{7,8,11,12} {2,10} {4,9,15} {1,6} {13,14} {3} {5}
{7,8,11,12} {2,10,13,14} {4,9,15} {1,6} {3} {5}
{3,7,8,11,12} {2,10,13,14} {4,9,15} {1,6} {5}
{3,7,8,11,12} {2,4,9,10,13,14,15} {1,6} {5}
{3,7,8,11,12} {1,2,4,6,9,10,13,14,15} {5}
{1,2,3,4,6,7,8,9,10,11,12,13,14,15} {5}
{1,2,3,4,5,6,7,8,9,10,11,12,13,14,15}

The complete process is shown graphically in the *dendogram* of Figure 12−5, a pictorial representation of the clustering.

As indicated, study 5 is a definite outlier. It becomes completely linked at the final step. Cluster {1,6} is also unique. It is origi-nally formed in the earlier stages of the clustering but does not become completely linked until the fourth to the last step in the clustering process. Examination of Figure 15−2 also supports the supposition that these two clusters should remain separate. At this point, subjective judgments need to be made as to where to complete the clustering. From an examination of Figure 15−2, a reasonable stopping point is provided in the four-cluster set:

{3,7,8,11,12} {2,4,9,10,13,14,15} {1,6} {5}

or in the five-cluster set:

{3,7,8,11,12} {2,10,13,14} {4,9,15} {1,6} {5}

In Figure 15−2, it appears that studies {4,9,15} cluster together. To make a rational judgment between these two possible cluster solutions the study classification schemes

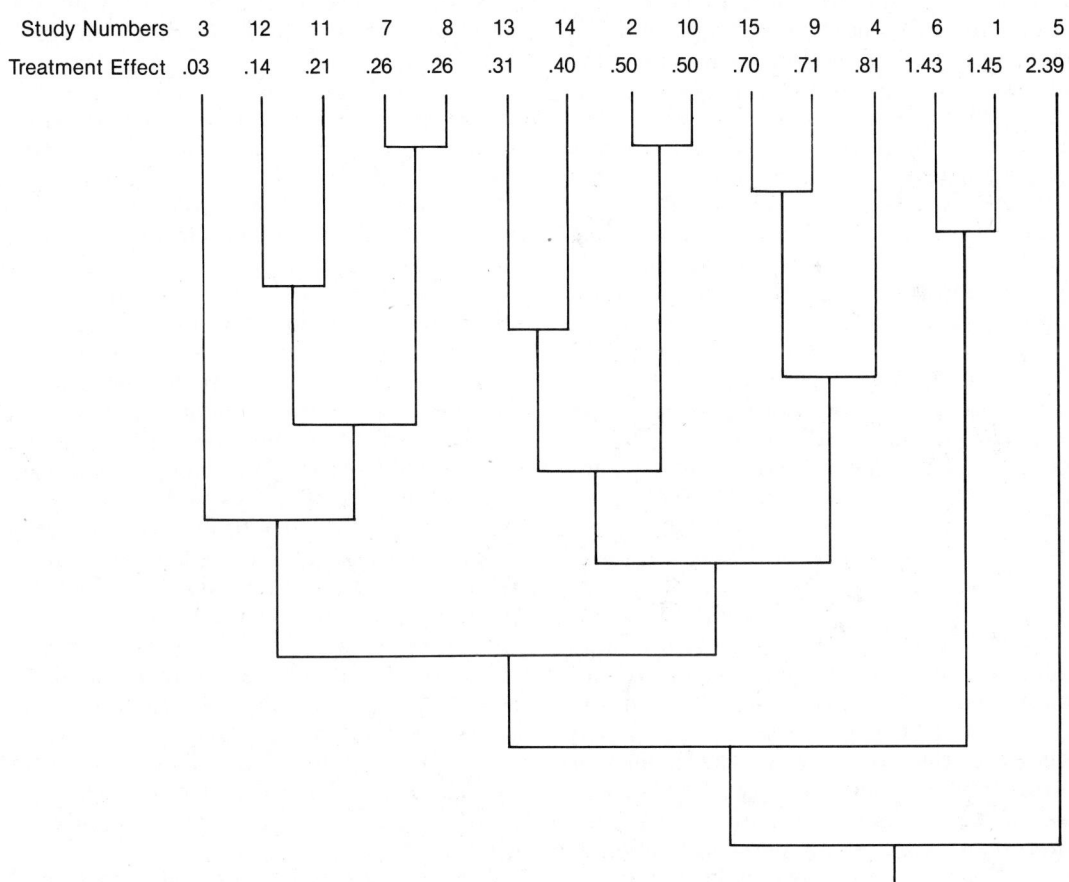

Figure 12−5. Dendogram for the proximity matrix of Table 15−1.

provided in Tables 15−5 and 15−6 can be used.

As illustrated, clustering is based on a set of rules for combining groups of similar objects. For example, when study 4 was joined with studies 9 and 15 the proximity measures were given as .10 and .11. All of the previous proximity measures had been used for the previous sets of clusters. Also, because clusters {9,15} and {4} are contained in cluster {4,9,15} the cluster method is referred to as a *hierarchical* clustering method. Hierarchical methods are most in use today. An advantage is that they generate dendograms that show how the clusters come together from clusters higher in the hierarchy.

The proximity measure used in this example is the simple euclidian distance between the objects measured on the scale of Figure 15−2. For multivariate data, the euclidian distance can be determined and used in a similar fashion. With euclidian distance, identity is measured by a proximity measure of zero, and so the proximity measure closest to zero is used as the starting point. With correlations used as proximity measures, the correlation closest to unity is used as the starting point. It is important for a researcher to choose the appropriate proximity measure because the final clustering is based on the arithmetic properties of such measures.

With large samples, the procedure for cluster analysis is very tedious. In such cases, computer programs are advised. BMDP (Dixon, 1983), SAS (SAS Institute, 1982), and SPSS[x] (1986) have cluster programs that produce useful and meaningful results, provided that the variables used pass tests of reliability and validity determinations. Ward's Method (1963) is recommended by Borgen and Barnett (1987).

Cluster analysis can be viewed as a competitor to factor analysis provided that proximity measures are correlation coefficients. Factor analysis is not recommended when sample sizes are small because of the large instability in measurements of correlation. For small samples, cluster analysis is probably preferred because the focus is more on rank order than on exact measurements of correlations between variables. Also, cluster analysis can be used for proximity measures other than correlation coefficients. Sometimes researchers use factor analysis in its reverse role and factor people rather than variables. This use of factor analysis is called *inverse* or *transposed factor analysis*. It is

also referred to as *Q type factor analysis* by Cattell (1966).

12−6 SUMMARY

In this chapter an introduction to four relatively new multivariate techniques that do not fit into the mainstream of more familiar multivariate methods was presented. These four methods are path analysis, structural equation modeling, multidimensional scaling, and cluster analysis. None of the methods has a basis in standard statistical theory and for that reason risks of type I errors are unknown. Although some computer programs provide probability measures, they must be used with caution and care. The methods make use of measurement principles, but the models themselves do not use classical measurement theory as their starting points. All are based on new ways of examining complex data sets. (For further discussion on these models see Hair, Anderson, and Tatham, 1987.)

Path analysis and structural equation modeling are used to study systems in which it is believed that known causal events operate. In path analysis, one dependent measure is present and multiple independent measures that are believed to impact on the dependent measures are required. The method can be extended to cover the case of multiple dependent measures. In the structural equation model, it is believed that unobservable variables relate to one another through observable variables that can be used to generate factors, concepts, or hypothetical constructs. The independent variables can be status variables, measured quantitative variables, or even manipulated treatment variables. These models were illustrated with two examples taken from the preoperative teaching study.

Multidimensional scaling is used to construct a pictorial representation of a set of objects or items in a space of two or more dimensions. It is used primarily to gain insight into the structure that exists among the items. This model was illustrated using the pain instrument development study in Chapter 3.

Cluster analysis is a method used to generate groupings of objects or persons for further study. It was illustrated using the meta-analytic study of Chapter 15.

Finally, it should be known that the use of these methods has been questioned by Cliff (1983), Marascuilo and Levin (1983), Rogosa (1980), and by Freedman (1987). The latter two critics propose the following two questions:

Are these valid methods for model building?
Are these methods scientifically sound?

They answer both questions with a resounding No!

It must be noted that goodness of fit tests are a statistical problem in the scientific analysis of data. Theories can never be proven. They can only be disproved. Thus, when a statistical goodness of fit test results in a nonsignificant finding a researcher has a complex philosophical and empirical problem. The null hypothesis can only be rejected. It can never be accepted. Thus, whenever a goodness of fit statistic is small it can mean that the theory is correct or it can mean that the deviations from theory are not large enough to generate a statistic that should lead to rejection. (See Fassinger, 1987, for more on this perplexing difficulty.)

REFERENCES

Aldenderfer, M.S., and Blashfield, R.K.: Cluster analysis. Beverly Hills, CA, Sage, 1984.

Bentler, P.M.: Theory and implementation of EQS: a structural equations program. Los Angeles, BMDP Statistical Software, Inc., 1985.

Bentler, P.M.: Bentler critiques structural equation modeling, The Score, 3: 3, 6, 1988.

Borgen, F.H., and Barnett, D.C.: Applying cluster analysis in counseling psychology research, Counseling Psychol., 34: 456–468, 1987.

Boyd, C.J., Frey, M.A., and Aaronson, L.S.: Structural equation models and nursing research: Part I, Nurs. Res., 37: 249–252, 1988.

Cattell, R.B.: The meaning and strategic use of factor analysis. In Cattell, R.B., ed: Handbook of Multivariate Experimental Psychology. Chicago, Rand McNally, 1966.

Cliff, N.: Some cautions concerning the applications of causal methods, Multivariate Behavior. Res., 18: 125–126, 1983.

Dixon, W.J., ed.: BMDP Statistical Software. Berkeley, CA, University of California Press, 1983.

Fassinger, R.: Use of structural equation modeling in counseling psychology research, Counseling Psychol., 34: 425–436, 1987.

Fitzgerald, L.F., and Hubert, L.J.: Multidimensional scaling: some possibilities for counseling psychology, Counseling Psychol., 34: 469–480, 1987.

Freedman, D.A.: As others see us: a case study in path analysis, J. Ed. Stat., 12: 101–128, 1987.

Hair, J.F., Anderson, R.E., and Tatham, R.L.: Multivariate Data Analysis, ed. 2. New York, Macmillan, 1987.

Hayduk, L.A.: Structural Equations Modeling with LISREL. Baltimore, Johns Hopkins University Press, 1987.

Hedges, L.V., and Olkin, I.: Statistical Methods for Meta-analysis. Orlando, FL, Academic Press, 1985.

Hubert, L., and Baker, F.B.: Data analysis by single-link and complete-link hierarchical clustering, J. Ed. Stat., 1: 87–111, 1976.

Hughes, M., Price, R., and Marrs, D.: Linking theory constructions and theory testing: models with multiple indicators of latent variables, Acad. Management Rev., 11: 128–144, 1986.

Joreskog, K., and Sorbom, D.: LISREL VI. Analysis of Linear Structural Relationships by Maximum Likelihood and Least Square Methods. Chicago, IL, National Education Resources, 1986.

Kruskal, J.B.: Nonmetric multidimensional scaling, Psychometrika, 29: 1–27; 115–129, 1966.

Linhart, H., and Zucchini, W.: Model Selection. New York, John Wiley & Sons, 1986.

Marascuilo, L.A., and Levin, J.: Multivariate Statistics in the Social Sciences: A Researcher's Guide. Belmont, CA, Wadsworth, 1983.

Popper, K.: The Logic of Scientific Discovery. New York, Basic Books, 1959.

Rock, D.L., Meyerowitz, B.E., Maisto, S.A., and Wallston, K.A.: The derivation and validation of six multidimensional health locus of control scale clusters, Res. Nurs. Health, 10: 185–195, 1987.

Rogosa, D.R.: A critique of cross-lagged correlation, Psychol. Bull., 88: 245–258, 1980.

Rounds, J.B., and Zevon, M.A.: Multidimensional scaling research in vocational psychology, Appl. Psychol. Measure., 7: 491–515, 1983.

SAS (SAS Institute): SAS User's Guide: Statistics. New York, Author, 1982.

SPSS, Inc.: SPSS^x User's Guide, ed. 2. New York, McGraw-Hill, 1986.

Ward, J.H.: Hierarchical grouping to optimize an objective function, J. Am. Stat. Assoc., 58: 236–244, 1963.

Chapter 13

STATISTICAL METHODS FOR CONTINGENCY TABLES

13-1 FREQUENCY COUNTS AND CONTINGENCY TABLES

In this chapter, the familiar Karl Pearson chi-square test for two-dimensional arrays of frequency data is reviewed, and the loglinear model is introduced and illustrated. The algorithms required for these data analytic models are not described in detail because of their complexity. The major use of these models for the nurse researcher is to provide statistical methods for testing hypotheses, estimating strengths of association, and estimating the effects of independent variables singly and together with frequency or enumeration data. The reason for examining these methods in this chapter is that qualitative measures such as frequency or enumeration data cannot be treated using statistical models like the analysis of variance, covariance, and multiple regression. Specialized methods are required for frequency or enumeration data.

The case of a two-dimensional contingency table with three rows and three columns is presented first. Next, procedures for multidimensional contingency tables are illustrated. Directions for testing hypotheses are presented. Planned and post hoc comparisons using contrasts are described and illustrated. Guidelines are presented on how to analyze frequency data more efficiently.

Frequency counts are probably the most often encountered quantitative variables of behavioral and health science research. If the results of the counts can be displayed in a two-dimensional frequency table, the Karl Pearson chi-square test can be used to test for (1) homogeneity of distributions across multiple groups and (2) independence between two possible explanatory qualitative variables.

Although the familiar chi-square test can be applied to multidimensional contingency tables, it is rarely used. In the past few years, a unifying theory is gaining popularity in the analysis of multidimensional contingency tables. This model is commonly referred to as the *loglinear model*. A two-dimensional contingency table can be formulated simply with the use of desk or hand calculator; however, the same is not true for contingency tables with three or more dimensions. Solutions have been programmed and are readily available at many computer facilities, and software is available for personal computer use by BMDP (Brown, 1981), SPSS[x] (Nie, Hull, Jenkins, et al., 1986), and SAS Institute (1985).

13-2 THE KARL PEARSON TEST FOR A TWO-DIMENSIONAL CONTINGENCY TABLE

As an example of a two-dimensional contingency table, consider the preoperative teaching study described earlier and consider classification of the 246 patients according to treatment and length of stay in hospital following surgery. The frequencies for this cross-tabulation are reported in Table 13-1. Here, the dependent variable, length of stay, has been redefined in terms of three mutually exclusive nonoverlapping categories given as

L_1— 2 and 3 days
L_2— 4 and 5 days
L_3— 6 or more days

The Karl Pearson chi-square test requires that theoretical cell frequencies exceed a minimal value of about 5 (Cochran, 1954). To satisfy this condition, it was necessary to reduce length of stay to three categories.

As shown in Table 13-1, 18 patients who were given treatment one had a length of stay of two to three days. At the same time, 26 remained in hospital for six or more days. Visual inspection of the data suggests that treatment one patients remained in hospital longer than treatment three patients. Treatment two patients remained in hospital for an intermediate period of time following operation.

The Karl Pearson chi-square test is used to test the hypothesis that the distribution of patients in the three length of stay categories (L_1, L_2, L_3) is independent or unrelated to the type of treatment (T_1, T_2, T_3) given before surgery. If the hypothesis is true, the numerical value of the chi-square statistic should be close to zero. If the hypothesis is false, the chi-square statistic can be large. The maximum value that the chi-square statistic can attain is $M \times N$, where N is the number of subjects and M is the minimum of $(R - 1)$ and $(C - 1)$ and where R is the number of rows in the table and C is the number of columns in the table. In this example, the chi-square statistic can range from a value of zero to a maximum value of $2(246) = 492$.

The Karl Pearson statistic is defined as

$$X^2_{RC} = \sum_{r=1}^{R} \sum_{c=1}^{C} \frac{(f_{rc} - F_{rc})^2}{F_{rc}}$$

where

f_{rc} = the observed frequency in the cell of the contingency table defined by the r-th row and the c-th column

and

F_{rc} = the estimated expected frequency for rc cell

Let

P_{rc} = the probability of appearing in the rc cell

with

$P_{r.}$ = the probability of appearing in the r-th row

and

$P_{.c}$ = the probability of appearing in the c-th column

TABLE 13-1 LENGTH OF STAY FOLLOWING SURGERY ACCORDING TO TREATMENT

Length of Stay	Treatment One	Treatment Two	Treatment Three	Total
L_1:2 and 3 days	18	21	50	89
L_2:4 and 5 days	38	39	25	102
L_3:6 or more days	26	22	7	55
Total	82	82	82	246

Under the hypothesis of independence or homogeneity of row probabilities the estimated expected frequencies are computed as

$$F_{rc} = f_{r.}f_{.c}/N$$

where

$f_{r.}$ = the total frequency in the r-th row
$f_{.c}$ = the total frequency in the c-th column

and

N = the total frequency for the entire table

For the data of Table 13−1,

$$F_{11} = 82 \times 89/246 = 29.67$$

The remaining expected frequencies are found in a similar manner. All expected frequencies are reported in Table 13−2. This table must be inspected to determine whether the chi-square test can be justified. If more than 20% of the cell frequencies are less than 5, the test should not be performed. This decision is based on a modification of Cochran's Rule (1954) for large contingency tables. In this case, all expected frequencies are greater than 5; therefore, the test can be performed. In practice, if expected cell frequencies are less than 5, neighboring cells need to be combined. With these estimated expected frequencies, the value of the Karl Pearson test is given as:

$$X_{RC}^2 = \frac{(18 - 29.67)^2}{29.67} + \frac{(38 - 34.00)^2}{34.00}$$
$$+ \cdots + \frac{(7 - 18.33)^2}{18.33} = 35.59$$

The sampling distribution of this statistic is chi-square with degrees of freedom given as $\nu = (R - 1)(C - 1)$. For the data of Table 13−1,

$$\nu = (3 - 1)(3 - 1) = 4$$

With the critical values reported in Table A-1, it is seen that the hypothesis of homogeneity in distribution for length of stay across the three treatments is rejected because $\chi_{4:0.95}^2 = 9.49$. The strength of the association is measured by Cramer's v^2 and is given as:

$$v^2 = X_{RC}^2/(M \times N) = 35.59/(2 \times 246) = 0.0723$$

Now that it is known that the distributions for the three treatments are not identical, it would be desirable to identify the cells that deviate from the hypothesis of homogeneity of distributions. Marascuilo and Serlin (1988) describe statistical procedures for achieving this goal. These methods are based on procedures derived by Goodman (1964, 1970).

An alternative method of making a post hoc investigation for very large samples is described. This method is based on a cell by cell comparison of the observed frequencies with the corresponding estimated frequencies. For example, 18 patients had treatment one with length of stay of 2 to 3 days. If the hypothesis of homogeneity had been true, the expected number of patients for this cell is given as 29.67. Thus, it is seen that the cell frequency is short by

$$f_{11} - F_{11} = (18 - 29.67) = -11.67$$

patients and the contribution to chi-square is given as

$$(f_{11} - F_{11})^2/F_{11} = (-11.67)^2/29.67 = 4.59$$

The remaining cell contributions are reported in Table 13−3, As shown, the chi-square value is inflated by (1) the large number of patients in the T_3 by L_1 cell under treatment three and (2) the small number of patients in the T_3 by L_3 cell under treatment three. Treatment three patients have the shortest length of stay in hospital following operation.

TABLE 13−2 ESTIMATED EXPECTED FREQUENCIES FOR THE DATA OF TABLE 13−1

Length of Stay	Treatment One	Treatment Two	Treatment Three	Total
L_1:2 and 3 days	29.67	29.67	29.67	89
L_2:4 and 5 days	34.00	34.00	34.00	102
L_3:6 or more days	18.33	18.33	18.33	55
Total	82	82	82	246

TABLE 13–3 CONTRIBUTIONS TO THE KARL PEARSON STATISTIC FOR THE DATA OF TABLE 13–1

Length of Stay	Treatment One	Treatment Two	Treatment Three	Total
L_1:2 and 3 days	4.59	2.53	13.93	
L_2:4 and 5 days	.47	.74	2.38	
L_3:6 or more days	3.21	.73	7.00	

A conservative rule of thumb when visually inspecting the frequency data is to identify the cells with chi-square contributions larger than the critical value of the test. These cells provide possible reasons for the rejected hypothesis. In this example, the critical value is equal to 9.49. Only the T_3 by L_1 cell has a contribution to chi-square that exceeds this value. On this basis it is concluded that treatment three patients tend to remain in the hospital for shorter periods than the patients of treatments one and two.

13–3 THE LOGLINEAR MODEL FOR A TWO-DIMENSIONAL CONTINGENCY TABLE

Consider an examination of the data of Table 13–1 from a loglinear model perspective. Under this model the same assumptions and hypotheses operate as that established for the Karl Pearson chi-square test. In this case, the familiar chi-square test statistic is replaced by the *likelihood ratio statistic*, which is defined as follows:

$$G_{RC}^2 = 2 \sum_{r=1}^{R} \sum_{c=1}^{C} f_{rc} \log_e \left(\frac{f_{rc}}{F_{rc}} \right)$$

The sampling distribution of this statistic can be approximated by a chi-square variable with degrees of freedom equal to $(R - 1)(C - 1)$. For the data of Table 13–1,

$$G_{RC}^2 = 2[18 \log_e(18/29.67) + 38 \log_e(38/34.00)$$
$$+ \cdots + 7 \log_e(7/18.33)]$$
$$= 36.19$$

The degrees of freedom for this statistic is given as $\nu = 4$ and the $\alpha = .05$ decision rule is given as:

Decision rule: Reject H_0 if $G^2 > 9.49$

Like the decision reached with the more familiar Karl Pearson statistic, the hypothesis of independence or homogeneity is rejected.

Note the similarity in values of $X^2 = 35.59$ and $G_{RC}^2 = 36.19$. This closeness in value almost always occurs. Thus, little seems to have been gained by this second analysis using G^2 instead of X^2, and this is true. Even so, the G^2 statistic has one major advantage not possessed by the X^2 statistic. Like the sum of squares total in the analysis of variance, the G^2 statistic can be partitioned into unique components which have the property of additivity. For two-dimensional tables, the partitioning property is not useful; however, this is not true for contingency tables based on the classification of subjects in terms of three or more variables, as shown in Section 13–5.

G^2 statistics can be partitioned in many ways. Marascuilo and Levin (1983) provide examples for partitioning the G^2 statistic for a single set of frequency data. In particular, they show how a two-factor design can be analyzed in terms of interactions or in terms of nested or simple effects factors. Agresti (1984) provides directions for partitioning the likelihood statistic for two-dimensional tables that can be extended to tables with more than two dimensions and for tables where one or both variables satisfy ordered relationships.

13–4 ODDS RATIOS AND CONTRASTS FOR CONTINGENCY TABLES

A statistical measure that is used in conjunction with the loglinear model is a measure of treatment effects called the *odds ratio*. This statistic is used to assess the joint effects of two variables that act together on a response variable. It plays the same role in contingency table analysis that interactions play in the analysis of variance. In fact, odds ratios have a structure very similar to that of the tetrad difference defined in Section 9–14. The ratios are used and interpreted in exactly the same way as described for tetrad differences in ANOVA. In this case, odds ratios are used to measure and interpret interactions for frequency or enumeration data.

As an example of how to compute and evaluate an odds ratio, reconsider the data of Table 13–1. The original three by three contingency table can be subdivided into 9 two by two tables. For example, consider the two by two factor contingency table taken from Table 13–1 consisting of patients assigned to T_1 (treatment one) and T_3 (treatment three) and patients whose length of stay was L_1 (2 or 3 days) and L_3 (6 or more days). The corresponding frequencies are as follows:

Length of Stay	Treatment One	Treatment Three
(2 or 3 days)	$f_{11} = 18$	$f_{13} = 50$
(6 or more days)	$f_{31} = 26$	$f_{33} = 7$

For treatment one, the frequencies are given as $f_{11} = 18$ and $f_{31} = 26$. For treatment three, the corresponding frequencies are given by $f_{13} = 50$ and $f_{33} = 7$.

Among the patients of treatment one the ratio of the number who stayed a short time to those who stayed a long time is given as

$$r_1 = f_{11}/f_{31} = 18/26 = (18/18) / (26/18)$$
$$= (1.00)/(1.44) = 0.69$$

For every patient whose length of stay was short, the number who remained a long time is equal to $1/0.69 = 1.44$. For the patients assigned to treatment three,

$$r_3 = f_{13}/f_{33} = 50/7 = (50/7) / (7/7)$$
$$= (7.14)/(1.00) = 7.14$$

For every one patient who stayed a long time, 7.14 stayed a short time. Certainly, the treatment assigned to the patients had a pronounced effect on the length of stay following surgery. Thus, the odds of staying a long time against the odds of staying a short time for patients in treatments one and three are .69 and 7.14, respectively. In other words, the odds favor a short stay in treatment three and a long stay in treatment one. For this example, the odds ratio is

$$\theta = r_1/r_3 = 0.69/7.14 = .0966$$

This number is hard to interpret. One way to simplify the interpretation is to report the ratios in terms of 100 patients for each group. In treatment one, the ratio of patients in L_1 relative to L_3 is given as 69 to 100. In treatment three, the corresponding ratio is 714 to 100. In treatment three, patients tend to stay for shorter periods of time than patients in treatment one.

If the treatments had equal effectiveness, then the odds for the two treatments should be equal and their ratios would be 1. This equality of odds would hold for all possible odds that could be generated for any two treatments and any two levels of length of stay. It can be shown that if the hypothesis of independence or homogeneity is true, then it is also true that the odds of success to failure in any two groups are identical. Note that in this illustration, the odds ratio was defined for a two by two contingency table. Odds ratios can be defined for tables with two or more rows or columns. They have their greatest applicability, however, in the two by two case.

If R_c and $R_{c'}$ represent the population odds in any two groups, G_c and $G_{c'}$, then the ratio of the two odds for categories r and r′ is defined as

$$\theta = R_c/R_{c'} = F_{rc}F_{r'c'}/F_{rc'}F_{r'c}$$

and can be estimated in the sample as

$$\hat{\theta} = r_c/r_{c'} = f_{rc}f_{r'c'}/f_{rc'}f_{r'c}$$

If the odds are equal to the same common value, their ratio is equal to *one* or *unity*. If the odds ratio equals unity, the treatment has no effect on the two levels of the dependent variable examined.

It can be shown that if the cell frequencies exceed five and if the logarithm of θ to the base $e = 2.7183$ is taken, then

$$g = \log_e \theta$$
$$= \log_e f_{rc} - \log_e f_{rc'} - \log_e f_{r'c} + \log_e f_{r'c'}$$

also can be used to measure the effects of the treatment effect. If the logarithm of the odds ratio to the base e is zero, the treatment is said to have no effect on the dependent variable. Because zero is associated with no association, it is customary to use this value when investigating treatment effects for qualitative data. Note that the structure of the logarithm of the odds ratio is identical with the structure of an interaction contrast in the analysis of variance presented in Section 9–14.

The similarity to the interaction contrast of the analysis of variance can be seen by dividing each frequency by the total sample size. If this is done, it follows that

$$g = \log_e \theta = [\log_e f_{rc}/N - \log_e f_{rc'}/N] - [\log_e f_{r'c}/N - \log_e f_{r'c'}/N]$$

The fractions in the brackets represent the proportion of persons who belong in each of the four cells of the original table. Thus, g can be written as

$$g = \log_e \theta = [\log_e P_{rc} - \log_e P_{rc'}] - [\log_e P_{r'c} - \log_e P_{r'c'}]$$

The contrast is now seen to represent an interaction measured in terms of the percentage of persons who belong to each of the four cells of the corresponding two by two contingency table. Thus, it is identical with the tetrad difference of the two by two analysis of variance measured in terms of the logarithms of the population percentages.

In terms of population odds and odds ratios, the null hypothesis for the two by two tables for treatments one and three and length of stay categories L_1: (2 or 3 days) and L_3: (6 or more days) can be stated as

$$H_0: R_1 = R_3$$

or

$$\text{as } H_0: g = 0$$

The alternative for either form of the null hypothesis is given as H_1: H_0 is false.

It can be shown that g has a sampling distribution that is approximately normal, with a mean of zero when the hypothesis of equal odds is true, and with squared standard error given as

$$SE^2(g) = 1/f_{rc} + 1/f_{rc'} + 1/f_{r'c} + 1/f_{r'c'}$$

For T_1 (treatment one) and T_3 (treatment three) at length of stay levels L_1: (2 or 3 days) and L_3: (6 or more days), the odds ratio is equal to

$$\hat{\theta} = 18(7)/26(50) = 0.0969$$

so that

$$g = \log_e \theta = -2.3338$$

The squared standard error for this contrast is given as

$$SE^2(g) = 1/18 + 1/7 + 1/26 + 1/50$$
$$= 0.2569 = (0.5069)^2$$

so that in terms of standard normal curve theory

$$Z = g/SE(g) = -2.3338/0.5069 = -4.60$$

As this number is in the $\alpha = 0.05$ two-tailed normal curve rejection region defined by $Z < -1.96$ and $Z > 1.96$, the null hypothesis of equal population odds is rejected. Treatment three is preferred to treatment one.

For this discussion, focus was placed on the contingency table defined by the frequencies f_{11}, f_{13}, f_{31}, and f_{33}. Other two by two contingency tables can be defined from the frequency data of Table 13–1. In fact, there are nine such tables (Table 13–4). As indicated, the four significant tables all involve T_3: (treatment three) and the patients whose length of stay following surgery was L_1: (2 or 3 days). This suggests that treatment three is the superior treatment. This finding agrees with that found using the method of looking at the contributions to chi-square illustrated in Section 13–2.

At this point in the discussion, type I error control has not been examined. It is informative to discuss in detail the exact hypothesis tested by the Karl Pearson statistic and the G^2 statistic. The null hypothesis tested by the Karl Pearson or the Likelihood Ratio test statistic is exceedingly complex. Goodman (1964) investigated the null hypothesis tested by these statistics. Goodman demonstrated that the alternative hypothesis is similar to that tested by the F test of the analysis of variance. In particular, the null and alternative hypotheses tested by the X^2 and G^2 statistics can be stated thus:

H_0: All contrasts or odds ratios in the logarithms of the frequency counts are equal to zero.

H_1: At least one contrast or odds ratio in the logarithms of the frequency counts exists that is not equal to zero.

TABLE 13–4 ALL POSSIBLE TWO BY TWO CONTINGENCY TABLES AND SAMPLE STATISTICS DERIVABLE FROM TABLE 13–1

	Treatment Group			$\hat{\theta}$	g	SE(g)	Z	Decision
	One	Two	Three					
L_1:	18	21						
L_2:	38	39		0.8797	−0.1282	0.3939	−0.33	NS
L_3:								
L_1:	18	21						
L_2:				0.7253	−0.3212	0.4325	−0.74	NS
L_3:	26	22						
L_1:								
L_2:	38	39		0.8245	−0.1930	0.3007	−0.64	NS
L_3:	26	22						
L_1:	18		50					
L_2:	38		25	0.2368	−1.4404	0.3767	−3.82	Sig.
L_3:								
L_1:	18		50					
L_2:				0.0969	−2.3338	0.5068	−4.60	Sig.
L_3:	26		7					
L_1:								
L_2:	38		25	0.4092	−0.8935	0.4976	−1.80	NS
L_3:	26		7					
L_1:		21	50					
L_2:		39	25	0.2692	−1.3122	0.3650	−3.59	Sig.
L_3:								
L_1:		21	50					
L_2:				0.1336	−2.0126	0.5059	−3.98	Sig.
L_3:		22	7					
L_1:								
L_2:		39	25	0.4964	−0.7004	0.5039	−1.39	NS
L_3:		22	7					

Result is significant at $\alpha = .05$, if $Z < -3.08$ or if $Z > +3.08$

Goodman also showed that each post hoc contrast can be tested for statistical significance in terms of the statistic,

$$Z = \hat{\psi} / SE(\hat{\psi})$$

and that the critical values for evaluating each contrast are given as

$$Z = -S \text{ and } Z = +S, \text{ where } S = \sqrt{\chi^2_{\nu:1-\alpha}}$$

The hypothesis tested H_0: *All* odds ratios are equal to zero. If this hypothesis is true, then the type of treatment has no relationship to the categories that define the dependent variable. After the omnibus test is performed, the researcher must decide on the reasons for the rejection. The best way to do this is to examine all the simple two by two odds ratios for statistical significance using S for the decision rule. If any ratios are found to be statistically different from zero, the researcher can stop and relate the significant findings to the research questions. If none of the two by two odds ratios is different from zero, post hoc data analysis becomes complicated. The null hypothesis that all odds ratios are zero includes odds ratios based on tables with two or more rows or columns. Thus, if no two by two odds ratios are significant, a researcher must make an analysis of the more complicated odds ratios by making a search among those defined by collapsing two rows or two columns. If none of these is significant, it may be necessary to examine more complicated odds ratios defined by collapsing three or more columns. In any case, the critical value necessary for this extensive post hoc investigation is not given as $Z = -1.96$ and $Z = +1.96$ but by Z values defined by the square root of the critical value required for the omnibus test. With $S = \sqrt{9.49} = 3.08$, four of the 2×2 tables are seen to be significant. The formula for determining the critical value was derived by Goodman (1964).

Other two by two contingency tables can be constructed by pooling two rows or columns. These other tables could be of interest to a researcher provided that the omnibus test of no interaction between the two variables is rejected. In this case, the omnibus null hypothesis of no interaction has been rejected. Thus, interest in other combined tables might be of theoretical or practical importance to the researcher. One such table is shown in Table 13–5. This table involves T_1: (treatment one) and T_2: (treatment two) and L_1: (2 or 3 days) with L_2 and L_3 combined to define the category L_{23}: (4 or more days). The associated odds ratio can be examined in terms of a linear contrast.

For this model, let f_{rc} equal the observed frequency for treatment c and length of stay level r. The generic form of a linear contrast is given as

$$\hat{\psi} = \sum_{r=1}^{R} \sum_{c=1}^{C} W_{rc} \log_e f_{rc}$$

where

$$\sum_{r=1}^{R} \sum_{c=1}^{C} W_{rc} = 0$$

The weights in each row and in each column sum to zero. The squared standard error for a contrast of this form is given as

$$SE(\hat{\psi})^2 = \sum_{r=1}^{R} \sum_{c=1}^{C} \frac{W_{rc}^2}{f_{rc}}$$

With large samples it can be shown that the sampling distribution of

$$Z = \hat{\psi}/SE(\hat{\psi})$$

is normal with a mean of zero and standard deviation of 1 if the hypothesis $H_0: \psi = 0$ is true.

Under this formulation of H_0 and H_1, all g $= \log_e \theta$ represent linear contrasts and can therefore be examined for statistical significance using this post hoc decision rule. Goodman (1964) showed that when the evaluation of a complex contrast is being made, the frequencies in the pooled cells are not summed. Each frequency is used separately when estimating the values of a contrast and when estimating the values of the squared standard errors.

The odds ratio associated with Table 13–5 is defined by the following sets of weights:

$$W_{11} = 1, W_{12} = -1, W_{21} = W_{31} = -\tfrac{1}{2}$$

and

$$W_{23} = W_{33} = -\tfrac{1}{2}$$

These weights are reported in Table 13–5. Note that the sum of the weights in each column is zero and that the sum of the weights in each row is also zero. Unless this condition is satisfied, the resulting linear combination of the logarithms of the frequencies is not a contrast. The g statistic for Table 13–5 is given as

$$\begin{aligned} g = {}& (1)\log_e 18 + (-1)\log_e 21 \\ &+ (-1/2)[\log_e 38 + \log_e 26] \\ &+ (1/2)[\log_e 39 + \log_e 22] \\ ={}& -0.2246 \end{aligned}$$

with squared standard error given as

$$\begin{aligned} SE^2(g) = {}& (1)^2/18 + (-1)^2/21 \\ &+ (-1/2)^2[1/38 + 1/26] \\ &+ (1/2)^2[1/39 + 1/22] \\ ={}& 0.1371 = (0.3703)^2 \end{aligned}$$

TABLE 13–5 A HIGHER ORDER TWO-DIMENSIONAL CONTINGENCY TABLE FORMED BY COMBINING ROWS L_2 AND L_3 OF TABLE 13–1

Length of Stay	Frequencies		Contrast Weights	
	Treatment One	Treatment Two	Treatment One	Treatment Two
L_1	18	21	1	−1
L_2 and L_3	38, 26	39, 22	−1/2, −1/2	1/2, 1/2

with

$$Z = -0.2246/0.3703 = -0.61$$

The critical values for evaluating this post hoc contrast are given as the Scheffé coefficients,

$$S = -\sqrt{9.49} = -3.08$$

and

$$S = +\sqrt{9.49} = 3.08$$

As indicated, the treatment differences are not significant for the comparison of T_1: (treatment one) to T_2: (treatment two) when the length of stay categories of L_2: (4 or 5 days) are combined with L_3: (6 or more days) and contrasted with the single category of L_1: (2 or 3 days). The null hypothesis associated with this post hoc defined contrast is not rejected.

This example shows that every cell frequency of the contingency table of interest enters into the computation of any contrast and associated standard error. This is true even for tables with three or more dimensions. Other rows or columns can be combined or collapsed and tested for statistical significance in a similar fashion.

13–5 LOGLINEAR ANALYSIS FOR A TWO BY THREE BY THREE CONTINGENCY TABLE

Consider the data of Table 13–6 which is an expanded version of Table 13–1 in that the 246 subjects are identified on the basis of their sex. It is with multidimensional contingency tables such as this that the loglinear model demonstrates its strength and usefulness. As indicated, 100 subjects are male and 146 are female. These subtables are referred to as *conditional* or *partial association tables* for gender, whereas Table 13–1 is often called the *unconditional* or *marginal association table*. Each set of subjects defines a three by three contingency table similar to that of Table 13–1. Each table could be analyzed separately to produce two sets of conditional decisions concerning treatment and length of stay following surgery. The disadvantage encountered in making such an analysis is that the impact of gender on treatment and length of stay would not be assessed directly. Their joint effect is meas-

ured in terms of a three-factor interaction involving the independent variables, gender and treatment, and the dependent variable, length of stay. The results of this type of analysis are summarized in Table 13–7. This table is typically included in a report or journal article. The similarity of this table to the source tables of the ANOVA makes it easy to read and interpret. As indicated, the important sources of variation are gender, length of stay following surgery, and the interaction of treatment with length of stay.

The first source of variance listed is that for treatment. This test is used to assess the following null hypothesis.

H_0: The distribution of patients to the three treatments is equal to the common value of 1/3.

If there were T treatments, the common value would be given by $P = 1/T$. As indicated,

$$G^2(T) = 0.00$$

Because three groups of patients are associated with this independent variable, the number of degrees of freedom for the test are given as $\nu = (T - 1) = (3 - 1) = 2$. The $\alpha = 0.05$ decision rule for rejecting the associated hypothesis is given as

Decision rule for treatment: Reject the hypothesis if the test statistic is larger than $\chi^2_{2:0.95} = 5.99$.

In this case the hypothesis is not rejected.

The nonrejection of this hypothesis should come as no surprise. By design, each treatment contains exactly 82 patients. The hypothesis tested by $G^2(T)$ is that the distribution of patients to the three treatments is *homogeneous* or that the proportion of cases distributed to the three treatments all are equal to 1/3. In this case, this hypothesis is true because it was decided to place 1/3 of the patients in each treatment group. Thus, the test of this hypothesis is not meaningful. Unfortunately, it appears in the Loglinear Analysis of Chi-Square Source Table generated by the computer program developed for the analysis. The program used is not able to distinguish independent variables from dependent variables. In practice, the test of this hypothesis should not be reported in a source table in reference to published research studies. (More on this test appears in Section 13–7.)

TABLE 13-6 TWO BY THREE BY THREE CONTINGENCY TABLE OF TREATMENT BY GENDER BY LENGTH OF STAY FOLLOWING SURGERY

Males

Length of Stay	Treatment One	Treatment Two	Treatment Three	Total
L_1:2 and 3 days	5	8	24	37
L_2:4 and 5 days	13	20	11	44
L_3:6 or more days	12	7	0	19
Total	30	35	35	100

Females

Length of Stay	Treatment One	Treatment Two	Treatment Three	Total
L_1:2 and 3 days	13	13	26	52
L_2:4 and 5 days	25	19	14	58
L_3:6 or more days	14	13	7	36
Total	52	47	47	146

The second listed source of variance is gender. This test is used to assess the following null hypothesis.

H_0: The distribution of male and female patients is equal to the common value of 1/2.

As indicated, $G^2(G) = 8.34$. The degrees of freedom for this test are given as $\nu = (G - 1) = (2 - 1) = 1$. The $\alpha = 0.05$ decision rule for rejecting the associated hypothesis is given as

Decision rule for gender: Reject the hypothesis if the test statistic is larger than $\chi^2_{1:0.95} = 3.84$.

In this case the hypothesis is rejected. The study contains more females than males.

The hypothesis tested by $G^2(G)$ is that the distribution of the two sexes is the same in the study or that the proportion of males is

equal to the proportion of females, and both are equal to 1/2. In most studies, testing this hypothesis is not very useful, and for this reason, this test is almost always ignored. What was said about the test of equal distribution of subjects to treatment applies equally well to the test of equal distribution of gender. (This is considered in Section 13-7.)

The third source of variance listed is the dependent variable, length of stay following surgery. This test is used to assess the following null hypothesis:

H_0: The distribution of patients to the three levels of length of stay is equal to the common value of 1/3

If there were L levels, the common value would be given as $P = 1/L$. In this case, rejection of this hypothesis is expected because most patients should leave within 4 or

TABLE 13-7 THE LOGLINEAR ANALYSIS OF CHI-SQUARE FOR THE DATA OF TABLE 13-6

Source of Variation	Degrees of Freedom	Test of Partial Association	Test of Marginal Association
Treatment	2	0.00	
Gender	1	8.34*	
Length of stay	2	14.60*	
T × G	2	0.65	0.82
T × L	4	34.49*	34.65*
G × L	2	0.88	1.04
T × G × L	4	9.13	

*$\chi^2_{1:.95} = 3.84$; $\chi^2_{2:.95} = 5.99$; $\chi^2_{4:.95} = 9.49$

5 days. Few should remain for more than 6 days. As indicated, $G^2(L) = 14.60$. The degrees of freedom for this test are given as $v = (L - 1) = (3 - 1) = 2$. The $\alpha = 0.05$ decision rule for the associated hypothesis is

Decision rule for length of stay: Reject the hypothesis if the test statistic is larger than $\chi^2_{2;0.95} = 5.99$

The hypothesis is rejected.

It is known that the distribution of patients to the categories L_1: (2 or 3 days), L_2: (4 or 5 days), and L_3: (6 or more days) are not all equal to one third. The sample statistics determined from the marginal frequencies of Table 13–1 are given as

$$\hat{P}_{1.} = 89/246 = 0.36$$
$$\hat{P}_{2.} = 102/246 = 0.41$$
$$\hat{P}_{3.} = 55/246 = 0.23$$

Thus, most patients remain in the hospital for 4 or 5 days following surgery. Fewer than one third stay for 6 or more days.

The fourth source of variance is represented by the interaction of treatment with gender. For the same reason that the test of treatment and the test of gender are meaningless, the test of this interaction hypothesis also is not helpful. For this source of variance,

$$G^2 \, (T \times G) = 0.65.$$

The degrees of freedom for this test are equal to

$$v = (T - 1) (G - 1) = (3 - 1) (2 - 1) = 2.$$

The $\alpha = 0.05$ decision rule is given as

Decision rule for the T × G interaction: Reject the hypothesis if the test statistic is larger than $\chi^2_{2;0.95} = 5.99$.

The hypothesis is not rejected.

The hypothesis under test with this statistic is that the distribution of men and women to the three treatments is identical. The proportions of males in the three different treatments are given as

$$\hat{P}_1 = 30/(30 + 52) = 0.37$$
$$\hat{P}_2 = 35/(35 + 47) = 0.42$$
$$\hat{P}_3 = 35/(35 + 47) = 0.42$$

The marginal proportion of males is given as

$$\hat{P} = 100/(100 + 146) = 0.41$$

None of the three treatment proportions is significantly different from the marginal value of 0.41. It is known that the study is not biased by having too many males or females assigned to any one of the three treatments. Although this test of hypothesis sheds little light on the effectiveness of the three treatments, it is at least known that the sexes are fairly represented across the three treatments. From a sampling point of view, the nonrejection of this hypothesis suggests that the systematic sampling scheme used in assigning subjects to the three treatments was successful.

The fifth source of variance is associated with the treatment by length of stay interaction. This is one of the major hypotheses of the preoperative teaching study. It is used to test the hypothesis that the distributions of the length of stay across the three treatments are homogeneous. Thus, it is identical with the test illustrated in Section 13–2 for the Karl Pearson chi-square test of homogeneity and in Section 13–3 for the Likelihood Ratio chi-square test. In this case, the null hypothesis can be stated as

H_0: The distributions of length of stay are identical for the three treatments.

This hypothesis should be rejected. For this test,

$$G^2(T \times L) = 34.49$$

The degrees of freedom for the test are given as

$$v = (T - 1) (L - 1) = (3 - 1) (3 - 1) = 4$$

and the $\alpha = 0.05$ decision rule is given as

Decision rule for the T × L interaction: Reject the hypothesis if the test statistic is larger than $\chi^2_{4;0.95} = 9.49$.

The hypothesis is rejected.

Note that this agrees with the decisions made in Sections 13–2 and 13–3 where the frequencies were collapsed across gender and where $X^2 = 35.59$ and $G^2 = 36.19$. The tests of those sections are referred to as *unconditional* or *marginal association tests*, whereas the test of this section is referred to as *conditional* or *partial association tests* (Bishop, Fienberg, and Holland, 1975). A comparison of these tests is presented in Section 13–6. The test for the two sets of tests are different because under the loglinear model, different algorithms are used for contingency tables of 2, 3, 4, . . . , dimensions. Because the null hypothesis is rejected, it is known that the distributions for length of stay following surgery are not the same for the three treatments. A post hoc investigation of the significant sources of variance is now in order. The procedure is illustrated in Section 13–8.

The sixth source of variance is associated with the gender by length of stay interaction. In this case, the null hypothesis under test can be written as

H_0: The distributions of length of stay are identical for men and women.

The value of the test statistic is given as

$$G^2(G \times L) = 0.88$$

The degrees of freedom for the test of homogeneity of the distribution of length of stay across the two sexes is given as

$$\nu = (S - 1)(L - 1) = (2 - 1)(3 - 1) = 2$$

The $\alpha = 0.05$ decision rule is given as

Decision rule for the gender by length of stay interaction: Reject the hypothesis if the test statistic is larger than $\chi^2_{2,0.95} = 5.99$.

The hypothesis of identical distribution of length of stay following surgery for males and females is retained. The proportions reported earlier for the main effect hypothesis for gender can be applied to both males and females.

The seventh and last source of variance is associated with the three-factor interaction. The null hypothesis can be stated as

H_0: The distributions of length of stay to the six cells defined by the treatment and gender interaction are homogeneous or identical.

For this hypothesis,

$$G^2(T \times S \times L) = 9.13$$

The degrees of freedom for this test are given as

$$\begin{aligned} \nu &= (T - 1)(G - 1)(L - 1) \\ &= (3 - 1)(2 - 1)(3 - 1) = 4 \end{aligned}$$

The $\alpha = 0.05$ decision rule is given as

Decision rule for the treatment by gender by length of stay interaction: Reject the hypothesis if the test statistic is larger than $\chi^2_{4,0.95} = 9.49$.

The null hypothesis is not rejected even though the value of the test statistic is very close to the critical value.

The hypothesis tested in the three-factor case, $T \times G \times L$, is complex. One way to view the hypothesis is in terms of the odds ratios defined in Section 13–4. If one considers each odds ratio that could be generated in the sample of males and the corresponding odds ratio in the sample of females, the hypothesis under tests states that corresponding odds ratios are equal. If they are not equal, it is concluded that the treatments have a different impact on the two sexes regarding the length of stay remaining in hospital following surgery. Another way to view the three-factor interaction is to consider the males and females assigned to treatment one and the distributions of length of stay following surgery. There is no interaction if the distributions by gender and length of stay are the same for the three different treatments. If such an interaction were to be identified as significant, a post hoc analysis would be in order to help identify reasons for the rejection of the hypothesis. These procedures are described in Section 13–8. (For further discussion on the loglinear model, see Agresti, 1984; Everitt, 1977; Fienberg, 1980; Knoke and Burk, 1980; Marascuilo and Busk, 1987. For an example of a five-dimensional loglinear analysis in nursing research, see Ihlenfeld, 1988.)

13–6 TESTS OF PARTIAL AND MARGINAL ASSOCIATION

The tests described in Section 13–5 are referred to as *partial tests of association*. The partial association test for the data of Table 13–6 and for treatment by length of stay is based on estimating the expected values in the contingency tables for the men and women separately. The test is similar to the F test used in multiple regression analysis to test the hypothesis that partial correlation coefficients are equal to zero. It is based on the assumption that the association pattern observed in the males for treatment and length of stay is identical with the association pattern observed in the females. If this condition were not satisfied, summing the data to produce a marginal table would not be justified. When the frequencies in the two tables are summed and tested for statistical significance, a second test, can be used which is referred to as a *marginal test of association.*

Both tests are necessary for analyzing higher order contingency tables. Both are required because of the meaning of *independence* for three or more variables. Whenever three variables are analyzed, all two-factor interaction tests are confounded by the possible appearance of a three-factor interaction. To protect the researcher against this possibility, the marginal tests are always performed. If the two tests lead to the same decision, no problem exists. If, however, the two tests lead to different conclusions, the researcher would have to use judgments about the variables and draw upon the research literature to come to final decisions. This does not happen often because the tests usually agree in the decisions they produce. A conservative rule of thumb is to retain the null hypothesis when the two tests disagree.

There are conditions in which the problem does not exist. As pointed out by Agresti (1984), the problem does not occur if either one of the two interacting variables has at least one nonsignificant conditional test with the remaining variables. For example, if T × G or L × G is not significant, then the tables for the males and females can be collapsed to produce a marginal table and a uniform conclusion.

13-7 THE PROBLEM OF CLASSIFYING INDEPENDENT AND DEPENDENT VARIABLES IN MULTIDIMENSIONAL CONTINGENCY TABLE ANALYSIS

Loglinear models can be encountered in a number of different contexts. For example, consider the three variable cases. For three variables, it is possible that

1. all three are interrelated dependent variables,
2. two are interrelated dependent variables and one is an independent variable or domain of study, or

3. only one is a dependent variable and the remaining two are independent variables.

The frequencies of Table 13-6 provide an example of the latter case. Treatment and gender are independent variables and length of stay is a dependent measure. The loglinear source tables for the three conditions are different from one another. Unfortunately, most computer programs are not written to make the distinction among the three different models. The distinction must be made by the individual researcher.

The computer analysis of Table 13-7 is based on the assumption that *one* sample has been classified according to treatment, gender, and length of stay. In this case, *three* separate samples of size 82 were set up for each treatment group. The correct way to view the study is as a fully crossed two-factor design with independent variables, treatment and gender, and dependent variable, length of stay. Under this model, the three main effect hypotheses are of little interest. The analysis would be as reported in Table 13-8. Here, the treatment by length of stay interaction is viewed as a main effect for treatment, the two-factor interaction of gender and length of stay is viewed as a main effect of gender, and the three-factor interaction is viewed as an interaction of treatment by gender. This is more in line with the classic ANOVA model for a quantitative dependent variable.

13-8 CONTRASTS FOR THREE-DIMENSIONAL CONTINGENCY TABLES

The contrast procedure illustrated for a two-dimensional contingency table applies to three-dimensional and higher order contingency tables directly. For this model, let f_{rcl} equal the observed frequency for

L: (length of stay) at level $\underline{r}$,
T: (treatment) at level $\underline{c}$,
G: (gender) at level $\underline{l}$.

The generic form of a linear contrast is given as

$$\hat{\psi} = \sum_{r=1}^{R} \sum_{c=1}^{C} \sum_{l=1}^{L} W_{rcl} \log_e f_{rcl}$$

TABLE 13–8 LOGLINEAR ANALYSIS FOR LENGTH OF STAY FOLLOWED BY SURGERY ACCORDING TO TREATMENT AND GENDER

Source of Variation	Degrees of Freedom	Test of Partial Association	Test of Marginal Association
Treatment	4	34.49*	34.65*
Gender	2	0.88	1.04
T × G	4	9.13	

*Significant at $\alpha = .05$

where

$$\sum_{r=1}^{R} \sum_{c=1}^{C} \sum_{l=1}^{L} W_{rcl} = 0$$

The weights sum to zero by row, column, and level. The squared standard error for contrast of this form is given as

$$SE(\hat{\psi})^2 = \sum_{r=1}^{R} \sum_{c=1}^{C} \sum_{l=1}^{L} \frac{W_{rcl}^2}{f_{rcl}}.$$

With large samples Goodman (1970) has shown that the sampling distribution of

$$Z = \hat{\psi} / SE(\hat{\psi})$$

is normal with a mean of zero and standard deviation of 1 if the hypothesis

$$H_0: \psi = 0$$

is true. For a post hoc analysis the critical values have been shown by Goodman (1970) to be given as

$Z = -S$ and $Z = +S$, where $S = \sqrt{\chi_{\nu:1-\alpha}^2}$

Let us reexamine the odds ratio defined by T_1: (treatment one) and T_3: (treatment three) and length of stay categories L_1: (2 and 3 days) and L_3: (6 or more days). In Section 13–4, the *marginal* odds ratio was examined by summing the frequencies for males and females. Here the corresponding *partial* odds ratio is examined. The frequencies that define the partial odds ratio are reported in Table 13–9. For the partial odds ratio, the frequencies of $f_{111} = 5$ and $f_{112} = 13$ are not collapsed as they were for the analysis of the marginal table. Instead, the frequencies are treated separately as are all frequencies in Table 13–9.

Note that one of the frequencies in Table 13–9 is given as $f_{331} = 0$. Cell frequencies of zero are a problem because division by zero and the logarithm of zero is undefined. One rule that seems to provide reasonable results is to add 1/2 to all of the cells of the contingency table before beginning the analysis. Many computer programs routinely do this. This substitution is called the *delta method*. In this example, each frequency f_{rcl}

TABLE 13–9 PARTIAL ODDS FOR TREATMENTS ONE AND THREE AND L_1 AND L_3 FOR MALES AND FEMALES

	Frequencies		Contrast Weights	
	Males			
LENGTH OF STAY*	TREATMENT ONE	TREATMENT THREE	TREATMENT ONE	TREATMENT THREE
L_1	5	24	1/2	−1/2
L_3	12	0	−1/2	1/2
	Females			
LENGTH OF STAY*	TREATMENT ONE	TREATMENT THREE	TREATMENT ONE	TREATMENT THREE
L_1	13	26	1/2	−1/2
L_3	14	7	−1/2	1/2

$L_1 = $ 2 and 3 days
$L_3 = $ 6 or more days

$$g = 1/2[\log_e 5.5 + \log_e 13.5] - 1/2[\log_e 24.5 + \log_e 26.5] - 1/2[\log_e 12.5 + \log_e 14.5]$$
$$+ 1/2[\log_e 0.5 + \log_e 7.5] = -3.0233$$

---

is replaced by $f_{rcl} + 1/2$. With this correction for frequencies of zero, the contrast for the evaluation of this odds ratio is given in the equation at the top of this page.

The squared standard error for this contrast is given as

$$SE^2(g) = (1/2)^2[\ 1/5.5 + 1/13.5 + \ldots + 1/7.5]$$
$$= (0.6542) = (0.8088)^2$$

Finally,

$$Z = g/SE(g) = -3.0233/0.8088 = -3.73$$

For the marginal odds ratio based on the same frequencies, the corresponding value of Z was shown to be $Z = -4.60$. The critical values for determining whether the hypothesis should be rejected are

$$-S = \sqrt{\chi^2_{4:0.95}} = -\sqrt{9.49} = -3.08$$

and

$$S = \sqrt{\chi^2_{4:0.95}} = \sqrt{9.49} = 3.08$$

Thus, the post hoc hypothesis is rejected. This is not surprising because it already has been seen that the partial and marginal tests led to the same decision.

Even though the three-factor interaction was not significant, a demonstration on how to perform a post hoc analysis on the odds ratios for three factors is provided. Three-factor odds ratios are used to test the hypothesis that the two-factor odds ratios across a third factor are all equal to the same value. Consider the two sets of data of Table 13−9. These figures represent the two by two tables for males and females classified according to T_1: (treatment one) and T_3: (treatment three) and length of stay after operation of L_1: (2 and 3 days) and L_3: (6 or more days). Again, the problem of a zero frequency exists and so the 1/2 correction is made. The log of the odds ratios and associated squared standard error for the males are given as

$$g_M = \log_e 5.5 - \log_e 24.5 - \log_e 12.5 + \log_e 0.5$$
$$= -4.7128$$

and

$$SE^2(g_M) = 1/5.5 + 1/24.5 + 1/12.5 + 1/0.5$$
$$= 2.3026$$

The corresponding statistics for the females are given as

$$g_F = \log_e 13.5 - \log_e 26.5 - \log_e 14.5 + \log_e 7.5$$
$$= -1.3337$$

and

$$SE^2(g_F) = 1/13.5 + 1/26.5 + 1/14.5 + 1/7.5$$
$$= 0.3141$$

These statistics are compared to determine whether the treatment by length of stay interaction is the same for the two sexes. This hypothesis can be tested by the contrast,

$$g = g_M - g_F = -4.7128 - (-1.3337)$$
$$= -3.3791$$

with squared standard error given as

$$SE^2(g) = SE^2(g_M) + SE^2(g_F)$$
$$= (2.3026) + (0.3141) = 2.6167$$
$$= (1.6176)^2$$

With these statistics,

$$Z = g/SE(g) = -3.3791/1.6176 = -2.09$$

The critical values for determining whether the hypothesis should be rejected are given as

$$-S = -\sqrt{\chi^2_{4:0.95}} = -\sqrt{9.49} = -3.08$$

and

$$S = \sqrt{\chi^2_{4:0.95}} = \sqrt{9.49} = 3.08$$

The hypothesis that the two odds ratios are not different from each other is not rejected and the statistics for the marginal table can be applied to males and females, equally. Remaining three-factor odds ratios may be tested for statistical significance in the same manner.

Similar to the analysis of variance, contrasts of the loglinear model can be examined as planned comparisons. If this is done, the critical values and the risks of making type II errors are reduced. Critical values for a planned analysis can be found in Marascuilo and Serlin (1988) or by counting the number of contrasts to be examined in each family. Let the number be C. If the family error rate is controlled at α, examine each contrast with $\alpha_o = \alpha/C$.

13–9 TREATMENT OF ORDERED CATEGORIES

Both the Karl Pearson chi-square test and the G^2 statistics are unaffected by permuting rows or columns in a contingency table. Thus, the order on scaled categories is ignored and the power that could be gained by incorporating that information into the model is lost—at least as present here. Agresti (1984) provides methods for capturing that information. In addition, Marascuilo and Levin (1983) show how the linear contrast of ANOVA trend analysis can be used to test for monotonicity and trend interactions.

13–10 EFFECT OF SAMPLE SIZE ON CONTINGENCY TABLE ANALYSIS

Like all sample statistics, the Karl Pearson chi-square statistic and the likelihood ratio statistics all are influenced by sample sizes. Extremely large samples have the potential for producing statistically significant results that are without theoretical or empirical meaning.

Increasing the number of variables in a study is bound to decrease the sample sizes in each of the cells of the resulting contingency table. With a decrease in sample size comes a decrease in power and an inflation in the numerical values of the standard errors of the parameter estimates and contrasts. When this happens, one might want to ignore the type I error control available when using the post hoc critical values. Many researchers consider any contrast that is more than 2 standard errors from zero as

representing a real population characteristic. Such a strategy makes sense. With small cell sizes many effects do not reach significance with the large values required for the post hoc analysis.

The assumptions required to justify the use of the Karl Pearson chi-square test and the loglinear model are minimal. The basic assumption is that all observations are independent of one another. Thus, one would not want to include in any contingency table brothers, spouses, litter mates, or any other type of matched pairs. In addition, a large enough sample should be chosen so that no more than 80% of estimated frequencies are less than 5. This is the Cochran Rule (1954) which helps ensure that the analysis remains conservative with respect to type I errors.

Because large samples can produce a statistically significant finding, measures of association are of importance in evaluating the effects of independent variables. Unlike the Karl Pearson model, the loglinear model does not have a clearly defined measure to represent the strength of the association. Marascuilo and Levin (1983) have proposed that measures of association be based on the ratio of the observed G^2 statistic to the maximum value that it can obtain in the sample. According to this formulation, a measure of association for any source of variation is given as

$$v^{2}* = G^2 / 2N\log_e M$$

where M is the minimum of the number of levels of the variables that are associated with G^2.

13–11 SUMMARY

The problems associated with the analysis of multidimensional contingency tables using categorical data have been solved through the development of loglinear models and user friendly computer programs. In this chapter, loglinear models were illustrated in terms of frequency or enumeration data using the preoperative teaching study. Examples from the preoperative teaching study were employed to illustrate the analysis of two-dimensional contingency tables using the chi-square statistic and the likelihood ratio statistic. Furthermore, odds ratios and contrasts for two by two contingency tables were depicted and their analysis was demonstrated. Next, the loglinear analysis for a two by two by three contingency table was presented. The distinctions between marginal tests of association and partial tests of association were offered and illustrated. Finally, post hoc contrasts for three-dimensional tables were demonstrated.

REFERENCES

Agresti, A.: Analysis of Ordinal Categorical Data. New York, John Wiley & Sons, 1984.

Bishop, Y.M.M, Fienberg, S.E., and Holland, P.V.: Discrete Multivariate Analysis: Theory and Practice. Cambridge, MA, MIT, 1975.

Brown, M.B.: BMDP Statistical Software. Berkeley, CA, University of California Press, 1981.

Cochran, W.G.: Some methods for strengthening the common chi-square test, Biometrics, 10: 417–451, 1954.

Everitt, B.S.: The Analysis of Contingency Tables. London, Chapmann and Hall, 1977.

Fienberg, S.E.: The Analysis of Cross-Classified Data, ed. 2. Cambridge, MA, MIT, 1980.

Goodman, L.A.: Simultaneous confidence limits for cross-product ratios in contingency tables, J. Roy. Stat. Soc., Series B, 26: 86–102, 1964.

Goodman, L.A.: The multivariate analysis of qualitative data: interactions among multiple classifications, J. Am. Stat. Assoc., 65: 226–256, 1970.

Ihlenfeld, J.T.: Log-linear contingency table analysis: an illustration, Nurs. Res. 37: 252–254, 1988.

Knoke, D., and Burke, P.J.: Log-linear Models. Beverly Hills, CA, Sage Publications, 1980.

Marascuilo, L.A., and Busk, P.L.: Loglinear models: a way to study main effects and interactions for multi-dimensional contingency tables with categorical data, J. Counseling Psychol., 34: 443–455, 1987.

Marascuilo, L.A., and Levin, J.: Multivariate Statistics in the Social Sciences. Belmont, CA, Wadsworth, 1983.

Marascuilo, L.A., and Serlin, R.C.: Statistical Methods for the Social and Behavioral Sciences. New York, Freeman, 1988.

Nie, N.H., Hull, C.H., Jenkins, J.G. et al.: Statistical Package for the Social Sciences. New York, McGraw Hill, 1985.

SAS, Inc.: SAS User's Guide: Statistics (Version 5). Carry, NC, Author, 1985.

Chapter 14

SINGLE SUBJECT RESEARCH

14–1 HISTORY OF AND ISSUES ASSOCIATED WITH SINGLE SUBJECT RESEARCH

In this chapter statistical methods for single subject research are provided. In particular, statistical models that are valid for the simplest designs (AB and ABAB) are described and illustrated for a single subject and for studies making use of a small number of persons.

Single subject research has had a long history in the behavioral and health sciences. The research on stimulus-response behavior of dogs by Pavlov, on the psychological state of patients by Freud, on behavior modification techniques with pigeons by Skinner, and the intellectual development of children by Piaget are well-known examples based on single subject research methodologies. In these investigations, researchers made use of single subjects to test theories and hypotheses about specific human and animal behavior. Because only one subject is used in these kinds of investigation, these studies are referred to as single subject research studies. Because the behaviors investigated in single subject research are so easily observable and readily measured, single subject research methods provide an excellent alternative to the restrictions imposed by experiments, surveys, and other multiple subject investi-

gation techniques with more diffuse types of dependent measures.

The high cost of sampling many subjects may compel a researcher to use one or a few subjects for investigation. An interest in unusual instances of behavior or rarely encountered subjects may further restrict an investigator to single subject designs. Single subject research provides methodological approaches that permit intensive observation or investigation with only one or with a very small number of subjects. For these primary reasons, single subject research has received increasing attention in recent years by researchers.

In clinical work, single subject designs provide an alternative to unsystematic case studies, which are the traditional means of evaluating treatments applied in settings where only one or a few patients, children, residents, or families may be the focus of the particular intervention. Unfortunately, the analytical procedures commonly used by many researchers for examining single subject data or data that have been reduced to a single criterion variable for a group of associated subjects are very weak and, from a statistical point of view, are often invalid.

The statistical problems associated with single subject research have been documented in the collected works edited by Kratochwill (1978). The most serious problems

317

are best illustrated by describing the most commonly used single subject design, referred to as the *two-phase (ABAB) design*. In this design, an observer takes measurements on a variable of interest or records the frequency of occurrence of a specific act over a randomly selected period of time.

For example, a client may be observed in a counseling session in which one of the objectives of a treatment is to help the client control and lower a normally high diastolic blood pressure. During the *A* or *baseline* phase of the study, when *no treatment* is administered, blood pressure readings may be taken electronically every 10 minutes for a total of five separate readings over a single counseling period. The A phase may extend over the first two or three counseling periods or, in other kinds of studies, until a stability in behavior is observed. During the *B* or *intervention* phase, the intervention may be introduced at a specific counseling period or at a randomly selected one. The purpose of the intervention is to provide training, guidelines, and reinforcement designed to help control and lower the diastolic blood pressure of the client. An example of a set of readings on a single patient is provided in Table 14–1.

As indicated by the mean values of Table 14–1, the diastolic blood pressure is high during the A phases when no treatment or help is provided to the patient on behaviors designed to lower the blood pressure; but, during the B phases the blood pressure readings are much lower, suggesting that the treatment is having an impact on this patient. The problem facing the nurse researcher is that of deciding on the basis of these data, that is, whether the intervention has produced a true reduction in the diastolic blood pressure readings. The null hypothesis to be tested is that the diastolic blood pressure remains constant over the A and B phases; that is, the treatment has no effect.

The temptation to perform a repeated measures analysis of variance (Winer, 1971) on the data of Table 14–1 is difficult to avoid. Some researchers have made the error of testing the null hypothesis of equal mean values across the four phase periods. Unfortunately, as shown by Toothaker, Banz, Noble, and colleagues (1983), the ANOVA test is not valid. In most single subject studies deviations from the phase mean in a given session are not statistically independent. In addition, in many studies errors between sessions may not be independent. In most situations they are correlated. In many single subject research studies, the correlations between the errors on adjacent trials or days are high, often exceeding .50 in value. As the time lag between observations increases, the correlations often decline rather slowly in value. This decline in correlation can be

TABLE 14–1 FIVE DIASTOLIC BLOOD PRESSURE READINGS OF A PATIENT DURING EIGHT COUNSELING SESSIONS

Session	Phase	Blood Pressure Readings					Session Mean	Phase Mean
		1	*2*	*3*	*4*	*5*		
1	A_1	92	90	90	88	90	90.0	
2	A_1	97	90	89	90	86	90.4	90.2
3	B_1	93	90	82	79	82	85.2	
4	B_1	86	80	79	83	80	81.6	83.4
5	A_2	92	90	89	90	86	89.4	
6	A_2	90	90	85	84	85	86.8	88.1
7	B_2	87	80	78	76	78	79.8	
8	B_2	82	79	80	79	82	80.4	80.1

used advantageously by the single subject researcher when analyzing data collected in a sound design.

The existence of a troublesome correlation is shown in Figure 14–1, which is a graphical display of the errors at time t correlated with the errors at time (t + 1). The errors, $e_t = Y_t - \overline{Y}$ where $\overline{Y}$ is the phase mean, are reported in Table 14–2. For session 1 at phase A_1, the first tabled error is given as

$$e_1 = 92.0 - 90.2 = 1.8$$

whereas the last tabled error is given as

$$e_{40} = 82.0 - 80.1 = 1.9$$

The lag correlations for the data of Table 14–2 are given as $r_{12} = .07$, $r_{13} = -.32$, $r_{14} = -.23$, and $r_{15} = -.01$. Except for sessions 1 and 3 with $r_{13} = -.32$, the errors tend to be uncorrelated. For the procedures described in this chapter, this is a desirable outcome.

An undesirable outcome is one in which high correlations exist between the errors close in time. Another undesirable state is the associated problem of carry-over effects

between phases so that the initial trials in the first B phase are frequently similar to the last trials in the first A phase. This type of carry-over is often seen between the first B phase and the second A phase and then finally between the second A phase and the second B phase. It should also be noted that both lack of normality and inequality of variances are not uncommon. For these reasons, procedures based on classic normal distribution models should not be used.

A solution to help alleviate the problems caused by lack of independence and carry-over effects is the adoption of *randomization tests*. These tests have been recommended for analyzing data from single subject (N = 1) and other small sample (N > 1) behavior change experiments by Edgington (1980a, 1980b, 1980c, and 1987), Kratochwill and Levin (1980), and Levin, Marascuilo, and Hubert (1978). Detailed discussions of the validity of randomization tests have been presented by Edgington (1980c) and Levin and coworkers (1978). In summary, Edgington (1980c, p. 246) specified the following three rules for valid use of randomization

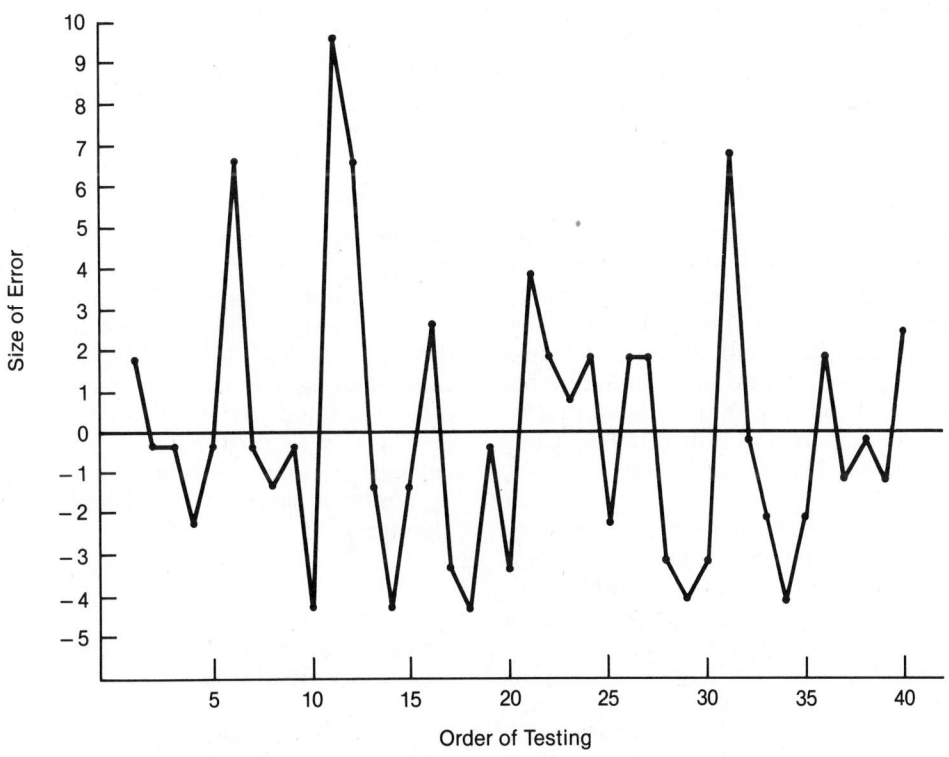

Figure 14–1. Time series representation of the errors of Table 14–2.

TABLE 14-2 ERRORS FOR THE DATA OF TABLE 14-1

Session	Error for Trial Number				
	1	*2*	*3*	*4*	*5*
1	1.8	−0.2	−0.2	−2.2	−0.2
2	6.8	−0.2	−1.2	−0.2	−4.2
3	9.6	6.6	−1.4	−4.4	−1.4
4	2.6	−3.4	−4.4	−0.4	−3.4
5	3.9	1.9	0.9	1.9	−2.1
6	1.9	1.9	−3.1	−4.1	−3.1
7	6.9	−0.1	−2.1	−4.1	−2.1
8	1.9	−1.1	−0.1	−1.1	1.9

tests. In most situations these steps can be easily followed:

1. There must be random assignment of treatment times to treatments.

2. The distribution of test statistic values must be based on data divisions that are appropriate for the type of random assignment used.

3. The test statistic value for a data division must be computed in the same way as it would be computed if that data division represented the obtained results.

Many researchers employing single subject designs still use only descriptive techniques to analyze data resulting from the application of designs described by Kratochwill and Brody (1978). Visual analysis of graphic presentations is the common procedure used to analyze *time-series data* resulting from single subject research. Several attempts have been made to describe how researchers should make visual inferences from the graphic presentations. Some authors concerned with this problem are Hersen and Barlow (1976), Kazdin (1982), and Kratochwill and Levin (1978). The guidelines are often ambiguous, and visual inference has been found to be an unreliable means of analysis. For arguments on this issue, see DeProspero and Cohen (1979), Gottman and Glass (1978), and Jones, Vaught, and Weinrott (1978).

Wampold and Furlong (1981) have examined the process of visual inference and empirically evaluated the subjects' ability to differentiate among graphs that demonstrate either a change in level, a change in trend, or a change in level and trend. A group of graduate students (n = 14), who were counselors-in-training and had completed a seminar in single subject research that emphasized visual inspection of data, along with a group of graduate students (n = 10), who had completed two of three quarter periods of study of a multivariate statistical course, sorted 4 graph sets of 36 graphs representing a two-phase (ABAB), single subject design. It was found that the counselor-in-training subjects, who were trained in visual inference, "appeared to use a scaling heuristic in which they attended to large changes between phases in a time series regardless of the relative variation" (p. 79). The counselor-in-training subjects ignored small intervention effects which the subjects who were trained in multivariate statistics were able to differentiate. "The subjects trained in multivariate statistics did not demonstrate this bias" (p. 79).

Gottman and Glass (1978) describe statistical procedures for single subject investigations. These methods, however, have not gained wide acceptance because they are difficult to apply and conclusions are even more difficult to interpret. As an attempt to provide easy to use and easy to understand methods, Levin, Marascuilo, and Hubert (1978) provided some randomization tests for the ABAB model, and Edgington (1980c) provided methods for an AB design with the random assignment to treatment. The methods described by Levin and colleagues (1978) and Edgington (1980c) are for one subject. These methods and their extensions to multiple samples are described in this chapter.

14-2 THE PHASE AS THE UNIT OF ANALYSIS

Single subject research rarely involves only one subject. Typically two, three, and sometimes even four subjects are in the study.

Methods for studying multiple subjects are the focus of this chapter. The methods are based on the use of the *phase periods* as the *units of analysis* and not the individual measurements made at each observation period. This adjustment is made to produce uncorrelated measures that may be used for the analysis. The justification for employing the phase as the unit of analysis had been provided by Levin and colleagues (1978).

Generally the observations within a phase are correlated so that each score cannot be used as an independent piece of datum. For this reason, the phase means are used for hypothesis testing. Even so, it should not be concluded that the phase means are necessarily statistically independent. Levin and colleagues (1978) have provided a table showing the values of the correlations between phase means if there were n observations per phase and if the correlation coefficient between adjacent observations were specified. The correlation coefficients between adjacent phase means are based on a model in which the lag correlations are given as

$$\rho_{ij} = \rho^{|i-j|}$$

The numbers in Table 14–3 are adapted from Table 3–1 of Levin and colleagues (1978). According to these figures, as long as the number of observations per phase is greater than 6 and as long as the correlation coefficient between adjacent observations does not exceed .40, the methods presented here should satisfy the assumptions of the statistical procedures. If the number of observations per phase equals 12 or less, the methods show promise provided that the correlation between adjacent trials does not exceed .60. With 18 observations per phase, correlations between adjacent trials can go as high as .70. If the phase means are based on 15 or more consecutive measurements,

large correlations should not invalidate the methods.

14–3 THE RANDOMIZATION TEST FOR AN ABAB DESIGN FOR ONE SUBJECT

The model for the randomization test is based on the use of the Fisher randomization test. Use of the randomization model has been recommended by Edgington (1980a) and illustrated for the ABAB design by Levin and colleagues (1978) for one and two subjects. In particular, the test described in this section provides an extension of the latter method to multiple subjects.

Consider the patient and data of Table 14–1. For convenience this patient is referred to as subject 1. To reduce the correlations between the mean values, the 10 observations of each phase are replaced by the mean diastolic blood pressure readings. The mean diastolic blood pressure for the four phases of subject 1 are given as 90.2, 83.4, 88.1, and 80.1, respectively. To generate the critical region to test the hypothesis that the mean values for phases A and B are equal, the four means, $(\overline{Y}_1, \overline{Y}_2, \overline{Y}_3, \overline{Y}_4)$, are randomly assigned to the phases by chance. The total number of possible assignments or combinations of these means to the A and B phases is given as the factorial expression,

$$\begin{aligned} m &= 4!/2!2! \\ &= (4 \times 3 \times 2 \times 1)/(2 \times 1)(2 \times 1) \\ &= 6 \end{aligned}$$

Let $\overline{Y}_1$ and $\overline{Y}_3$ be the values of the means in phases 1 and 3. The data for the two phases are pooled and summed using,

$$T_1 = \overline{Y}_1 + \overline{Y}_3$$

TABLE 14–3 LAG CORRELATIONS FOR PHASE SAMPLE SIZES FOR THE MODEL $\rho_{ij} = \rho^{|i-j|}$

Phase Sample Size	Value of the First Lag Correlation								
	0.10	0.20	0.30	0.40	0.50	0.60	0.70	0.80	0.90
6	0.02	0.04	0.06	0.09	0.14	0.20	0.30	0.44	0.67
12	0.01	0.02	0.03	0.04	0.06	0.09	0.14	0.25	0.47
18	0.01	0.01	0.02	0.03	0.04	0.06	0.09	0.16	0.34

The sum of the means for the A phase is reported in Table 14–4. The numbers in this table are used to define a rejection rule and critical region that is used to decide when the hypothesis

$$H_0: \mu_A = \mu_B$$

should be rejected in favor of the alternative hypothesis

$$H_1: \mu_A > \mu_B$$

The values of T_1 that are more in agreement with H_1 than they are with H_0 are used to define the rejection rule and the critical region.

The possible values for T_1 are given by the ordered values, 163.5, 168.1, 170.3, 171.5, 173.6, and 178.3. If the null hypothesis is true, each of these values has an equal probability of being observed. Thus, the probability of each value is

$$P = 1/m = 1/6 = 0.1667$$

The value of T_1 that is most in agreement with the alternative hypothesis is 178.3. Thus, it is seen that for a one-tailed test with $\alpha = 0.1667$, the decision rule is given as

Decision rule: Reject the hypothesis of no treatment effect if $T_1 = 178.3$.

In this case the actual value of T_1 is given as

$$T_1 = 90.2 + 88.1 = 178.3$$

The hypothesis is rejected at $\alpha = 0.1667$.

Because the risk of a type I error is greater than 0.05, very few researchers would be satisfied with this test. As can be seen, it is not possible to generate a test with a risk of a type I error less than or equal to .05 and so a one subject ABAB research scheme is not de-fensible. If, however, a study based on two subjects is performed, a test with a value close to 0.05 can be obtained.

Suppose a second subject is exposed to the same behavior modification treatment and suppose the four phase means for subject 2 are as follows: 98.2, 82.6, 84.0, and 78.8. The six random assignments of means to the A phase for this subject and the corresponding values of T_2 are shown in Table 14–5.

The results for these two subjects are combined into a single criterion, which is used to obtain a single probability distribution that can then be used to make a decision rule for assessing the effectiveness of the intervention. To generate a decision rule for two subjects, the information for the two subjects is summed to give a single index of treatment effect. For this,

$$T = T_1 + T_2$$

is determined. To obtain the probability distributions of T, the scheme illustrated in Table 14–6 can be used. The first row of Table 14–6 provides an ordered list of the six possible T_1 values. The first column is the ordered list of the six possible T_2 values. The complete set of T values is found by adding the marginal column values, T_1, with the intersecting marginal row values, T_2. For example, if

$$T_1 = 163.5 \text{ and } T_2 = 161.4$$

then

$$T = 163.5 + 161.4 = 324.9$$

The remaining values are found using the same rule. All values are reported in Table 14–6. From this tabulation, the decision rule for rejecting H_0 is obtained.

TABLE 14–4 DISTRIBUTION OF $T_1 = \bar{Y}_1 + \bar{Y}_3$ FOR SUBJECT 1

Possible Values		Value of	Probability
$\bar{Y}_1$	$\bar{Y}_3$	T_1	of T_1
90.2	83.4	173.6	0.1667
90.2	88.1	178.3*	0.1667
90.2	80.1	170.3	0.1667
83.4	88.1	171.5	0.1667
83.4	80.1	163.5	0.1667
88.1	80.1	168.2	0.1667

*Observed value of T_1

TABLE 14–5 DISTRIBUTION OF $T_1 = \bar{Y}_1 + \bar{Y}_3$ FOR SUBJECT 2

Possible Values		Value of	Probability
$\bar{Y}_1$	$\bar{Y}_3$	T_2	of T_2
98.2	82.6	180.8	0.1667
98.2	84.0	182.2*	0.1667
98.2	78.8	177.0	0.1667
82.6	84.0	166.6	0.1667
82.6	78.8	161.4	0.1667
84.0	78.8	162.8	0.1667

*Observed value of T_2

TABLE 14-6 DISTRIBUTION OF T = T₁ + T₂

Value of T₂	Value of T₁					
	163.5	*168.2*	*170.3*	*171.5*	*173.6*	*178.3**
161.4	324.9	329.6	331.7	332.9	335.0	339.7
162.8	326.3	331.0	333.1	334.3	336.4	341.1
166.6	330.1	334.8	336.9	338.1	340.2	344.9
177.0	340.5	345.2	347.3	348.5	350.6	355.3
180.8	344.3	349.0	351.1	352.3	354.4	359.1
182.2*	356.3	351.0	353.1	354.3	356.4	361.1*

*Observed values

For H_1: $\mu_A > \mu_B$, the one-tailed decision rule is given as

Decision rule: Reject the hypothesis if T = 361.1 or if T = 359.1.

The risk of a type I error for this rule is

$$\alpha = 2/36 = 0.0555$$

For the example, the observed value of T is given as

$$T = 178.3 + 182.8 = 361.1$$

Thus, the hypothesis is rejected for the one-tailed test of H_0: $\mu_A > \mu B$.

As mentioned earlier, single subject research is actually multiple sample research in which the sample sizes are truly small. Although the distributions for three or four subjects could be generated to give exact probabilities, such excessive labor is not necessary. Examination of the distribution for just two subjects shows that the probability distribution is symmetrical and in appearance roughly approximates the normal distribution. The distributions based on three or more subjects can be approximated adequately with the normal distribution. The procedure for 3 or more subjects proceeds as follows.

Let the four-phase mean values for subject i be denoted by $\overline{Y}_{i1}$, $\overline{Y}_{i2}$, $\overline{Y}_{i3}$, and $\overline{Y}_{i4}$, respectively. For this model, we have the following relationships for the i-th subject:

1. The observed value of the sum of the two-phase means for subject number i is given as

$$T_i = \overline{Y}_{i1} + \overline{Y}_{i3}$$

2. The expected value of the mean for subject i is given as

$$E(\overline{Y}_i) = [\overline{Y}_{i1} + \overline{Y}_{i2} + \overline{Y}_{i3} + \overline{Y}_{i4}]/4$$

3. The expected value for the sum of the two means for subject i is given as

$$E(T_i) = 2\, E(\overline{Y}_i) = 2\, \mu_i$$

4. The variance of the means for subject i is given as

$$Var(\overline{Y}_i) = \sum_{p=1}^{4} (\overline{Y}_{ip} - \mu_i)^2/4$$

5. The variance of the sum of the two means for subject i is given as

$$Var(T_i) = 4/3\, Var(\overline{Y}_i)$$

As an example of the use of this model, suppose that five subjects are tested and give rise to the figures reported in Table 14-7.

TABLE 14-7 SAMPLE STATISTICS FOR FIVE SUBJECTS OBSERVED IN AN ABAB DESIGN

Subject	Phase A₁	Phase B₁	Phase A₂	Phase B₂	T₁	E(Ȳ₁)	E(T₁)	Var(Ȳ₁)	Var(T₁)
1	90.2	83.4	88.1	80.1	178.3	85.450	170.90	15.6025	20.8033
2	98.2	82.6	84.0	78.8	182.2	85.900	171.80	54.0500	72.0667
3	99.2	76.3	80.7	77.9	179.9	83.525	167.05	84.3819	112.5092
4	95.3	88.3	90.2	82.3	185.5	89.025	178.05	21.6269	28.8358
5	97.6	90.2	89.3	84.7	186.9	90.450	180.90	21.3925	28.5233

The arithmetic for subject 1 is shown as follows:

1. $T_1 = 90.2 + 88.1 = 178.3$

2. $E(\overline{Y}_1) = [90.2 + 83.4 + 88.1 + 80.1]/4$
$= 85.45$

3. $E(T_1) = 2(85.45) = 170.90$

4. $Var(\overline{Y}_1) = [(90.2 - 85.45)^2 + \ldots + (80.1 - 85.45)^2]/4$
$= 15.6025$

5. $Var(T_1) = (4/3)(15.6025) = 20.8033$

The statistics for the remaining four subjects are found in a similar fashion (reported in Table 14–7). With these values, the summary measure for all five subjects is found by pooling the data. The pooling is done with

$$T = T_1 + T_2 + T_3 + T_4 + T_5$$

For this example,

$$T = 178.3 + 182.2 + 179.9 + 185.5$$
$$+ 186.9$$
$$= 912.8$$

The expected value of T is found by summing the separate expected values associated with each subject. In this case,

$$E(T) = E(T_1) + E(T_2) + E(T_3) + E(T_4)$$
$$+ E(T_5)$$

For the 5 subjects of this study,

$$E(T) = 170.90 + 171.80 + 167.05 + 178.05$$
$$+ 180.90$$
$$= 868.7$$

For five subjects, the variance of T is given as

$$Var(T) = Var(T_1) + Var(T_2) + Var(T_3)$$
$$+ Var(T_4) + Var(T_5)$$

For the example,

$$Var(T) = 20.8033 + 72.0667 + 112.5092$$
$$+ 28.8358 + 28.5233$$
$$= 262.7383$$

Using these values, the form of the test based on normal curve theory is as follows:

$$Z = [T - E(T)]/\sqrt{Var(T)}$$

For the example,

$$Z = [912.8 - 868.7]/\sqrt{262.7383}$$
$$= 2.72$$

The $\alpha = .05$ decision rule for this example is given by reading values from the last row of Table A–5.

Decision rule: Reject H_0 if $Z > + 1.645$.

The null hypothesis H_0: $\mu_A = \mu_B$ is rejected in favor of the alternative hypothesis H_1: $\mu_A > \mu_B$ because $Z > +1.645$, the $\alpha = .05$ value of the standard normal distribution. It is concluded that the mean values for the A phase are higher than the mean values for the B phase. In addition, it is concluded that the intervention has been successful in assisting patients in the control and lowering of their diastolic blood pressure.

A confidence interval for $\mu_D = \mu_A - \mu_B$ is available as

$$\mu_D = \overline{D} \pm Z_{\alpha/2}\sigma_{\overline{D}}$$

where

$$\overline{D} = \overline{Y}_A - \overline{Y}_B$$

with S equal to the number of subjects and P equal to the number of phases

$$\sigma_{\overline{D}}^2 = \frac{4}{S^2P^2} Var(T)$$

For this example,

1. $\overline{Y}_A = \dfrac{90.2 + 88.1 + \ldots + 89.3}{10} = 91.28$

2. $\overline{Y}_B = \dfrac{83.4 + 80.1 + \ldots + 84.7}{10} = 82.46$

3. $\overline{D} = 91.28 - 82.46 = 8.82$

and

4. $\sigma_{\overline{D}}^2 = \dfrac{4}{5^2 4^2} (262.7383) = 2.6274$

so that

$$\mu_{\overline{D}} = 8.82 \pm 1.96\sqrt{2.6274}$$
$$= 8.82 \pm 3.18$$

or

$$5.64 \leq \mu_{\overline{D}} \leq 12.00$$

Thus, the mean reduction in diastolic blood pressure can be as low as 5.64 mm of mercury or as high as 12.00 mm of mercury. Because a one-tailed alternative hypothesis was investigated, a justification for a one-tailed confidence interval is easy to obtain. In this case, the one-tailed confidence interval is given as

$$\mu \geq 8.82 - 1.645 \ \sqrt{2.6274} = 6.15$$

Thus, the intervention tends to lower the diastolic blood pressure by about 6 mm of mercury.

14−4 THE WILCOXON RANK TEST FOR MULTIPLE SINGLE SUBJECT DESIGNS

One of the disadvantages of using the original data for the analysis of multiple single subject designs as described in Section 14−3 is the lengthy arithmetic. This can be avoided by using the Wilcoxon model and ranks as described in Section 9−17. That application of the Wilcoxon statistic is described here.

If T_i is the Wilcoxon statistic for the i-th subject, it follows that for the five subjects of Table 14−7,

$$T_1 = 4 + 3 = 7,$$
$$T_2 = 3 + 4 = 7,$$
$$T_3 = 4 + 3 = 7,$$
$$T_4 = 4 + 3 = 7, \text{ and}$$
$$T_5 = 4 + 2 = 6,$$

so that

$$T = T_1 + T_2 + T_3 + T_4 + T_5$$
$$= 7 + 7 + 7 + 7 + 6 = 34$$

On the basis of T = 34, a decision must be made regarding whether H_0 should be rejected or retained.

If P represents the number of phases, with $N_1 = P/2$ at A and $N_2 = P/2$ at B and if S equals the number of subjects, then the formulas for the large sample form of the Wilcoxon statistic of Section 9−17 reduce to

$$E(T) = S\{P(P + 1)/4\}$$
$$Var(T) = S\{P^2(P + 1)/48\}$$

and

$$Z = [T \pm 1/2 - E(T)]/\sqrt{Var(T)}$$

If T < E(T), +1/2 is used and if T > E(T), −1/2 is used. For the example,

$$E(T) = 5\{(4)(4 + 1)/4\} = 25$$
$$Var(T) = 5\{(4^2)(4 + 1)/48\} = 8.3333$$

and

$$Z = [33.5 - 25]/\sqrt{8.3333} = 2.94$$

The hypothesis is rejected at $\alpha = .05$ because Z > 1.645. (For more discussion about this procedure, see Marascuilo and Busk, 1988.)

14−5 MONOTONIC TRENDS IN PHASE MEANS

One of the problems encountered in single subject research is the not uncommon carry-over effects from one phase to another in the ABAB design. For example, in the study described in Table 14−1, the phase means of the diastolic blood pressures might be expected to parallel the following pattern

$$A_1 > A_2 > B_1 > B_2$$

and thereby trace a *monotonically* decreasing trend. A monotonic trend is a continuous increase or decrease in the phase mean values. In this example, the expected direction of the trend is downward. When such an outcome is expected, a researcher can increase the statistical power of the tests of Sections 14−3 and 14−4 by using a test for monotonicity. The coefficients for evaluating monotonic trends are reported in Table A−10. When the number of phases is equal to four, the weights for a monotonic trend are given as

$$W_1 = 4, \ W_2 = 3, \ W_3 = 2, \text{ and } W_4 = 1$$

Under this model, $T = \overline{Y}_1 + \overline{Y}_3$ would be replaced by the criterion:

$$M = 4\overline{Y}_1 + 3\overline{Y}_2 + 2\overline{Y}_3 + 1\overline{Y}_4$$

If it were thought that the means would increase, then the coefficients are used in reverse order and the test criterion is given as

$$M = 1\overline{Y}_1 + 2\overline{Y}_2 + 3\overline{Y}_3 + 4\overline{Y}_4$$

With this criterion the randomization distribution of M is determined and the corresponding decision rule is specified. From this distribution a decision rule for rejecting the hypothesis can be defined as

$$H_0: \mu_{A_1} = \mu_{A_2} = \mu_{B_1} = \mu_{B_2}$$

against the alternative hypothesis,

$$H_1: \mu_{A_1} > \mu_{A_2} > \mu_{B_1} > \mu_{B_2}$$

For the model using the five subjects of the previous section, order was not considered important; it was necessary only to examine combinations of phase values to generate the distribution of T. For examining monotonicity, order is important. For P phases, the number of unique values of M is given by the factorial expression,

$$m = P! = P(P - 1)(P - 2) \ldots (4)(3)(2)(1)$$

In practice the complete distribution of M does not need to be determined; only the critical region is needed. For the data of Table 14–1, the value of

$$m = 4! = (4)(3)(2)(1) = 24$$

1. For one subject, the $\alpha = 0.05$ critical region consists of the $0.05(24) = 1.2$ the largest possible value of M. Because this must be an integer, the number is rounded to 1.

2. For two subjects, the total number of permutations is given as $m = 24(24) = 576$ so that the $\alpha = .05$ critical region consists of the $(.05)(576) = 28.8$ extreme values, which is rounded to the 28 most extreme values.

3. For three subjects, the $\alpha = .05$ critical region consists of the $0.05(24)^3 = 691.2$ most extreme values, which is rounded to the 691 most extreme outcomes.

As the number of subjects increases, the number of outcomes in the critical region increases in a geometric fashion. With such a large number of extreme outcomes, the determination of the exact critical regions be-

comes a formidable task. Fortunately, large sample normal curve theory can be used to approximate the exact critical region.

With m = 24 possible permutations, the α = 0.05 decision rule is given as the most extreme value. In this case the most extreme value is given as

$$M = 4(90.2) + 3(88.1) + 2(83.4) + 1(80.1) = 872.0$$

Thus, the decision rule for rejection of H_0 is

Decision rule: Reject H_0 if M = 872.0

Because the observed value of M = 872.0, the hypothesis of no monotonic trend is rejected. It is concluded that the means for the A phases are larger than the means for the B phases. In addition, it is concluded that the intervention designed to reduce and control diastolic blood pressure in the single subject of this study was successful.

For two or more subjects, normal curve theory can be used to approximate the exact critical region. That model is now illustrated for the five subjects of the previous section.

The expected value of M_i is

$$E(M_i) = [1 + 2 + 3 + 4]E(\overline{Y}_i) = 10\,E(\overline{Y}_i)$$

and the variance of M_i is

$$Var(M_i) = (20/3)Var(\overline{Y}_i)$$

The summary statistics for the five subjects of Table 14–7 are reported in Table 14–8. With these values, the pooled statistic across the five subjects is

$$M = M_1 + M_2 + M_3 + M_4 + M_5$$
$$= 872.0 + 888.8 + 869.4 + 910.7$$
$$+ 923.2$$
$$= 4464.1$$

TABLE 14–8 SAMPLE STATISTICS FOR FIVE SUBJECTS IN AN ABAB DESIGN USING THE MONOTONICITY MODEL

Subject	Phase A_1	Phase A_2	Phase B_1	Phase B_2	M_i	$E(\overline{Y}_i)$	$E(M_i)$	$Var(\overline{Y}_i)$	$Var(M_i)$
1	90.2	88.1	83.4	80.1	872.0	85.450	854.50	15.6025	104.0167
2	98.2	84.0	82.6	78.8	888.8	85.900	859.00	54.0500	360.3333
3	99.2	80.7	76.3	77.9	869.4	83.525	535.25	84.3819	562.5460
4	95.3	90.2	88.3	82.3	910.7	89.025	890.25	21.6269	144.1793
5	97.6	89.3	90.2	84.7	923.2	90.450	904.50	21.3925	142.6167

with

$$E(M) = E(M_1) + E(M_2 + E(M_3) + E(M_4)$$
$$+ E(M_5)$$
$$= 854.50 + 859.00 + 835.25 +$$
$$890.25 + 904.50$$
$$= 4343.5$$

and

$$Var(M) = Var(M_1) + Var(M_2) + Var(M_3)$$
$$+ Var(M_4) + Var(M_5)$$
$$= 104.0167 + 360.3333 + 562.5460$$
$$+ 144.1793 + 142.6167$$
$$= 1313.6920$$

Using these values, the large sample form of the test based on normal curve theory is as follows:

$$Z = [M - E(M)]/\sqrt{Var(M)}$$
$$= [4464.1 - 4343.5]/\sqrt{1313.6920}$$
$$= 3.33$$

The critical value read from the last row of Table A−5 for this test at $\alpha = .05$ is given by the upper end tail value of $Z = 1.645$. The null hypothesis is rejected at $\alpha = 0.05$. It is concluded that the mean values for the A phase are larger than the mean values for the B phase and that the intervention was effective in reducing and controlling the diastolic blood pressure of the five experimental subjects.

If ranks are used, then we have the following for subject 1:

$$M_1 = 4(4) + 3(3) + 2(2) + 1(1) = 30$$

with $M_2 = 30$, $M_3 = 29$, $M_4 = 30$, and $M_5 = 29$, so that

$$M = M_1 + M_2 + M_3 + M_4 + M_5$$
$$= 148$$

In this case,

$$E(M) = S[P(P + 1)^2/4]$$
$$Var(M) = S[P^2(P^2 - 1)(P + 1)/144]$$

and

$$Z = [(M \pm 1/2) - E(M)]/\sqrt{Var(M)}$$

If $M < E(M)$, $+1/2$ is used and if $M > E(M)$, $-1/2$ is used. For the example,

$$E(M) = 5[(4)(4 + 1)^2/4] = 125$$
$$Var(M) = 5[(4^2(4^2 - 1)(4 + 1)/144] = 41.6667$$

so that

$$Z = [147.5 - 125]/\sqrt{41.6667} = 3.48$$

H_0 is rejected.

14−6 INCREASING THE NUMBER OF PHASES TO OBTAIN GREATER STATISTICAL POWER

In addition to increasing the number of subjects to gain greater statistical power, another way to increase power is to increase the number of phases. For example, a single subject design for one subject using three sets of AB phases gives rise to m = 20 different values of

$$T = T_{i1} + T_{i3} + T_{i5}$$

for each subject so that for two subjects the critical region can be based on the 0.05 (20)(20) = 20 most extreme values. In addition, normal curve approximations are more than satisfactory for three or more independent subjects. For the test based on a monotonic trend among the means measured by

$$M = 1\overline{Y}_{i1} + 2\overline{Y}_{i3} + 3\overline{Y}_{i5} +$$
$$4\overline{Y}_{i2} + 5\overline{Y}_{i4} + 6Y_{i6}$$

the number of different permutations for one subject is given as m = 720 so that for two subjects, the number of possible outcomes is given as m = 720(720) = 518400. The normal approximation is excellent for this situation.

If the design is increased to P phases with P/2 at A and P/2 at B, the extended formulas are

$$T_i = \overline{Y}_{i1} + \overline{Y}_{i3} + \ldots + \overline{Y}_{i(P-1)}$$
$$E(\overline{Y}_i) = [\overline{Y}_{i1} + \overline{Y}_{i2} + \ldots + \overline{Y}_{iP}]/P = \mu_i$$
$$E(T_i) = (P/2) E(\overline{Y}_i) = (P/2) \mu_i$$
$$Var(\overline{Y}_i) = \sum_{i=1}^{P} (\overline{Y}_{iP} - \mu_i)^2/P$$

and

$$Var(T_i) = [(P/2)^2/(P - 1)] Var(\overline{Y}_i)$$

For S subjects,

$$T = T_1 + T_2 + \ldots + T_S$$

The null hypothesis is rejected if

$$Z = [T - E(T)]/\sqrt{Var(T)}$$

is in the rejection region defined under the standard normal distribution.

In the general case for P phases with P/2 at A and P/2 at B, the test statistic and its corresponding expected value and variance for the test of monotonicity are given as

$$M_1 = [1\overline{Y}_{i1} + 2\overline{Y}_{i3} + \ldots$$
$$+ (P/2)\overline{Y}_{i(P-1)}] + [(P/2 + 1)\overline{Y}_{i2}$$
$$+ (P/2 + 2)\overline{Y}_{i4} + \ldots + P\overline{Y}_{iP}]$$

$$E(M_i) = [P(P + 1)/2] E(\overline{Y}_i),$$

$$Var(M_i) = [P^2(P + 1)/12] Var(\overline{Y}_i)$$

For S subjects,

$$M = M_1 + M_2 + \ldots + M_S$$

The null hypothesis is rejected if

$$Z = [M - E(M)]/\sqrt{Var(M)}$$

is in the rejection region defined under the standard normal distribution.

14−7 THE AB DESIGN WITH A RANDOM STARTING POINT FOR THE B PHASE

In this section, the randomization model for the AB design described by Edgington (1987) is presented. As an example of this test's applicability, consider a study in which a patient in a mental health program was observed on 20 consecutive days and in which the dependent variable is the amount of restful sleep at night. Because the patient was exhibiting poor sleeping ability, it was decided to increase his physical activity during the day to see whether the extra activity would help increase nighttime sleep. For the treatment, the patient was placed in a daily activity program. The total exercise regimen was 2 hours a day. The daily sleep in quarter hours is shown in Table 14−9 for 20 observation periods.

Edgington (1987) described a simple AB model where the initiation of the B phase is selected at random. During the A phase, the single subject researcher collects data and when the series stabilizes, the B phase is introduced at a time selected at random. The

TABLE 14−9 NUMBER OF RESTFUL HOURS OF SLEEP FOR PATIENT ONE

Block	Phase	Hours
1	A	5.25
2	A	5.00
3	A	4.75
4	A	6.00
5	A	6.25
6	A	5.00
7	A	6.50
8	B	9.00
9	B	8.00
10	B	7.25
11	B	8.25
12	B	7.00
13	B	9.25
14	B	8.00
15	B	7.75
16	B	8.00
17	B	7.75
18	B	8.00
19	B	7.00
20	B	8.00

observation periods are called *blocks* and are denoted by A or B.

For the example, suppose it was decided that there should be 20 observation periods. Edgington (1987) recommends no less than 5 blocks for both A and B. For 20 observation periods, this latter constraint means that the B phase cannot begin before the 6th block and cannot appear for the first time after the 16th block. Thus, the introduction of the treatment must occur on block numbers 6, 7, . . . , or 16. The single subject researcher chooses one of these numbers by referring to Table A−11 of random numbers. Suppose that the number chosen is 8 and the results of the study are as reported in Table 14−9.

The criterion variable for the Edgington test is the difference in the mean values for the A and B phases. The problem is to decide when the difference is larger than could be expected on the basis of chance. To make this decision, the distribution in the differences in the means needs to be determined for all possible outcomes that could be generated by the randomization process used to initiate the intervention.

Table 14−10 is a list of the 11 possible mean values and differences in mean values that could have been generated for the A and B phases if the B phase was initiated at block numbers 6, 7, . . . , 16. Under the hypothesis that the treatment has no effect, all

TABLE 14–10 DISTRIBUTION OF $\overline{D} = \overline{Y}_B - \overline{Y}_A$ FOR THE EDGINGTON MODEL

Intervention Block	Mean of B	Mean of A	Difference
6	7.65	5.45	2.20
7	7.84	5.38	2.46
8*	7.94	5.54	2.40
9	7.85	5.97	1.88
10	7.84	6.19	1.65
11	7.90	6.30	1.60
12	7.86	6.48	1.38
13	7.97	6.52	1.45
14	7.79	6.73	1.06
15	7.75	6.82	0.97
16	7.75	6.88	0.87

*Intervention block

assignments are equally likely and the differences in the means each have a probability of 1/11. If the intervention had taken place in block number 6, the mean values would be the following numbers:

$$\overline{Y}_A = 1/5(5.25 + 5.00 + \ldots + 6.25)$$
$$= 5.45$$

and

$$\overline{Y}_B = 1/15(5.00 + 6.50 + \ldots + 8.00)$$
$$= 7.65$$

so that

$$\overline{D} = 7.65 - 5.45 = 2.20$$

The remaining values are found in a similar way by increasing the number of outcomes in the A phase by one and decreasing the number of outcomes in the B phase by one. The observed value of $\overline{D}$ is given as

$$\overline{D}_0 = 2.40$$

With a one-tailed test at $\alpha = 1/11 = 0.0909$, the hypothesis of equal mean values cannot be rejected because the critical region consists of the single extreme value $\overline{D} = 2.46$.

Even if the hypothesis is not rejected, the results suggest that the addition of more subjects should be promising. Thus, consider the addition of two more subjects to the design. Data for these subjects are reported in Table 14–11. The B phase is introduced at the randomly selected block 12 for subject 2 and at the randomly selected block 11 for subject 3. Summary statistics for these three subjects are shown in Table 14–12.

For these data,

$$T = \overline{D}_1 + \overline{D}_2 + \overline{D}_3$$
$$= 2.40 + 2.79 + 2.28$$
$$= 7.47$$

TABLE 14–11 NUMBER OF HOURS OF RESTFUL SLEEP FOR THREE PATIENTS

Block	Patient One Phase	Patient One Hours	Patient Two Phase	Patient Two Hours	Patient Three Phase	Patient Three Hours
1	A	5.25	A	6.25	A	5.25
2	A	5.00	A	6.00	A	5.00
3	A	4.75	A	4.00	A	3.00
4	A	6.00	A	6.25	A	4.75
5	A	6.25	A	7.00	A	8.00
6	A	5.00	A	6.00	A	6.00
7	A	6.50	A	5.00	A	7.50
8	B	9.00	A	5.25	A	5.00
9	B	8.00	A	4.00	A	3.50
10	B	7.25	A	4.00	A	4.50
11	B	8.25	A	6.00	B	7.00
12	B	7.00	B	7.00	B	6.00
13	B	9.25	B	8.00	B	7.50
14	B	8.00	B	9.00	B	5.00
15	B	7.75	B	8.25	B	8.00
16	B	8.00	B	8.00	B	8.25
17	B	7.75	B	7.50	B	7.50
18	B	8.00	B	9.00	B	8.50
19	B	7.00	B	8.75	B	9.00
20	B	8.00	B	8.50	B	8.50

TABLE 14–12 SUMMARY STATISTICS FOR THE THREE SUBJECTS OF TABLE 14–11

Possible Intervention Point	Subject One	Subject Two	Subject Three
6	2.20	1.05	1.58
7	2.46	1.10	1.51
8	2.40*	1.38	1.15
9	1.88	1.61	1.38
10	1.65	2.11	1.83
11	1.60	2.62	2.28*
12	1.38	2.79*	2.17
13	1.45	2.82	2.32
14	1.06	2.67	2.20
15	0.97	2.35	2.72
16	0.87	2.22	2.62
Mean value of $\overline{D}$	1.63	2.07	1.98
Variance of $\overline{D}$	0.2821	0.3953	0.2454

*Intervention point

$$E(T) = E(\overline{D}_1) + E(\overline{D}_2) + E(\overline{D}_3)$$
$$= 1.63 + 2.07 + 1.98$$
$$= 5.68$$

and

$$Var(T) = Var(\overline{D}_1) + Var(\overline{D}_2) + Var(\overline{D}_3)$$
$$= 0.2821 + 0.3953 + 0.2454$$
$$= 0.9228$$

Using these values, the large sample normal curve statistic is

$$Z = [T - E(T)]/\sqrt{Var(T)}$$
$$= [7.47 - 5.68]/\sqrt{0.9228}$$
$$= 1.86$$

The hypothesis that $\mu_A = \mu_B$ is rejected at $\alpha = 0.05$ because $Z > 1.645$.

The Edgington model can be extended to provide a confidence interval for $\mu_D = \mu_A - \mu_B$. The $(1 - \alpha)\%$ confidence interval is given as

$$\mu_D = \overline{D} \pm Z_{\alpha/2}\sigma_{\overline{D}}$$

where $\overline{D} = T/Sc$ and

$$\sigma_{\overline{D}}^2 = (1/S)Var(T)$$

For the example,

$$\overline{D} = (1/3)(7.47) = 2.49$$

and

$$\sigma_{\overline{D}}^2 = (1/3)(.9228) = .3076$$

so that the 95% confidence interval for the mean increase in restful sleep is given as

$$\mu_D = 2.49 \pm 1.96 \sqrt{0.3076}$$
$$= 2.49 \pm 1.08$$

Thus, the mean increase in the number of hours of sleep ranges from a low of 1.4 hours to a high of 3.6 hours. Because a one-tailed test was used, a one-tailed confidence interval can be justified. In this case,

$$\mu_D > 2.49 - 1.645 \sqrt{0.3076} = 1.58$$

14–8 SINGLE SUBJECT RESEARCH IN NURSING SCIENCE

An advantage offered by single subject studies is the unique opportunity for the nurse researcher to study unusual or atypical types of patient behaviors, pathophysiological processes, and environmental circumstances. In health care, a nurse frequently encounters situations which are limited to particular types of patients or unusual disease processes. Consequently, the opportunities for obtaining a large sample in these circumstances are completely beyond the realm of feasibility. Infrequently observed or noted events must be captured at the time of their occurrence. Therefore, the selection of one or two individual patients to observe and try alternative nursing interaction or treatment approaches must be measured and evaluated at the time of occurrence. If it is reasonable to assume that no similar occasions may arise in the near future, the opportunity to do a single subject study must not be lost.

Another advantage of single subject methods is the ability to capture the particular responses of selected persons to treatments or nursing interventions. When large groups are studied, as in experiments involving multiple groups, individual differences are certain to be masked. Unique responses are lost by the statistical treatment of aggregate summary measurements of multiple patient behaviors. Not all patients respond similarly to a given set of independent variables in multiple treatment group research. The nurse investigator may be particularly concerned about individual differences among patients rather than collective responses to alternative intervention strategies. Single subject designs may best portray particular understanding of the internal processes experienced by patients given different treatments.

In the current cultural concerns for protecting individual freedom and a person's rights and privileges, a research design using each person as a unit of study may best address the issue of protecting the particularistic attributes of each person in current society. A design fashioned to a particular patient truly recognizes the sole or separate characteristics of the individual under study. It is well known in medical research that persons have different responses to specific medical treatments, medications, and health care therapeutics. Frequently, it is very difficult to predict the behavior or responses of one person to a given or particular medical regimen based on what is learned from responses of groups of subjects to similar protocols. Single subject investigations may afford greater insight into and more comprehensive understanding of the unique characteristics of patients undergoing a range of alternative intervention strategies.

Another advantage of single subject designs is that they provide workable models for undergraduate and graduate students of nursing to gain an appreciation and understanding of the research process. The ease of selecting one or two subjects as the unit of study circumvents the odious requirements of getting access to large samples in multiple institutions for more traditional statistical analyses. A group of students could study a single clinical phenomenon, such as pain modification strategies, with different subsets of clients. A uniform literature review could be conducted minimizing disperse efforts among different students to fashion a substantive literature base for conducting an individual study. Each student could use the identical research and clinical literature as a base on which to justify and interpret the specific single subject pain study.

Furthermore, if the identical ABAB design for pain modification were used by each student, the data could be pooled using the Wilcoxon model described in Sections 14–4 and 14–5. Although the models were illustrated for a common measure across all subjects, this is not a restriction of the models. The method of pooling across subjects is valid, provided that the underlying construct under study is the same for all individual single subject investigations. In some cases, the use of meta-analytic techniques (described in Chapter 15) can also be used to combine information across subjects.

14–9 SUMMARY

In this chapter, single subject designs have been illustrated in the case of the AB and ABAB design. Other designs are used in single subject research. The most typical pattern is found in the ABAB research protocol. Use of appropriate statistical methods were described in terms of randomization test procedures and the Wilcoxon test based on ranks. Methods for treating carry-over phase effects also were described. Examples from clinical research were used to exemplify the application of single subject designs to clinical nursing research issues.

Single subject designs are apparently strong in possessing aspects of internal validity but singularly weak in attaining attributes of external validity. The investigator's ability to generalize from individual persons under study to a population at large is the outstanding weakness of single subject research. Generalizations from instances of *one* case are *always* suspect. Consequently, the investigator using a single subject design must exercise extreme caution and circumspection when presenting the results. The problem of generalizability is not necessarily eliminated by the inclusion of additional subjects representing the construct under investigation. Atypical cases or unusual instances of clinical phenomena are usually selected for investigation. The ability to extrapolate findings from infrequently noted or specialized occurrences greatly constrains the investigator's ability to move from single instances to generic conclusions.

REFERENCES

DeProspero, A., and Cohen, S.: Inconsistent visual analysis of intersubject data, J. Appl. Behav. Anal., *12:* 315–319, 1979.

Edgington, E.S.: Random assignment and statistical tests for one-subject experiments, Behav. Assess., *2:* 19–28, 1980a.

Edgington, E.S.: Randomization Tests. New York, Dekker, 1980b.

Edgington, E.S.: Validity of randomization tests for one-subject experiments, J. Ed. Stat., *5:* 235–251, 1980c.

Edgington, E.S.: Randomized single-subject experiments and statistical tests, J. Consult. Psych., *34:* 437–442, 1987.

Gottman, J.M., and Glass, G.V.: Analysis of interrupted time-series experiments. In Kratochwill, T.R., ed., Single Subject Research: Strategies for Evaluating Change. New York, Academic Press, 1978.

Hersen, M., and Barlow, D.H. Single-Case Experimental Designs: Strategies for Studying Behavior Change. Oxford, Pergamon, 1976.

Jones, R.R., Vaught, R.S., and Weinrott, M.: Effects of serial dependency on the agreement between visual and statistical inference, J. Appl. Behav. Anal., *11:* 277–283, 1978.

Kazdin, A.E.: Single-Case Research Designs: Methods for Clinical and Applied Settings. New York, Oxford University Press, 1982.

Kratochwill, T.R., ed.: Single-Subject Research: Strategies for Evaluating Change. New York, Academic Press, 1978.

Kratochwill, T.R., and Brody, G.H.: Single subject designs: a perspective on the controversy over employing statistical inference and implications for research and training in behavior modification, Behav. Modif., *2:* 291–307, 1978.

Kratochwill, T.R., and Levin, J.: On the applicability of behavior therapy research, Behav. Assess., *2:* 353–360, 1980.

Levin, J.R., Marascuilo, L.A., and Hubert, L.J.: N = 1 nonparametric randomization tests. In Kratochwill, T.R., ed., Single-Subject Research: Strategies for Evaluating Change: New York, Academic Press, 1978.

Marascuilo, L.A., and Busk, P.L.: Combining statistics for multiple-baseline AB and replicated ABAB designs across subjects, Behav. Assess., *10:* 1–28, 1988.

Toothaker, L.E., Banz, M., Noble, C., et al.: N = 1 designs: the failure of ANOVA-based tests, J. Ed. Stat., *8:* 289–309, 1983.

Wampold, B.E., and Furlong, M.J.: Randomization tests in single-subject designs: illustrative examples, J. Behavioral Assess., *3:* 329–341, 1981.

Winer, B.J.: Statistical Principles in Experimental Design, ed. 2. New York, McGraw-Hill, 1971.

Chapter 15

METHODS FOR META-ANALYSIS

15−1 SYNTHESIZING TOPICS IN NURSING RESEARCH

One of the first tasks that an investigator must complete before attacking a new research question is a thorough review of the literature. Until recently, there was little to guide a researcher in this task. It would be seen that review articles and the research reviews of proposed investigations vary in style, tone, and methodologies. In the past, there were few acceptable guidelines to assist a researcher in reviewing the literature. Recently, the scene has changed.

Smith and Glass (1977) published a review of psychotherapy research in which they introduced to behavioral science a new model named *meta-analysis*. It is used for reviewing, evaluating, and synthesizing research findings across a large number of studies that relate to a single hypothesis. Meta-analysis involves the statistical treatment of a large collection of results abstracted from individual studies with the purpose of integrating the findings into a summary statement of the effects of an independent variable on a dependent measure or measures. It thus provides methods and techniques for organizing, describing, and collating data from an array of studies. In meta-analysis, knowledge is aggregated and summarized from diverse investigation of the same phenomena. It was used in the Devine and Cook (1983) and the Hathaway (1986) studies of different psycho-educational and preoperative teaching programs for persons undergoing surgery (referred to repeatedly in earlier chapters). In this chapter, an introduction to meta-analysis is provided for nursing science.

The major emphasis of a meta-analysis is to determine the magnitude of an effect size of a particular treatment. With two or more treatments, an added component of meta-analysis is deciding which treatment is best. According to Glass (1976), effect size is defined as the mean difference on the dependent variable between experimental and control subjects measured relative to the

333

within group standard deviation. After quantification of each study with respect to effect sizes, aggregate data are summarized by:

1. determining the average of the effect sizes across studies for each treatment under investigation and
2. comparing the average effect size across treatments for each variable or variables.

In the first meta-analytic study reported in the professional literature, Smith and Glass (1977) examined published articles and unpublished doctoral dissertations on the effectiveness of psychotherapy. They tested the hypothesis that psychotherapy has no effect on clients. The investigators demonstrated that psychotherapy does have an impact and, more important, they provided a quantitative measurement of the effects of psychotherapy. For this study, an extensive literature search produced 375 controlled evaluations of the effects of psychotherapy. Over 800 measurements of effect size were ascertained from the 375 controlled evaluation studies. Aggregate summary statistics were gathered and used for the analysis. The average effect size over the 800 measures was estimated to be about .68 standard deviations units. This indicates that on the average the typical therapy group mean was found to be about two thirds of a standard deviation above the mean of a typical untreated control group. In addition, the effect sizes of four different types of psychotherapy were compared with those of untreated control groups. The effect sizes for the four types of psychotherapy were estimated and found not to be different in their average impact.

Before a presentation of specific meta-analytic procedures, the general steps required to conduct a fruitful meta-analysis are listed as follows:

1. A treatment or intervention program is identified as worthy of summarization or aggregation.
2. The criteria are established for the identification and selection of materials to be included or excluded from the analysis.
3. A thorough search of the literature is conducted for all published articles and fugitive unpublished research or program evaluation reports relating to the research questions or hypotheses of interest.
4. The estimates are made of the treatment

effects for all the research studies retained for the analysis.
5. The estimates of treatment effects are tested for homogeneity and differences are noted.
6. The estimates shown to be homogeneous are pooled to provide individual treatment effect statistics for all the conditions or treatments under investigation.
7. The pooled estimates are tested for homogeneity, and differences in the pooled estimates are noted and evaluated for empirical or theoretical significance.
8. The other analyses examining possible confounding or intervening variables are performed on the homogeneous measures of the treatment effects to shed further light on the findings.
9. A report is written summarizing the findings of the meta-analysis.

15–2 TREATMENT EFFECT IN META-ANALYSIS

The *treatment effect* of a meta-analysis is a standardized measure of treatment versus control mean differences in a dependent variable or aggregate of a set of dependent variables. The measure is closely related to the two-sample t test described in Section 9–6 and is defined as follows:

$$\hat{\delta} = \frac{\overline{Y}_E - \overline{Y}_C}{\sqrt{MSW}}$$

where

$\overline{Y}_E$ = the mean score for the experimental group

$\overline{Y}_C$ = the mean score for the control group

and

MSW = the mean square within or the estimate of the common variance associated with the two-sample t test

If the assumption of equal variance is not satisfied, Glass, McGaw, and Smith (1981) recommend that the standard deviation of the control group be used in place of the pooled estimate of the common variance. The connection between the treatment effect and the two-sample t test is given as

$$t = \frac{\hat{\delta}}{\sqrt{\dfrac{1}{N_E} + \dfrac{1}{N_C}}}$$

where

N_E = the number in the experimental group

and

N_C = the number in the control group

Because $\hat{\delta}$ is a simple function of the t test, the test of the null hypothesis that the treatment effect is equal to zero is performed by doing the t test of Section 9–6. Thus, the test of the null hypothesis $H_0 : \delta = 0$ is identical with the two-sample t test null hypothesis $H_0 : \mu_C = \mu_E$. If the null hypothesis of the t test is rejected, it is known immediately that the treatment effect is statistically different from zero.

15–3 APPLICATION OF THE TREATMENT EFFECT MODEL TO A NURSING RESEARCH TOPIC

Throughout chapters in this text, a variety of research strategies and quantitative techniques have been used to evaluate three preoperative teaching programs based on measures of subjective levels of pain. This body of scientific and professional literature offers many opportunities for the application of meta-analytic techniques to assess the impact of intervention programs concerned with pain management. This means that nurse investigators who are interested in different treatment approaches to assist persons to cope with pain can turn to the general behavioral and health science literature to identify successful attempts to treat pain. If, for instance, an investigator is interested in the management and treatment of pain in nonhospitalized persons, a variety of cognitive/behavioral pain reduction analog models found in the professional literature can be studied. In any case, a thorough search of the literature is a precursor to a valid analysis and in turn meta-analysis.

As a first step, a meta-analysis of studies concerned with reducing pain in persons with migraine symptoms, upper torso, and skeletal pain was selected. As a second step, general overall criteria for inclusion and exclusion of studies were developed. Key search terms were identified to initiate a computer search process on both *Medline* and *ERIC* professional literature computerized data bases. A very large number of citations were listed for different cognitive and behavioral treatment methods for different types of pain. As the literature search strategy proceeded, the criteria had to be refined because specific problems in article selection emerged. Furthermore, various types of pain were depicted.

The bulk of the studies identified involved college students who were participants in different laboratory-induced pain experiences. This suggested an overabundance of artificially conducted pain studies. There was a lack of clinically relevant, staged laboratory or hospital short-term pain studies. A nursing study in which college women were told to simulate having a baby and imagine themselves in active labor illustrates the unreality of a contrived pain experience (Gedden, Beck, Hauge, and Pohlman, 1984).

A new literature search was initiated, restricting the selection of investigations to those involving persons in the community who were actually experiencing short-term or long-term pain and persons who subsequently initiated actions seeking pain relief from a variety of professional care takers. Furthermore, it was decided that located studies had to contain at least one control group and one experimental (treatment) group. In addition, the experimental group had to be exposed to a clearly explicated cognitive or behavioral treatment designed to relieve the client's pain.

About 20 studies were located which met the above criteria. A principal difference between the persons seeking pain relief emerged. Either they were referred by other professionals, or they responded to requests for volunteers which appeared in newspapers or radio or television solicitations. It was found that a vast array of services were offered, including biofeedback, meditation, sensory imagery exercises, relaxation procedures, and other like modalities.

Each study was examined to determine

whether it should be included in the final analysis. On the basis of this investigation together with use of the above criteria, a number of articles were excluded. The 15 studies that were retained are summarized in Table 15–1. As indicated, the treatment effects ranged from a low of 0.03 to a high of 2.39, which suggests heterogeneous effects across the studies.

Another example of a meta-analytic study of nonmedical treatment of chronic pain was performed by Malone and Strube (1988). These investigators located 109 published studies covering a 28-year period. Of the studies located, only 48 provided sufficient information on which to determine effect sizes. They were able to demonstrate the importance of using a multidimensional framework for pain assessment and to demonstrate that a vast variety of nonmedical treatments proved effective for pain management.

The sample sizes for the studies are relatively small, ranging from a low of 10 to a high of 52. It is also important to note that some studies involved a large number of variables. For example, studies 5, 6, and 8 made 12 treatment versus control group comparisons. Study number 12 used 36 different comparisons on a total of 16 subjects. Both of these sample characteristics provide problems in the execution of a metaanalysis. Small samples generate weak power properties for statistical tests of ho-

mogeneity of treatment effects. With small samples, large variance in treatment effects may lead to nonrejected null hypotheses of treatment effects. As a consequence, the pooling of treatment effect estimates that are disperse, like those of Table 15–1, may result. Multiple dependent measures also reduce the power of the statistical tests of homogeneity because multiple correlated variables tend to contain redundant information. Here, the effects of the redundancy can be reduced by using only one or a small number of variables that capture the salient dimensions of the treatment effects.

None of the treatment effects of Table 15–1 is negative. This is by design. In any meta-analysis, a researcher must read carefully how a positive treatment effect is defined in each study. Some dependent measures show positive effects when the treatment difference is negative. This is a function of how the individual researcher has established outcome criteria. In this meta-analysis, a number of the outcome variables in some studies were expected to show a decrease in value provided that the treatment was successful. For such variables, the treatment effects should be negative. To make beneficial effects uniform or comparable across studies, reported negative treatment effects were made positive, so that only positive treatment effects are reported.

TABLE 15–1 FIFTEEN STUDIES USED FOR A META-ANALYSIS ON PAIN AND THE REQUIRED SUMMARY STATISTICS

Study	Authors	Treatment Effect	Sample Size	Squared Standard Error (SE^2)	Number of Variables
1	Brown (1984)	1.45	26	0.1156	8
2	Cox et al. (1975)	0.50	18	0.1250	6
3	Engstrom (1983)	0.03	32	0.0616	8
4	Haynes et al. (1975)	0.81	13	0.2226	6
5	Kaplan et al. (1983)	2.39	20	0.0838	12
6	Larsson and Melin (1986)	1.43	18	0.1084	12
7	Lin et al. (1985)	0.26	52	0.0777	4
8	Moore and Chaney (1985)	0.26	23	0.0794	12
9	Nocella and Kaplan (1982)	0.71	20	0.2126	2
10	Nouwen (1983)	0.50	20	0.2063	4
11	Philips (1977)	0.21	10	0.4022	3
12	Scott and Clum (1984)	0.14	16	0.0913	36
13	Surman et al. (1974)	0.31	40	0.1024	3
14	Tan and Poser (1982)	0.40	24	0.0781	8
15	Turner (1982)	0.70	23	0.1987	5

15-4 VOTE COUNTING PROCEDURES

The researcher conducting a meta-analysis frequently discovers that authors do not provide sufficient information that permits the estimation of the treatment effects. Often, the mean values of the dependent measures of the control group, the experimental group, or both groups are not provided. More often it is observed that no information concerning variation in the dependent measure is reported. Inexplicably, standard deviations are not reported. Because the treatment effect is defined in terms of the control and experimental group means and the within group standard deviation, a researcher may be tempted to discard these studies from the meta-analysis. This introduces a bias into the meta-analysis. When many studies have incomplete data, one can resort to a *vote counting procedure* for the meta-analysis. In this model, the number of statistically significant results which favor the treatment under assessment are counted.

The vote counting model was first described by Light and Smith (1971). If most of the results are statistically significant, it is concluded that the treatment conditions are the winners. The model can be modified to include three different outcomes, that is, statistically significant in the positive direction, statistically significant in the negative direction, and not statistically significant. The set that contains more than one third of all analyzed studies is declared the winner.

The vote counting method is flawed because it ignores different sample sizes and differences in the qualities of the various treatment conditions. Also, the method ignores sites, types of patients, ages of clients, gender differences, and an array of other study characteristics. Unfortunately, sometimes only statements of significance are available and the meta-analyst must approach the task constructively. Hedges and Olkin (1985) have modified the vote counting meta-analytic model to provide estimates of the treatment effects, given only knowledge of the number of statistically significant studies. The proposed method is nonparametric and provides estimates with large standard errors. The method is illustrated here.

Let the number of studies be denoted by K and let the number of statistically positive results be denoted by X. Thus, the proportion of positive results is given as $\hat{P} = X/K$. The $(1 - \alpha)\%$ confidence interval for P is given in equation 1 below.

Consider a meta-analysis based on K = 25 studies and suppose that the number with positive results is given as X = 19 so that

$$\hat{P} = 19/25 = 0.76$$

Thus, the 95% confidence interval for the proportion of successful treatment studies is given in equation 2 below.

Thus, the proportion of studies that favor the treatment conditions ranges from a low of 0.59 to a high of 0.93. The end points of the interval and the point estimate of P are used to estimate the treatment effect.

To estimate the treatment effects, the figures of Table 15-2 are used. This table was prepared by Hedges and Olkin (1985). The table is entered with two indices. One is the average size of the control and experimental samples. The other is the estimates of the proportions of favorable studies. Suppose for the example that the average sample size is N = 20. With $\hat{P} = 0.76$, the value for

①
$$\hat{P} + Z_{(\alpha/2)} \sqrt{\frac{\hat{P}(1 - \hat{P})}{K}} < P < \hat{P} + Z_{(1-\alpha/2)} \sqrt{\frac{\hat{P}(1 - \hat{P})}{K}}$$

②
$$0.76 - 1.96 \sqrt{\frac{(0.76)(0.24)}{25}} < P < 0.76 + 1.96 \sqrt{\frac{(0.76)(0.24)}{25}}$$

$$0.76 - 0.17 < P < 0.76 + 0.17$$

$$0.59 < P < 0.93$$

TABLE 15-2 PROBABILITY THAT THE SAMPLE MEAN OF THE EXPERIMENTAL GROUP EXCEEDS THE SAMPLE MEAN OF THE CONTROL GROUP*

N						Size of δ							
	0.00	0.02	0.04	0.06	0.08	0.10	0.20	0.40	0.50	0.60	0.80	0.90	1.00
5	0.50	0.51	0.52	0.54	0.55	0.56	0.62	0.74	0.78	0.87	0.90	0.92	0.94
10	0.50	0.52	0.54	0.55	0.57	0.59	0.67	0.81	0.87	0.91	0.96	0.98	0.99
15	0.50	0.52	0.54	0.57	0.59	0.61	0.71	0.86	0.91	0.95	0.99	0.99	1.00
20	0.50	0.52	0.55	0.58	0.60	0.63	0.74	0.90	0.94	0.97	0.99	1.00	
25	0.50	0.53	0.56	0.58	0.61	0.64	0.76	0.92	0.96	0.98	1.00		
50	0.50	0.54	0.58	0.62	0.66	0.69	0.84	0.98	0.99	1.00			
100	0.50	0.56	0.61	0.66	0.71	0.76	0.92	0.99	1.00				
200	0.50	0.58	0.66	0.73	0.79	0.84	0.98	1.00					
400	0.50	0.61	0.71	0.80	0.87	0.92	1.00						

*Average sample size = N
  Treatment effect = δ

Abstract from Table 2 of Hedges, L. V., and Olkin, I.: *Statistical Method for Meta-Analysis*, pp. 58–59. Orlando, FL, Academic Press, 1985. By permission of the authors.

the treatment effect is found by *interpolation* to be

$$\hat{\delta} = 0.225$$

The interpolation is performed between the following numbers taken from Table 15–2.

Treatment effect	0.20	δ	0.40
Probability	0.74	0.76	0.90

The 95% confidence interval for δ is found by entering Table 15–2 with the upper and lower bounds of the confidence interval for P and the average sample size of N = 20. In this case the interpolation is performed between the sets of numbers at the bottom of the page.

With these interpolations, the 95% confidence interval for δ is given as

$$0.07 < \delta < 0.475.$$

Note that the probabilities of Table 15–2 begin at 0.50, not at 0.00. Probabilities below 0.50 are associated with negative values of the treatment effect. For example, if N = 20 and $\hat{\delta} = -0.40$, the corresponding probability is given as $1.00 - 0.90 = 0.10$.

15–5 INTERPRETING THE TREATMENT EFFECT USING PROBABILITY MEASURES ASSOCIATED WITH VOTE COUNTING PROCEDURES

In this section, an alternative way to interpret a treatment effect is provided. The interpretation is based on the following model. Consider selecting at random a subject from the experimental condition and comparing this subject to a typical subject from the control condition. One way to measure the effectiveness of the experimental condition is to determine the probability of the experimental subject having a value on the dependent measure which is higher than that of the control subject. If the treatment effect is zero, the probability of a subject in the experimental group having a dependent measure value which exceeds the mean value of the control group is one half. Neither program is superior to the other under this condition.

For the example of the previous section, the worst possible scenario estimate of the treatment effect is given as $\delta = 0.07$, the lower value of the 95% confidence interval. Because the treatment effects are measured

	Lower Limit			Upper Limit		
Treatment effect	0.06	δ	0.08	0.40	δ	0.50
Probability	0.58	0.59	0.60	0.90	0.93	0.94

in standard deviation units, the proportion of subjects in the experimental group who have higher variable measures than the mean performance of the subjects in the control group can be determined. This is accomplished by assuming that the underlying variables are normally distributed and making use of the fact that the scale of $\hat{\delta}$ is equal to one. Under these conditions, the probabilities under the normal curve reported in Table A-5 can be used directly. Under these assumptions, the proportion of subjects who score higher than the mean of the control group is given as

$$P(Z > 0.00|\mu = 0.07) = P(Z > -0.07)$$
$$= 0.53$$

Thus, the proportion of patients who score above the control condition average can be as low as 3%, as shown in Figure 15–1. For the best possible scenario, $\delta = 0.475$. For this condition,

$$P(Z > 0.00|\mu = 0.475) = P(Z > -0.475)$$
$$= 0.68$$

For the best possible treatment effect, 68% of the patients do better than the mean of the control patients. This 18% excess above the chance value of 50% is large for behavioral and health research data. For the average scenario, the proportion of the treatment patients who do better than the mean of the control patients is given as

$$P(Z > 0.00|\mu = 0.225)$$
$$= P(Z > -0.225) = 0.59$$

Here, the excess over .50 is equal to .09. Nine percent of the patients in the experimental group do better than the average subject in the control group. These three situations are shown graphically in Figure 15–1.

15–6 TREATMENT EFFECTS FOR A SINGLE STUDY

As an example of a single study for which a measurement of the treatment effect is desired, consider the data of Table 15–3. These data have been extracted from the study by Brown (1984). As indicated, there are eight different comparisons involving two treatments and one control. In this section only

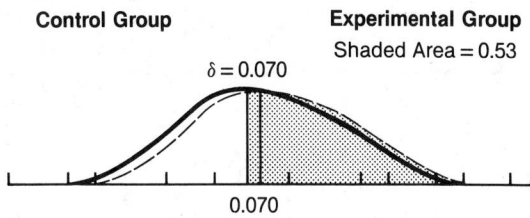
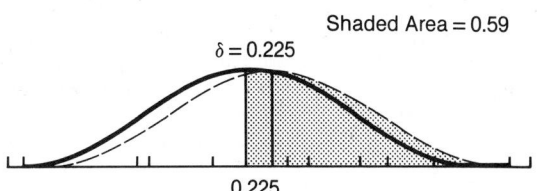
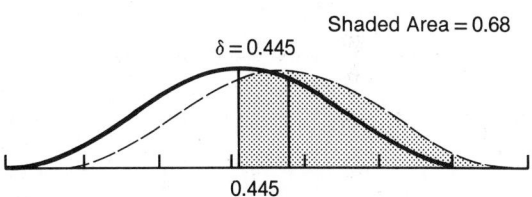

Figure 15–1. Three possible treatment differences showing the proportion of cases in the treatment group that exceed the mean value in the control group. The treatment effect sizes are $\delta = 0.070$, 0.225, and 0.475.

the comparison of the control to treatment one is made.

The analysis begins with an examination of the *headache index*. For this variable, the mean change from pretest to posttest for the control group is given as $\overline{Y}_C = -5.62$ and for the treatment group the mean change is given as $\overline{Y}_E = 33.85$. The standard deviation of the control group is given as $S_C = 35.17$ and the standard deviation of the experimental group is given as $S_E = 22.63$. The latter figures are not reported in Table 15–3. In terms of these standard deviations, the pooled estimate of the variance is

$$MSW = \frac{(13 - 1)(35.17)^2 + (13 - 1)(22.63)^2}{(13 - 1) + (13 - 1)}$$
$$= \sqrt{874.5229}$$

The pooled standard deviation is equal to $MSW = 29.57$ so that the treatment effect is given as

TABLE 15-3 SAMPLE STATISTICS, TREATMENT EFFECTS, AND 95% CONFIDENCE INTERVALS*

Control Group Versus Experimental Group One

Variable	$\overline{Y}_C$	$\overline{Y}_E$	MSW	N_C	N_E	Treatment Effect	SE^2	Confidence Interval	
HEADACHE INDEX									
Baseline to treatment	−5.62	33.85	29.57	13	13	1.34	0.1881	0.49	2.19
Baseline to follow-up	−6.85	49.77	29.02	13	13	1.95	0.2271	1.02	2.88
HEADACHE DURATION									
Baseline to treatment	−28.38	13.00	24.28	13	13	1.70	0.2097	0.80	2.60
Baseline to follow-up	−34.69	12.07	49.98	13	13	0.93	0.1707	0.12	1.74

Control Group Versus Experimental Group Two

Variable	$\overline{Y}_C$	$\overline{Y}_E$	MSW	N_C	N_E	Treatment Effect	SE^2	Confidence Interval	
HEADACHE INDEX									
Baseline to treatment	−5.62	45.23	26.29	13	13	1.93	0.2258	1.00	2.86
Baseline to follow-up	−6.85	53.69	30.64	13	13	1.98	0.2289	1.04	2.92
HEADACHE DURATION									
Baseline to treatment	−28.38	4.54	27.53	13	13	1.20	0.1814	0.36	2.04
Baseline to follow-up	−34.69	−1.77	51.17	13	13	0.64	0.1615	−0.15	1.43

*Data taken from Brown, J. M.: Imagery coping strategies in the treatment of migraine, Pain, *18*: 157–167, 1984.

$$\hat{\delta} = \frac{\overline{Y}_E - \overline{Y}_C}{\sqrt{MSW}}$$

$$= \frac{(33.85) - (-5.62)}{29.57} = 1.34$$

The squared standard error of this estimate is given as

$$SE^2(\hat{\delta}) = \frac{1}{N_C} + \frac{1}{N_E} + \frac{\hat{\delta}^2}{2(N_C + N_E)}$$

$$= \frac{1}{13} + \frac{1}{13} + \frac{(1.34)^2}{2(13 + 13)} = 0.1881$$

The 95% confidence interval for the treatment effect is given in the equation below. The interval is very wide because of the small sample sizes.

Small samples are a problem for the meta-analyst because they generate wide and generally less than meaningful confidence intervals. Another problem with small samples is that treatment effects are biased, and the bias is most pronounced for small samples. This problem is discussed in Section 15–12. Notice in the denominator of the squared standard error the presence of the algebraic expression $2(N_C + N_E)$. This expression provides a general form for the standard error. If the standard deviation of the control group is used, the denominator is replaced by $2N_C$. If the sample sizes are large, the formula for the standard error can be simplified and the term involving $\hat{\delta}$ can be dropped from arithmetic computations. This luxury is not available for the illustrated example.

15–7 TREATMENT EFFECTS FOR MULTIPLE VARIABLES WITHIN A SINGLE STUDY

Another problem that the meta-analyst must face is that of multivariate measures within a single study. The Brown study has many.

$$1.34 - 1.96\sqrt{0.1881} \leq \delta \leq 1.34 + 1.96\sqrt{0.1881}$$

$$1.34 - 0.85 \leq \delta \leq 1.34 + 0.85$$

$$0.49 \leq \delta \leq 2.19$$

The most important eight treatment effects have been selected for the meta-analysis. One of the objects of meta-analysis is to use data reduction techniques that pool many treatment effects to a single measure. This is achieved by replacing all treatment effects with a mean value. For K treatment effects the average value is given by

$$\bar{\delta} = \frac{\hat{\delta}_1 + \hat{\delta}_2 + \ldots + \hat{\delta}_K}{P}$$

This estimate of the treatment effect is called the *pooled estimate*. For the Brown study the pooled estimate is given as

$$\bar{\delta} = \frac{1.34 + 1.95 + 1.70 + 0.93}{4} = 1.48$$

Another problem for the meta-analyst is that the standard error for the pooled treatment effect depends upon a knowledge of all correlation coefficients among all summarized variables. Invariably, the standard error cannot be computed because authors rarely provide the numerical values of the correlation coefficients needed to perform the computations.

To complete this exposition, a model is provided for determining the standard error of a pooled estimate of a treatment effect. Unfortunately, the necessary summary statistics often are not printed, and the opportunities for using this estimate are infrequent. Because of this infrequent opportunity, a second solution is offered that can be used, provided that a researcher assumes a numerical value for the average of the correlation coefficients. The formula for the squared standard error for the pooled estimate of the treatment effect is given in the equation at the bottom of this page. In this formula,

$$SE^2(\hat{\delta}_P) = \left(\frac{1}{N_C} + \frac{1}{N_E}\right) + \frac{\hat{\delta}_P^2}{2(N_C + N_E)}$$

and

$$Cov(\hat{\delta}_P, \hat{\delta}_{P'}) = r_{PP'}\left(\frac{1}{N_C} + \frac{1}{N_E}\right) + r_{PP'}^2 \frac{\hat{\delta}_P \hat{\delta}_{P'}}{2(N_C + N_E)}$$

For the example, the correct squared standard error cannot be computed because the necessary correlation coefficients are unknown. An approximation to the correct standard error can be obtained by making some assumptions. These formulas are described by Marascuilo, Busk, and Serlin (1988).

For the first simplification, note in Table 15−3 that the squared standard errors of the P = 4 treatment effects are very similar to one another. Their average is given as 0.1989. This average value is used for the approximation. For the second simplification, all correlation coefficients are set equal to a common value by making a rational good guess of the average value of all of the correlation coefficients. With many social science variables, a good guess for the average value is to set $\bar{r}$ equal to 0.5. For the third simplification, each $\hat{\delta}_P$ is replaced by the average $\bar{\delta} = 1.48$. With these substitutions

$$SE^2(\hat{\delta}_P) = 0.1989$$

and

$$Cov(\hat{\delta}_P, \hat{\delta}_{P'}) = (0.50)\left(\frac{1}{13} + \frac{1}{13}\right)$$
$$+ (0.50)^2 \frac{(1.48)^2}{2(13 + 13)} = 0.0875$$

so that

$$SE^2(\bar{\delta}) = (1/4)^2[4(0.1989) + 4(4 − 1)(0.0875)]$$
$$= 0.1154$$

With this value, a 95% confidence interval for $\bar{\delta}$ is given as

$$\bar{\delta} = 1.48 \pm 1.96\sqrt{0.1154} = 1.48 \pm 0.67$$

or equivalently

$$0.81 < \bar{\delta} < 2.15.$$

If one averages the limits of the four intervals of group one in Table 15−3, it is seen that the average limits are given by 0.61 and 2.35. Thus, an average 95% confidence interval is given as

$$0.61 < \bar{\delta} < 2.35$$

$$SE^2(\bar{\delta}) = (1/P)^2\{[SE^2(\hat{\delta}_1) + SE^2(\hat{\delta}_2) + \ldots + SE^2(\hat{\delta}_P)] + 2[\hat{Cov}(\hat{\delta}_1, \hat{\delta}_2) + \hat{Cov}(\hat{\delta}_1, \hat{\delta}_3) + \ldots$$
$$+ \hat{Cov}(\hat{\delta}_{(P-1)}, \hat{\delta}_P)]\}$$

In some cases, a meta-analyst can do better by making a search of relevant literature and estimating the average correlation coefficient. Also, if the sample sizes are large, a fourth simplification can be adopted. All terms involving the treatment effects are eliminated for this simplification. A large sample approximation formula for the squared standard error is given as

$$SE^2(\bar{\delta}) = (1/P) [1 + \bar{r}(P - 1)]SE^2(\hat{\delta})$$

If $M = (1/P) [1 + \bar{r}(P - 1)]$, then the approximate squared standard error is given as

$$SE^2(\bar{\delta}) = M[SE^2(\hat{\delta})]$$

Values of M are listed in Table 15−4. For the example, $P = 4$. When the average correlation coefficient is set equal to $\bar{r} = 0.40$, the value of M read in Table 15−4 is given as M $= .8500$. Thus,

$$SE^2(\bar{\delta}) = .8500(.1154) = .0973$$

With this value, a 95% confidence interval for the average treatment effect is

$$\bar{\delta} = 1.48 \pm 1.96\sqrt{0.0973} = 1.48 \pm 0.61$$
$$\bar{\delta} = 1.48 \pm 0.61,$$

which is slightly more efficient than that of the previous example in which the correlation coefficients were set equal to .50.

It is illuminating to examine Table 15−4 in detail. Note that if the correlation coefficients are less than .50 the multiplying factor is less than unity. The standard error of the pooled estimate tends to be smaller than the standard error for any of the variables. This was demonstrated for the average correlation coefficient of .40. This should be expected. When correlations are close to zero, the information obtained from each treatment effect is unrelated to the information obtained from any other measure of the same treatment effect. As more data are accumulated, better estimates are produced; however, if the variables are highly correlated, the information from each variable concerning the treatment effect is redundant. Pooling similar information about the treatment effect is not going to improve the precision of the estimate by a large amount.

15−8 POOLING TREATMENT EFFECTS WITHIN A STUDY

In the previous section, it was shown how multiple treatment effects can be pooled across different variables to obtain a single estimate of a specific treatment. Sometimes, a researcher includes two or more different treatment groups in a study, which are compared with the same treatment conditions. When this happens, the meta-analyst occasionally may wish to pool the various treatment effects. The techniques described in the previous section can be modified to solve this problem.

For the data of Table 15−3, the treatment

TABLE 15−4 ADJUSTMENT FACTORS FOR ESTIMATING SQUARED STANDARD ERROR OF A TREATMENT EFFECT WHEN THE EXACT VALUES OF THE CORRELATION COEFFICIENTS ARE UNKNOWN

Number of Variables	Average Value of the Correlation Coefficients								
	0.00	0.20	0.30	0.40	0.50	0.60	0.70	0.80	1.00
1	1.0000	1.0000	1.0000	1.0000	1.0000	1.0000	1.0000	1.0000	1.0000
2	.5000	.7000	.8000	.9000	1.0000	1.1000	1.2000	1.3000	1.5000
3	.3333	.6000	.7333	.8667	1.0000	1.1333	1.2667	1.4000	1.6667
4	.2500	.5500	.7000	.8500	1.0000	1.1500	1.3000	1.4500	1.7500
5	.2000	.5200	.6800	.8400	1.0000	1.1600	1.3200	1.4800	1.8000
6	.1667	.5000	.6667	.8333	1.0000	1.1667	1.3333	1.5000	1.8333
7	.1428	.4857	.6571	.8286	1.0000	1.1714	1.3429	1.5143	1.8573
8	.1250	.4750	.6500	.8250	1.0000	1.1750	1.3500	1.5250	1.8750
9	.1111	.4667	.6444	.8222	1.0000	1.1778	1.3556	1.5334	1.8890
10	.1000	.4600	.6400	.8200	1.0000	1.1800	1.3600	1.5400	1.9000
20	.0500	.4300	.6200	.8100	1.0000	1.1900	1.3800	1.5700	1.9500
40	.0250	.4150	.6100	.8050	1.0000	1.1950	1.3900	1.5850	1.9750
Limit	.0000	.4000	.6000	.8000	1.0000	1.2000	1.4000	1.6000	2.0000

①
$$SE^2(\bar{\delta}) = \frac{M}{W^2}\left(\sum_q^Q W_q^2\left(\frac{1}{N_C} + \frac{1}{N_E}\right) + 2\sum_{q<q'}^Q\sum^Q W_q W_{q'}\left(\frac{1}{N_C}\right)\right)$$

②
$$SE^2(\bar{\delta}) = \frac{1.0000}{(17.3763)^2}\left((8.6655)^2\left(\frac{1}{13} + \frac{1}{13}\right)\right.$$
$$\left. + (8.7108)^2\left(\frac{1}{13} + \frac{1}{13}\right) + 2(8.6655)(8.7108)\left(\frac{1}{13}\right)\right) = 0.1154$$

effect and standard error for treatment one are given as

$$\bar{\delta}_1 = 1.48$$

and

$$SE^2(\bar{\delta}_1) = 0.1154$$

The corresponding measures for treatment two are given as

$$\bar{\delta}_2 = 0.143$$

and

$$SE^2(\bar{\delta}_2) = 0.1148$$

For Q treatments, the pooled treatment effect is given as

$$\bar{\delta} = \frac{W_1\bar{\delta}_1 + W_2\bar{\delta}_2 + \ldots + W_Q\bar{\delta}_Q}{W_1 + W_2 + \ldots + W_Q}$$

The appropriate weights to use for this pooling are the reciprocals of the squared standard errors of each treatment effect that are pooled. For the example,

$$W_1 = 1/0.1154 = 8.6655$$

and

$$W_2 = 1/0.1148 = 8.7108$$

so that

$$\bar{\delta} = \frac{8.6655(1.48) + 8.7108(1.43)}{8.6655 + 8.7108}$$

$$= \frac{25.2814}{17.3763} = 1.45$$

As before, the standard error of $\bar{\delta}$ cannot be computed because the correlation coefficients are unknown. A large sample approximation to the squared standard error is available by using the coefficients of Table 15−4 and dropping from all formulas the terms involving the treatment effects. Under these conditions, the equation 1 above applies. For the example, $Q = 2$ and $M = 1.0000$ so that equation 2 above is true.

This is the value reported in Table 15−1. The remaining squared standard errors reported in Table 15−1 were established in the same way. With this large sample estimate, the 95% confidence interval for the average treatment effect is given as

$$\bar{\delta} = 1.45 \pm 1.96\sqrt{0.1154} = 1.45 \pm 0.67$$

As this example illustrates, correlation coefficients of .50 neither increase nor decrease the width of a confidence interval. This suggests that when the correlation coefficients fluctuate around .50, it is advisable for a researcher to choose only one important variable for the analysis.

15−9 TESTS OF HOMOGENEITY OF TREATMENT EFFECTS ACROSS STUDIES

As suggested earlier, the numerical values of the treatment effects for the 15 studies of Table 15−1 vary over a broad range. This is not a favorable condition for a meta-analytic study in which the main goal is to obtain a summary or pooled estimate of the treatment effect. Thus, before data can be pooled, it should be ascertained that the estimates are not statistically different from one another. A test of this hypothesis has been proposed by Hedges and Olkin (1985). The test statistic is

$$U = \sum_{k=1}^{K} W_k(\hat{\delta}_k - \bar{\delta})^2$$

where

$$W_k = \frac{1}{SE^2(\hat{\delta}_k)}$$

and

$$\bar{\delta} = \frac{W_1\hat{\delta}_1 + W_2\hat{\delta}_2 + \ldots + W_K\hat{\delta}_K}{W_1 + W_2 + \ldots + W_K}$$

Under H_0 the sampling distribution of U is chi-square with degrees of freedom given as $\nu = (K - 1)$. The definitional formula is rarely used to determine the value of U. Instead, the following computational form is preferred:

$$U = A - \frac{B^2}{C}$$

where

$$A = \sum_{k=1}^{K} W_k\hat{\delta}_k^2$$

$$B = \sum_{k=1}^{K} W_k\hat{\delta}_k$$

and

$$C = \sum_{k=1}^{K} W_k$$

In terms of this notation, the pooled estimate of the treatment effects is given simply as

$$\bar{\delta} = B/C$$

and its squared standard error is given as

$$SE^2(\bar{\delta}) = 1/C$$

The statistic U is used to test the hypothesis that all of the treatment effects are equal to a common value. The hypothesis under test can be written as

$$H_0: \delta_1 = \delta_2 = \ldots = \delta_K$$

An equivalent form of H_0 is given as

H_0: All contrasts in the treatment effect are equal to zero.

For this form of H_0, a contrast is defined as

$$\psi = a_1\delta_1 + a_2\delta_2 + \ldots + a_K\delta_K$$

with

$$a_1 + a_2 + \ldots + a_K = 0$$

In this form, it is seen that contrasts can be examined on a post hoc basis provided that the hypothesis of homogeneity has been rejected. The critical values for a post hoc analysis are given as

$$S = \pm\sqrt{\chi^2_{(K-1:1-\alpha)}}$$

For the data of Table 15–1,

$$A = 121.1960$$
$$B = 88.6930$$

and

$$C = 134.5920$$

The pooled treatment effect for the 15 studies is given as

$$\bar{\delta} = B/C = 88.6930/134.5920 = 0.66$$

and the squared standard error is given as

$$SE^2(\bar{\delta}) = 1/C = 1/134.5920 = 0.0074$$

The 95% confidence interval for the treatment effect is

$$\delta = \bar{\delta} \pm 1.96 \; SE(\bar{\delta})$$
$$= 0.66 \pm 1.96\sqrt{(0.0074)}$$
$$= 0.66 \pm 0.17.$$

This means that the treatment effect could be as small as 0.49 or as large as 0.83. This represents a large treatment effect. On the basis of these 15 studies, it can be concluded that on the average the difference in the dependent measures for the experimental groups versus those of the control groups is about two thirds of a standard deviation, favoring the experimental groups. The minimal difference could be as small as one-half of a standard deviation and the maximal difference could be as large as eight-tenths of a standard deviation. In any case, it must be concluded that any difference that exceeds a .50 standard deviation is a large difference as far as health variables are concerned.

Although the treatment effect across all 15 studies is large, the question remains as to whether the effects are homogeneous across the 15 studies, so that the treatment effects can be pooled to provide a single estimate. The hypothesis of homogeneity can be tested by examining the value of U. The numerical value of U is given as

$$U = 121.1960 - (88.6930)^2/134.5920$$
$$= 62.75$$

Because K = 15, the number of degrees of freedom for the test is given as $\nu = (K - 1)$ = (15 − 1) = 14 . With α = 0.05, the 95% decision rule read from Table A-1 is given as

Decision rule: Reject H_0 if U>23.68.

The hypothesis is rejected. Because H_0 has been rejected, post hoc comparisons would be made with

$$S = \pm\sqrt{23.68} = \pm 4.87$$

In this case, study 5 differs from studies 3, 7, 8, and 12. Study 11 was not included in the rejection set because it has the largest standard error.

Statistical methods are tools for a research worker that should be used to better understand the relationships that exist among variables. Statistical methods are not ends unto themselves. They should be used as adjuncts to data analysis. Here, study 11 was excluded because of being statistically significant from study 5 and yet, studies 7 and 8 have larger treatment effects. From an empirical inspection of Figure 15−2 it, too, should be included in the set of significant differ-

ences. Figure 15−2 provides a visual display of the studies according to treatment effect sizes ranging from zero to 3 standard deviations. As can be seen, 12 of the 15 studies cluster between zero and 1 standard deviation, two of the studies cluster about 1.44 standard deviations, and one stands as an outlier at 2.39 standard deviations. The outlier is study 5.

If one adheres strictly to the decisions made by the post hoc analysis of the treatment effect differences, two strategies appear. The conservative strategy suggests that study 5 should be excluded from the summary measure. The liberal strategy suggests that studies 3, 7, 8, and 12 be excluded from the analysis. Both strategies are examined here.

With study 5 excluded, the numerical value of U is given as

$$U = 53.0325 - (60.1727)^2/122.6588$$
$$= 23.52$$

This is considerably smaller than the U = 62.75 reported for all 15 studies. The null hypothesis for these 14 studies is not rejected because the critical value for this test is also given as U>23.68. With its exclusion, the 95% confidence interval for δ is

$$\delta = 0.49 \pm 1.96\sqrt{0.0082} = 0.49 \pm 0.18$$

Thus the population value of δ could be as low as 0.31 or as high as 0.63. Note that the estimate is smaller in value and the width of the confidence is slightly larger with the exclusion of study 5.

With studies 3, 7, 8, and 12 excluded, the numerical value of

$$U = 119.2453 - (80.0518)^2/81.9409$$
$$= 41.04$$

This is smaller than the U = 62.75 reported for all 15 studies but not small enough to produce a nonsignificant finding. This strategy is not useful in identifying homogeneous studies. The critical value for this test is also

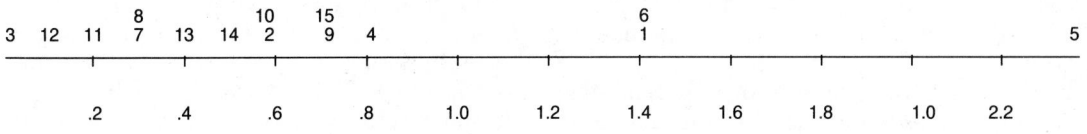

Figure 15−2. Ranking of the 15 studies of Table 15−1 according to treatment effect size.

given as U >23.68. With the exclusion of these four studies, the 95% confidence interval is given as

$$\delta = 0.98 \pm 1.96\sqrt{0.0122} = 0.98 \pm 0.22$$

Without a doubt this strategy is liberal. The point estimate of the treatment effect is almost 1 standard deviation, with the lower end of the confidence interval at about three-fourths of a standard deviation and the upper limit at about one and one and a quarter standard deviations. These conclusions do not correspond to the visual image presented in Figure 15−2.

A third strategy based on the post hoc analysis is to exclude studies 3, 7, 8, and 12 and study 5. With this analysis, the 15 investigations are partitioned into three disjointed sets of studies. One set contains 10 studies with the remaining 2 sets consisting of 4 studies and 1 study, respectively. With this strategy the U statistic for the 10 pooled studies is given as

$$U = 51.0818 - (51.5315)^2/70.0077 = 13.15$$

This is considerably smaller than the U = 62.75 reported for all 15 studies. The critical value for this test is also given as U > 23.68. With the exclusion of these 5 studies, the hypothesis of homogeneity is not rejected for the remaining studies. The 95% confidence interval for δ is given as

$$\delta = 0.74 \pm 1.96\sqrt{0.0143} = 0.74 \pm 0.23$$

On the basis of this analysis, the best estimate of the treatment effect for these 10 studies is about three-fourths of a standard deviation. In addition, the population value of δ could be as low as 0.51 (about one-half of a standard deviation) or as high as 0.97 (about 1 standard deviation).

A similar analysis would be made for the four pooled studies and for the one study that stands alone. This three-group analysis is the one recommended for the data of Table 15−1 because it removes the extreme studies from either end of the scale of treatment effects and because it produces nonsignificant values for the corresponding three U statistics.

A nonstatistical method for clustering the 15 studies is illustrated in Section 12−5 and shown graphically in the dendogram of Figure 12−5.

15−10 TESTS OF HOMOGENEITY IN RESEARCH DOMAINS

If the initial test of the hypothesis of homogeneity leads to rejection, a researcher may wish to group the studies into nonoverlapping sets and then make tests of homogeneity in the resulting groups. We have classified the 15 studies of Table 15−1 into a set of various subgroups. The classifications are of two types. One is a qualitative classification of the studies according to methodological indices, the other is a classification according to substantive indices. The qualitative classifications are reported in Table 15−5. The columns of this table represent a classification of the 15 studies according to criteria established by the meta-analyst. The classification was made by two independent judges in terms of the following criteria:

1. The random assignment of clients to either an experimental or control condition is described.
2. The investigator established a priori criteria for determination of client eligibility for entrance into the study.
3. The professional therapists with identifiable experience and credentials were clearly described as the treatment agent in the study.
4. The author(s) of the particular study were identifiable as also serving as one or more treatment agents in the study.
5. The therapist(s) did not know the hypotheses underlying the specific pain study.
6. The clarity of information given to clients about the particular study and the exact nature of the treatment provided was reported.
7. The description of the treatment assured clients that their pain would be relieved.
8. The clarity of information provided about the client's prior history and treatment of pain was adequate.
9. The data that addressed the psychometric properties of reliability contained in study research instruments was adequate.
10. The data that addressed the psychometric properties of validity contained in study research instruments was adequate.
11. The manner in which clients were selected or referred to the study was described.
12. A medical examination was used as a screening and evaluation device.

TABLE 15-5 EVALUATIONS OF 16 CRITERION QUALITY INDICES USED TO JUDGE THE 15 PAIN STUDIES OF TABLE 15-1*

Study Number	Criterion Quality Index															
	1	2	3	4	5	6	7	8	9	10	11	12	13	14	15	16
1	Y	Y	NK	N	N	Y	N	Y	NA	NA	Y	Y	Y	Y	Y	NA
2	Y	Y	Y	N	N	Y	N	Y	NA	NA	Y	N	Y	Y	Y	NA
3	Y	N	Y	N	N	Y	N	N	N	N	N	N	Y	Y	Y	NA
4	Y	Y	Y	N	N	N	Y	Y	NA	NA	Y	N	Y	Y	Y	NA
5	Y	Y	N	Y	N	Y	N	NA	NA	NA	N	NA	Y	Y	Y	Y
6	Y	Y	Y	N	N	Y	N	Y	NA	NA	Y	Y	Y	Y	Y	NA
7	Y	Y	Y	NA	Y	Y	N	Y	NA	NA	Y	Y	Y	Y	N	NA
8	Y	Y	N	N	N	Y	N	Y	NA	NA	N	Y	Y	N	N	Y
9	Y	Y	Y	N	N	N	N	Y	NA	NA	N	N	Y	Y	Y	Y
10	Y	Y	N	Y	N	Y	N	Y	NA	NA	Y	Y	Y	Y	Y	NA
11	Y	Y	Y	N	N	N	Y	Y	NA	NA	N	Y	N	Y	Y	NA
12	Y	Y	Y	N	N	N	N	N	N	N	N	Y	Y	Y	Y	N
13	Y	Y	Y	N	N	N	Y	Y	Y	NK	N	Y	Y	Y	Y	Y
14	Y	Y	Y	N	N	Y	N	Y	N	N	N	Y	Y	Y	Y	Y
15	Y	Y	N	N	N	Y	N	Y	NK	NK	N	Y	Y	Y	N	NA

*Y = yes; N = no; NA = not applicable; NK = not known

13. The theoretical and empirical bases for the use of dependent (outcome) measures were explicated.

14. The research report was thorough and would enable the replication of the study by other researchers.

15. The presence of confounding variables was recognized or was clearly present in the design of the investigation.

16. The external raters used to measure one or more dependent variables did not know study hypotheses.

The second classification of the 15 studies is based on substantive dimensions of treatment method, type of pain, and conceptual basis of intervention. These classifications are summarized in Table 15-6. The variables for these classifications are the following:

1. Length of treatment
2. Location and type of pain
3. Modality of therapy
4. Number and type of clients in therapy
5. Clarity of the conceptual basis of the treatment
6. Types of dependent measures
7. Sex ratio of women to men in the study
8. Age of clients reported as the mean or median of the group
9. Types of control groups

Tests of homogeneity can be performed within each set of similar studies. With post

hoc investigations, a number of treatment effects may be identified which can help provide a better understanding of the entire collection of studies. In the example, the overall test of homogeneity led to the decision to reject the hypothesis of homogeneity. Thus, a researcher would make further investigations among the grouped studies. Hedges and Olkin (1985) provide information about some interesting methods of conducting such post hoc investigations. The meta-analyst must remember that each post hoc test should use the *same critical value* as the original test based on all of the studies of the meta-analysis.

As an example of the test of homogeneity for a particular characteristic, consider criterion 6 of Table 15-5. The 15 studies can be divided into two groups. Clients in studies 1, 2, 3, 5, 6, 7, 8, 10, 14, and 15 were given information about their particular treatment. The homogeneity statistic for these 10 studies is given as $U = 57.13$, which is considerably larger than the critical value of 23.68. For these 10 studies, the treatment effect is given as $\hat{\delta} = 0.75$. The most likely reason for the rejection of the hypothesis of homogeneity is that studies 1, 5, and 6 have very large treatment effects relative to the remaining 7 studies. For the 5 studies, 4, 9, 11, 12, and 13, in which clients were not given information about the precise nature of the treatment, the homogeneity statistic is given as $U = 2.09$. This value is well below the critical

TABLE 15-6 EVALUATIONS OF 9 CRITERION SUBSTANTIVE INDICES USED TO JUDGE THE 15 PAIN STUDIES OF TABLE 15-1

Study	1	2	3	4	5	6	7	8	9
1	L	U	C, E	A	H	C	35/4	< 45*	A
2	L	U	A, E	A	H	C	20/7	< 45*	A
3	L	B	C, D, E	A, B	H	C, D	NK/NK	NK	A
4	L	U	A, E	A	M	C	14/7	< 45*	A
5	S	O	C, E, F	A	H	A, C, E	0/40	NK	A
6	L	U	D, E	B	M	C	30/2	< 45*	B
7	L	U	F	A	H	C	55/46	< 45*	A
8	L	O	C, E	B, C	M	A, C	1/42	> 45*	B
9	S	U	C, E	A	L	A	NK/NK	< 45*	B, D
10	L	B	A	A	H	C, D	10/10	> 45*	B
11	L	U	A	A	M	E	NK/NK	NK	D
12	S	S	D, E	A	H	D, E	55/9	NK/NK	D
13	S	S	B, E, F	A	M	A	27/13	> 45*	C
14	S	O	C, D, E	A	M	A, D	0/36	> 45*†	A, B
15	L	B	C, E	B	H	C, D	33/3	< 45*	B

NOTE. See text for explanation of each variable.
Variable 1—Long-term(L), short-term(S)
Variable 2—Upper torso(U), back(B), orthopedic(O), surgical(S)
Variable 3—Biofeedback(A), hypnosis(B), imagery/visualization(C), information/instruction(D), relaxation(E), other(F)
Variable 4—Individual(A), group(B), with spouse(C), other(D)
Variable 5—High(H), medium(M), low(L)
Variable 6—Observer ratings(A), psychosocial(B), subjective self-report(C), standardized self-report(D), other(E)
Variable 7—Gender, number of females to number of males
Variable 8—Mean age (*), median age (†)
Variable 9—Placebo(A), waiting list(B), traditional(C), other(D)

value of 23.68. For these 5 studies, the treatment effect is given as $\hat{\delta} = 0.37$.

In practice, tests of homogeneity would be made for all of the groupings suggested in Tables 15-5 and 15-6. Treatment effects would be estimated from all sets of studies that were homogeneous and conceptually related to one another, as indicated by the classifications of Tables 15-5 and 15-6. The total set of findings would constitute the basis for the report.

15-11 COMPARISONS WITHIN STUDIES

The treatment effects reported for each study of Table 15-1 are based on pooling treatment effects within studies. Of course, the pooling is justified only if the treatment effects are not statistically different from one another. Thus, the meta-analyst should test the hypothesis of homogeneity of treatment

effects within each study before attempting to pool across studies. Unfortunately, this is a very difficult problem and is not solvable in most situations. As stated before, many authors do not provide the necessary correlation coefficients. One way around the problem is to replace each correlation coefficient with $\bar{r} = 0.50$ and then perform a pairwise multiple comparison test similar to that of Tukey's test for sample means across the treatment effects. The test statistic is given as

$$Z = \frac{\hat{\delta}_L - \hat{\delta}_S}{SE(\hat{\delta}_L - \hat{\delta}_S)}$$

where $\hat{\delta}_L$ and $\hat{\delta}_S$ are the largest and smallest treatment effects and where the equation at the bottom of this page applies.

The hypothesis,

$$H : \delta_1 = \delta_2 = \ldots = \delta_K$$

is rejected if $Z < Z_L$ or if $Z > Z_U$. The critical values are read from Table A-8 with

$$SE^2(\hat{\delta}_L - \hat{\delta}_S) = SE^2(\hat{\delta}_L) + SE^2(\hat{\delta}_S) - SE(\hat{\delta}_L)SE(\hat{\delta}_S)$$

$C = \binom{K}{2}$ and $\alpha = 0.05$ or 0.01. For the data of Table 15–3

$$\hat{\delta}_L = 1.98, \hat{\delta}_S = 0.64$$

$$SE^2(\hat{\delta}_L) = 0.2289$$

and

$$SE^2(\hat{\delta}_S) = 0.1615$$

so that

$$Z = \frac{1.98 - 0.64}{\sqrt{0.2289 + 0.1615 - (0.4784)(0.4019)}}$$

$$= \frac{1.34}{0.4451}$$

$$= 3.01$$

Because $K = 8$, the number of pairwise comparisons is given as $C = 28$. With $\alpha = 0.05$, critical values read from the last column of Table A–8 are given as $Z_L = -3.12$ and $Z_U = +3.12$. Thus, it is concluded that the treatment effects can be pooled.

Other tests exist for testing this hypothesis. They are described by Hedges and Olkin (1985). For the omnibus test they describe, the critical values for a post hoc analysis are given as

$$S = \pm \sqrt{\chi^2_{(K-1):(1-\alpha)}}$$

For $K = 8$ and $\alpha = 0.05$,

$$S = \pm \sqrt{15.51} = \pm 3.92$$

With these critical values, even the largest pairwise difference is not statistically different from zero.

15–12 BIAS IN THE ESTIMATION OF TREATMENT EFFECTS

Hedges and Olkin (1985) have shown that the sample treatment effect provides a biased estimate of the population value. In addition, they have provided correction factors for removing the bias, which are reported in Table 15–7. The numbers in this table, $J(m)$, are used to correct for bias. Table 15–7 is entered with the index $m = N - 2$, where N is the total sample size. In terms of $J(m)$,

TABLE 15–7 EXACT VALUES OF THE BIAS CORRECTION FACTOR J(m)

m	J(m)	m	J(m)
2	0.5642	17	0.9551
3	0.7236	18	0.9577
4	0.7979	19	0.9599
5	0.8408	20	0.9619
6	0.8686	21	0.9638
7	0.8882	22	0.9655
8	0.9027	23	0.9670
9	0.9139	24	0.9684
10	0.9228	25	0.9699
11	0.9300	26	0.9708
12	0.9359	27	0.9719
13	0.9410	28	0.9728
14	0.9453	29	0.9739
15	0.9490	30	0.9748
16	0.9523	40	0.9811
		50	0.9849
		100	0.9925

Abstracted from Table 2 of Hedges, L. V., and Olkin, I.: *Statistical Method for Meta-Analysis*, p. 80. Orlando, FL, Academic Press, 1985. By permission of the author.

the correction for bias treatment effect is given as

$$\hat{\delta}_C = J(m)\hat{\delta}$$

In general, the bias is not corrected if the total sample sizes exceed 20. However, for completeness the method is illustrated for the first row of values in Table 15–3. For these data $\hat{\delta} = 1.34$. In this case $N = 13 + 13 = 26$, so that $m = 26 - 2 = 24$. With this value the correction for bias is given as

$$J(m) = 0.9684$$

so that the unbiased estimate of the treatment effect is

$$\hat{\delta}_C = (0.9684)(1.34) = 1.30$$

As indicated, the correction for bias has a minimal effect on the estimation of the population treatment effect. It should be noted that the standard error also is affected by small sample sizes. For the unbiased estimate of the treatment effect, the corresponding standard error is given as

$$SE(\hat{\delta}_C) = J(m)SE(\hat{\delta})$$
$$= (0.9684)(0.4337)$$
$$= 0.4200$$

These corrected values would be used in all the formulas presented in the previous sections of this chapter. Because the corrections generally are small, they were not included in the examples presented.

15–13 SUMMARY

In this chapter the basic statistical procedures required for meta-analysis were presented. From the point of view presented in this chapter, meta-analysis is an analysis of studies and a way to combine information across studies bearing on a single research hypothesis. The typical meta-analysis begins with an exhaustive search of the literature for all published journal articles, technical reports, doctoral dissertations, and masters' theses. After the articles are collected, they are examined to determine the appropriateness for inclusion in the meta-analytic study. In the critical review of these studies, the investigator establishes a typology of methodological criteria and substantive dimensions. The review is performed in light of the overall general hypotheses tested within the full collection of retained manuscripts. These classifications are used for a priori or post hoc comparisons across studies.

The statistical analysis begins with a manuscript by manuscript summarization of the findings in terms of treatment effects and standard errors. This process was described and illustrated in this chapter. In most situations, each manuscript gives rise to more than one treatment effect because studies rarely involve only one dependent measure. Because of this, each investigator has to call upon specialized knowledge of the field and of the theories on which the research is based in order to make informed decisions about the grouping of studies.

Upon completion of the analysis within each manuscript, the investigator embarks upon the main purposes of the study and tests for homogeneity of treatment effects across all the studies included in the meta-analysis. This procedure was described in Section 15–7. The hypothesis of homogeneity is rejected if $U > \chi^2_{(K-1):(1-\alpha)}$. In most meta-analytic studies, the hypothesis of homogeneity is rejected. When this happens, post hoc comparisons should be made to determine which studies may be pooled together to provide multiple estimates of the treatment effect (see Section 15–9).

Upon completion of the latter analysis, use is made of various classifications of the manuscripts. Tests of homogeneity are performed on manuscripts with common characteristics. If the hypothesis of homogeneity is not rejected, a single measure of treatment effect is obtained. But if the hypothesis is rejected, post hoc comparisons are made with the purpose of dividing the manuscripts into disjointed but homogeneous sets. The critical value for all post hoc tests is also given by the critical value used for the omnibus test of homogeneity,

$$S = \pm\sqrt{\chi^2_{(K-1):(1-\alpha)}}$$

From these analyses, a final research report is prepared.

Other aspects of meta-analysis were considered. If sample sizes are small, estimates of treatment effects are biased. Directions were provided on correcting for the bias. Also, the most rudimentary form of meta-analysis, vote counting, was described. This method can be used when all studies are simply classified as providing a significant or nonsignificant treatment effect.

As a final comment for the nurse researcher, the carrying out of a meta-analysis is not easy. In most situations, expert advice and discerning counsel is mandatory. In this chapter, the basic tools that should help one get started on this exciting and imaginative research strategy have been described and illustrated.

REFERENCES

Brown, J.M.: Imagery coping strategies in the treatment of migraine, Pain, 18: 157–167, 1984.

Cox, D.J., Freundlich, A., and Meyer, R.G.: Differential effectiveness of electromyograph feedback, verbal relaxation instructions, and medication placebo with tension headaches, J. Consult. Clin. Psychol., 43: 892–898, 1975.

Devine, E.C., and Cook, T.D.: A meta-analysis of effects of psychoeducational interventions on length of post surgical hospital stay, Nurs. Res., 32: 267–274, 1983.

Engstrom, D.: Cognitive behavioral therapy methods in chronic pain treatment. In Bonica, J.J., ed.: Advances in Pain Research and Therapy. New York, Raven Press, 829–835, 1983.

Gedden, E., Beck, N., Hauge, G., and Pohlman, S.: Self-reports and psychophysiological effects of five pain-coping strategies, Nurs. Res., 33: 260–265, 1984.

Glass, G.V.: Primary, secondary, and meta-analysis of research, Ed. Res., 5: 3–8, 1976.

Glass, G.V., McGaw, B., and Smith, M.L.: Meta-analysis in Social Research. Beverly Hills, CA, Sage Publications, 1981.

Hathaway, D.: Effects of preoperative instruction in postoperative outcomes: a meta-analysis, Nurs. Res., 35: 269–275. 1986.

Haynes, S.N., Griffin, P., Mooney, D., and Parise, M.: Electromyographic biofeedback and relaxation instructions in the treatment of muscle contraction headaches, Behav. Ther., 6: 672–678, 1975.

Hedges, L.V., and Olkin, I.: Statistical Methods for Meta-analysis. Orlando, FL, Academic Press, 1985.

Kaplan, R.M., Metzger, G., and Jablecki, C.: Brief cognitive and relaxation training increases tolerance for a painful clinical electromyographic examination, Psychosom. Med., 46: 155–162, 1983.

Larsson, B., and Melin, L.: Chronic headaches in adolescents: Treatment in a school setting with relaxation training as compared with information-contact and self-regulation, Pain, 25: 325–336, 1986.

Light, R.J., and Smith, P.V.: Accumulating evidence: procedures for resolving contradictions among different research studies, Harvard Ed. Rev., 41: 429–471, 1971.

Lin, J.C., Singleton, G.W., Schaeffer, J.N., et al.: Geophysical variables and behavior: XXVII. Magnetic Necklace: Its therapeutic effectiveness on neck and shoulder pain: 2. Psychological assessment, Psychol. Rep., 56: 639–649, 1985.

Malone, M.D., and Strube, M.J.: Meta-analysis of nonmedical treatments for chronic pain, Pain, 34: 231–244, 1988.

Marascuilo, L.A., Busk, P.L., and Serlin, R.C.: Large sample multivariate procedures for comparing and combining effect sizes within a single study, J. Exp. Ed., 57: 69–85, 1988.

Moore, J.E., and Chaney, E.F.: Outpatient group treatment of chronic pain: effects of spouse involvement, J. Consult. Clin. Psychol., 53: 326–334, 1985.

Nocella, J., and Kaplan, R.: Training children to cope with dental treatment, J. Pediat. Psychol., 7: 175–178, 1982.

Nouwen, A.: EMG biofeedback used to reduce standing levels of paraspinal muscle tension in chronic low back pain, Pain, 17: 353–360, 1983.

Philips, C.: The modification of tension headache pain using EMG biofeedback, Behav. Res. Ther., 15: 118–129, 1977.

Scott, L.E., and Clum, G.A.: Examining the interaction effects of coping style and brief interventions in the treatment of postsurgical pain, Pain, 20: 279–291, 1984.

Smith, M.L., and Glass, G.V.: Meta-analysis of psychotherapy outcome studies, Am. Psychol., 32: 752–760, 1977.

Surman, O.S., Hackett, T.P., Silverberg, E.L., and Behrendt, D.M.: Usefulness of psychiatric interventions in patients undergoing cardiac surgery, Arch. Gen. Psychiatry, 30: 830–835, 1974.

Tan, S.Y., and Poser, E.G.: Acute pain in a clinical setting: Effects of cognitive-behavioral skills training, Behav. Res. Ther., 20: 535–545, 1982.

Turner, J.A.: Comparison of group progressive-relaxation training and cognitive-behavioral group therapy for chronic low back pain, J. Consulting Clin. Psychol., 50: 757–765, 1982.

APPENDICES

TABLE A–1   CRITICAL VALUES OF THE CHI-SQUARE DISTRIBUTION

df	$P_{.005}$	$P_{.01}$	$P_{.025}$	$P_{.05}$	$P_{.10}$	$P_{.90}$	$P_{.95}$	$P_{.97.5}$	$P_{.99}$	$P_{.99.5}$
1	0.000039	0.00016	0.00098	0.0039	0.0158	2.71	3.84	5.02	6.63	7.88
2	0.0100	0.0201	0.0506	0.1026	0.2107	4.61	5.99	7.38	9.21	10.60
3	0.0717	0.115	0.216	0.352	0.584	6.25	7.81	9.35	11.34	12.84
4	0.207	0.297	0.484	0.711	1.064	7.78	9.49	11.14	13.28	14.86
5	0.412	0.554	0.831	1.15	1.61	9.24	11.07	12.83	15.09	16.75
6	0.676	0.872	1.24	1.64	2.20	10.64	12.59	14.45	16.81	18.55
7	0.989	1.24	1.69	2.17	2.83	12.02	14.07	16.01	18.48	20.28
8	1.34	1.65	2.18	2.73	3.49	13.36	15.51	17.53	20.09	21.95
9	1.73	2.09	2.70	3.33	4.17	14.68	16.92	19.02	21.67	23.59
10	2.16	2.56	3.25	3.94	4.87	15.99	18.31	20.48	23.21	25.19
11	2.60	3.05	3.82	4.57	5.58	17.28	19.68	21.92	24.72	26.76
12	3.07	3.57	4.40	5.23	6.30	18.55	21.03	23.34	26.22	28.30
13	3.57	4.11	5.01	5.89	7.04	19.81	22.36	24.74	27.69	29.82
14	4.07	4.66	5.63	6.57	7.79	21.06	23.68	26.12	29.14	31.32
15	4.60	5.23	6.26	7.26	8.55	22.31	25.00	27.49	30.58	32.80
16	5.14	5.81	6.91	7.96	9.31	23.54	26.30	28.85	32.00	34.27
18	6.26	7.01	8.23	9.39	10.86	25.99	28.87	31.53	34.81	37.16
20	7.43	8.26	9.59	10.85	12.44	28.41	31.41	34.17	37.57	40.00
24	9.89	10.86	12.40	13.85	15.66	33.20	36.42	39.36	42.98	45.56
30	13.79	14.95	16.79	18.49	20.60	40.26	43.77	46.98	50.89	53.67
40	20.71	22.16	24.43	26.51	29.05	51.81	55.76	59.34	63.69	66.77
60	35.53	37.48	40.48	43.19	46.46	74.40	79.08	83.30	88.38	91.95
120	83.85	86.92	91.57	95.70	100.62	140.23	146.57	152.21	158.95	163.65

From Dixon, W. J., and Massey, Jr., F. J.: Introduction to Statistical Analysis, ed. 3. New York, McGraw-Hill, Inc., 1969. Used with permission of McGraw-Hill Book Company.

TABLE A–2 CRITICAL VALUES OF THE WALD-WOLFOWITZ RUN TEST

N_1	N_2	$w_{.005}$	$w_{.01}$	$w_{.025}$	$w_{.05}$	$w_{.10}$	$w_{.90}$	$w_{.95}$	$w_{.975}$	$w_{.9}$	$w_{.995}$
2	5	—	—	—	—	3	—	—	—	—	—
	8	—	—	—	3	3	—	—	—	—	—
	11	—	—	—	3	3	—	—	—	—	—
	14	—	—	3	3	3	—	—	—	—	—
	17	—	—	3	3	3	—	—	—	—	—
	20	—	3	3	3	4	—	—	—	—	—
5	5	—	3	3	4	4	8	8	9	9	—
	8	3	3	4	4	5	9	10	10	—	—
	11	4	4	5	5	6	10	—	—	—	—
	14	4	4	5	6	6	—	—	—	—	—
	17	4	5	5	6	7	—	—	—	—	—
	20	5	5	6	6	7	—	—	—	—	—
8	8	4	5	5	6	6	12	12	13	13	14
	11	5	6	6	7	8	13	14	14	15	15
	14	6	6	7	8	8	14	15	15	16	16
	17	6	7	8	8	9	15	15	16	—	—
	20	7	7	8	9	10	15	16	16	—	—
11	11	6	7	8	8	9	15	16	16	17	18
	14	7	8	9	9	10	16	17	18	19	19
	17	8	9	10	10	11	17	18	19	20	21
	20	9	9	10	11	12	18	19	20	21	21
14	14	8	9	10	11	12	18	19	20	21	22
	17	9	10	11	12	13	20	21	22	23	23
	20	10	11	12	13	14	21	22	23	24	24
17	17	11	11	12	13	14	22	23	24	25	25
	20	12	12	14	14	16	23	24	25	26	27
20	20	13	14	15	16	17	25	26	27	28	29

For n or m greater than 20, the quantile w_p of T may be approximated by

$$w_p = \frac{2mn}{m+n} + 1 + x_p \sqrt{\frac{2mn(2mn - m - n)}{(m+n)^2(m+n-1)}}$$

where x_p is the p quantile of a standard normal random variable. The entries in this table are quantiles w_p of the Wald-Wolfowitz test statistic T. To enter the table let N_1 be the smaller sample size and N_2 the larger. If the exact values of N_1 and N_2 are not listed below, use the nearest values given as an approximation. This approximation will be exact in most cases. Reject H_0 at the level α if T is less than w_α (or greater than $w_{1-\alpha}$) for the one-tailed test, or, in the two-tailed test, if either $T < w_{\alpha/2}$ or $T > w_{1-\alpha/2}$. The test statistic is discrete, so the exact α will be less than or equal to the apparent α used in the test. For sample sizes greater than 20, the normal approximation given at the end of the tables may be used.

TABLE A-3 CRITICAL VALUES OF THE GRUBBS TEST

Number of observations n	5% Significance level	2.5% Significance level	1% Significance level
3	1.15	1.15	1.15
4	1.46	1.48	1.49
5	1.67	1.71	1.75
6	1.82	1.89	1.94
7	1.94	2.02	2.10
8	2.03	2.13	2.22
9	2.11	2.21	2.32
10	2.18	2.29	2.41
11	2.23	2.36	2.48
12	2.29	2.41	2.55
13	2.33	2.46	2.61
14	2.37	2.51	2.66
15	2.41	2.55	2.71
16	2.44	2.59	2.75
17	2.47	2.62	2.79
18	2.50	2.65	2.82
19	2.53	2.68	2.85
20	2.56	2.71	2.88
21	2.58	2.73	2.91
22	2.60	2.76	2.94
23	2.62	2.78	2.96
24	2.64	2.80	2.99
25	2.66	2.82	3.01
30	2.75	2.91	
35	2.82	2.98	
40	2.87	3.04	
45	2.92	3.09	
50	2.96	3.13	
60	3.03	3.20	
70	3.09	3.26	
80	3.14	3.31	
90	3.18	3.35	
100	3.21	3.38	

$$T_n = \frac{x_n - \bar{x}}{s} \qquad s = \left\{ \frac{\sum (x_i - \bar{x})^2}{n - 1} \right\}^{\frac{1}{2}}$$

$$= \left\{ \frac{n \sum x_i^2 - (\sum x_i)^2}{n(n - 1)} \right\}^{\frac{1}{2}}$$

$$T_1 = \frac{\bar{x} - x_1}{s} \qquad x_1 \leqslant x_2 \leqslant \cdots \leqslant x_n$$

For $n > 25$, the values of T are approximated. All values have been adjusted for division by $n - 1$ instead of n in calculating s.

By permission from *Technometrics* and Dr. Frank E. Grubbs, in *Technometrics*, February 1969.

TABLE A–4 RANDOM NORMAL DEVIATIONS

01	02	03	04	05	06	07	08	09	10
0.464	0.137	2.455	−0.323	−0.068	0.296	−0.288	1.298	0.241	−0.957
0.060	−2.526	−0.531	−0.194	0.543	−1.558	0.187	−1.190	0.022	0.525
1.486	−0.354	−0.634	0.697	0.926	1.375	0.785	−0.963	−0.853	−1.865
1.022	−0.472	1.279	3.521	0.571	−1.851	0.194	1.192	−0.501	−0.273
1.394	−0.555	0.046	0.321	2.945	1.974	−0.258	0.412	0.439	−0.035
0.906	−0.513	−0.525	0 595	0.881	−0.934	1.579	0.161	−1.885	0.371
1.179	−1.055	0.007	0.769	0.971	0.712	1.090	−0.631	−0.255	−0.702
−1.501	−0.488	−0.162	−0.136	1.033	0.203	0.448	0.748	−0.423	−0.432
−0.690	0.756	−1.618	−0.345	−0.511	−2.051	−0.457	−0.218	0.857	−0.465
1.372	0.225	0.378	0.761	0.181	−0.736	0.960	−1.530	−0.260	0.120
−0.482	1.678	−0.057	−1.229	−0.486	0.856	−0.491	−1.983	−2.830	−0.238
−1.376	−0.150	1.356	−0.561	−0.256	−0.212	0.219	0.779	0.953	−0.869
−1.010	0.598	−0.918	1.598	0.065	0.415	−0.169	0.313	−0.973	−1.016
−0.005	−0.899	0.012	−0.725	1.147	−0.121	1.096	0.481	−1.691	0.417
1.393	−1.163	−0.911	1.231	−0.199	−0.246	1.239	−2.574	−0.558	0.056
−1.787	−0.261	1.237	1.046	−0.508	−1.630	−0.146	−0.392	−0.627	0.561
−0.105	−0.357	−1.384	0.360	−0.992	−0.116	−1.698	−2.832	−1.108	−2.357
−1.339	1.827	−0.959	0.424	0.969	−1.141	−1.041	0.362	−1.726	1.956
1.041	0.535	0.731	1.377	0.983	−1.330	1.620	−1.040	0.524	−0.281
0.279	−2.056	0.717	−0.873	−1.096	−1.396	1.047	0.089	−0.573	0.932
−1.805	−2.008	−1.633	0.542	0.250	−0.166	0.032	0.079	0.471	−1.029
−1.186	1.180	1.114	0.882	1.265	−0.202	0.151	−0.376	−0.310	0.479
0.658	−1.141	1.151	−1.210	−0.927	0.425	0.290	−0.902	0.610	2.709
−0.439	0.358	−1.939	0.891	−0.227	0.602	0.873	−0.437	−0.220	−0.057
−1.399	−0.230	0.385	−0.649	−0.577	0.237	−0.289	0.513	0.738	−0.300
0.199	0.208	−1.083	−0.219	−0.291	1.221	1.119	0.004	−2.015	−0.594
0.159	0.272	−0.313	0.084	−2.828	−0.439	−0.792	−1.275	−0.623	−1.047
2.273	0.606	0.606	−0.747	0.247	1.291	0.063	−1.793	−0.699	−1.347
0.041	−0.307	0.121	0.790	−0.584	0.541	0.484	−0.986	0.481	0.996
−1.132	−2.098	0.921	0.145	0.446	−1.661	1.045	−1.363	−0.586	−1.023
0.768	0.079	−1.473	0.034	−2.127	0.665	0.084	−0.880	−0.579	0.551
0.375	−1.658	−0.851	0.234	−0.656	0.340	−0.086	−0.158	−0.120	0.418
−0.513	−0.344	0.210	−0.736	1.041	0.008	0.427	−0.831	0.191	0.074
0.292	−0.521	1.266	−1.206	−0.899	0.110	−0.528	−0.813	0.071	0.524
1.026	2.990	−0.574	−0.491	−1.114	1.297	−1.433	−1.345	−3.001	0.479
−1.334	1.278	−0.568	−0.109	−0.515	−0.566	2.923	0.500	0.359	0.326
−0.287	−0.144	−0.254	0.574	−0.451	−1.181	−1.190	−0.318	−0.094	1.114
0.161	−0.886	−0.921	−0.509	1.410	−0.518	0.192	−0.432	1.501	1.068
−1.346	0.193	−1.202	0.394	−1.045	0.843	0.942	1.045	0.031	0.772
1.250	−0.199	−0.288	1.810	1.378	0.584	1.216	0.733	0.402	0.226
0.630	−0.537	0.782	0.060	0.499	−0.431	1.705	1.164	0.884	−0.298
0.375	−1.941	0.247	−0.491	0.665	−0.135	−0.145	−0.498	0.457	1.064
−1.420	0.489	−1.711	−1.186	0.754	−0.732	−0.066	1.006	−0.798	0.162
−0.151	−0.243	−0.430	−0.762	0.298	1.049	1.810	2.885	−0.768	−0.129
−0.309	0.531	0.416	−1.541	1.456	2.040	−0.124	0.196	0.023	−1.204
0.424	−0.444	0.593	0.993	−0.106	0.116	0.484	−1.272	1.066	1.097
0.593	0.658	−1.127	−1.407	−1.579	−1.616	1.458	1.262	0.736	−0.916
0.862	−0.885	−0.142	−0.504	0.532	1.381	0.022	−0.281	−0.342	1.222
0.235	−0.628	−0.023	−0.463	−0.899	−0.394	−0.538	1.707	−0.188	−1.153
−0.853	0.402	0.777	0.833	0.410	−0.349	−1.094	0.580	1.395	1.298

From tables of the RAND Corporation, by permission.

TABLE A–5 CRITICAL VALUES OF THE STANDARD NORMAL DISTRIBUTION

Z	Y	Cumulative probability
−3.25	$\mu - 3.25\sigma$	.0006
−3.20	$\mu - 3.20\sigma$	.0007
−3.15	$\mu - 3.15\sigma$	.0008
−3.10	$\mu - 3.10\sigma$	.0010
−3.05	$\mu - 3.05\sigma$	.0011
−3.00	$\mu - 3.00\sigma$	.0013
−2.95	$\mu - 2.95\sigma$	.0016
−2.90	$\mu - 2.90\sigma$	.0019
−2.85	$\mu - 2.85\sigma$	.0022
−2.80	$\mu - 2.80\sigma$	.0026
−2.75	$\mu - 2.75\sigma$	.0030
−2.70	$\mu - 2.70\sigma$	.0035
−2.65	$\mu - 2.65\sigma$	.0040
−2.60	$\mu - 2.60\sigma$	.0047
−2.55	$\mu - 2.55\sigma$	.0054
−2.50	$\mu - 2.50\sigma$	.0062
−2.45	$\mu - 2.45\sigma$	.0071
−2.40	$\mu - 2.40\sigma$	.0082
−2.35	$\mu - 2.35\sigma$	.0094
−2.30	$\mu - 2.30\sigma$	.0107
−2.25	$\mu - 2.25\sigma$	.0122
−2.20	$\mu - 2.20\sigma$	.0139
−2.15	$\mu - 2.15\sigma$	.0158
−2.10	$\mu - 2.10\sigma$	.0179
−2.05	$\mu - 2.05\sigma$	.0202
−2.00	$\mu - 2.00\sigma$	.0228
−1.95	$\mu - 1.95\sigma$	.0256
−1.90	$\mu - 1.90\sigma$	.0287
−1.85	$\mu - 1.85\sigma$	.0322
−1.80	$\mu - 1.80\sigma$	.0359
−1.75	$\mu - 1.75\sigma$	.0401
−1.70	$\mu - 1.70\sigma$	.0446
−1.65	$\mu - 1.65\sigma$	.0495
−1.60	$\mu - 1.60\sigma$	.0548
−1.55	$\mu - 1.55\sigma$	.0606
−1.50	$\mu - 1.50\sigma$	.0668
−1.45	$\mu - 1.45\sigma$	.0735
−1.40	$\mu - 1.40\sigma$	.0808
−1.35	$\mu - 1.35\sigma$	.0885
−1.30	$\mu - 1.30\sigma$	.0968
−1.25	$\mu - 1.25\sigma$	.1056
−1.20	$\mu - 1.20\sigma$	.1151
−1.15	$\mu - 1.15\sigma$	.1251
−1.10	$\mu - 1.10\sigma$	.1357
−1.05	$\mu - 1.05\sigma$	.1469
−1.00	$\mu - 1.00\sigma$	.1587
−0.95	$\mu - 0.95\sigma$	.1711
−0.90	$\mu - 0.90\sigma$	.1841
−0.85	$\mu - 0.85\sigma$	.1977
−0.80	$\mu - 0.80\sigma$	.2119
−0.75	$\mu - 0.75\sigma$	.2266
−0.70	$\mu - 0.70\sigma$	.2420

Table continued on the following page

TABLE A–5 *Continued*

Z	Y	Cumulative probability
−0.65	$\mu - 0.65\sigma$	.2578
−0.60	$\mu - 0.60\sigma$	.2743
−0.55	$\mu - 0.55\sigma$	.2912
−0.50	$\mu - 0.50\sigma$	.3085
−0.45	$\mu - 0.45\sigma$	.3264
−0.40	$\mu - 0.40\sigma$	.3446
−0.35	$\mu - 0.35\sigma$	.3632
−0.30	$\mu - 0.30\sigma$	.3821
−0.25	$\mu - 0.25\sigma$	.4013
−0.20	$\mu - 0.20\sigma$	.4207
−0.15	$\mu - 0.15\sigma$	.4404
−0.10	$\mu - 0.10\sigma$	.4602
−0.05	$\mu - 0.05\sigma$	.4801
0.00	μ	.5000
0.05	$\mu + 0.05\sigma$	.5199
0.10	$\mu + 0.10\sigma$	.5398
0.15	$\mu + 0.15\sigma$	.5596
0.20	$\mu + 0.20\sigma$	.5793
0.25	$\mu + 0.25\sigma$	.5987
0.30	$\mu + 0.30\sigma$	.6179
0.35	$\mu + 0.35\sigma$	.6368
0.40	$\mu + 0.40\sigma$	.6554
0.45	$\mu + 0.45\sigma$	.6736
0.50	$\mu + 0.50\sigma$	.6915
0.55	$\mu + 0.55\sigma$	.7088
0.60	$\mu + 0.60\sigma$	.7257
0.65	$\mu + 0.65\sigma$	.7422
0.70	$\mu + 0.70\sigma$	.7580
0.75	$\mu + 0.75\sigma$	.7734
0.80	$\mu + 0.80\sigma$	.7881
0.85	$\mu + 0.85\sigma$	.8023
0.90	$\mu + 0.90\sigma$	.8159
0.95	$\mu + 0.95\sigma$	.8289
1.00	$\mu + 1.00\sigma$	.8413
1.05	$\mu + 1.05\sigma$	.8531
1.10	$\mu + 1.10\sigma$	.8643
1.15	$\mu + 1.15\sigma$	.8749
1.20	$\mu + 1.20\sigma$	.8849
1.25	$\mu + 1.25\sigma$	.8944
1.30	$\mu + 1.30\sigma$	.9032

TABLE A–5 *Continued*

Z	Y	Cumulative probability
1.35	$\mu + 1.35\sigma$	.9115
1.40	$\mu + 1.40\sigma$	.9192
1.45	$\mu + 1.45\sigma$	.9265
1.50	$\mu + 1.50\sigma$	.9332
1.55	$\mu + 1.55\sigma$	.9394
1.60	$\mu + 1.60\sigma$	.9452
1.65	$\mu + 1.65\sigma$	.9505
1.70	$\mu + 1.70\sigma$	.9554
1.75	$\mu + 1.75\sigma$	.9599
1.80	$\mu + 1.80\sigma$	.9641
1.85	$\mu + 1.85\sigma$	.9678
1.90	$\mu + 1.90\sigma$	.9713
1.95	$\mu + 1.95\sigma$	.9744
2.00	$\mu + 2.00\sigma$	.9772
2.05	$\mu + 2.05\sigma$	.9798
2.10	$\mu + 2.10\sigma$	.9821
2.15	$\mu + 2.15\sigma$	.9842
2.20	$\mu + 2.20\sigma$	.9861
2.25	$\mu + 2.25\sigma$	.9878
2.30	$\mu + 2.30\sigma$	.9893
2.35	$\mu + 2.35\sigma$	.9906
2.40	$\mu + 2.40\sigma$	.9918
2.45	$\mu + 2.45\sigma$	.9929
2.50	$\mu + 2.50\sigma$	.9938
2.55	$\mu + 2.55\sigma$	.9946
2.60	$\mu + 2.60\sigma$	.9953
2.65	$\mu + 2.65\sigma$	.9960
2.70	$\mu + 2.70\sigma$	.9965
2.75	$\mu + 2.75\sigma$	.9970
2.80	$\mu + 2.80\sigma$	.9974
2.85	$\mu + 2.85\sigma$	.9978
2.90	$\mu + 2.90\sigma$	.9981
2.95	$\mu + 2.95\sigma$	.9984
3.00	$\mu + 3.00\sigma$	.9987
3.05	$\mu + 3.05\sigma$	.9989
3.10	$\mu + 3.10\sigma$	.9990
3.15	$\mu + 3.15\sigma$	.9992
3.20	$\mu + 3.20\sigma$	.9993
3.25	$\mu + 3.25\sigma$	.9994

TABLE A-6 CRITICAL VALUES OF THE t DISTRIBUTION

df	.005	.01	.025	.05	.10	.90	.95	.975	.99	.995
1	−63.657	−31.821	−12.706	−6.314	−3.078	3.078	6.314	12.706	31.821	63.657
2	−9.925	−6.965	−4.303	−2.920	−1.886	1.886	2.920	4.303	6.965	9.925
3	−5.841	−4.541	−3.182	−2.353	−1.638	1.638	2.353	3.182	4.541	5.841
4	−4.604	−3.747	−2.776	−2.132	−1.533	1.533	2.132	2.776	3.747	4.604
5	−4.032	−3.365	−2.571	−2.015	−1.476	1.476	2.015	2.571	3.365	4.032
6	−3.707	−3.143	−2.447	−1.943	−1.440	1.440	1.943	2.447	3.143	3.707
7	−3.499	−2.998	−2.365	−1.895	−1.415	1.415	1.895	2.365	2.998	3.499
8	−3.355	−2.896	−2.306	−1.860	−1.397	1.397	1.860	2.306	2.896	3.355
9	−3.250	−2.821	−2.262	−1.833	−1.383	1.383	1.833	2.262	2.821	3.250
10	−3.169	−2.764	−2.228	−1.812	−1.372	1.372	1.812	2.228	2.764	3.169
11	−3.106	−2.718	−2.201	−1.796	−1.363	1.363	1.796	2.201	2.718	3.106
12	−3.055	−2.681	−2.179	−1.782	−1.356	1.356	1.782	2.179	2.681	3.055
13	−3.012	−2.650	−2.160	−1.771	−1.350	1.350	1.771	2.160	2.650	3.012
14	−2.977	−2.624	−2.145	−1.761	−1.345	1.345	1.761	2.145	2.624	2.977
15	−2.947	−2.602	−2.131	−1.753	−1.341	1.341	1.753	2.131	2.602	2.947
16	−2.921	−2.583	−2.120	−1.746	−1.337	1.337	1.746	2.120	2.583	2.921
17	−2.898	−2.567	−2.110	−1.740	−1.333	1.333	1.740	2.110	2.567	2.898
18	−2.878	−2.552	−2.101	−1.734	−1.330	1.330	1.734	2.101	2.552	2.878
19	−2.861	−2.539	−2.093	−1.729	−1.328	1.328	1.729	2.093	2.539	2.861
20	−2.845	−2.528	−2.086	−1.725	−1.325	1.325	1.725	2.086	2.528	2.845
21	−2.831	−2.518	−2.080	−1.721	−1.323	1.323	1.721	2.080	2.518	2.831
22	−2.819	−2.508	−2.074	−1.717	−1.321	1.321	1.717	2.074	2.508	2.819
23	−2.807	−2.500	−2.069	−1.714	−1.319	1.319	1.714	2.069	2.500	2.807
24	−2.797	−2.492	−2.064	−1.711	−1.318	1.318	1.711	2.064	2.492	2.797
25	−2.787	−2.485	−2.060	−1.708	−1.316	1.316	1.708	2.060	2.485	2.787
26	−2.779	−2.479	−2.056	−1.706	−1.315	1.315	1.706	2.056	2.479	2.779
27	−2.771	−2.473	−2.052	−1.703	−1.314	1.314	1.703	2.052	2.473	2.771
28	−2.763	−2.467	−2.048	−1.701	−1.313	1.313	1.701	2.048	2.467	2.763
29	−2.756	−2.462	−2.045	−1.699	−1.311	1.311	1.699	2.045	2.462	2.756
30	−2.750	−2.457	−2.042	−1.697	−1.310	1.310	1.697	2.042	2.457	2.750
40	−2.704	−2.423	−2.021	−1.684	−1.303	1.303	1.684	2.021	2.423	2.704
60	−2.660	−2.390	−2.000	−1.671	−1.296	1.296	1.671	2.000	2.390	2.660
120	−2.617	−2.358	−1.980	−1.658	−1.289	1.289	1.658	1.980	2.358	2.617
∞	−2.576	−2.326	−1.960	−1.645	−1.282	1.282	1.645	1.960	2.326	2.576

TABLE A-7 CRITICAL VALUES OF THE F DISTRIBUTION

Denom. df	Cum. prop	v_1, Degrees of freedom for numerator 1	2	3	4	5	6	7	8	9	10	11	12	15	20	24	30	40	60	120	∞	Cum. prop
1	.005	$.0^{6}62$	$.0^{5}51$	.018	.032	.044	.054	.062	.068	.073	.078	.082	.085	.093	.101	.105	.109	.113	.118	.122	.127	.005
	.010	$.0^{5}25$	.010	.029	.047	.062	.073	.082	.089	.095	.100	.104	.107	.115	.124	.128	.132	.137	.141	.146	.151	.01
	.025	$.0^{4}15$	.026	.057	.082	.100	.113	.124	.132	.139	.144	.149	.153	.161	.170	.175	.180	.184	.189	.194	.199	.025
	.05	$.0^{2}62$	.054	.099	.130	.151	.167	.179	.188	.195	.201	.207	.211	.220	.230	.235	.240	.245	.250	.255	.261	.05
	.95	161	200	216	225	230	234	237	239	241	242	243	244	246	248	249	250	251	252	253	254	.95
	.975	648	800	864	900	922	937	948	957	963	969	973	977	985	993	997	100^{1}	101^{1}	101^{1}	101^{1}	102^{1}	.975
	.99	405^{1}	500^{1}	540^{1}	562^{1}	576^{1}	586^{1}	593^{1}	598^{1}	602^{1}	606^{1}	608^{1}	611^{1}	616^{1}	621^{1}	623^{1}	626^{1}	629^{1}	631^{1}	634^{1}	637^{1}	.99
	.995	162^{2}	200^{2}	216^{2}	225^{2}	231^{2}	234^{2}	237^{2}	239^{2}	241^{2}	242^{2}	243^{2}	244^{2}	246^{2}	248^{2}	249^{2}	250^{2}	251^{2}	253^{2}	254^{2}	255^{2}	.995
2	.005	$.0^{5}50$	$.0^{5}50$	.020	.038	.055	.069	.081	.091	.099	.106	.112	.118	.130	.143	.150	.157	.165	.173	.181	.189	.005
	.01	$.0^{5}20$	.010	.032	.056	.075	.092	.105	.116	.125	.132	.139	.144	.157	.171	.178	.186	.193	.201	.209	.217	.01
	.025	$.0^{3}13$	.026	.062	.094	.119	.138	.153	.165	.175	.183	.190	.196	.210	.224	.232	.239	.247	.255	.263	.271	.025
	.05	$.0^{2}50$	.053	.105	.144	.173	.194	.211	.224	.235	.244	.251	.257	.272	.286	.294	.302	.309	.317	.326	.334	.05
	.95	18.5	19.0	19.2	19.2	19.3	19.3	19.4	19.4	19.4	19.4	19.4	19.4	19.4	19.4	19.5	19.5	19.5	19.5	19.5	19.5	.95
	.975	38.5	39.0	39.2	39.2	39.3	39.3	39.4	39.4	39.4	39.4	39.4	39.4	39.4	39.4	39.5	39.5	39.5	39.5	39.5	39.5	.975
	.99	98.5	99.0	99.2	99.2	99.3	99.3	99.4	99.4	99.4	99.4	99.4	99.4	99.4	99.4	99.5	99.5	99.5	99.5	99.5	99.5	.99
	.995	198	199	199	199	199	199	199	199	199	199	199	199	199	199	199	199	199	199	199	200	.995
3	.005	$.0^{4}46$	$.0^{5}50$	.021	.041	.060	.077	.092	.104	.115	.124	.132	.138	.154	.172	.181	.191	.201	.211	.222	.234	.005
	.01	$.0^{3}19$	.010	.034	.060	.083	.102	.118	.132	.143	.153	.161	.168	.185	.203	.212	.222	.232	.242	.253	.264	.01
	.025	$.0^{2}12$	.026	.065	.100	.129	.152	.170	.185	.197	.207	.216	.224	.241	.259	.269	.279	.289	.299	.310	.321	.025
	.05	$.0^{2}46$	.052	.108	.152	.185	.210	.230	.246	.259	.270	.279	.287	.304	.323	.332	.342	.352	.363	.373	.384	.05
	.95	10.1	9.55	9.28	9.12	9.01	8.94	8.89	8.85	8.81	8.79	8.76	8.74	8.70	8.66	8.63	8.62	8.59	8.57	8.55	8.53	.95
	.975	17.4	16.0	15.4	15.1	14.9	14.7	14.6	14.5	14.5	14.4	14.4	14.3	14.3	14.2	14.1	14.1	14.0	14.0	13.9	13.9	.975
	.99	34.1	30.8	29.5	28.7	28.2	27.9	27.7	27.5	27.3	27.2	27.1	27.1	26.9	26.7	26.6	26.5	26.4	26.3	26.2	26.1	.99
	.995	55.6	49.8	47.5	46.2	45.4	44.8	44.4	44.1	43.9	43.7	43.5	43.4	43.1	42.8	42.6	42.5	42.3	42.1	42.0	41.8	.995
4	.005	$.0^{4}44$	$.0^{5}50$	.022	.043	.064	.083	.100	.114	.126	.137	.145	.153	.172	.193	.204	.216	.229	.242	.255	.269	.005
	.01	$.0^{3}18$	.010	.035	.063	.088	.109	.127	.143	.156	.167	.176	.185	.204	.226	.237	.249	.261	.274	.287	.301	.01
	.025	$.0^{2}11$	.026	.066	.104	.135	.161	.181	.198	.212	.224	.234	.243	.263	.284	.296	.308	.320	.332	.346	.359	.025
	.05	$.0^{2}44$	.052	.110	.157	.193	.221	.243	.261	.275	.288	.298	.307	.327	.349	.360	.372	.384	.396	.409	.422	.05
	.95	7.71	6.94	6.59	6.39	6.26	6.16	6.09	6.04	6.00	5.96	5.94	5.91	5.86	5.80	5.77	5.75	5.72	5.69	5.66	5.63	.95
	.975	12.2	10.6	9.98	9.60	9.36	9.20	9.07	8.98	8.90	8.84	8.79	8.75	8.66	8.56	8.51	8.46	8.41	8.36	8.31	8.26	.975
	.99	21.2	18.0	16.7	16.0	15.5	15.2	15.0	14.8	14.7	14.5	14.4	14.4	14.2	14.0	13.9	13.8	13.7	13.7	13.6	13.5	.99
	.995	31.3	26.3	24.3	23.2	22.5	22.0	21.6	21.4	21.1	21.0	20.8	20.7	20.4	20.2	20.0	19.9	19.8	19.6	19.5	19.3	.995
5	.005	$.0^{4}43$	$.0^{5}50$	.022	.045	.067	.087	.105	.120	.134	.146	.156	.165	.186	.210	.223	.237	.251	.266	.282	.299	.005
	.01	$.0^{3}17$	.010	.035	.064	.091	.114	.134	.151	.165	.177	.188	.197	.219	.244	.257	.270	.285	.299	.315	.332	.01
	.025	$.0^{2}11$	.025	.067	.107	.140	.167	.189	.208	.223	.236	.248	.257	.280	.304	.317	.330	.344	.359	.374	.390	.025
	.05	$.0^{2}43$	.052	.111	.160	.198	.228	.252	.271	.287	.301	.313	.322	.345	.369	.382	.395	.408	.422	.437	.452	.05
	.95	6.61	5.79	5.41	5.19	5.05	4.95	4.88	4.82	4.77	4.74	4.71	4.68	4.62	4.56	4.53	4.50	4.46	4.43	4.40	4.36	.95
	.975	10.0	8.43	7.76	7.39	7.15	6.98	6.85	6.76	6.68	6.62	6.57	6.52	6.43	6.33	6.28	6.23	6.18	6.12	6.07	6.02	.975
	.99	16.3	13.3	12.1	11.4	11.0	10.7	10.5	10.3	10.2	10.1	9.96	9.89	9.72	9.55	9.47	9.38	9.29	9.20	9.11	9.02	.99
	.995	22.8	18.3	16.5	15.6	14.9	14.5	14.2	14.0	13.8	13.6	13.5	13.4	13.1	12.9	12.8	12.7	12.5	12.4	12.3	12.1	.995

Denominator degrees of freedom

Read $.0^{3}56$ as .00056, 200^{1} as 2,000, 162^{4} as 1,620,000, and so on.

Table continued on the following page

363

TABLE A-7 CRITICAL VALUES OF THE F DISTRIBUTION Continued

v_1, Degrees of freedom for numerator

Denominator degrees of freedom

Denom df	Cum. prop.	1	2	3	4	5	6	7	8	9	10	11	12	15	20	24	30	40	60	120	∞	Cum. prop.
6	.005	$0^4$43	$0^3$50	.022	.045	.069	.090	.109	.126	.140	.153	.164	.174	.197	.224	.238	.253	.269	.286	.304	.324	.005
	.01	$0^3$17	.010	.036	.066	.094	.118	.139	.157	.172	.186	.197	.207	.232	.258	.273	.288	.304	.321	.338	.357	.01
	.025	$0^3$11	.025	.068	.109	.143	.172	.195	.215	.231	.246	.258	.268	.293	.320	.334	.349	.364	.381	.398	.415	.025
	.05	$0^2$43	.052	.112	.162	.202	.233	.259	.279	.296	.311	.324	.334	.358	.385	.399	.413	.428	.444	.460	.476	.05
	.95	5.99	5.14	4.76	4.53	4.39	4.28	4.21	4.15	4.10	4.06	4.03	4.00	3.94	3.87	3.84	3.81	3.77	3.74	3.70	3.67	.95
	.975	8.81	7.26	6.60	6.23	5.99	5.82	5.70	5.60	5.52	5.46	5.41	5.37	5.27	5.17	5.12	5.07	5.01	4.96	4.90	4.85	.975
	.99	13.7	10.9	9.78	9.15	8.75	8.47	8.26	8.10	7.98	7.87	7.79	7.72	7.56	7.40	7.31	7.23	7.14	7.06	6.97	6.88	.99
	.995	18.6	14.5	12.9	12.0	11.5	11.1	10.8	10.6	10.4	10.2	10.1	10.0	9.81	9.59	9.47	9.36	9.24	9.12	9.00	8.88	.995
7	.005	$0^4$42	$0^3$50	.023	.046	.070	.093	.113	.130	.145	.159	.171	.181	.206	.235	.251	.267	.285	.304	.324	.345	.005
	.01	$0^3$17	.010	.036	.067	.096	.121	.143	.162	.178	.192	.205	.216	.241	.270	.286	.303	.320	.339	.358	.379	.01
	.025	$0^3$10	.025	.068	.110	.146	.176	.200	.221	.238	.253	.266	.277	.304	.333	.348	.364	.381	.399	.418	.437	.025
	.05	$0^2$42	.052	.113	.164	.205	.238	.264	.286	.304	.319	.332	.343	.369	.398	.413	.428	.445	.461	.479	.498	.05
	.95	5.59	4.74	4.35	4.12	3.97	3.87	3.79	3.73	3.68	3.64	3.60	3.57	3.51	3.44	3.41	3.38	3.34	3.30	3.27	3.23	.95
	.975	8.07	6.54	5.89	5.52	5.29	5.12	4.99	4.90	4.82	4.76	4.71	4.67	4.57	4.47	4.42	4.36	4.31	4.25	4.20	4.14	.975
	.99	12.2	9.55	8.45	7.85	7.46	7.19	6.99	6.84	6.72	6.62	6.54	6.47	6.31	6.16	6.07	5.99	5.91	5.82	5.74	5.65	.99
	.995	16.2	12.4	10.9	10.0	9.52	9.16	8.89	8.68	8.51	8.38	8.27	8.18	7.97	7.75	7.65	7.53	7.42	7.31	7.19	7.08	.995
8	.005	$0^4$42	$0^3$50	.023	.047	.072	.095	.115	.133	.149	.164	.176	.187	.214	.244	.261	.279	.299	.319	.341	.364	.005
	.01	$0^3$17	.010	.036	.068	.097	.123	.146	.166	.183	.198	.211	.222	.250	.281	.297	.315	.334	.354	.376	.398	.01
	.025	$0^3$10	.025	.069	.111	.148	.179	.204	.226	.244	.259	.273	.285	.313	.343	.360	.377	.395	.415	.435	.456	.025
	.05	$0^2$42	.052	.113	.166	.208	.241	.268	.291	.310	.326	.339	.351	.379	.409	.425	.441	.459	.477	.496	.516	.05
	.95	5.32	4.46	4.07	3.84	3.69	3.58	3.50	3.44	3.39	3.35	3.31	3.28	3.22	3.15	3.12	3.08	3.04	3.01	2.97	2.93	.95
	.975	7.57	6.06	5.42	5.05	4.82	4.65	4.53	4.43	4.36	4.30	4.24	4.20	4.10	4.00	3.95	3.89	3.84	3.78	3.73	3.67	.975
	.99	11.3	8.65	7.59	7.01	6.63	6.37	6.18	6.03	5.91	5.81	5.73	5.67	5.52	5.36	5.28	5.20	5.12	5.03	4.95	4.86	.99
	.995	14.7	11.0	9.60	8.81	8.30	7.95	7.69	7.50	7.34	7.21	7.10	7.01	6.81	6.61	6.50	6.40	6.29	6.18	6.06	5.95	.995
9	.005	$0^4$42	$0^3$50	.023	.047	.073	.096	.117	.136	.153	.168	.181	.192	.220	.253	.271	.290	.310	.332	.356	.382	.005
	.01	$0^3$17	.010	.037	.068	.098	.125	.149	.169	.187	.202	.216	.228	.257	.289	.307	.326	.346	.368	.391	.415	.01
	.025	$0^3$10	.025	.069	.112	.150	.181	.207	.230	.248	.265	.279	.291	.320	.352	.370	.388	.408	.428	.450	.473	.025
	.05	$0^2$42	.052	.113	.167	.210	.244	.272	.296	.315	.331	.345	.358	.386	.418	.435	.452	.471	.490	.510	.532	.05
	.95	5.12	4.26	3.86	3.63	3.48	3.37	3.29	3.23	3.18	3.14	3.10	3.07	3.01	2.94	2.90	2.86	2.83	2.79	2.75	2.71	.95
	.975	7.21	5.71	5.08	4.72	4.48	4.32	4.20	4.10	4.03	3.96	3.91	3.87	3.77	3.67	3.61	3.56	3.51	3.45	3.39	3.33	.975
	.99	10.6	8.02	6.99	6.42	6.06	5.80	5.61	5.47	5.35	5.26	5.18	5.11	4.96	4.81	4.73	4.65	4.57	4.48	4.40	4.31	.99
	.995	13.6	10.1	8.72	7.96	7.47	7.13	6.88	6.69	6.54	6.42	6.31	6.23	6.03	5.83	5.73	5.62	5.52	5.41	5.30	5.19	.995

Denominator degrees of freedom																						
	.005	$.0^{4}41$	$.0^{2}50$	.023	.048	.073	.098	.119	.139	.156	.171	.185	.197	.226	.260	.279	.299	.321	.344	.370	.397	.005
	.01	$.0^{3}17$	.010	.037	.069	.100	.127	.151	.172	.190	.206	.220	.233	.263	.297	.316	.336	.357	.380	.405	.431	.01
	.025	$.0^{2}10$	.025	.069	.113	.151	.183	.210	.233	.252	.269	.283	.296	.327	.360	.379	.398	.419	.441	.464	.488	.025
	.05	$.0^{2}41$	.052	.114	.168	.211	.246	.275	.299	.319	.336	.351	.363	.393	.426	.444	.462	.481	.502	.523	.546	.05
10	.95	4.96	4.10	3.71	3.48	3.33	3.22	3.14	3.07	3.02	2.98	2.94	2.91	2.85	2.77	2.74	2.70	2.66	2.62	2.58	2.54	.95
	.975	6.94	5.46	4.83	4.47	4.24	4.07	3.95	3.85	3.78	3.72	3.66	3.62	3.52	3.42	3.37	3.31	3.26	3.20	3.14	3.08	.975
	.99	10.0	7.56	6.55	5.99	5.64	5.39	5.20	5.06	4.94	4.85	4.77	4.71	4.56	4.41	4.33	4.25	4.17	4.08	4.00	3.91	.99
	.995	12.8	9.43	8.08	7.34	6.87	6.54	6.30	6.12	5.97	5.85	5.75	5.66	5.47	5.27	5.17	5.07	4.97	4.86	4.75	4.64	.995
	.005	$.0^{4}40$	$.0^{2}50$	.023	.048	.074	.099	.121	.141	.158	.174	.188	.200	.231	.266	.286	.308	.330	.355	.382	.412	.005
	.01	$.0^{3}16$	.010	.037	.069	.100	.128	.153	.175	.193	.210	.224	.237	.268	.304	.324	.344	.366	.391	.417	.444	.01
	.025	$.0^{2}10$	.025	.069	.114	.152	.185	.212	.236	.256	.273	.288	.301	.332	.368	.386	.407	.429	.450	.476	.503	.025
	.05	$.0^{2}41$	.052	.114	.168	.212	.248	.278	.302	.323	.340	.355	.368	.398	.433	.452	.469	.490	.513	.535	.559	.05
11	.95	4.84	3.98	3.59	3.36	3.20	3.09	3.01	2.95	2.90	2.85	2.82	2.79	2.72	2.65	2.61	2.57	2.53	2.49	2.45	2.40	.95
	.975	6.72	5.26	4.63	4.28	4.04	3.88	3.76	3.66	3.59	3.53	3.47	3.43	3.33	3.23	3.17	3.12	3.06	3.00	2.94	2.88	.975
	.99	9.65	7.21	6.22	5.67	5.32	5.07	4.89	4.74	4.63	4.54	4.46	4.40	4.25	4.10	4.02	3.94	3.86	3.78	3.69	3.60	.99
	.995	12.2	8.91	7.60	6.88	6.42	6.10	5.86	5.68	5.54	5.42	5.32	5.24	5.05	4.86	4.76	4.65	4.55	4.45	4.34	4.23	.995
	.005	$.0^{4}41$	$.0^{2}50$	.023	.048	.075	.100	.122	.143	.161	.177	.191	.204	.235	.272	.292	.315	.339	.365	.393	.424	.005
	.01	$.0^{3}16$	.010	.037	.070	.101	.130	.155	.176	.196	.212	.227	.241	.273	.310	.330	.352	.375	.401	.428	.458	.01
	.025	$.0^{2}10$	.025	.070	.114	.153	.186	.214	.238	.259	.276	.292	.305	.337	.374	.394	.416	.437	.461	.487	.514	.025
	.05	$.0^{2}41$	.052	.114	.169	.214	.250	.280	.305	.325	.343	.358	.372	.404	.439	.458	.478	.499	.522	.545	.571	.05
12	.95	4.75	3.89	3.49	3.26	3.11	3.00	2.91	2.85	2.80	2.75	2.72	2.69	2.62	2.54	2.51	2.47	2.43	2.38	2.34	2.30	.95
	.975	6.55	5.10	4.47	4.12	3.89	3.73	3.61	3.51	3.44	3.37	3.32	3.28	3.18	3.07	3.02	2.96	2.91	2.85	2.79	2.72	.975
	.99	9.33	6.93	5.95	5.41	5.06	4.82	4.64	4.50	4.39	4.30	4.22	4.16	4.01	3.86	3.78	3.70	3.62	3.54	3.45	3.36	.99
	.995	11.8	8.51	7.23	6.52	6.07	5.76	5.52	5.35	5.20	5.09	4.99	4.91	4.72	4.53	4.43	4.33	4.23	4.12	4.01	3.90	.995
	.005	$.0^{4}41$	$.0^{2}50$	.023	.049	.076	.102	.125	.147	.166	.183	.198	.212	.246	.286	.308	.333	.360	.389	.422	.457	.005
	.01	$.0^{3}16$	.010	.037	.070	.103	.132	.158	.181	.202	.219	.235	.249	.284	.324	.346	.370	.397	.425	.456	.490	.01
	.025	$.0^{2}10$	.025	.070	.116	.156	.190	.219	.244	.265	.284	.300	.315	.349	.389	.410	.433	.458	.485	.514	.546	.025
	.05	$.0^{2}41$	.051	.115	.170	.216	.254	.285	.311	.333	.351	.368	.382	.416	.454	.474	.496	.519	.545	.571	.600	.05
15	.95	4.54	3.68	3.29	3.06	2.90	2.79	2.71	2.64	2.59	2.54	2.51	2.48	2.40	2.33	2.29	2.25	2.20	2.16	2.11	2.07	.95
	.975	6.20	4.76	4.15	3.80	3.58	3.41	3.29	3.20	3.12	3.06	3.01	2.96	2.86	2.76	2.70	2.64	2.59	2.52	2.46	2.40	.975
	.99	8.68	6.36	5.42	4.89	4.56	4.32	4.14	4.00	3.89	3.80	3.73	3.67	3.52	3.37	3.29	3.21	3.13	3.05	2.96	2.87	.99
	.995	10.8	7.70	6.48	5.80	5.37	5.07	4.85	4.67	4.54	4.42	4.33	4.25	4.07	3.88	3.79	3.69	3.59	3.48	3.37	3.26	.995
	.005	$.0^{4}39$	$.0^{2}50$	.023	.050	.077	.104	.129	.151	.171	.190	.206	.221	.258	.301	.327	.354	.385	.419	.457	.500	.005
	.01	$.0^{3}16$	.010	.037	.071	.105	.135	.162	.187	.208	.227	.244	.259	.297	.340	.365	.392	.422	.455	.491	.532	.01
	.025	$.0^{2}10$	.025	.071	.117	.158	.193	.224	.250	.273	.292	.310	.325	.363	.406	.430	.456	.484	.514	.548	.585	.025
	.05	$.0^{2}40$	.051	.115	.172	.219	.258	.290	.318	.340	.360	.377	.393	.430	.471	.493	.518	.544	.572	.603	.637	.05
20	.95	4.35	3.49	3.10	2.87	2.71	2.60	2.51	2.45	2.39	2.35	2.31	2.28	2.20	2.12	2.08	2.04	1.99	1.95	1.90	1.84	.95
	.975	5.87	4.46	3.86	3.51	3.29	3.13	3.01	2.91	2.84	2.77	2.72	2.68	2.57	2.46	2.41	2.35	2.29	2.22	2.16	2.09	.975
	.99	8.10	5.85	4.94	4.43	4.10	3.87	3.70	3.56	3.46	3.37	3.29	3.23	3.09	2.94	2.86	2.78	2.69	2.61	2.52	2.42	.99
	.995	9.94	6.99	5.82	5.17	4.76	4.47	4.26	4.09	3.96	3.85	3.76	3.68	3.50	3.32	3.22	3.12	3.02	2.92	2.81	2.69	.995
	.005	$.0^{4}40$	$.0^{2}50$	.023	.050	.078	.106	.131	.154	.175	.193	.210	.226	.264	.310	.337	.367	.400	.437	.479	.527	.005
	.01	$.0^{3}16$	.010	.038	.072	.106	.137	.165	.189	.211	.231	.249	.264	.304	.350	.376	.405	.437	.473	.513	.558	.01
	.025	$.0^{2}10$	.025	.071	.117	.159	.195	.227	.253	.277	.297	.315	.331	.370	.415	.441	.468	.498	.531	.568	.610	.025
	.05	$.0^{2}40$	.051	.116	.173	.221	.260	.293	.321	.345	.365	.383	.399	.437	.480	.504	.530	.558	.588	.622	.659	.05
24	.95	4.26	3.40	3.01	2.78	2.62	2.51	2.42	2.36	2.30	2.25	2.21	2.18	2.11	2.03	1.98	1.94	1.89	1.84	1.79	1.73	.95
	.975	5.72	4.32	3.72	3.38	3.15	2.99	2.87	2.78	2.70	2.64	2.59	2.54	2.44	2.33	2.27	2.21	2.15	2.08	2.01	1.94	.975
	.99	7.82	5.61	4.72	4.22	3.90	3.67	3.50	3.36	3.26	3.17	3.09	3.03	2.89	2.74	2.66	2.58	2.49	2.40	2.31	2.21	.99
	.995	9.55	6.66	5.52	4.89	4.49	4.20	3.99	3.83	3.69	3.59	3.50	3.42	3.25	3.06	2.97	2.87	2.77	2.66	2.55	2.43	.995

Read $.0^{3}56$ as .00056, 200^{1} as 2,000, 162^{4} as 1,620,000, and so on.

Table continued on the following page

TABLE A-7 CRITICAL VALUES OF THE F DISTRIBUTION Continued

v_1, Degrees of freedom for numerator

Denom. df	Cum. prop.	1	2	3	4	5	6	7	8	9	10	11	12	15	20	24	30	40	60	120	∞	Cum. prop.
30	.005	$.0^440$	$.0^550$	.024	.050	.079	.107	.133	.156	.178	.197	.215	.231	.271	.320	.349	.381	.416	.457	.504	.559	.005
	.01	$.0^416$	.010	.038	.072	.107	.138	.167	.192	.215	.235	.254	.270	.311	.360	.388	.419	.454	.493	.538	.590	.01
	.025	$.0^510$	.025	.071	.118	.161	.197	.229	.257	.281	.302	.321	.337	.378	.426	.453	.482	.515	.551	.592	.639	.025
	.05	$.0^440$	.051	.116	.174	.222	.263	.296	.325	.349	.370	.389	.406	.445	.490	.516	.543	.573	.606	.644	.685	.05
	.95	4.17	3.32	2.92	2.69	2.53	2.42	2.33	2.27	2.21	2.16	2.13	2.09	2.01	1.93	1.89	1.84	1.79	1.74	1.68	1.62	.95
	.975	5.57	4.18	3.59	3.25	3.03	2.87	2.75	2.65	2.57	2.51	2.46	2.41	2.31	2.20	2.14	2.07	2.01	1.94	1.87	1.79	.975
	.99	7.56	5.39	4.51	4.02	3.70	3.47	3.30	3.17	3.07	2.98	2.91	2.84	2.70	2.55	2.47	2.39	2.30	2.21	2.11	2.01	.99
	.995	9.18	6.35	5.24	4.62	4.23	3.95	3.74	3.58	3.45	3.34	3.25	3.18	3.01	2.82	2.73	2.63	2.52	2.42	2.30	2.18	.995
40	.005	$.0^440$	$.0^550$	.024	.051	.080	.108	.135	.159	.181	.201	.220	.237	.279	.331	.362	.396	.436	.481	.534	.599	.005
	.01	$.0^416$	.010	.038	.073	.108	.140	.169	.195	.219	.240	.259	.276	.319	.371	.401	.435	.473	.516	.567	.628	.01
	.025	$.0^599$	.025	.071	.119	.162	.199	.232	.260	.285	.307	.327	.344	.387	.437	.466	.498	.533	.573	.620	.674	.025
	.05	$.0^440$	.051	.116	.175	.224	.265	.299	.329	.354	.376	.395	.412	.454	.502	.529	.558	.591	.627	.669	.717	.05
	.95	4.08	3.23	2.84	2.61	2.45	2.34	2.25	2.18	2.12	2.08	2.04	2.00	1.92	1.84	1.79	1.74	1.69	1.64	1.58	1.51	.95
	.975	5.42	4.05	3.46	3.13	2.90	2.74	2.62	2.53	2.45	2.39	2.33	2.29	2.18	2.07	2.01	1.94	1.88	1.80	1.72	1.64	.975
	.99	7.31	5.18	4.31	3.83	3.51	3.29	3.12	2.99	2.89	2.80	2.73	2.66	2.52	2.37	2.29	2.20	2.11	2.02	1.92	1.80	.99
	.995	8.83	6.07	4.98	4.37	3.99	3.71	3.51	3.35	3.22	3.12	3.03	2.95	2.78	2.60	2.50	2.40	2.30	2.18	2.06	1.93	.995
60	.005	$.0^440$	$.0^550$	.024	.051	.081	.110	.137	.162	.185	.206	.225	.243	.287	.343	.376	.414	.458	.510	.572	.652	.005
	.01	$.0^416$	.010	.038	.073	.109	.142	.172	.199	.223	.245	.265	.283	.328	.383	.416	.453	.495	.545	.604	.679	.01
	.025	$.0^599$	.025	.071	.120	.163	.202	.235	.264	.290	.313	.333	.351	.396	.450	.481	.515	.555	.600	.654	.720	.025
	.05	$.0^440$	.051	.116	.176	.226	.267	.303	.333	.359	.382	.402	.419	.463	.514	.543	.575	.611	.652	.700	.759	.05
	.95	4.00	3.15	2.76	2.53	2.37	2.25	2.17	2.10	2.04	1.99	1.95	1.92	1.84	1.75	1.70	1.65	1.59	1.53	1.47	1.39	.95
	.975	5.29	3.93	3.34	3.01	2.79	2.63	2.51	2.41	2.33	2.27	2.22	2.17	2.06	1.94	1.88	1.82	1.74	1.67	1.58	1.48	.975
	.99	7.08	4.98	4.13	3.65	3.34	3.12	2.95	2.82	2.72	2.63	2.56	2.50	2.35	2.20	2.12	2.03	1.94	1.84	1.73	1.60	.99
	.995	8.49	5.80	4.73	4.14	3.76	3.49	3.29	3.13	3.01	2.90	2.82	2.74	2.57	2.39	2.29	2.19	2.08	1.96	1.83	1.69	.995
120	.005	$.0^339$	$.0^550$	.024	.051	.081	.111	.139	.165	.189	.211	.230	.249	.297	.356	.393	.434	.484	.545	.623	.733	.005
	.01	$.0^416$	.010	.038	.074	.110	.143	.174	.202	.227	.250	.271	.290	.338	.397	.433	.474	.522	.579	.652	.755	.01
	.025	$.0^398$	.025	.072	.120	.165	.204	.238	.268	.295	.318	.340	.359	.406	.464	.498	.536	.580	.633	.698	.789	.025
	.05	$.0^339$	.051	.117	.177	.227	.270	.306	.337	.364	.388	.408	.427	.473	.527	.559	.594	.634	.682	.740	.819	.05
	.95	3.92	3.07	2.68	2.45	2.29	2.18	2.09	2.02	1.96	1.91	1.87	1.83	1.75	1.66	1.61	1.55	1.50	1.43	1.35	1.25	.95
	.975	5.15	3.80	3.23	2.89	2.67	2.52	2.39	2.30	2.22	2.16	2.10	2.05	1.95	1.82	1.76	1.69	1.61	1.53	1.43	1.31	.975
	.99	6.85	4.79	3.95	3.48	3.17	2.96	2.79	2.66	2.56	2.47	2.40	2.34	2.19	2.03	1.95	1.86	1.76	1.66	1.53	1.38	.99
	.995	8.18	5.54	4.50	3.92	3.55	3.28	3.09	2.93	2.81	2.71	2.62	2.54	2.37	2.19	2.09	1.98	1.87	1.75	1.61	1.43	.995
∞	.005	$.0^339$	$.0^550$	.024	.052	.082	.113	.141	.168	.193	.216	.236	.256	.307	.372	.412	.460	.518	.592	.699	1.00	.005
	.01	$.0^416$	.010	.038	.074	.111	.145	.177	.206	.232	.256	.278	.298	.349	.413	.452	.499	.554	.625	.724	1.00	.01
	.025	$.0^398$	.025	.072	.121	.166	.206	.241	.272	.300	.325	.347	.367	.418	.480	.517	.560	.611	.675	.763	1.00	.025
	.05	$.0^339$	.051	.117	.178	.229	.273	.310	.342	.369	.394	.417	.436	.484	.543	.577	.617	.663	.720	.797	1.00	.05
	.95	3.84	3.00	2.60	2.37	2.21	2.10	2.01	1.94	1.88	1.83	1.79	1.75	1.67	1.57	1.52	1.46	1.39	1.32	1.22	1.00	.95
	.975	5.02	3.69	3.12	2.79	2.57	2.41	2.29	2.19	2.11	2.05	1.99	1.94	1.83	1.71	1.64	1.57	1.48	1.39	1.27	1.00	.975
	.99	6.63	4.61	3.78	3.32	3.02	2.80	2.64	2.51	2.41	2.32	2.25	2.18	2.04	1.88	1.79	1.70	1.59	1.47	1.32	1.00	.99
	.995	7.88	5.30	4.28	3.72	3.35	3.09	2.90	2.74	2.62	2.52	2.43	2.36	2.19	2.00	1.90	1.79	1.67	1.53	1.36	1.00	.995

Denominator degrees of freedom

Read $.0^356$ as .00056, 200^1 as 2,000, 162^4 as 1,620,000, and so on.

TABLE A-8 CRITICAL VALUES OF THE DUNN MULTIPLE COMPARISON TEST

Number of comparisons C	α	Error df 5	7	10	12	15	20	24	30	40	60	120	∞
2	.05	3.17	2.84	2.64	2.56	2.49	2.42	2.39	2.36	2.33	2.30	2.27	2.24
	.01	4.78	4.03	3.58	3.43	3.29	3.16	3.09	3.03	2.97	2.92	2.86	2.81
3	.05	3.54	3.13	2.87	2.78	2.69	2.61	2.58	2.54	2.50	2.47	2.43	2.39
	.01	5.25	4.36	3.83	3.65	3.48	3.33	3.26	3.19	3.12	3.06	2.99	2.94
4	.05	3.81	3.34	3.04	2.94	2.84	2.75	2.70	2.66	2.62	2.58	2.54	2.50
	.01	5.60	4.59	4.01	3.80	3.62	3.46	3.38	3.30	3.23	3.16	3.09	3.02
5	.05	4.04	3.50	3.17	3.06	2.95	2.85	2.80	2.75	2.71	2.66	2.62	2.58
	.01	5.89	4.78	4.15	3.93	3.74	3.55	3.47	3.39	3.31	3.24	3.16	3.09
6	.05	4.22	3.64	3.28	3.15	3.04	2.93	2.88	2.83	2.78	2.73	2.68	2.64
	.01	6.15	4.95	4.27	4.04	3.82	3.63	3.54	3.46	3.38	3.30	3.22	3.15
7	.05	4.38	3.76	3.37	3.24	3.11	3.00	2.94	2.89	2.84	2.79	2.74	2.69
	.01	6.36	5.09	4.37	4.13	3.90	3.70	3.61	3.52	3.43	3.34	3.27	3.19
8	.05	4.53	3.86	3.45	3.31	3.18	3.06	3.00	2.94	2.89	2.84	2.79	2.74
	.01	6.56	5.21	4.45	4.20	3.97	3.76	3.66	3.57	3.48	3.39	3.31	3.23
9	.05	4.66	3.95	3.52	3.37	3.24	3.11	3.05	2.99	2.93	2.88	2.83	2.77
	.01	6.70	5.31	4.53	4.26	4.02	3.80	3.70	3.61	3.51	3.42	3.34	3.26
10	.05	4.78	4.03	3.58	3.43	3.29	3.16	3.09	3.03	2.97	2.92	2.86	2.81
	.01	6.86	5.40	4.59	4.32	4.07	3.85	3.74	3.65	3.55	3.46	3.37	3.29
15	.05	5.25	4.36	3.83	3.65	3.48	3.33	3.26	3.19	3.12	3.06	2.99	2.94
	.01	7.51	5.79	4.86	4.56	4.29	4.03	3.91	3.80	3.70	3.59	3.50	3.40
20	.05	5.60	4.59	4.01	3.80	3.62	3.46	3.38	3.30	3.23	3.16	3.09	3.02
	.01	8.00	6.08	5.06	4.73	4.42	4.15	4.04	3.90	3.79	3.69	3.58	3.48
25	.05	5.89	4.78	4.15	3.93	3.74	3.55	3.47	3.39	3.31	3.24	3.16	3.09
	.01	8.37	6.30	5.20	4.86	4.53	4.25	4.1*	3.98	3.88	3.76	3.64	3.54
30	.05	6.15	4.95	4.27	4.04	3.82	3.63	3.54	3.46	3.38	3.30	3.22	3.15
	.01	8.68	6.49	5.33	4.95	4.61	4.33	4.2*	4.13	3.93	3.81	3.69	3.59
35	.05	6.36	5.09	4.37	4.13	3.90	3.70	3.61	3.52	3.43	3.34	3.27	3.19
	.01	8.95	6.67	5.44	5.04	4.71	4.39	4.3*	4.26	3.97	3.84	3.73	3.63
40	.05	6.56	5.21	4.45	4.20	3.97	3.76	3.66	3.57	3.48	3.39	3.31	3.23
	.01	9.19	6.83	5.52	5.12	4.78	4.46	4.3*	4.1*	4.01	3.89	3.77	3.66
45	.05	6.70	5.31	4.53	4.26	4.02	3.80	3.70	3.61	3.51	3.42	3.34	3.26
	.01	9.41	6.93	5.60	5.20	4.84	4.52	4.3*	4.2*	4.1*	3.93	3.80	3.69
50	.05	6.86	5.40	4.59	4.32	4.07	3.85	3.74	3.65	3.55	3.46	3.37	3.29
	.01	9.68	7.06	5.70	5.27	4.90	4.56	4.4*	4.2*	4.1*	3.97	3.83	3.72
100	.05	8.00	6.08	5.06	4.73	4.42	4.15	4.04	3.90	3.79	3.69		3.48
	.01	11.04	7.80	6.20	5.70	5.20	4.80	4.7*	4.4*	4.5*		4.00	3.89
250	.05	9.68	7.06	5.70	5.27	4.90	4.56	4.4*	4.2*	4.1*	3.97	3.83	3.72
	.01	13.26	8.83	6.9*	6.3*	5.8*	5.2*	5.0*	4.9*	4.8*			4.11

*Obtained by graphical interpolation. Permission granted by the American Statistical Association to reproduce the table of percentage points of the Dunn multiple comparison test from Dunn, O. J.: Multiple comparisons among means, J. Am. Stat. Assoc., 56: 52–64, 1961.

TABLE A–9 FISHER'S z TRANSFORMATION FOR CORRELATION COEFFICIENTS

r	z	r	z
.01	0.010	.50	0.549
.02	0.020	.51	0.563
.03	0.030	.52	0.577
.04	0.040	.53	0.590
.05	0.050	.54	0.604
.06	0.060	.55	0.618
.07	0.070	.56	0.633
.08	0.080	.57	0.648
.09	0.090	.58	0.663
.10	0.100	.59	0.678
.11	0.110	.60	0.693
.12	0.121	.61	0.709
.13	0.131	.62	0.725
.14	0.141	.63	0.741
.15	0.151	.64	0.758
.16	0.161	.65	0.775
.17	0.172	.66	0.793
.18	0.182	.67	0.811
.19	0.192	.68	0.829
.20	0.203	.69	0.848
.21	0.213	.70	0.867
.22	0.224	.71	0.887
.23	0.234	.72	0.908
.24	0.245	.73	0.929
.25	0.255	.74	0.950
.26	0.266	.75	0.973
.27	0.277	.76	0.996
.28	0.288	.77	1.020
.29	0.299	.78	1.045
.30	0.310	.79	1.071
.31	0.321	.80	1.099
.32	0.332	.81	1.127
.33	0.343	.82	1.157
.34	0.354	.83	1.188
.35	0.365	.84	1.221
.36	0.377	.85	1.256
.37	0.389	.86	1.293
.38	0.400	.87	1.333
.39	0.412	.88	1.376
.40	0.424	.89	1.422
.41	0.436	.90	1.472
.42	0.448	.91	1.528
.43	0.460	.92	1.589
.44	0.472	.93	1.658
.45	0.485	.94	1.738
.46	0.497	.95	1.832
.47	0.510	.96	1.946
.48	0.523	.97	2.092
.49	0.536	.98	2.298
		.99	2.647

TABLE A–10 CONTRAST WEIGHTS FOR MONOTONIC TRENDS

Number of Groups or Conditions	Contrast Weights									
2	1	2								
3	1	2	3							
4	1	2	3	4						
5	1	2	3	4	5					
6	1	2	3	4	5	6				
7	1	2	3	4	5	6	7			
8	1	2	3	4	5	6	7	8		
9	1	2	3	4	5	6	7	8	9	
10	1	2	3	4	5	6	7	8	9	10

TABLE A-11 RANDOM NUMBERS

10	09	73	25	33	76	52	01	35	86	34	67	35	48	76	80	95	90	91	17	39	29	27	49	45
37	54	20	48	05	64	89	47	42	96	24	80	52	40	37	20	63	61	04	02	00	82	29	16	65
08	42	26	89	53	19	64	50	93	03	23	20	90	25	60	15	95	33	47	64	35	08	03	36	06
99	01	90	25	29	09	37	67	07	15	38	31	13	11	65	88	67	67	43	97	04	43	62	76	59
12	80	79	99	70	80	15	73	61	47	64	03	23	66	53	98	95	11	68	77	12	17	17	68	33
66	06	57	47	17	34	07	27	68	50	36	69	73	61	70	65	81	33	98	85	11	19	92	91	70
31	06	01	08	05	45	57	18	24	06	35	30	34	26	14	86	79	90	74	39	23	40	30	97	32
85	26	97	76	02	02	05	16	56	92	68	66	57	48	18	73	05	38	52	47	18	62	38	85	79
63	57	33	21	35	05	32	54	70	48	90	55	35	75	48	28	46	82	87	09	83	49	12	56	24
73	79	64	57	53	03	52	96	47	78	35	80	83	42	82	60	93	52	03	44	35	27	38	84	35
98	52	01	77	67	14	90	56	86	07	22	10	94	05	58	60	97	09	34	33	50	50	07	39	98
11	80	50	54	31	39	80	82	77	32	50	72	56	82	48	29	40	52	42	01	52	77	56	78	51
83	45	29	96	34	06	28	89	80	83	13	74	67	00	78	18	47	54	06	10	68	71	17	78	17
88	68	54	02	00	86	50	75	84	01	36	76	66	79	51	90	36	47	64	93	29	60	91	10	62
99	59	46	73	48	87	51	76	49	69	91	82	60	89	28	93	78	56	13	68	23	47	83	41	13
65	48	11	76	74	17	46	85	09	50	58	04	77	69	74	73	03	95	71	86	40	21	81	65	44
80	12	43	56	35	17	72	70	80	15	45	31	82	23	74	21	11	57	82	53	14	38	55	37	63
74	35	09	98	17	77	40	27	72	14	43	23	60	02	10	45	52	16	42	37	96	28	60	26	55
69	91	62	68	03	66	25	22	91	48	36	93	68	72	03	76	62	11	39	90	94	40	05	64	18
09	89	32	05	05	14	22	56	85	14	46	42	75	67	88	96	29	77	88	22	54	38	21	45	98
91	49	91	45	23	68	47	92	76	86	46	16	28	35	54	94	75	08	99	23	37	08	92	00	48
80	33	69	45	98	26	94	03	68	58	70	29	73	41	35	53	14	03	33	40	42	05	08	23	41
44	10	48	19	49	85	15	74	79	54	32	97	92	65	75	57	60	04	08	81	22	22	20	64	13
12	55	07	37	42	11	10	00	20	40	12	86	07	46	97	96	64	48	94	39	28	70	72	58	15
63	60	64	93	29	16	50	53	44	84	40	21	95	25	63	43	65	17	70	82	07	20	73	17	90
61	19	69	04	46	26	45	74	77	74	51	92	43	37	29	65	39	45	95	93	42	58	26	05	27
15	47	44	52	66	95	27	07	99	53	59	36	78	38	48	82	39	61	01	18	33	21	15	94	66
94	55	72	85	73	67	89	75	43	87	54	62	24	44	31	91	19	04	25	92	92	92	74	59	73
42	48	11	62	13	97	34	40	87	21	16	86	84	87	67	03	07	11	20	59	25	70	14	66	70
23	52	37	83	17	73	20	88	98	37	68	93	59	14	16	26	25	22	96	63	05	52	28	25	62
04	49	35	24	94	75	24	63	38	24	45	86	25	10	25	61	96	27	93	35	65	33	71	24	72
00	54	99	76	54	64	05	18	81	59	96	11	96	38	96	54	69	28	23	91	23	28	72	95	29
35	96	31	53	07	26	89	80	93	54	33	35	13	54	62	77	97	45	00	24	90	10	33	93	33
59	80	80	83	91	45	42	72	68	42	83	60	94	97	00	13	02	12	48	92	78	56	52	01	06
46	05	88	52	36	01	39	09	22	86	77	28	14	40	77	93	91	08	36	47	70	61	74	29	41
32	17	90	05	97	87	37	92	52	41	05	56	70	70	07	86	74	31	71	57	85	39	41	18	38
69	23	46	14	06	20	11	74	52	04	15	95	66	00	00	18	74	39	24	23	97	11	89	63	38
19	56	54	14	30	01	75	87	53	79	40	41	92	15	85	66	67	43	68	06	84	96	28	52	07
45	15	51	49	38	19	47	60	72	46	43	66	79	45	43	59	04	79	00	33	20	82	66	95	41
94	86	43	19	94	36	16	81	08	51	34	88	88	15	53	01	54	03	54	56	05	01	45	11	76
98	08	62	48	26	45	24	02	84	04	44	99	90	88	96	39	09	47	34	07	35	44	13	18	80
33	18	51	62	32	41	94	15	09	49	89	43	54	85	81	88	69	54	19	94	37	54	87	30	43
80	95	10	04	06	96	38	27	07	74	20	15	12	33	87	25	01	62	52	98	94	62	46	11	71
79	75	24	91	40	71	96	12	82	96	69	86	10	25	91	74	85	22	05	39	00	38	75	95	79
18	63	33	25	37	98	14	50	65	71	31	01	02	46	74	05	45	56	14	27	77	93	89	19	36
74	02	94	39	02	77	55	73	22	70	97	79	01	71	19	52	52	75	80	21	80	81	45	17	48
54	17	84	56	11	80	99	33	71	43	05	33	51	29	69	56	12	71	92	55	36	04	09	03	24
11	66	44	98	83	52	07	98	48	27	59	38	17	15	39	09	97	33	34	40	88	46	12	33	56
48	32	47	79	28	31	24	96	47	10	02	29	53	68	70	32	30	75	75	46	15	02	00	99	94
69	07	49	41	38	87	63	79	19	76	35	58	40	44	01	10	51	82	16	15	01	84	87	69	38

From tables of the RAND Corporation, by permission.

TABLE B–1 DATA FOR THE 246 PATIENTS IN THE HYPOTHETICAL PREOPERATIVE TEACHING STUDY

V_1	V_2	V_3	V_4	V_5	V_6	V_7	V_8	V_9	V_{10}	V_{11}	V_{12}	V_{13}	V_{14}	V_{15}	V_{16}	V_{17}	V_{18}	V_{19}	V_{20}	V_{21}
245	1	1001	1	39	2	11	1	2	2	134	1	1	0	0	50	4	8	3	0	6
2	2	1002	0	51	3	8	2	2	1	145	4	1	0	0	45	6	5	2	0	7
236	3	1003	1	51	1	12	3	2	1	155	2	2	0	0	46	6	5	1	1	4
240	1	1004	1	63	2	8	1	1	3	149	4	2	0	0	50	6	6	3	2	8
5	2	1005	1	50	1	12	2	2	2	145	3	2	0	1	47	4	1	0	0	3
156	3	1006	1	61	3	12	3	1	2	173	4	1	0	0	70	6	9	5	3	8
7	1	1007	0	51	1	14	1	2	4	144	1	2	0	1	55	5	7	4	2	4
163	2	1008	1	50	1	16	2	2	5	113	2	2	0	0	32	4	5	3	0	3
229	3	1009	1	42	1	12	3	2	3	156	1	2	0	0	44	2	1	0	3	1
10	1	1010	0	53	2	8	1	2	1	163	3	1	0	0	53	6	7	2	2	7
160	2	1011	1	53	1	16	2	2	4	137	1	1	0	0	57	6	4	2	2	5
228	3	1012	1	50	1	12	3	2	4	153	1	2	0	0	47	2	3	0	0	2
225	1	1013	1	71	3	8	1	1	2	185	4	1	0	0	73	5	10	4	2	12
16	2	1014	0	38	2	9	2	2	1	132	1	3	0	1	44	4	5	0	0	4
14	3	1015	0	48	1	14	3	2	3	163	2	1	0	0	47	4	3	0	0	1
15	1	1016	0	44	1	12	1	2	3	176	1	1	0	0	45	3	4	0	0	2
119	2	1017	1	48	1	16	2	2	5	145	2	1	0	1	45	7	6	3	3	4
222	3	1018	1	34	3	12	3	2	2	141	2	1	0	0	70	5	7	2	0	6
20	1	1019	0	67	1	12	1	2	1	188	3	2	0	0	57	9	5	4	0	7
19	2	1020	0	63	2	5	2	1	4	168	3	1	0	0	47	3	4	2	1	4
153	3	1021	1	39	1	12	3	2	2	138	1	1	0	0	54	4	2	1	1	2
144	1	1022	1	44	1	12	1	2	4	166	1	1	0	0	57	4	6	1	0	2
215	2	1023	1	47	1	12	2	2	4	150	2	1	0	0	53	5	4	0	0	2
25	3	1024	0	39	3	16	3	2	4	155	3	2	0	1	67	5	6	2	0	2
24	1	1025	0	54	1	13	1	1	3	176	2	1	0	0	49	7	6	0	3	7
151	2	1026	1	62	3	8	2	1	2	191	4	1	0	0	52	7	6	3	3	9
211	3	1027	1	40	2	12	3	2	4	146	1	1	0	0	50	3	7	1	0	4
148	1	1028	1	58	1	20	1	1	1	183	3	2	0	0	48	7	7	3	3	6
205	2	1029	1	59	2	12	2	2	5	169	2	3	0	0	48	3	4	0	0	3
202	3	1030	1	43	3	10	3	2	3	146	4	3	0	0	62	5	7	4	0	8
199	1	1031	1	45	2	12	1	1	4	132	1	2	0	0	47	3	6	3	0	8
33	2	1032	0	36	1	12	2	2	1	126	1	1	0	1	42	3	3	0	0	2
32	3	1033	0	51	2	16	3	1	4	146	1	2	1	0	46	2	3	0	0	2
110	1	1034	1	35	1	8	1	2	5	165	1	1	0	0	44	2	6	1	0	1
139	2	1035	1	40	2	12	2	2	2	132	1	1	0	0	46	4	5	0	0	6
196	3	1036	1	40	2	12	3	2	4	120	3	1	1	0	58	6	3	2	2	5
39	1	1037	0	69	3	8	1	1	1	218	3	2	0	0	57	5	7	2	1	7
37	2	1038	0	57	1	21	2	2	4	150	1	1	0	0	46	2	4	0	0	1
38	3	1039	0	42	2	10	3	2	1	170	3	1	0	0	47	5	5	1	0	6
136	1	2001	1	61	3	8	1	1	1	147	4	2	0	0	58	5	9	2	1	7
41	2	2002	0	47	2	12	2	2	3	157	3	2	0	1	49	6	7	3	0	4
130	3	2003	1	54	1	9	3	1	1	164	2	1	0	0	51	5	4	3	0	3
127	1	2004	1	55	1	14	1	2	5	127	2	2	0	0	48	7	7	3	2	6
102	2	2005	1	25	1	17	2	2	4	129	1	1	0	1	31	3	4	0	0	1
46	3	2006	0	60	1	8	3	1	1	206	3	1	0	0	47	3	2	0	0	6
45	1	2007	0	48	3	16	1	2	2	224	3	1	1	0	60	9	10	6	3	10
125	2	2008	1	47	1	16	2	2	3	119	2	2	0	0	44	6	6	3	1	4
48	3	2009	0	43	2	12	3	2	2	170	1	3	0	0	45	3	2	0	0	1
178	1	2010	1	28	1	9	1	2	1	138	1	1	0	0	41	4	8	2	0	2
182	2	2011	1	45	3	3	2	1	2	163	4	1	0	0	64	6	8	4	3	8
175	3	2012	1	35	2	12	3	2	3	139	1	3	0	0	49	2	6	1	0	3
53	1	2013	0	61	1	8	1	2	2	169	3	1	0	0	51	7	7	4	1	9
52	2	2014	0	29	1	14	2	2	1	147	1	2	0	1	42	4	5	0	0	2
108	3	2015	1	38	1	9	3	1	1	156	1	3	1	0	44	4	5	2	0	3
171	1	2016	1	31	1	12	1	2	3	122	1	1	0	1	44	4	6	3	0	2
168	2	2017	1	45	1	12	2	2	2	158	1	2	0	0	45	3	4	0	0	1
57	3	2018	0	31	3	13	3	2	3	174	2	2	0	0	55	4	3	2	0	2
105	1	2019	1	52	3	8	1	2	1	145	1	3	0	0	55	5	9	2	1	6
60	2	2020	0	53	2	16	2	1	5	162	3	1	0	0	46	4	4	0	0	2
59	3	2021	0	64	3	5	3	1	2	169	4	1	1	0	67	5	6	4	1	6
104	1	2022	1	49	2	16	1	2	4	136	3	1	0	0	58	6	6	4	1	7
1	2	2023	0	47	2	16	2	2	3	160	1	3	0	0	47	4	4	0	0	3
246	3	2024	1	27	1	12	3	1	3	138	1	3	1	0	43	3	4	4	0	1
244	1	2025	1	54	1	8	1	2	1	158	2	2	0	0	49	7	8	3	3	6

Table continued on the following page

V₁	V₂	V₃	V₄	V₅	V₆	V₇	V₈	V₉	V₁₀	V₁₁	V₁₂	V₁₃	V₁₄	V₁₅	V₁₆	V₁₇	V₁₈	V₁₉	V₂₀	V₂₁
65	2	2026	0	33	1	16	2	1	4	136	1	1	0	0	39	3	3	0	0	1
12	3	2027	0	44	2	14	3	2	3	156	3	3	0	0	46	3	4	0	1	4
227	1	2028	1	32	2	12	1	1	1	109	1	1	0	0	49	3	5	0	0	2
116	2	2029	1	45	1	8	2	1	2	119	1	1	0	0	41	3	1	0	0	2
18	3	2030	0	37	1	16	3	2	3	164	2	2	0	0	40	3	3	0	0	3
223	1	2031	1	31	2	17	1	1	4	120	1	2	0	0	55	5	6	4	0	7
221	2	2032	1	42	1	15	2	2	4	110	3	2	0	0	49	5	5	3	2	4
216	3	2033	1	28	1	16	3	1	5	150	1	1	0	1	47	2	2	0	0	1
214	1	2034	1	37	2	12	1	2	1	131	1	1	0	0	48	3	4	0	0	3
207	2	2035	2	42	2	12	2	2	5	144	1	1	0	0	49	3	4	0	0	1
35	3	2036	0	40	1	18	3	2	3	145	1	1	0	0	36	3	4	2	0	1
36	1	2037	0	45	1	16	1	2	4	164	2	1	0	0	43	5	7	3	1	8
198	2	2038	1	35	1	12	2	2	3	129	1	2	0	0	48	3	3	0	0	3
42	3	2039	0	38	1	19	3	2	5	128	1	2	0	0	31	2	1	0	0	1
194	1	2040	1	51	2	10	1	2	1	161	3	1	0	0	51	7	9	5	3	12
192	2	2041	1	38	2	14	2	1	3	146	1	2	0	0	45	4	5	2	0	2
47	3	2042	0	29	1	12	3	2	3	143	1	1	0	1	42	2	0	0	0	1
187	1	2043	1	51	1	16	1	2	4	181	1	1	0	0	49	7	8	4	2	6
190	2	2044	1	50	2	8	2	1	1	214	3	3	0	0	49	7	10	5	2	8
55	3	2045	0	30	1	16	3	2	2	151	1	2	0	0	44	2	2	0	0	0
172	1	2046	1	44	1	12	1	2	3	146	1	1	0	0	46	2	4	2	0	2
167	2	2047	1	50	1	22	2	2	5	155	3	2	0	0	39	6	6	4	2	6
62	3	2048	0	54	2	10	3	1	1	150	3	1	0	0	47	5	4	0	0	6
63	1	2049	0	63	1	17	1	2	4	162	2	3	0	1	45	6	6	2	3	7
164	2	2050	1	50	1	16	2	2	3	150	2	1	0	0	45	3	4	1	1	4
69	3	2051	0	54	2	11	3	1	2	166	4	1	0	0	52	2	3	1	0	3
71	1	2052	0	55	1	22	1	2	3	177	2	3	0	0	47	5	6	2	2	4
152	2	2053	1	37	2	20	2	2	3	147	1	1	0	0	50	3	2	0	0	2
84	3	2054	0	48	2	12	3	1	2	163	4	3	0	0	46	4	3	2	0	6
124	1	2055	1	46	1	16	1	2	4	155	2	1	0	0	42	7	9	4	2	8
86	2	2056	0	27	1	16	2	2	3	141	1	1	0	1	46	3	3	0	0	0
117	3	2057	1	42	2	12	3	2	2	150	1	2	0	0	40	2	3	2	0	5
95	1	2058	0	46	2	12	1	2	5	160	2	2	0	0	58	5	7	5	1	7
96	2	2059	0	41	1	14	2	2	4	153	3	2	0	1	35	5	5	2	2	6
98	3	2060	0	49	2	16	3	1	3	152	1	1	0	0	41	2	3	0	0	3
99	1	2061	0	59	2	19	1	2	5	201	1	3	1	0	38	3	2	3	1	2
100	2	2062	0	53	1	8	2	1	2	188	2	3	0	0	50	7	6	4	2	6
101	3	2063	1	67	1	14	3	1	4	163	2	2	0	0	53	5	5	3	1	3
97	1	2064	0	32	3	12	1	1	3	149	1	1	0	1	54	5	9	3	3	2
103	2	2065	1	48	1	12	2	2	5	139	2	1	0	0	50	3	4	1	0	4
94	3	2066	0	44	1	18	3	2	3	133	3	1	0	0	49	3	3	1	0	1
93	1	2067	0	51	2	12	1	2	5	170	4	3	0	1	63	7	8	1	2	4
106	2	2068	1	48	2	10	2	1	2	150	1	3	0	0	54	5	5	4	0	3
107	3	2069	1	32	1	16	3	2	5	142	1	1	0	0	44	2	3	2	0	0
91	1	2070	0	47	1	16	1	2	3	167	1	1	0	0	36	5	7	3	2	4
109	2	2071	1	45	2	12	2	2	4	127	2	1	0	0	49	4	5	1	0	3
90	3	2072	0	61	2	8	3	1	1	164	4	1	1	0	49	2	2	0	0	0
111	1	3001	1	54	3	8	1	1	1	156	1	1	0	0	68	5	8	3	3	4
112	2	3002	1	44	2	12	2	1	2	128	1	2	0	0	44	4	6	2	0	3
92	3	3003	0	55	3	12	3	2	3	225	3	1	0	0	50	5	5	3	2	5
114	1	3004	1	39	1	13	1	2	4	138	2	1	0	1	40	4	6	1	0	2
89	2	3005	0	52	3	7	2	2	1	200	4	3	0	0	54	6	7	4	3	7
115	3	3006	1	40	1	12	3	2	2	145	1	1	1	0	40	2	4	0	0	0
88	1	3007	0	65	3	5	1	1	5	180	2	1	0	1	63	9	8	3	3	13
118	2	3008	1	46	2	12	2	2	4	135	1	2	0	0	51	4	7	2	0	5
87	3	3009	1	55	2	20	3	1	4	190	4	3	0	0	52	4	5	3	0	6
120	1	3010	0	46	3	3	1	1	1	147	2	1	0	0	53	4	7	2	2	4
121	2	3011	1	52	3	12	2	2	5	142	3	1	0	0	54	4	5	2	0	4
85	3	3012	0	38	1	12	3	2	2	137	1	1	0	1	47	2	3	0	0	0
123	1	3013	1	45	3	16	1	2	5	158	4	2	0	0	45	5	7	3	3	6
82	2	3014	0	42	1	8	2	2	1	153	1	3	0	0	51	2	5	0	0	3
80	3	3015	0	66	3	14	3	1	3	217	4	3	0	0	49	5	4	3	2	6
126	1	3016	1	54	1	3	1	1	1	127	3	1	0	0	51	3	4	2	1	4
79	2	3017	0	42	2	12	2	2	5	150	1	2	0	1	46	5	8	3	0	2
128	3	3018	1	42	2	16	3	2	2	136	1	3	0	0	45	2	5	1	0	1
129	1	3019	1	42	3	11	1	2	1	155	2	2	1	0	71	6	10	2	2	6

V₁	V₂	V₃	V₄	V₅	V₆	V₇	V₈	V₉	V₁₀	V₁₁	V₁₂	V₁₃	V₁₄	V₁₅	V₁₆	V₁₇	V₁₈	V₁₉	V₂₀	V₂₁
81	2	3020	0	46	1	8	2	2	1	149	2	1	0	0	57	4	5	0	0	6
131	3	3021	1	56	3	13	3	2	4	154	1	1	0	0	65	5	4	2	1	4
132	1	3022	1	61	3	8	1	1	4	191	4	1	0	0	58	6	9	4	1	6
78	2	3023	0	36	1	12	2	2	5	140	1	1	0	1	45	4	5	0	0	2
134	3	3024	1	42	1	12	3	2	2	155	1	2	0	0	46	2	4	1	0	2
135	1	3025	1	30	1	8	1	2	1	135	2	2	0	0	42	4	7	4	0	5
133	2	3026	1	56	3	22	2	2	2	201	3	2	0	0	50	7	9	3	2	9
76	3	3027	0	52	2	12	3	2	4	166	3	3	0	0	50	3	4	2	0	2
138	1	3028	1	43	1	16	1	1	3	173	2	3	0	0	44	4	7	3	3	6
75	2	3029	0	58	3	10	2	2	1	150	4	1	0	0	51	4	4	2	0	4
140	3	3030	1	58	3	9	3	2	1	135	3	1	0	0	51	3	4	0	0	4
141	1	3031	1	45	1	16	1	2	4	154	2	1	0	0	47	3	6	0	0	1
73	2	3032	0	50	1	16	2	2	2	162	2	1	0	0	56	4	4	1	1	6
143	3	3033	1	48	1	21	3	2	5	142	1	2	1	0	45	5	6	3	0	5
74	1	3034	0	65	3	5	1	1	1	152	4	3	0	0	58	5	7	0	1	4
145	2	3035	1	44	2	20	2	2	3	136	3	3	0	0	46	3	3	0	0	4
146	3	3036	1	51	1	12	3	2	5	154	1	1	0	0	44	2	4	1	0	3
147	1	3037	1	41	1	12	1	2	2	124	1	1	0	0	47	4	7	4	0	2
72	2	3038	0	38	3	16	2	1	1	144	4	1	1	0	56	5	4	2	2	3
149	3	3039	1	50	2	15	3	2	4	152	1	3	0	0	39	3	4	2	0	2
150	1	3040	1	58	3	11	1	2	3	214	4	2	0	0	57	8	10	5	3	10
137	2	3041	1	46	1	16	2	2	4	112	1	1	0	0	47	2	3	0	0	1
70	3	3042	0	42	1	22	3	2	2	145	1	3	0	0	45	2	4	0	0	0
66	1	3043	0	48	3	12	1	1	4	161	2	2	1	1	51	6	7	6	2	9
154	3	3044	1	40	1	12	2	2	3	147	1	1	0	0	46	3	4	0	0	0
155	3	3045	1	41	2	6	3	1	1	132	1	1	1	0	52	3	7	0	0	2
68	1	3046	0	64	3	8	1	2	4	164	4	1	0	0	55	5	7	2	1	2
157	2	3047	1	43	1	14	2	2	2	158	1	2	0	0	47	6	6	4	2	6
158	3	3048	1	37	1	12	3	2	3	145	1	3	0	1	52	4	5	2	1	7
159	1	3049	1	55	3	10	1	1	1	155	2	1	0	0	64	3	8	1	1	8
64	2	3050	0	52	1	8	2	1	1	158	1	3	1	0	51	3	5	2	1	4
161	3	3051	1	44	3	8	3	2	4	138	3	1	0	0	57	3	3	2	0	4
162	1	3052	1	53	3	12	1	2	4	157	4	1	0	0	54	5	7	2	1	7
113	2	3053	1	43	1	12	2	1	1	134	1	3	0	0	46	4	5	0	0	2
61	3	3054	0	50	2	8	3	2	3	154	1	1	0	0	48	2	4	1	0	2
165	1	3055	1	46	3	12	1	2	2	133	3	2	0	0	46	7	9	4	1	8
122	2	3056	1	51	2	16	2	2	5	204	3	1	0	0	54	7	7	5	3	6
58	3	3057	0	36	1	16	3	1	2	126	1	3	0	1	39	2	4	2	0	0
56	1	3058	0	38	1	15	1	2	3	143	1	1	0	0	45	3	6	0	0	2
169	2	3059	1	62	3	12	2	1	1	137	4	2	0	0	54	5	7	3	1	6
170	3	3060	1	41	3	18	3	2	2	135	1	1	0	0	69	6	6	2	0	2
166	1	3061	1	49	1	9	1	2	4	165	1	2	0	0	55	4	7	2	0	3
54	2	3062	0	27	1	16	2	1	5	134	1	3	0	0	44	4	5	3	0	4
173	3	3063	1	50	1	17	3	2	4	154	2	1	0	0	43	4	5	2	0	3
174	1	3064	1	36	2	12	1	1	3	143	3	1	0	1	44	4	6	5	0	5
51	2	3065	0	41	3	17	2	2	2	157	2	3	1	0	58	4	4	2	2	9
176	3	3066	1	40	1	12	3	2	4	137	1	2	0	0	41	3	4	4	0	2
177	1	3067	1	39	1	12	1	2	3	119	1	1	0	0	46	3	5	2	0	2
83	2	3068	0	49	3	16	2	2	4	149	4	1	0	0	51	5	5	1	1	5
179	3	3069	1	59	2	14	3	1	1	168	4	2	0	0	38	6	6	6	2	6
180	1	3070	1	42	3	16	1	2	2	165	3	1	0	0	64	5	6	2	1	6
181	2	3071	1	34	1	12	2	2	4	140	1	1	0	0	48	3	3	0	0	0
50	3	3072	0	38	1	12	3	2	3	153	1	3	0	1	47	2	2	0	0	1
183	1	3073	1	53	3	16	1	1	5	172	3	3	0	0	70	7	7	4	2	9
184	2	3074	1	54	3	8	2	2	1	145	3	2	0	0	62	8	9	4	1	12
49	3	3075	0	40	2	16	3	2	2	156	1	1	0	0	50	2	3	1	0	2
186	1	3076	1	37	1	17	1	2	4	127	1	1	0	0	47	4	7	2	0	4
185	2	3077	1	35	1	16	2	2	4	137	1	1	1	0	46	4	6	3	2	6
188	3	3078	1	37	1	12	3	2	3	122	1	2	0	0	47	4	4	2	0	3
189	1	3079	1	54	3	9	1	1	1	157	4	2	0	0	45	6	11	4	3	6
44	2	3080	0	55	1	16	2	1	4	180	3	3	0	0	43	7	5	4	2	5
191	3	3081	1	38	1	13	3	2	2	133	1	1	0	0	47	2	6	2	0	0
43	1	3082	0	39	1	12	1	2	3	120	1	3	1	0	54	3	5	2	1	4
193	2	3083	1	36	2	2	2	2	1	125	1	1	0	0	65	4	6	3	0	2
40	3	3084	0	63	3	8	3	1	1	205	2	3	0	0	62	5	4	2	3	4
195	1	3085	1	49	3	12	1	2	4	155	4	2	0	0	62	5	7	2	1	7

Table continued on the following page

TABLE B-1 Continued

V₁	V₂	V₃	V₄	V₅	V₆	V₇	V₈	V₉	V₁₀	V₁₁	V₁₂	V₁₃	V₁₄	V₁₅	V₁₆	V₁₇	V₁₈	V₁₉	V₂₀	V₂₁
77	2	3086	0	50	1	8	2	1	2	153	3	1	0	0	52	4	4	1	0	2
197	3	3087	1	34	1	16	3	1	4	121	1	1	0	0	47	3	6	3	0	1
34	1	3088	0	48	1	12	1	1	3	155	3	1	0	1	47	4	4	2	0	3
142	2	3089	1	55	3	16	2	1	4	146	2	1	0	0	59	6	5	1	1	8
200	3	3090	1	43	2	12	3	1	2	162	4	2	0	0	66	6	9	5	2	1
31	1	3091	0	43	2	16	1	2	4	154	3	3	0	0	54	6	4	4	1	6
201	2	3092	1	52	2	12	2	1	4	154	2	3	0	0	46	4	5	5	1	5
203	3	3093	1	35	1	16	3	2	3	142	1	3	1	0	53	2	5	0	0	0
30	1	3094	0	47	1	8	1	1	2	166	2	1	0	0	47	4	5	2	0	5
204	2	3095	1	48	1	16	2	2	4	159	3	1	0	0	60	6	6	2	2	4
206	3	3096	1	38	1	16	3	1	5	130	2	1	0	0	52	7	3	2	1	1
29	1	3097	0	46	1	17	1	1	3	120	1	1	1	1	45	3	4	2	1	6
208	2	3098	1	41	3	12	2	2	2	149	3	3	0	0	62	5	5	1	0	7
209	3	3099	1	44	1	12	3	1	1	122	1	2	0	0	44	2	3	0	0	2
210	1	3100	1	62	2	8	1	1	4	170	3	2	0	0	48	4	5	3	1	7
27	2	3101	0	39	1	16	2	2	2	155	2	3	0	0	49	5	5	2	0	2
212	3	3102	1	62	3	22	3	1	5	135	4	1	0	0	50	3	3	1	0	6
213	1	3103	1	45	1	9	1	1	1	144	3	1	0	0	43	3	6	0	0	5
26	2	3104	0	49	1	13	2	2	4	158	3	3	0	0	46	4	3	0	0	3
28	3	3105	0	47	2	12	3	2	4	137	1	1	0	0	51	2	2	1	0	3
22	1	3106	0	43	2	20	1	2	4	172	3	3	0	1	49	6	6	3	1	6
23	2	3107	0	55	1	8	2	1	3	153	2	3	0	0	52	7	5	2	0	5
218	3	3108	1	40	2	16	3	2	2	166	4	3	0	0	52	4	3	2	0	1
219	1	3109	1	43	1	12	1	2	1	120	1	3	0	0	41	3	5	2	0	5
220	2	3110	1	59	3	9	2	1	4	153	4	1	0	0	62	5	4	1	0	9
21	3	3111	0	42	1	19	3	2	5	144	1	1	0	1	47	2	3	1	0	2
217	1	3112	1	50	2	15	1	2	4	212	1	2	0	0	53	4	6	3	3	6
17	2	3113	0	42	1	1	2	2	3	188	3	3	0	0	69	7	6	2	2	4
224	3	3114	1	56	2	12	3	1	4	156	2	1	0	0	62	3	4	2	0	5
67	1	3115	0	42	2	12	1	2	4	149	4	3	1	0	42	4	85	3	1	8
226	2	3116	1	53	1	16	2	2	2	139	4	1	0	0	65	6	7	5	1	3
13	3	3117	0	50	1	16	3	2	2	168	3	1	0	0	59	3	2	0	0	2
11	1	3118	0	41	3	16	1	1	4	204	1	1	0	0	60	5	6	3	3	7
9	2	3119	0	54	2	8	2	2	1	217	2	3	0	0	51	5	6	2	2	6
230	3	3120	1	46	1	18	3	2	4	152	1	3	0	0	55	2	3	1	0	2
8	1	3121	0	66	3	5	1	1	3	187	2	1	0	0	60	6	6	4	2	10
232	2	3122	1	39	1	16	2	2	4	160	3	3	0	1	38	4	6	2	0	3
233	3	3123	1	48	2	12	3	2	2	156	1	2	0	0	56	4	6	2	0	4
231	1	3124	1	39	2	17	1	1	2	139	1	1	0	0	48	4	7	3	1	5
6	2	3125	0	47	2	12	2	2	4	137	3	3	0	0	64	4	7	2	0	7
234	3	3126	1	42	1	13	3	2	5	137	3	3	0	0	52	5	4	1	0	0
237	1	3127	1	47	1	16	1	1	4	154	2	3	0	0	57	4	5	2	2	4
238	2	3128	1	47	1	12	2	2	3	127	4	2	0	0	39	6	6	2	1	4
239	3	3129	1	45	2	10	3	2	1	137	1	1	0	1	50	3	4	0	0	1
235	1	3130	1	40	1	12	1	2	4	146	1	1	0	0	42	3	6	2	0	5
241	2	3131	1	46	2	14	2	1	2	139	1	1	0	0	49	4	4	2	0	6
4	3	3132	0	42	1	16	3	2	4	148	2	1	0	0	47	2	4	1	0	2
242	1	3133	1	37	1	12	1	2	5	125	1	2	0	0	51	3	5	1	0	4
3	2	3134	0	36	1	15	2	1	3	121	1	1	1	1	40	3	4	2	1	5
243	3	3135	1	30	1	12	3	1	3	117	2	1	0	1	38	2	4	0	0	1

Of the 21 variables, the first column (V_1) is the sequence of patients in the study—the patient number. V_2 is an assignment to one of three preoperative teaching programs. V_3 is the code number of patients in the study: Hospital 1—1001, 1002, . . . 1039, Hospital 2—2001, 2002, . . . 2072, Hospital 3—3001, 3002, . . . 3135. Variable V_4 is gender—0 = male; 1 = female. V_5 is age at last birthday. V_6 is severity—1 = mild, 2 = moderate, 3 = severe. V_7 is completed years of education. V_8 is hospital—1 = rural, 2 = suburban, 3 = central city. V_9 is provider 1. Private. 2. Public. V_{10} is family income—1 = less than $5,000, 2 = $5,000 to $15,000. 3 = $15,000 to $30,000, 4 = $30,000 to $50,000, 5 = more than $50,000. V_{11} is weight in pounds. V_{12} is smoking—1 = never smoked, 2 = less than one pack per week, 3 = less than one pack per day but more than one pack per week, 4 = one or more packs per day. V_{13} is alcohol use—1 = never used alcohol, 2 = less than one drink per day, 3 = more than one drink per day. V_{14} is drug use—0 = never used drugs, 1 = has used drugs. V_{15} is exercise—0 = never exercises, 1 = exercises. V_{16} is uncertainty—20, 21, . . . 80. V_{17} is length of stay—number of days in hospital following surgery. V_{18} is painmed1—number of medications administered following the first twenty-four hours after surgery. V_{19} is painmed2—number of medications administered following the second twenty-four hours after surgery. V_{20} is popcomps—number of postoperative complications. V_{21} is dayspdch—number of days at home before leaving residence.

INDEX

Page numbers followed by the letter "t" indicate the reference is to a table.
Page numbers in italic type indicate a reference to a figure.